NUTRITION ESSENTIALS
A Personal Approach

WENDY J. SCHIFF

EDITION

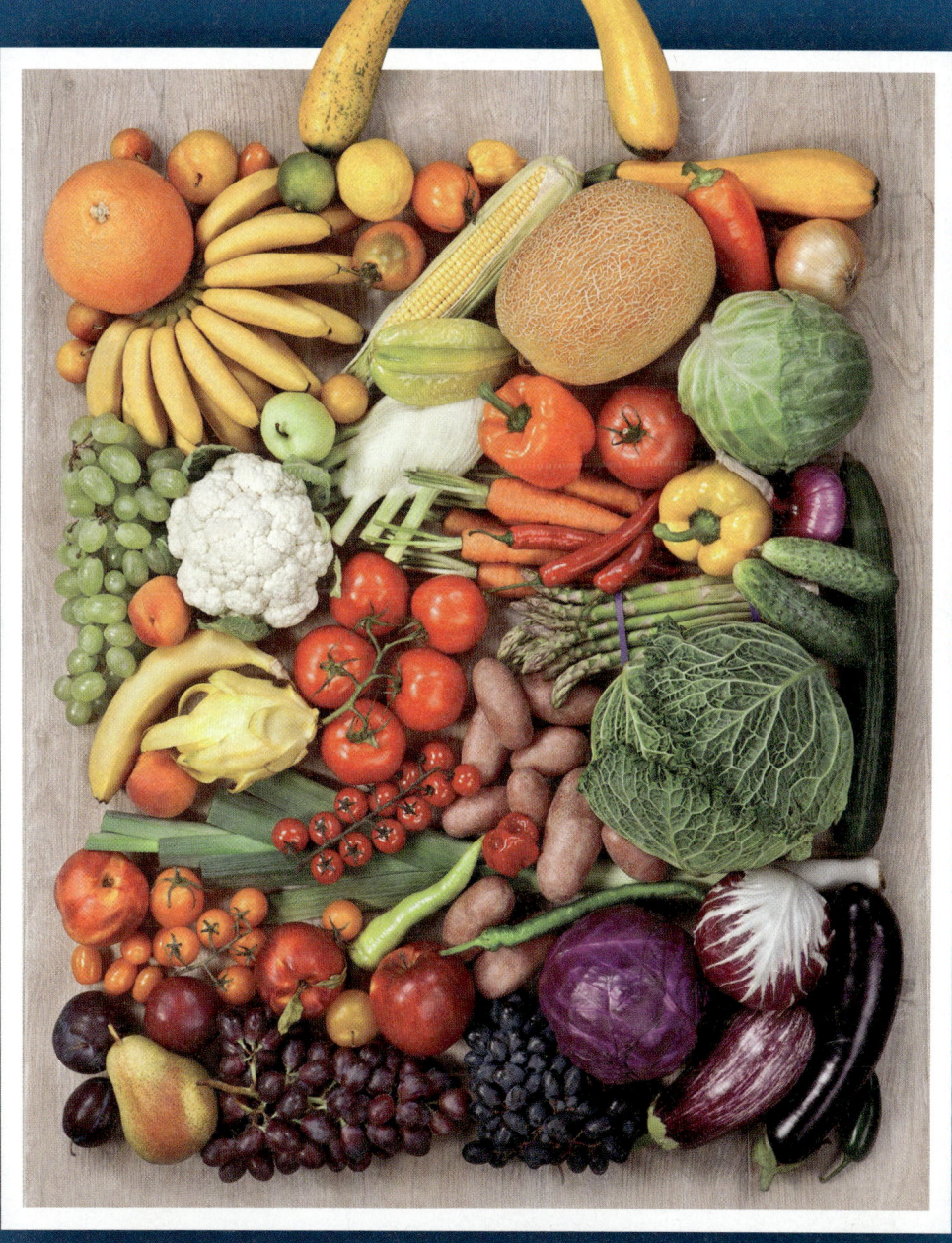
Roman legoshyn/123RF

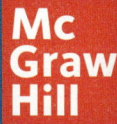
McGraw Hill

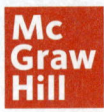

NUTRITION ESSENTIALS

Published by McGraw-Hill Education, 2 Penn Plaza, New York, NY 10121. Copyright © 2021 by McGraw-Hill Education. All rights reserved. Printed in the United States of America. No part of this publication may be reproduced or distributed in any form or by any means, or stored in a database or retrieval system, without the prior written consent of McGraw-Hill Education, including, but not limited to, in any network or other electronic storage or transmission, or broadcast for distance learning.

Some ancillaries, including electronic and print components, may not be available to customers outside the United States.

This book is printed on acid-free paper.

1 2 3 4 5 6 7 8 9 LKV 24 23 22 21 20

ISBN 978-1-260-57149-3
MHID 1-260-57149-1

Cover Image: ©Roman Iegoshyn/123RF

All credits appearing on page or at the end of the book are considered to be an extension of the copyright page.

The Internet addresses listed in the text were accurate at the time of publication and McGraw-Hill Education does not guarantee the accuracy of the information presented at these sites. The inclusion of a website, photo, or mention of a specific product does not indicate an endorsement by the authors or McGraw-Hill Education.

mheducation.com/highered

Brief Contents

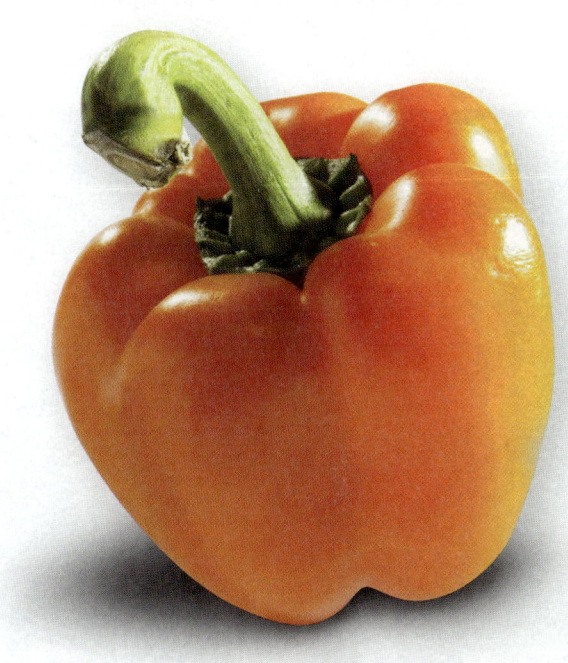

1 **Food *Is* More Than Something to Eat**   2

2 **Nutrition Information: Fact or Fiction?**   22

3 **Making More Nutritious Choices**   40

4 **How Food Becomes You**   70

5 **Carbohydrates: Fuel and Fiber**   100

6 **Lipids: Focusing on Fats and Cholesterol**   128

7 **Proteins: Life's Building Blocks**   160

8 **Vitamins: Nutrients That Multitask**   186

9 **Key Minerals, Water, and the Nonnutrient Alcohol**   228

10 **Nutrition for a Healthy Weight and Fit Body**   276

11 **Nutrition for Your Life, Environment, and World**   320

© Purestock/SuperStock RF

Appendixes

A   English-Metric Conversion and Metric-to-Household Units   A-2
B   Daily Values (DVs) Table   A-3
C   The Basics of Energy Metabolism   A-4
D   References   A-6
E   Dietary Reference Intake (DRI) Tables   A-21
F   Modifying Recipes for Healthy Living   A-27

Meet the Author

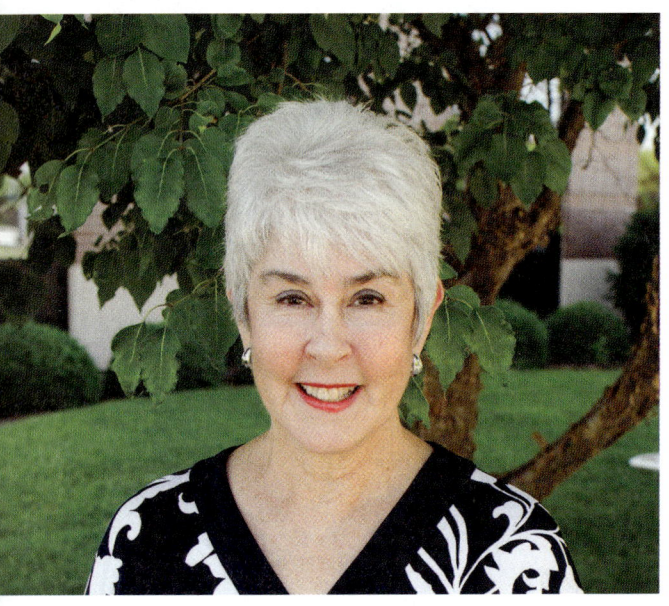
© McGraw-Hill Education. Mark Dierker, photographer.

Wendy J. Schiff, MS, RDN, received her BS in biological health/medical dietetics and MS in human nutrition from The Pennsylvania State University. She has taught introductory food and nutrition courses at the University of Missouri–Columbia, as well as nutrition, human biology, and personal health courses at St. Louis Community College–Meramec. She has worked as a public health nutritionist at the Allegheny County Health Department (Pittsburgh, Pennsylvania) and State Food and Nutrition Specialist for Missouri Extension at Lincoln University in Jefferson City, Missouri. In addition to authoring *Nutrition Essentials: A Personal Approach,* she is author of *Nutrition for Healthy Living* and coauthor of *Human Nutrition: Science for Healthy Living.* Wendy has authored or coauthored many other nutrition- and health-related educational materials as well. She is a registered dietitian nutritionist and a member of the Academy of Nutrition and Dietetics.

To Kevin and Bill

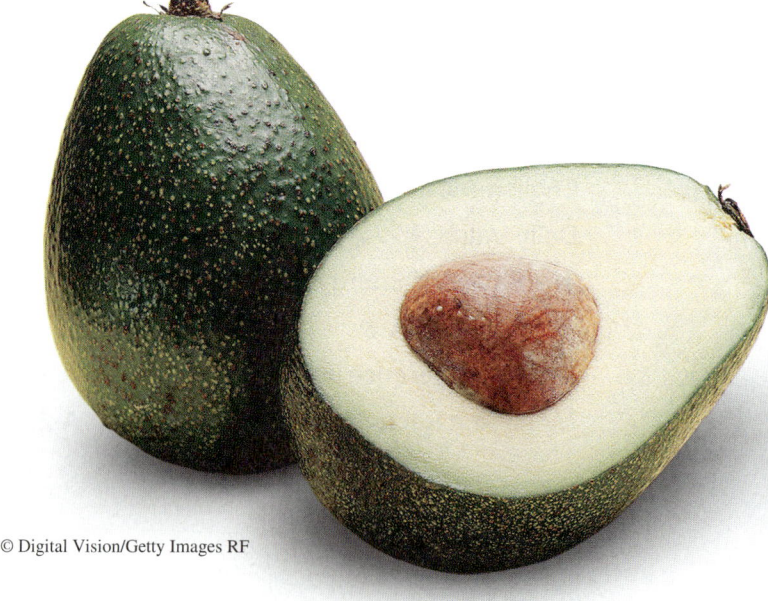
© Digital Vision/Getty Images RF

A Note from the Author

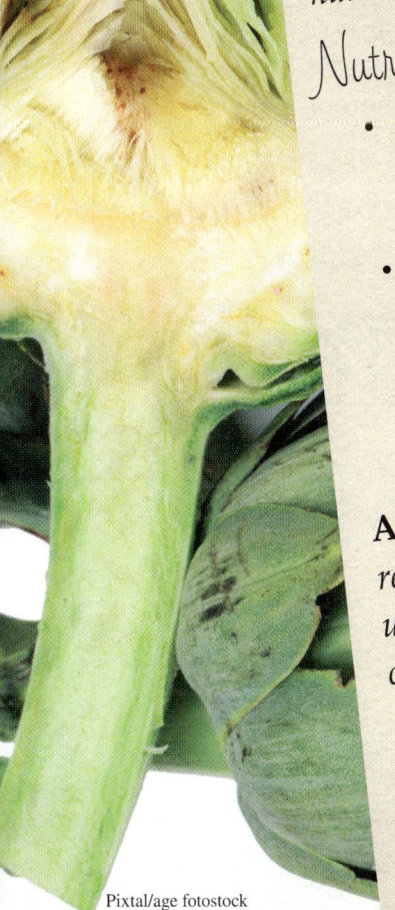

Pixtal/age fotostock

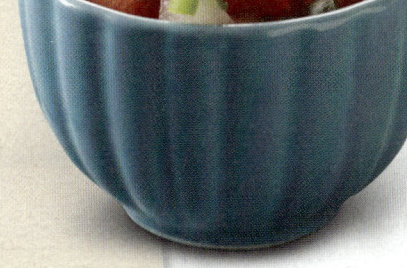

© Heather Winters/Getty Images RF

A few years ago, I decided that none of the college-level personal nutrition textbooks available was "right" for most students who wanted to learn about nutrition but weren't interested in majoring in the field of nutrition and dietetics.

My goal was to create a fresh approach and prepare a personal nutrition book that was less rigorous but would still cover the essentials of nutrition science. This book would be written in a style that was engaging and easy to read and understand. To facilitate learning, the text would include relevant and interesting photos and other visuals as well as superb illustrations to help explain basic but often challenging concepts. The textbook would also include personal perspectives about diets, foods, and nutrition from real college students, and practical food and nutrition tips to help students become more informed consumers.

Nutrition Essentials: A Personal Approach

- has a consumer-oriented focus, providing practical tips for applying concepts such as ways to prepare foods to make them safer and healthier, and ways to become a savvy consumer of nutrition-related information; and
- provides non-nutrition majors with the basic scientific principles of nutrition in a highly visual, engaging context. For example, the major steps involved in complex physiological processes, such as protein digestion and glucose regulation, are realistically illustrated and featured as Essential Concepts.

As I prepared the third edition of **Nutrition Essentials: A Personal Approach**, new blood pressure guidelines and physical activity recommendations were introduced. The third edition has been extensively updated to reflect these and other significant advances in the constantly changing field of nutrition.

The previous editions of **Nutrition Essentials: A Personal Approach** met all of my goals for a personal nutrition textbook. Now, the instructors who teach and the students who take personal nutrition courses have a new edition of this textbook to enjoy!

Best wishes,

Wendy J Schiff

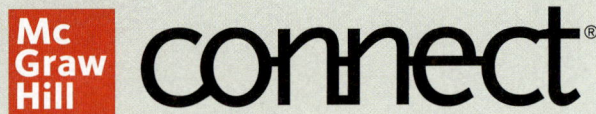

FOR INSTRUCTORS

You're in the driver's seat.

Want to build your own course? No problem. Prefer to use our turnkey, prebuilt course? Easy. Want to make changes throughout the semester? Sure. And you'll save time with Connect's auto-grading too.

65%
Less Time Grading

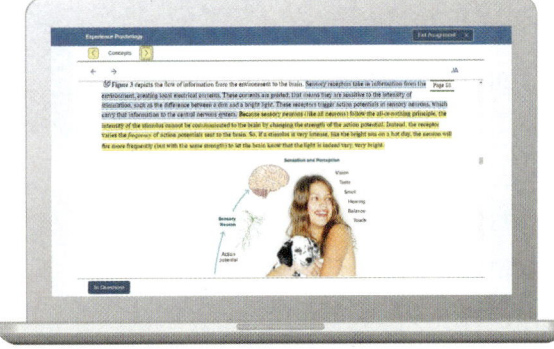

Laptop: McGraw-Hill; Woman/dog: George Doyle/Getty Images

They'll thank you for it.

Adaptive study resources like SmartBook® 2.0 help your students be better prepared in less time. You can transform your class time from dull definitions to dynamic debates. Find out more about the powerful personalized learning experience available in SmartBook 2.0 at **www.mheducation.com/highered/connect/smartbook**

Make it simple, make it affordable.

Connect makes it easy with seamless integration using any of the major Learning Management Systems—Blackboard®, Canvas, and D2L, among others—to let you organize your course in one convenient location. Give your students access to digital materials at a discount with our inclusive access program. Ask your McGraw-Hill representative for more information.

Padlock: Jobalou/Getty Images

Solutions for your challenges.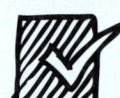

A product isn't a solution. Real solutions are affordable, reliable, and come with training and ongoing support when you need it and how you want it. Our Customer Experience Group can also help you troubleshoot tech problems—although Connect's 99% uptime means you might not need to call them. See for yourself at **status.mheducation.com**

Checkmark: Jobalou/Getty Images

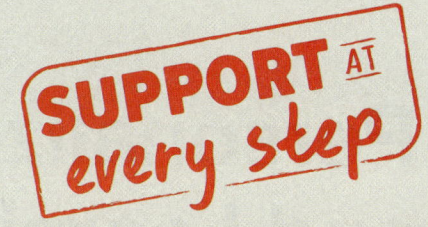

FOR STUDENTS

Effective, efficient studying.

Connect helps you be more productive with your study time and get better grades using tools like SmartBook 2.0, which highlights key concepts and creates a personalized study plan. Connect sets you up for success, so you walk into class with confidence and walk out with better grades.

Study anytime, anywhere.

Download the free ReadAnywhere app and access your online eBook or SmartBook 2.0 assignments when it's convenient, even if you're offline. And since the app automatically syncs with your eBook and SmartBook 2.0 assignments in Connect, all of your work is available every time you open it. Find out more at **www.mheducation.com/readanywhere**

> "I really liked this app—it made it easy to study when you don't have your textbook in front of you."
>
> - Jordan Cunningham, Eastern Washington University

No surprises.

The Connect Calendar and Reports tools keep you on track with the work you need to get done and your assignment scores. Life gets busy; Connect tools help you keep learning through it all.

Calendar: owattaphotos/Getty Images

Learning for everyone.

McGraw-Hill works directly with Accessibility Services Departments and faculty to meet the learning needs of all students. Please contact your Accessibility Services office and ask them to email accessibility@mheducation.com, or visit **www.mheducation.com/about/accessibility** for more information.

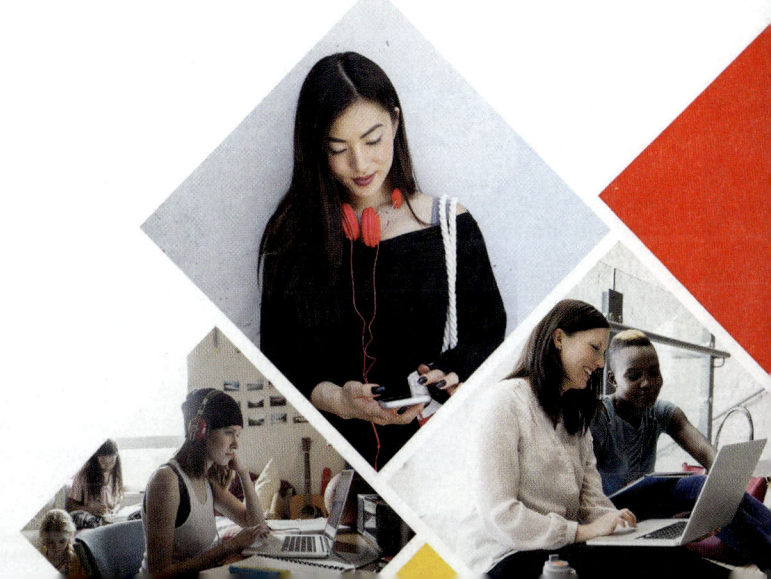

Top: Jenner Images/Getty Images, Left: Hero Images/Getty Images, Right: Hero Images/Getty Images

Personalized Teaching and Learning Environment

Saves students and instructors time while improving performance.

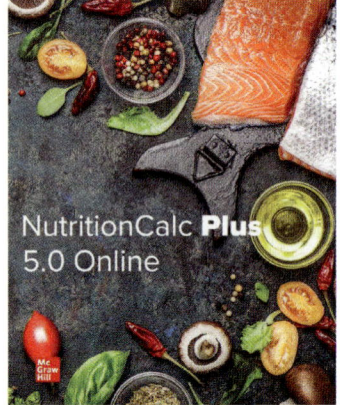
vicushka/123RF

NutritionCalc Plus

NutritionCalc Plus is a **powerful dietary analysis tool** featuring more than 30,000 foods from the reliable and accurate ESHA Research nutrient database, which is comprised of data from the latest USDA Standard Reference database, manufacturer's data, restaurant data, and data from literature sources. NutritionCalc Plus allows users to track food and activities, and then analyze their choices with a robust selection of intuitive reports. The interface was updated to accommodate ADA requirements and modern mobile experience native to today's students.

Dietary Analysis Case Studies in Connect®

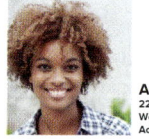
Ava Ponce
22 year old, Female, 5'6", 145 lbs
Weight gain/loss: 0 lbs/week
Activity level: Active
pkchai/Shutterstock

One of the challenges instructors face with teaching nutrition classes is having time to grade individual dietary analysis projects. To help overcome this challenge, assign auto-graded dietary analysis case studies. These tools require students to use NutritionCalc Plus to analyze dietary data, generate reports, and answer questions to **apply their nutrition knowledge to real-world situations**. These assignments were developed and reviewed by faculty who use such assignments in their own teaching. They are designed to be relevant, current, and interesting!

> "The case studies provide a neutral way for my students to explore dietary analysis. My students are engaged by the case study assignments and find them easy to use. The fact that they are auto-graded gives me more time to focus on content development and instruction for my course."
>
> —Hannah Thornton, Texas State University

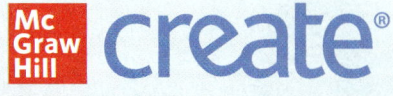

McGraw-Hill Create® is a self-service website that allows you to create customized course materials using McGraw-Hill's comprehensive, cross-disciplinary content and digital products.

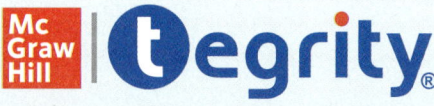

Tegrity in Connect is a tool that makes class time available 24/7 by automatically capturing every lecture. With a simple one-click start-and-stop process, you capture all computer screens and corresponding audio in a format that is easy to search, frame by frame. Students can replay any part of any class with easy-to-use, browser-based viewing on a PC, Mac, or other mobile device.

Educators know that the more students can see, hear, and experience class resources, the better they learn. Tegrity's unique search feature helps students efficiently find what they need, when they need it, across an entire semester of class recordings. Help turn your students' study time into learning moments immediately supported by your lecture. With Tegrity, you also increase intent listening and class participation by easing students' concerns about note taking.

Source: Jill Paisley

Assess My Diet

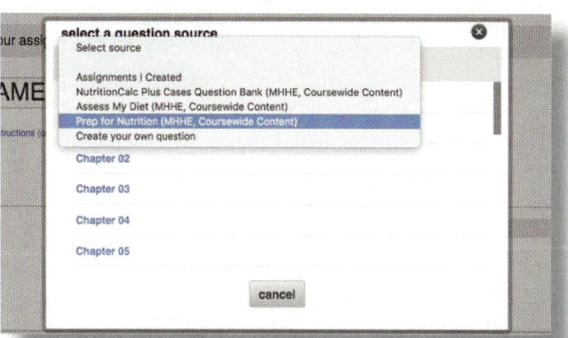

Auto-graded personalized dietary analysis. Students are using NutritionCalc Plus to analyze their own dietary patterns. But how can instructors integrate that information into a meaningful learning experience? With Assess My Diet, instructors can now assign auto-graded, personalized dietary analysis questions within Connect. These questions refresh their memory on the functions and food sources of each nutrient and prompt the students to evaluate their own eating behaviors. Students can evaluate their own nutrient intakes compared to current Dietary Reference Intakes and demonstrate their ability to perform calculations on their own data, such as percent of calories from saturated fat. They can compare the nutrient density of their own food selections to see which of their food choices provides the most fiber or iron. A benefit of the Assess My Diet question bank is that it offers assignable content that is personalized to the students' data, yet still auto graded. It **saves time** and keeps all assignments in one place.

Prep for Nutrition

To help you **level-set your classroom**, we've created Prep for Nutrition. This question bank highlights a series of questions, including Basic Chemistry, Biology, Dietary Analysis, Mathematics, and Student Success, to give students a refresher on the skills needed to enter and be successful in their course! By having these foundational skills, you will feel more confident your students can begin class, ready to understand more complex concepts and topics. Prep for Nutrition is **course-wide for ALL nutrition titles** and can be found in the Question Bank dropdown within Connect.

Campus

McGraw-Hill Campus® is a groundbreaking service that puts world-class digital learning resources just a click away for all your faculty and students. All your faculty—whether or not they use a McGraw-Hill title—can instantly browse, search, and access the entire library of McGraw-Hill instructional resources and services, including eBooks, test banks, PowerPoint slides, animations, and learning objects—from any Learning Management System (LMS), at no additional cost to your institution. Users also have single-on access to McGraw-Hill digital platforms, including Connect, ALEKS®, Create, and Tegrity.

A Visual Approach

Highly visual; designed with today's college students in mind.

Nutrition Essentials: A Personal Approach was developed with a magazine-like design and today's student in mind. The many photos and appealing page layouts entice students to explore and read further. Furthermore, the highly visual nature of the book's layout reduces anxiety sometimes associated with large blocks of text.

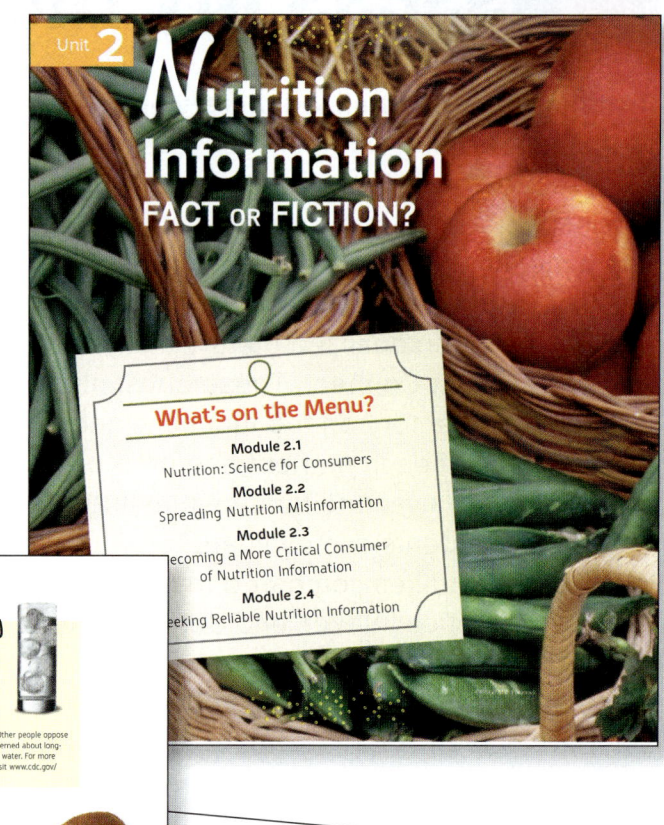

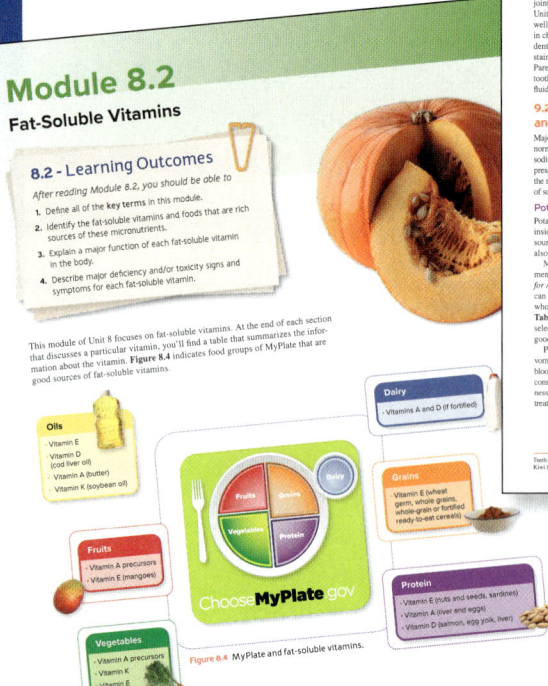

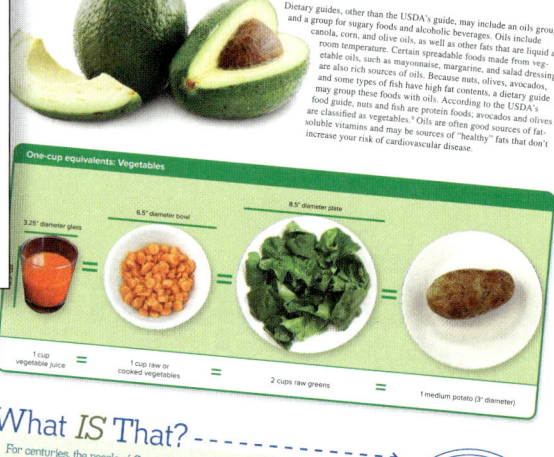

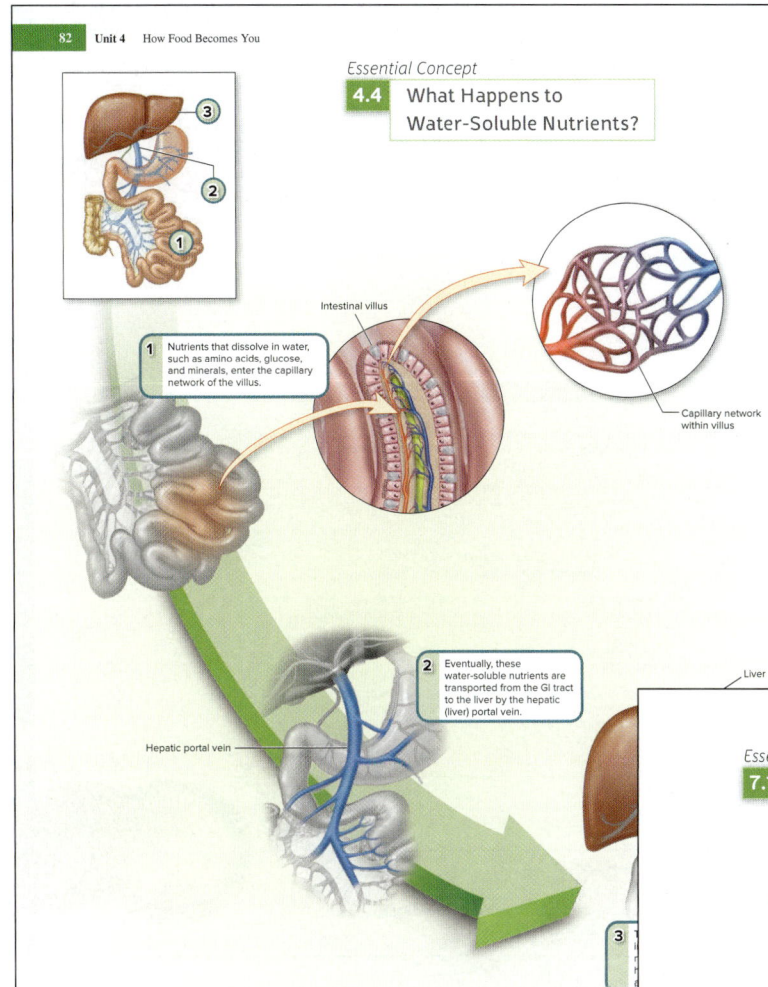

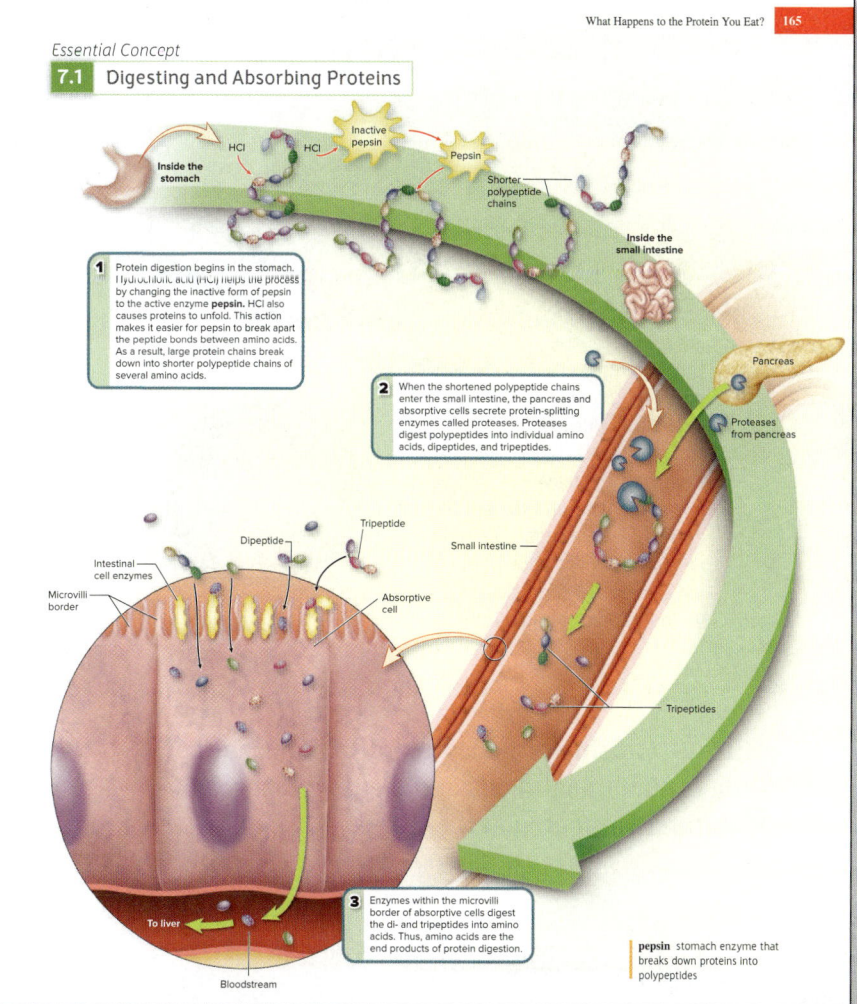

Essential Concept takes a complex scientific process and illustrates it in a unique, step-by-step manner to facilitate learning, especially for students who are not science majors. Topics include the scientific method, how the body digests proteins, and the role of hormones in regulating blood glucose levels. Numbered boxes contain points that relate to a particular portion of the illustration, while the large green arrows help students visualize stepping through the process.

What's In Your Diet?!, found at the end of most units, is a personal dietary analysis activity that offers many ways for students to apply nutrition-related concepts to their daily lives immediately.

Tasty Tidbits, interesting bits of information about food or nutrition, provide students with practical ways to be more savvy consumers and to make healthier choices.

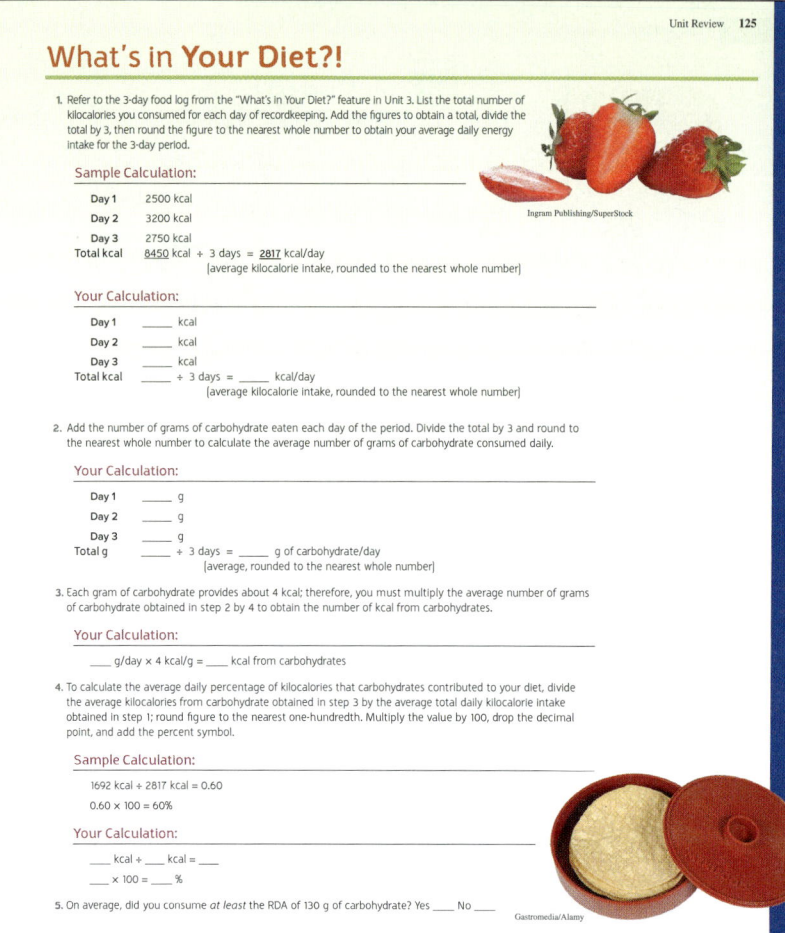

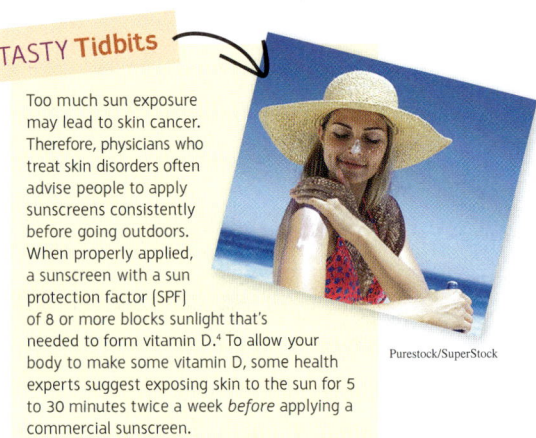

TASTY Tidbits

Too much sun exposure may lead to skin cancer. Therefore, physicians who treat skin disorders often advise people to apply sunscreens consistently before going outdoors. When properly applied, a sunscreen with a sun protection factor (SPF) of 8 or more blocks sunlight that's needed to form vitamin D.[4] To allow your body to make some vitamin D, some health experts suggest exposing skin to the sun for 5 to 30 minutes twice a week *before* applying a commercial sunscreen.

Purestock/SuperStock

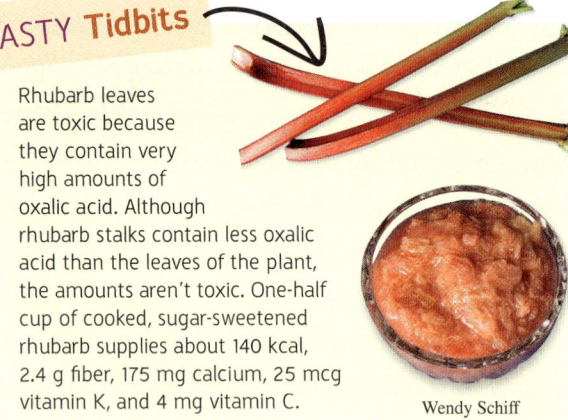

TASTY Tidbits

Rhubarb leaves are toxic because they contain very high amounts of oxalic acid. Although rhubarb stalks contain less oxalic acid than the leaves of the plant, the amounts aren't toxic. One-half cup of cooked, sugar-sweetened rhubarb supplies about 140 kcal, 2.4 g fiber, 175 mg calcium, 25 mcg vitamin K, and 4 mg vitamin C.

Wendy Schiff

Culture & Cuisine provides a brief but intriguing discussion of traditional foods and dietary practices of various cultures from around the world.

Culture & Cuisine

Throughout the world, populations rely on three starchy foods—rice, corn, and wheat—to supply the majority of their food energy intake. Other starchy foods, especially millet, sorghum, cassava, taro, potatoes, and yams, are often consumed along with the three starchy *staple* foods. A staple food forms the foundation of a population's diet and provides a large share of their calorie and nutrient needs. Rice, for example, is a staple food for almost 50% of the world's population.

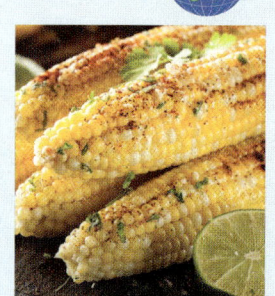

Brent Hofacker/Alamy Stock Photo
Mexican street corn

What IS That?

Foods that contain live and active probiotics may be beneficial to your health, particularly your intestinal health. Kefir is a "cultured" milk. Cultured milks, such as kefir and cultured buttermilk, have probiotics added to them. The probiotic bacteria ferment the natural carbohydrate in milk for energy, and produce acid and carbon dioxide as a result. The acid curdles the milk and gives it a distinctive taste; the carbon dioxide provides some "fizz," like a carbonated soft drink. A 1-cup serving of kefir that's made from 2% milk supplies about the same energy and nutrient contents as 1 cup of 2% milk.

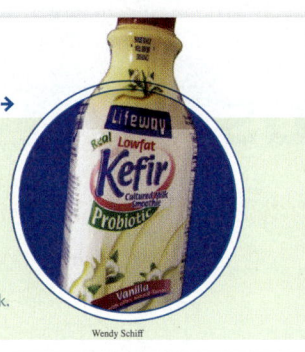
Wendy Schiff

What *IS* That? highlights foods that are often unfamiliar to Americans and provides nutrition information about the foods. Exposing students to new food items expands their options as a consumer.

Nutrition Fact or Fiction? dispels popular food and nutrition myths such as "sugar causes hyperactivity," "the 5-second rule," and the "freshman 15."

Nutrition Fact or Fiction?
Sugar makes children hyperactive.

If you've ever attended a child's birthday party, you can understand why people often blame sugary foods for causing "hyper" behavior. The results of scientific studies, however, don't indicate that sugar is a cause of *attention-deficit/hyperactivity disorder*, also known as *ADHD*.[2] There are a few different types of ADHD, but affected children generally have difficulty paying attention, following instructions, sitting quietly, and controlling their impulses. The cause of ADHD is uncertain, but genetic factors play an important role. Other risk factors include premature birth (being born too soon), low birth weight, and brain injury. Furthermore, pregnant women who smoke or drink alcohol increase their risk of having children with ADHD.

When children attend parties, their excitement and lower self-control are

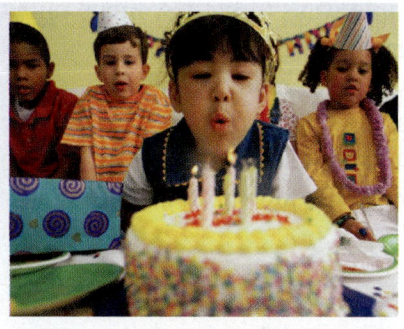
Ryan McVay/Getty Images

Answer This questions give students opportunities to practice using basic skills, including math, graph reading, and critical thinking, to answer questions relating to the unit's content. The correct response to an Answer This is located on the last page of the unit.

Answer This

If your total calorie intake is 2400 kcal per day and fat provides 30% of your calories, how many grams of fat do you consume? You'll find the answer on the last page of this unit.

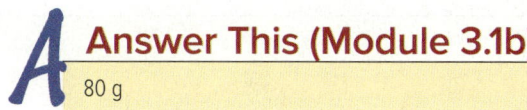**Answer This (Module 3.1b)**

80 g

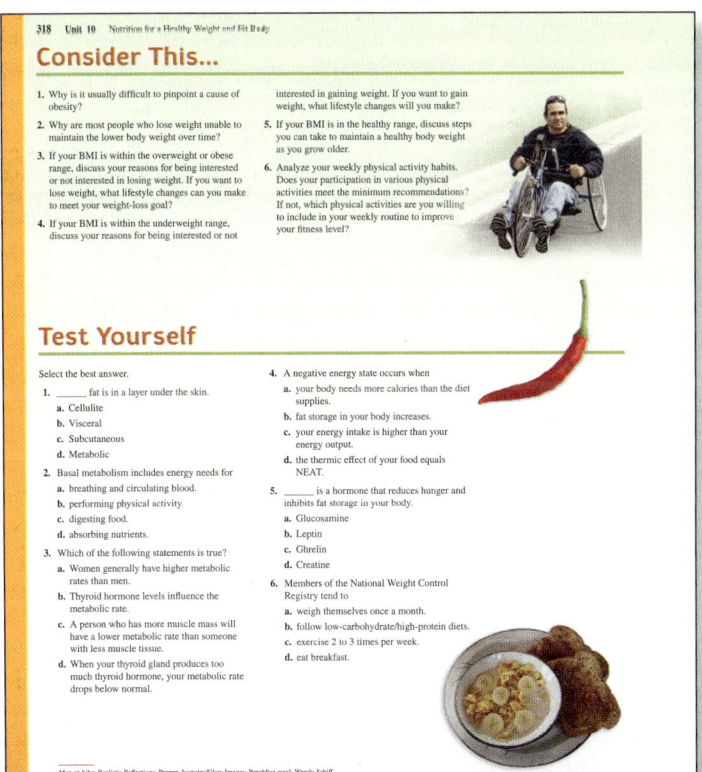

Consider This… presents critical thinking questions related to the unit's content that help students apply what they read.

Test Yourself at the end of each unit features multiple-choice questions designed to help students check their knowledge and prepare for exams. Answers are provided in small, upside-down print at the end of each test.

Consumer Focus

Teaches students how to better evaluate nutrition information for a healthier life.

Nutrition Essentials: A Personal Approach is consumer focused, providing students with ample ways to both evaluate nutrition information as well as apply practical tips for healthier living. An entire unit, Nutrition Information: Fact or Fiction? (Unit 2), is devoted to understanding the scientific method and evaluating nutrition information.

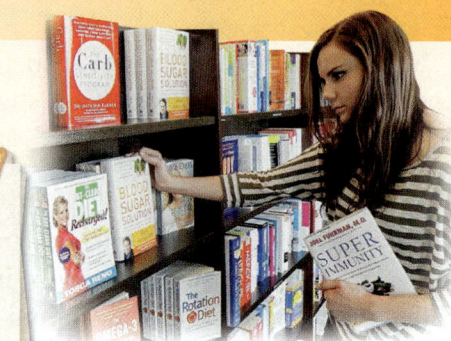

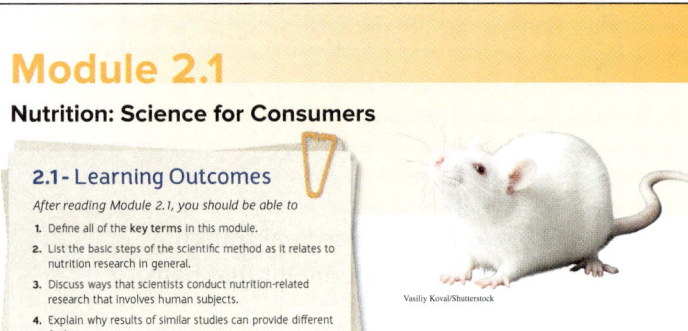

Personalized Focus

The nutrition textbook that's written for YOU!

- The personalized, consumer focus gives plenty of practical examples to help you choose and prepare nutritious foods as well as make nutrition-related decisions that are good for your health.

- The proven successful Connect for *Nutrition Essentials: A Personal Approach* digital program, including Question Bank, Test Bank, Prep for Nutrition, LearnSmart/SmartBook adaptive reading, and NutritionCalc Plus dietary analysis, gives you access to one of the most effective and successful adaptive learning resources available on the market today.

Nutrition Essentials: A Personal Approach is uniquely designed to provide non-science majors with the basic scientific principles of nutrition in a highly visual, engaging framework focused on their personal choices and experiences. Adaptive learning resources LearnSmart and SmartBook create an individualized study plan to help you achieve success in understanding nutrition.

Each unit highlights an actual college student's or recent college graduate's nutrition concerns. These relatable accounts in a student's own words help frame the content of that unit and encourage you to think about your own dietary choices.

"I was born in Madras (Chennai), India . . . I moved to the United States with my family when I was nine years old. I love Indian food. When I visit India, my diet is very different than what I eat here. You can buy a variety of spicy foods, such as peppery corn-on-the-cob and vazhakkai bajji (banana slices that are fried after being dipped in besan flour mixed with chili powder), that are cooked in stalls that line city streets. The variety of fresh, tropical fruits is amazing. I love fresh jackfruit! I can't find fresh jackfruit where I now live."

"My mom makes naan (nahn) and roti from scratch. Naan and roti are flatbreads that are often served with a spicy lentil and/or curry gravy. I like sticky white rice with meals, and I eat all types of vegetables, beans, and lentils. I'll also eat poultry, eggs, dairy foods, and seafood, but I don't eat red meat because I think it's unhealthy. My parents don't eat foods from animals."

Sachin Raghothaman

Josh Kuennen

What's New in This Edition

Earlier editions of this textbook included visually stimulating and creative page layouts, and beautifully rendered, pedagogically based illustrations that were designed to engage students' interest in the narrative's topics and facilitate learning. The third edition maintains this energetic, colorful, and appealing design. We have retained many of the interesting photos and replaced others. Photos help draw students' attention to the narrative and enable them to relate content to the real world. It's important to note that the use of products in photos is for example representation only and does not constitute an endorsement.

The third edition of *Nutrition Essentials: A Personal Approach* has been extensively updated with new information and its sources. The following points highlight some of the major revisions:

- Each unit has a Culture & Cuisine feature (new to this edition) that discusses traditional foods or dietary practices from around the world. Such features include information about popular Asian Indian foods, traditional Mexican foods, and the use of insects for a protein source.
- Additional Test Yourself (end-of-unit quiz) and Consider This… questions have been incorporated into most of the units.
- Many of the diagrams and illustrations throughout the textbook have been modified to increase their clarity. For example, Essential Concept 7.2 (What Can Happen to Unneeded Amino Acids?) has been revised to help students better follow steps involved in an aspect of amino acid metabolism.
- The food composition tables that contain information about amounts of specific nutrients in commonly eaten foods have been updated.
- Three of the unit openers have been revised to feature a new college student or recent college graduate who shares personal reflections about his or her dietary choices. These openers help draw readers into the unit's content.
- Answers to Test Yourself are included at the end of each quiz but upside down, so students don't need to search for them in the appendixes.

The following points highlight some significant revisions that have been made to specific units:

- The opener of Unit 4 (How Food Becomes You) features a young woman with celiac disease. The unit also includes a new Essential Concept that illustrates the process of absorbing fat-soluble nutrients from the digestive tract and transporting them to other cells in the body.
- Unit 5 (Carbohydrates: Fuel and Fiber) has a new section that's about non-alcoholic fatty liver disease (NAFLD), which affects millions of adult Americans. Furthermore, a new Essential Concept that illustrates carbohydrate digestion, absorption, and elimination has been added to replace Figure 5.3 in the previous edition. The new Figure 5.3 illustrates the fate of glucose after absorption.
- Unit 7 (Proteins: Life's Building Blocks) has a new module (7.6 Stretching Your Food Dollars).

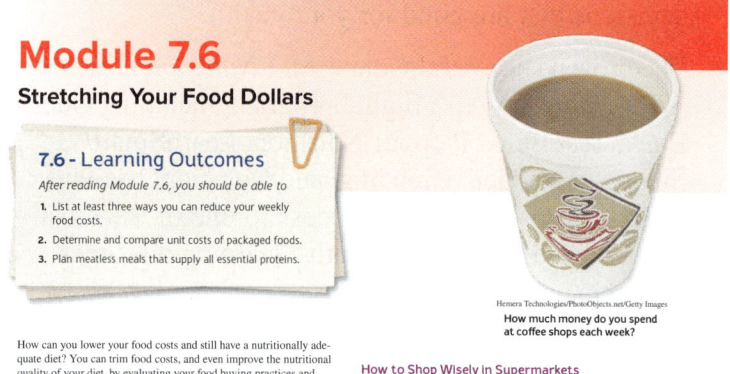

- Unit 8 (Vitamins: Nutrients That Multitask) has a new Nutrition Fact or Fiction? that features a case study about a young man who took toxic levels of niacin. Two new Essential Concepts have been added to replace figures in the previous edition. One of the new Essential Concepts illustrates major steps in the body's use of vitamins B-12 and folate for red blood cell production. The other new Essential Concept shows major steps involved in the body's use of vitamin K for blood clotting.
- Unit 9 (Key Minerals, Water, and the Nonnutrient Alcohol) has revised blood pressure guidelines (Table 9.6) and new information about the ULs for sodium and potassium (Table 9.7).

TABLE 9.6 CLASSIFYING BLOOD PRESSURE LEVELS (ADULTS)*

Blood Pressure Classification	Systolic mm Hg	And/Or	Diastolic mm Hg
Normal	< 120	and	< 80
Elevated	120–129	and	< 80
Hypertension: Stage 1	130–139	or	80–89
Hypertension: Stage 2	≥ 140	or	≥ 90

*Key: < is "less than"; ≥ is "more than or equal to."
Source: American Heart Association: Monitoring your blood pressure at home. 2017. www.heart.org/en/health-topics/high-blood-pressure/understanding-blood-pressure-readings/monitoring-your-blood-pressure-at-home Accessed: July 6, 2019

- Unit 10 (Nutrition for a Healthy Weight and Fit Body) highlights recommendations of the U.S. Department of Health and Human Services' latest physical activity guidelines (2018). Information about intermittent fasting has been added to the information about weight-loss diets.
- Unit 11 has two new What *IS* That? features that discuss kiwano and bioengineered foods.
- Appendix E (Dietary Reference Intake [DRI] Tables) has been updated to reflect the 2019 DRIs for sodium and potassium.

Acknowledgments

The development of an accurate and current manuscript for *Nutrition Essentials: A Personal Approach,* Third Edition, was facilitated with the help of numerous college nutrition instructors. I offer my sincere thanks to the following colleagues who reviewed the second edition and provided a wide range of valuable feedback.

Reviewers

Allison Childress
Texas Tech University

Maryann Eastep
University of Delaware

Meghan Garrett
Reynolds Community College

Paula Inserra
John Tyler Community College

Traci Keck
University of Texas at San Antonio

Tory Keeter
University of Oklahoma

Fran Lukacik
Community College of Philadelphia

Ricky Nelson
Century College

Caroline West Passerrello
University of Pittsburgh

Laurie Runk
Coastline Community College

Stephen P. Sowulewski
Reynolds Community College

Ka Wong
J. Sargeant Reynolds Community College

My heartfelt thanks extends to everyone at McGraw-Hill Education who helped in the development and production of the third edition of *Nutrition Essentials: A Personal Approach.* I also owe a great deal of gratitude to Marisa Moreno, Damian Nguyen, Mary Wester, Amanda Croker, McKenzie Frey, Karlin West, Sachin Raghothaman, Olivia Coomes, Nancy Scott, Neill Warrington, and Theresa Washington. These current and former college students helped make *Nutrition Essentials* a more personal approach by contributing their quotations and photos to unit openers.

Members of my McGraw-Hill Education team deserve to be recognized for their hard work and commitment to the development and production of the third edition of *Nutrition Essentials: A Personal Approach.* Lauren Vondra, Portfolio Manager, took the necessary steps to move forward with the new edition. I am grateful for her guidance and willingness to continue developing the features of this unique textbook. My Senior Content Production Manager, Vicki Krug, had one of the most difficult jobs as a member of the team. She had to make sure that production deadlines were met. Vicki also forwarded instructions for art and corrections to staff at the outside companies that prepared illustrations for and printed the textbook. Each year, she has to juggle the production of several textbooks at one time, and she did an amazing job of successfully managing the production of *Nutrition Essentials.*

Jim Connely, Marketing Director, and Kristine Rellihan, Market Development Manager, did a great job of helping me analyze the needs of students taking personal nutrition courses so I could build on the success of the first and second editions. Jim and Kristine, thanks so much! David Hash, Lead Designer, developed the amazing cover and new design features for this new edition; Abbey Jones, Content Licensing Specialist, handled the securing of permissions and releases; and Rachael Hillebrand, Assessment Content Project Manager, oversaw the digital program. Such "behind-the-scenes" staff are critical players in the production of a high-quality textbook. My special thanks also extend to David, Abbey, and Rachael.

I also want to thank Lynn Breithaupt, Executive Director, for providing the support that was necessary for developing, publishing, and marketing the new edition of this textbook. Last, but not least, my Senior Product Developer, Darlene Schueller, deserves my sincerest gratitude for the hard work, long hours, and extraordinary dedication she invested in the production of the third edition of *Nutrition Essentials: A Personal Approach* and the Connect and LearnSmart resources that support the textbook. Meeting deadlines can be very challenging for an author, but Darlene made the revision process flow smoothly. For over 20 years, I've written college-level textbooks and related educational material for different publishers. I've worked with several product developers, but there's no doubt in my mind: Darlene is the best!

Wendy J Schiff

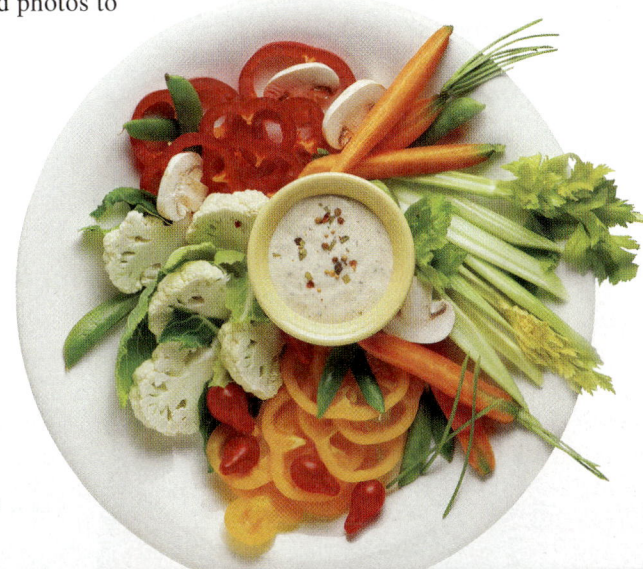

© C Squared Studios/Getty Images RF

Contents

Preface viii

Unit 1 Food *Is* More Than Something to Eat 2

- Module 1.1 Why Learn About Nutrition? 4
- Module 1.2 Nutrition Basics 6
- Module 1.3 Key Nutrition Concepts 13

Unit 2 Nutrition Information: Fact or Fiction? 22

- Module 2.1 Nutrition: Science for Consumers 24
- Module 2.2 Spreading Nutrition Misinformation 30
- Module 2.3 Becoming a More Critical Consumer of Nutrition Information 32
- Module 2.4 Seeking Reliable Nutrition Information 36

Unit 3 Making More Nutritious Choices 40

- Module 3.1 Requirements and Recommendations 42
- Module 3.2 Planning Nutritious Meals and Snacks 45
- Module 3.3 Making Sense of Food Labels 57
- Module 3.4 Should I Take Dietary Supplements? 60

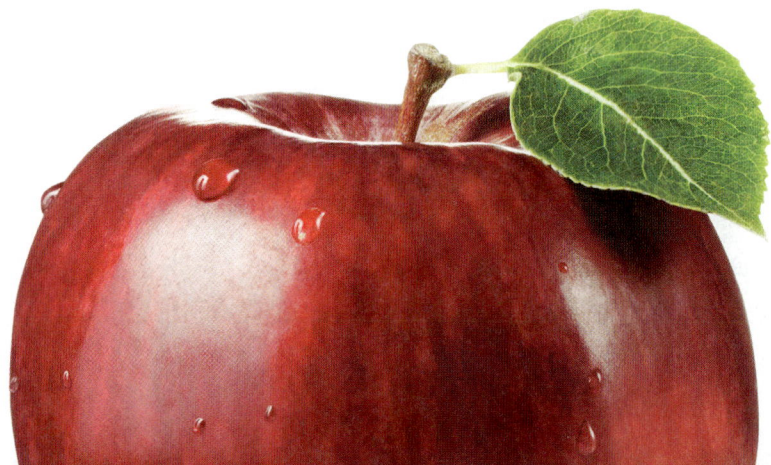

© Lauren Burke/Getty Images RF

Unit 4 How Food Becomes You 70

Module 4.1 From Cells to Systems 72
Module 4.2 Digestive System 75
Module 4.3 Common Digestive System Disorders 87
Module 4.4 Metabolism Basics 95

Unit 5 Carbohydrates: Fuel and Fiber 100

Module 5.1 Sugars, Sweeteners, Starches, and Fiber 102
Module 5.2 What Happens to the Carbohydrates You Eat? 113
Module 5.3 Carbohydrates and Health 117

Unit 6 Lipids: Focusing on Fats and Cholesterol 128

Module 6.1 What Are Lipids? 130
Module 6.2 What Happens to the Fat and Cholesterol You Eat? 138
Module 6.3 Cardiovascular Disease: Major Killer of Americans 142

Unit 7 Proteins: Life's Building Blocks 160

Module 7.1 What Are Proteins? 162
Module 7.2 What Happens to the Protein You Eat? 164
Module 7.3 Proteins in Foods 169
Module 7.4 What's Vegetarianism? 172
Module 7.5 Proteins and Health 174
Module 7.6 Stretching Your Food Dollars 179

Unit 8 Vitamins: Nutrients That Multitask 186

Module 8.1 Introducing Vitamins 188
Module 8.2 Fat-Soluble Vitamins 193
Module 8.3 Water-Soluble Vitamins 205
Module 8.4 Vitamins and Cancer 221

© Clover/SuperStock RF

xx   Contents

Unit 9 Key Minerals, Water, and the Nonnutrient Alcohol 228

Module 9.1   Minerals for Life   230
Module 9.2   Key Minerals and Your Health   234
Module 9.3   Water: Liquid of Life   257
Module 9.4   Drink to Your Health?   263

Unit 10 Nutrition for a Healthy Weight and Fit Body 276

Module 10.1   Overweight or Obese?   278
Module 10.2   Factors That Influence Your Body Weight   286
Module 10.3   Managing Your Weight Safely   293
Module 10.4   Disordered Eating and Eating Disorders   301
Module 10.5   Get Moving; Get Healthy!   304

Unit 11 Nutrition for Your Life, Environment, and World 320

Module 11.1   Nutrition for a Lifetime   322
Module 11.2   How Safe Is My Food?   338
Module 11.3   Dietary Adequacy: A Global Concern   349

Appendixes   A-1

A   English-Metric Conversion and Metric-to-Household Units   A-2
B   Daily Values (DVs) Table   A-3
C   The Basics of Energy Metabolism   A-4
D   References   A-6
E   Dietary Reference Intake (DRI) Tables   A-21
F   Modifying Recipes for Healthy Living   A-27

Glossary   G-1
Index   I-1

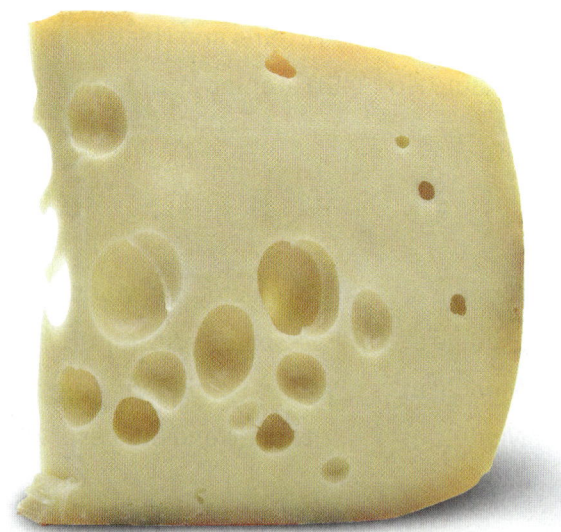

© ballyscanlon/Getty Images RF

NUTRITION ESSENTIALS

Third Edition

A Personal Approach

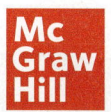

Unit 1
Food *Is* More Than Something to Eat

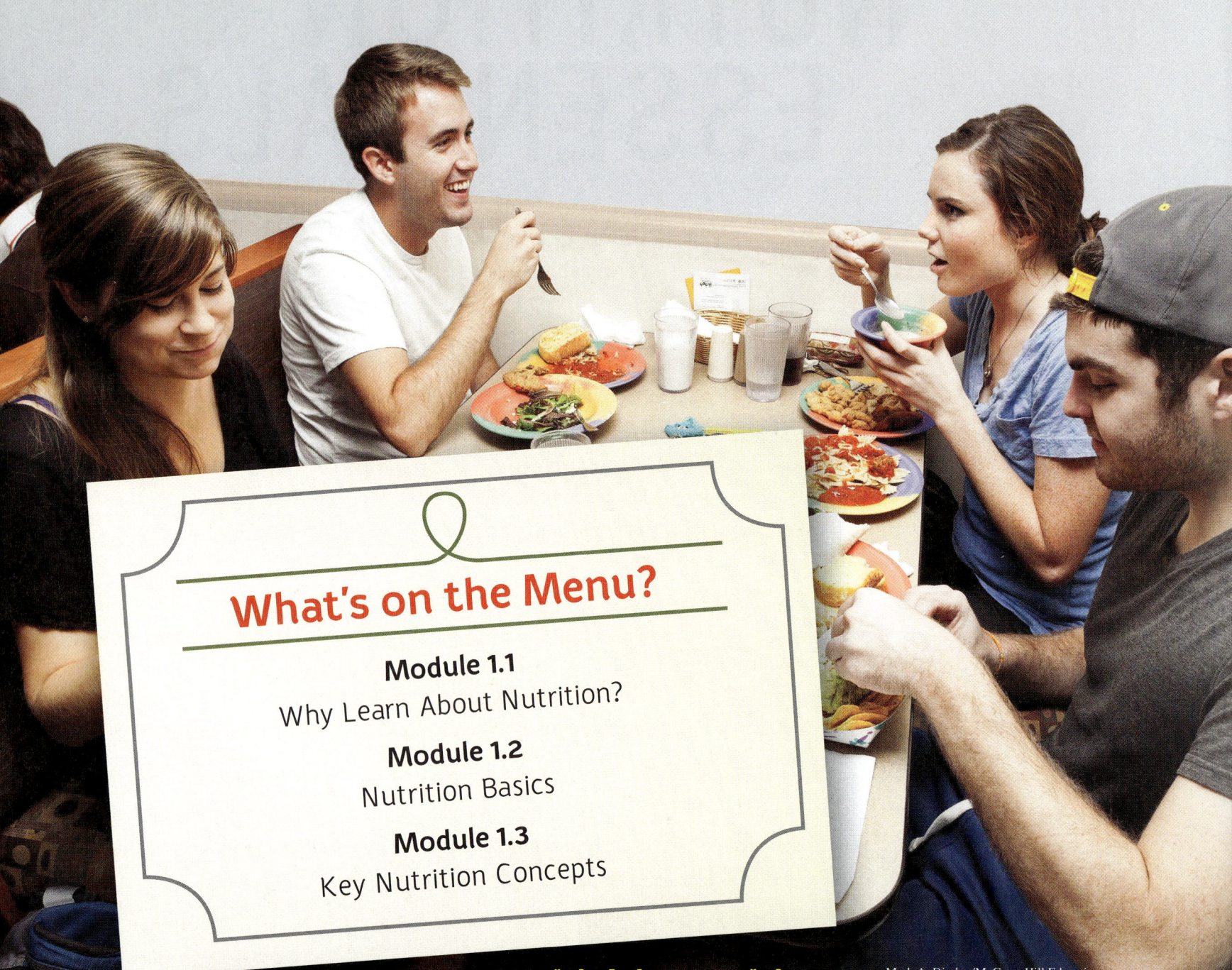

What's on the Menu?

Module 1.1
Why Learn About Nutrition?

Module 1.2
Nutrition Basics

Module 1.3
Key Nutrition Concepts

Mark A. Dierker/McGraw-Hill Education

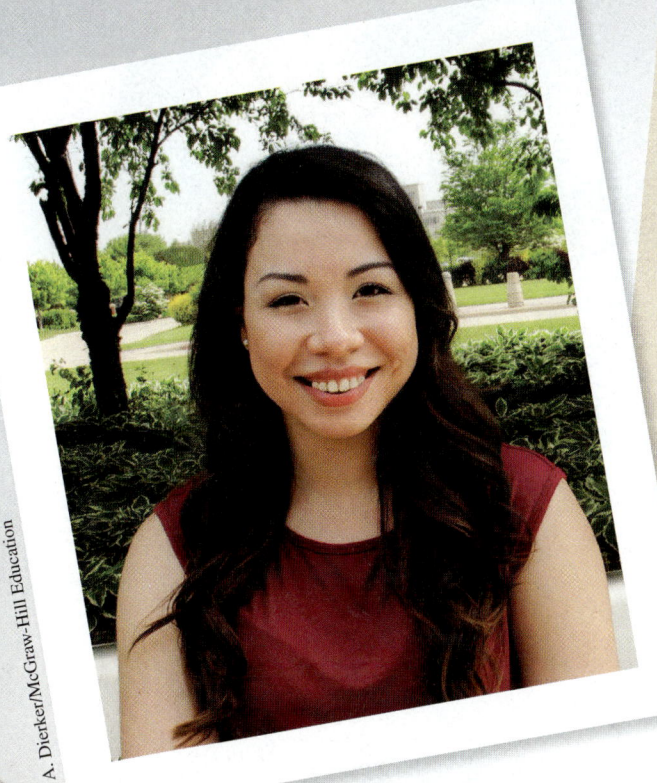

"My family's Hispanic, and most of my family was born in Texas, so I grew up helping my mother and grandmother cook 'Tex-Mex' food, using recipes passed down generation to generation. Now my diet isn't limited to Tex-Mex, but it's still my favorite type of food. I always associate this food with family gatherings."

Marisa Moreno

Pico de gallo
Wendy Schiff

Marisa Moreno is a recent graduate of Loras College. Her Hispanic ethnic background greatly influences her favorite food choices, which she describes as "Tex-Mex." According to Marisa, "Tex-Mex dishes are similar to traditional Mexican dishes, such as tacos, tostadas, burritos, tamales, fajitas, and enchiladas, but Tex-Mex food preparation uses some different ingredients. Mexican tacos, for example, typically include crumbly white goat cheese, whereas Tex-Mex tacos have shredded yellow American cheese. Tex-Mex dishes are often served with *pico de gallo* on top. *Pico de gallo* is a salsalike topping that is made from fresh diced tomatoes, jalapeño and serrano peppers, chopped green onions and fresh cilantro (a leafy herb that looks like fresh parsley), lemon juice, and a little salt. Also, Tex-Mex recipes often incorporate sauces made with hot chili peppers that are popular in the southwestern United States. Cumin is the southwestern spice generally used in Tex-Mex dishes . . . hot chili sauce is added on nearly everything."

Regardless of your ethnic/cultural background, your body needs **nutrients,** the life-sustaining chemicals in food, to function properly. **Nutrition** is the scientific study of nutrients and how the body uses these chemicals.

Eating supplies your body with nutrients and satisfies your hunger, but it also can be comforting, especially if eating certain foods soothes your anxiety or ends your boredom. The foods you choose to eat can have social and religious meaning. For example, lobster and prime rib steak are often associated with people who have high incomes. Other foods, such as a frosted layer cake topped with lit candles, stuffed roasted turkey, and communion wafers, are associated with birthday celebrations, seasonal holidays, and religious rites. Thus, food *is* more than just something to eat.

nutrients life-sustaining chemicals in food that are necessary for proper body functioning

nutrition study of nutrients and how the body uses these substances

Module 1.1

Why Learn About Nutrition?

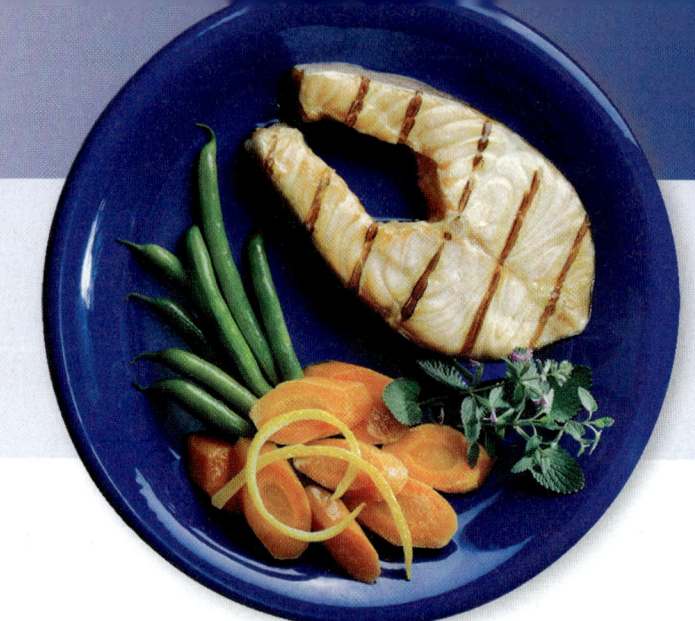

Purestock/SuperStock

1.1 - Learning Outcomes

After reading Module 1.1, you should be able to

1. Define all of the **key terms** in this module.
2. Discuss various factors that can influence a person's food selections.
3. Identify the leading causes of death in the United States and lifestyle factors that contribute to the risk of these diseases.

Have you ever thought about why you eat certain foods and not others? To what extent does your ethnic/cultural background influence your food choices? Overall, how would you rate the nutritional quality of the food that you eat—good, just OK, or poor?

Many factors, including your ethnic/cultural background, influence what you eat (**Fig. 1.1**). Your usual food choices are likely to be foods that you can afford, that you can prepare easily or obtain quickly, and that taste good. Your **diet** is your usual pattern of food choices. Why should you care about your diet? In the United States, poor eating habits contribute to several leading causes of death, including heart disease, some types of cancer, stroke, and diabetes (**Fig. 1.2**). Conditions such as heart disease, cancer, and diabetes are *chronic diseases*—health problems that usually take many years to develop and have complex causes.

Unfortunately, you weren't born with the ability to select a diet with the proper mix of nutrients. To eat *well*, you need to learn about nutrition and the effects that your food selections can have on your health.

A **risk factor** is a personal characteristic that increases your chances of developing a chronic disease. Some risk factors, such as having damaged or missing genes, being an older adult, and being a biological male or female, cannot be changed. Family

diet usual pattern of food choices

risk factor personal characteristic that increases a person's chances of developing a disease

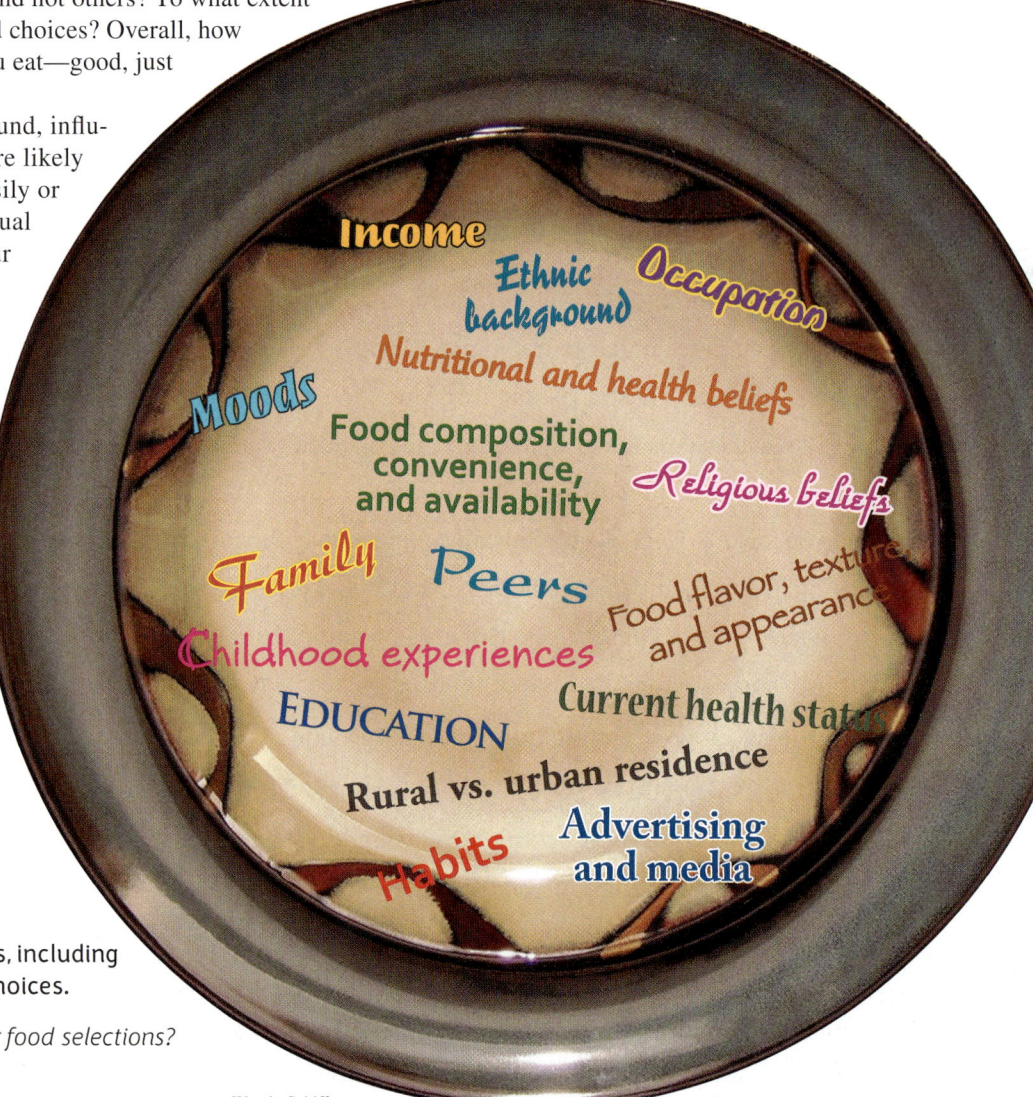

Figure 1.1 Many factors, including these, influence food choices.

■ *What influences your food selections?*

Wendy Schiff

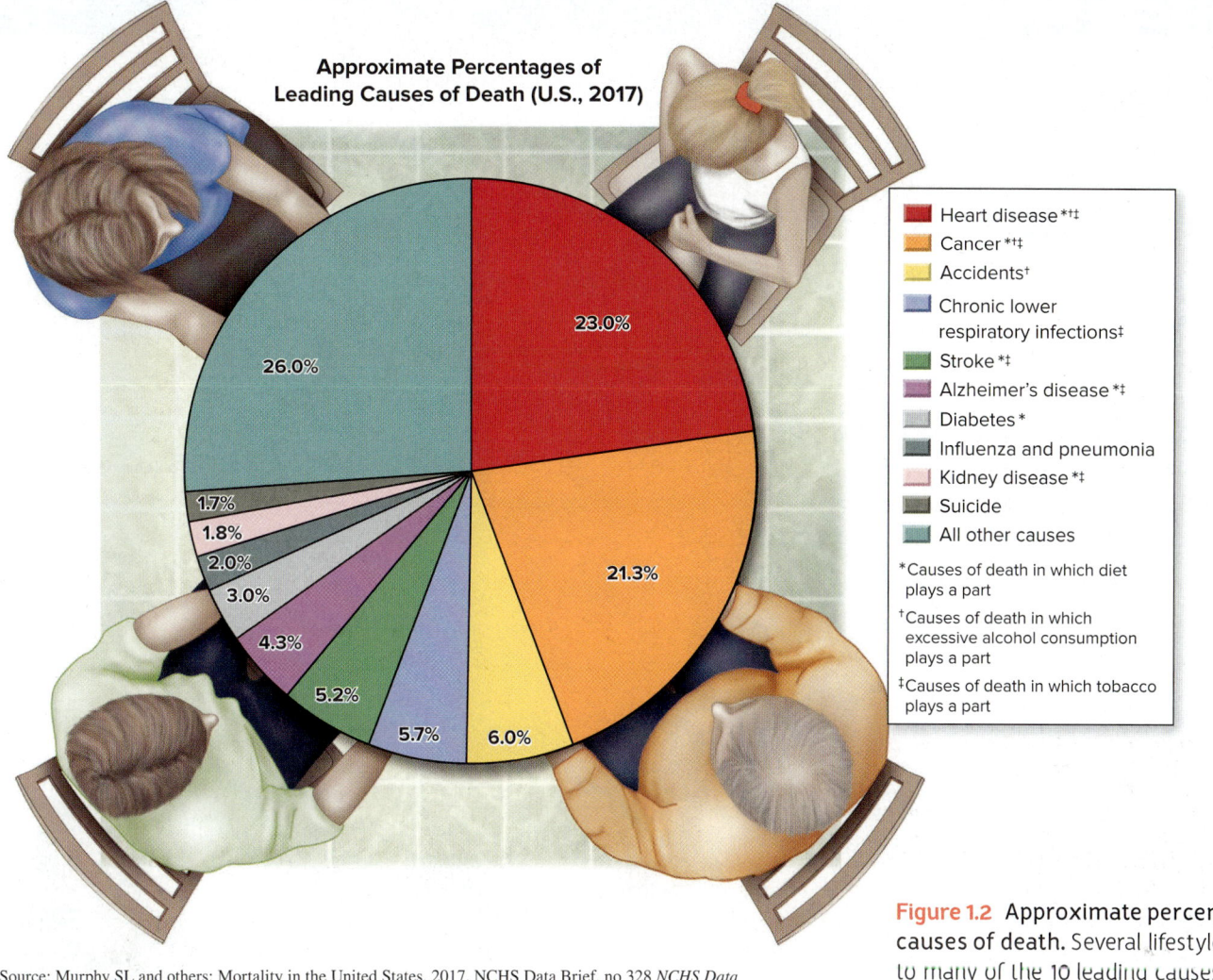

Figure 1.2 Approximate percentages of leading causes of death. Several lifestyle factors contribute to many of the 10 leading causes of death in the United States.

Source: Murphy SL and others: Mortality in the United States, 2017. NCHS Data Brief, no 328 *NCHS Data Brief.* Hyattsville, MD: National Center for Health Statistics. 2018

■ *Are any of these diseases in your family history?*

medical history, for example, is an important risk factor for heart disease. Your family's medical history can reveal disorders that were or can be passed down from generation to generation. Such disorders are often linked to faulty genetic information. If your father's father had a heart attack before he was 55 years old and your mother is being treated for having high blood pressure and a high blood cholesterol level (risk factors for heart disease), your family history indicates you have a higher-than-average risk of having a heart attack. For many people, however, having a family history of a chronic disease does not mean that they definitely will develop the condition. Other risk factors that contribute to health problems include age, environmental conditions, and lifestyle practices.

Lifestyle is a person's way of living that includes diet, physical activity habits, use of drugs such as tobacco and alcohol, and other typical patterns of health-related behavior. Your lifestyle may increase or reduce your chances of developing a chronic disease or delay its occurrence for years, even decades. Many people die prematurely because of their lifestyle practices. Fortunately, lifestyle-related risk factors usually can be changed to make them less risky. Smoking, for example, is a lifestyle. If you smoke, stopping can greatly reduce the likelihood that you will develop serious chronic diseases, especially lung cancer and premature heart disease. In the United States, cigarette smoking is the leading cause of preventable deaths.[1]

Reading this textbook can help you evaluate your diet and decide if it needs to be changed. You may be able to increase your chances of living a long and healthy life by consuming more fruits, vegetables, unsalted nuts, fat-free or low-fat dairy products, seafood, dried beans and peas, and whole-grain cereals, as well as exercising regularly.[2] Furthermore, reducing your intake of fatty meats, refined grain products, and sugar-sweetened foods, particularly beverages, may also improve your health.

lifestyle way of living that includes diet, physical activity habits, use of tobacco and alcohol, and other typical patterns of behavior

Module 1.2
Nutrition Basics

1.2 - Learning Outcomes

After reading Module 1.2, you should be able to

1. Define all of the **key terms** in this module.
2. List the six classes of nutrients, and identify a major role of each class of nutrient in the body.
3. Calculate the caloric value of a serving of food based on its macronutrient (and alcohol) contents.
4. Provide examples of essential nutrients, nonnutrients, phytochemicals, and dietary supplements.
5. Explain the importance of supplying the body with antioxidants.

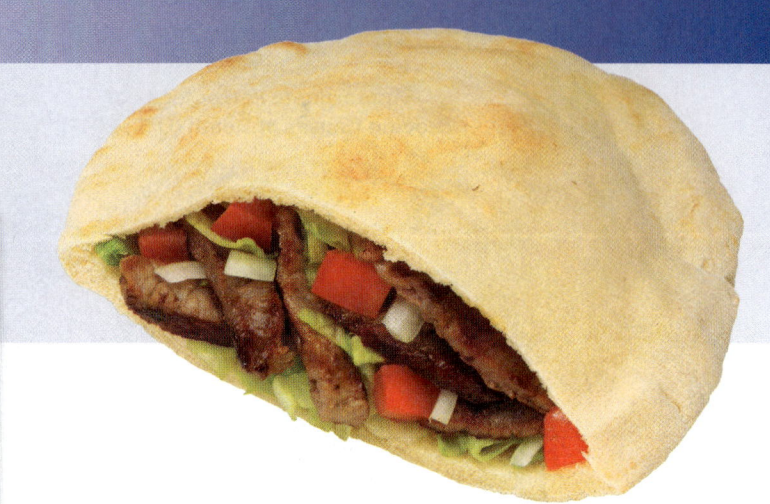

Ingram Publishing/Alamy

1.2a Nutrients and Their Major Functions

There are six classes of nutrients: carbohydrates, fats and other lipids, proteins, vitamins, minerals, and water. Carbohydrates, lipids, proteins, and vitamins are **organic nutrients** because they have the element carbon in their chemical structures.

Table 1.1 presents major roles of nutrients in your body. Note that most nutrients have more than one function and some nutrients have similar roles in your body. In general, you need certain nutrients for energy, growth and development, and regulation of cellular functions, including the repair and maintenance of cells. In many instances, several nutrients work together to keep your body healthy.

Although average healthy young men and women have similar amounts of vitamins, minerals, and carbohydrates in their bodies, young women have less water and protein and more fat (**Fig. 1.3**).

organic nutrients nutrients that have carbon in their chemical structures

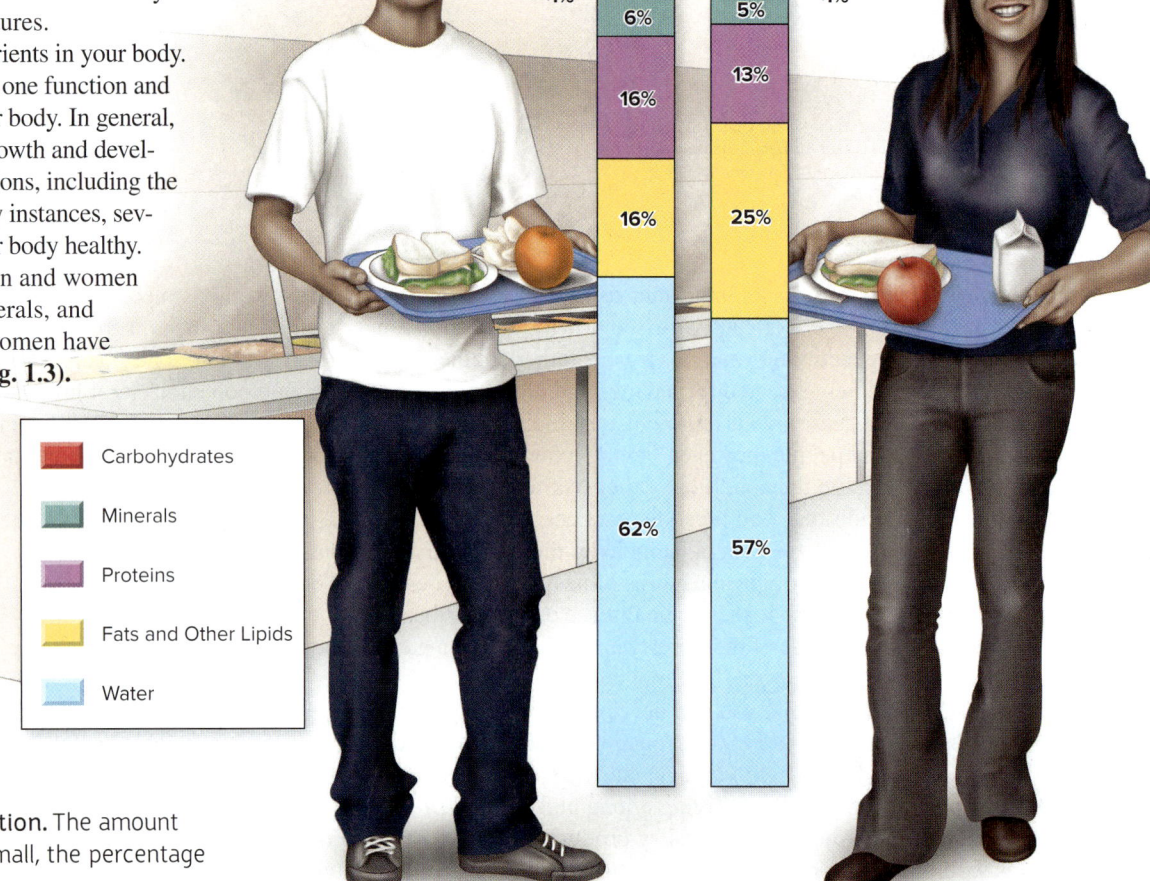

Figure 1.3 **Comparing body composition.** The amount of vitamins in the human body is so small, the percentage isn't shown.

6

TABLE 1.1 NUTRIENTS AND THEIR MAJOR FUNCTIONS IN THE BODY

Nutrient	Major Functions
Carbohydrates	Source of energy (most forms)
Lipids	Source of energy (fats), cellular development, physical growth and development, regulation of body processes, absorption of fat-soluble vitamins
Proteins	Production of structural and functional components; cellular development, growth, and maintenance; regulation of body processes; immune function; fluid balance; source of energy
Vitamins	Regulation of body processes, maintenance of immune function, production and maintenance of tissues, protection against agents that can damage cellular components
Minerals	Regulation of body processes, including fluid balance; formation of certain chemical messengers; structural and functional components of various substances and tissues; necessary for physical growth, maintenance, and development
Water	Maintenance of fluid balance, regulation of body temperature, elimination of wastes, transportation of substances, participant in many chemical reactions

Cutting board: Mark A. Dierker/McGraw-Hill Education; Red onion: Burke Triolo Productions/Getty Images USA, Inc.; Cut peppers: I. Rozenbaum & F. Cirou/PhotoAlto

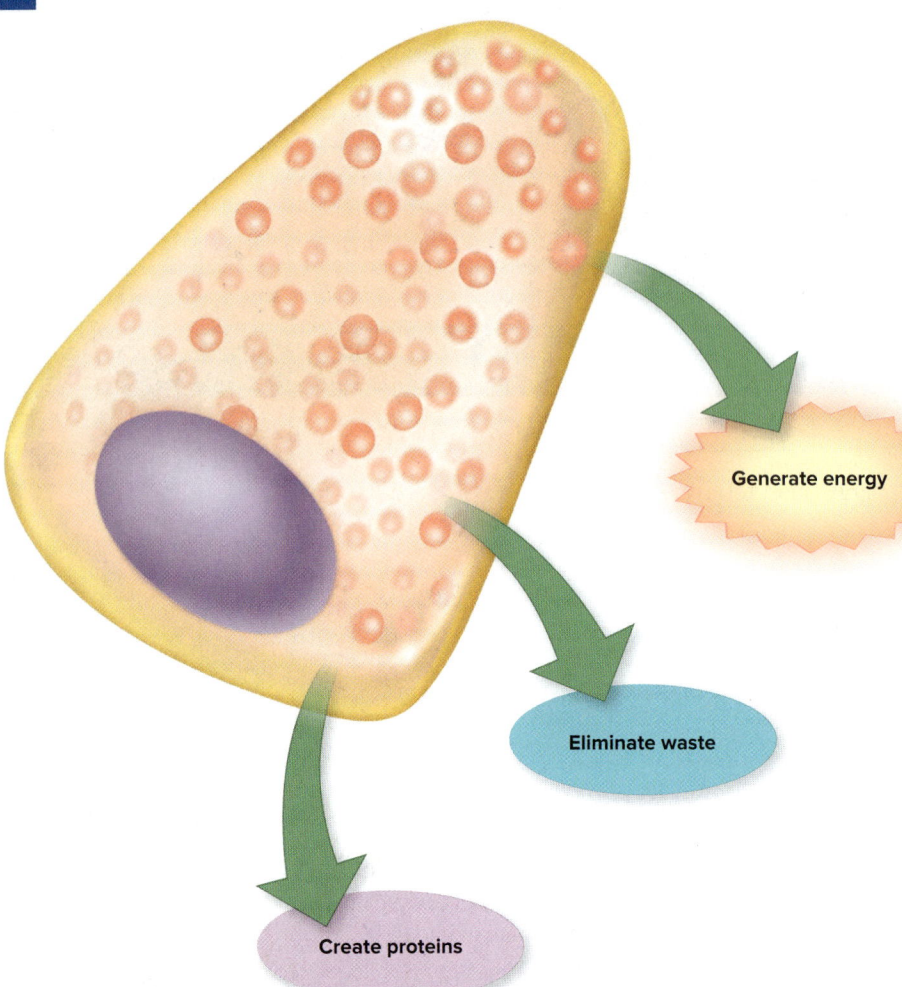

Figure 1.4 Some functions of a typical human cell.

A **cell** is the smallest functional unit in a living organism, including a human being **(Fig. 1.4)**. Cells do not need food to survive, but they do need the nutrients in food to carry out their metabolic activities. **Metabolism** is the total of all chemical reactions (changes) that occur in living cells, including reactions involved in generating energy, making proteins, and eliminating waste products.

1.2b Food Energy

Every cell in your body uses energy to carry out its various activities, whether you're running, sitting, or studying, and even while you're sleeping. As long as you're alive, you're constantly using energy. Foods and beverages that contain fat, carbohydrate, protein, and/or alcohol supply energy for your body. You'll learn how your cells obtain energy in Unit 4.

You're probably familiar with the term *calorie*, the unit that describes the energy content of food. The amount of energy in food is reported in 1000-calorie units called **kilocalories (kcal)**, or **Calories**. If no number of kilocalories is specified, it's appropriate to use "calories." In this textbook, the term "kilocalories" is interchangeable with "food energy" or simply "energy."

cell smallest living functional unit in an organism

metabolism total of all chemical processes that take place in living cells

kilocalorie (kcal) or Calorie unit of measuring food energy

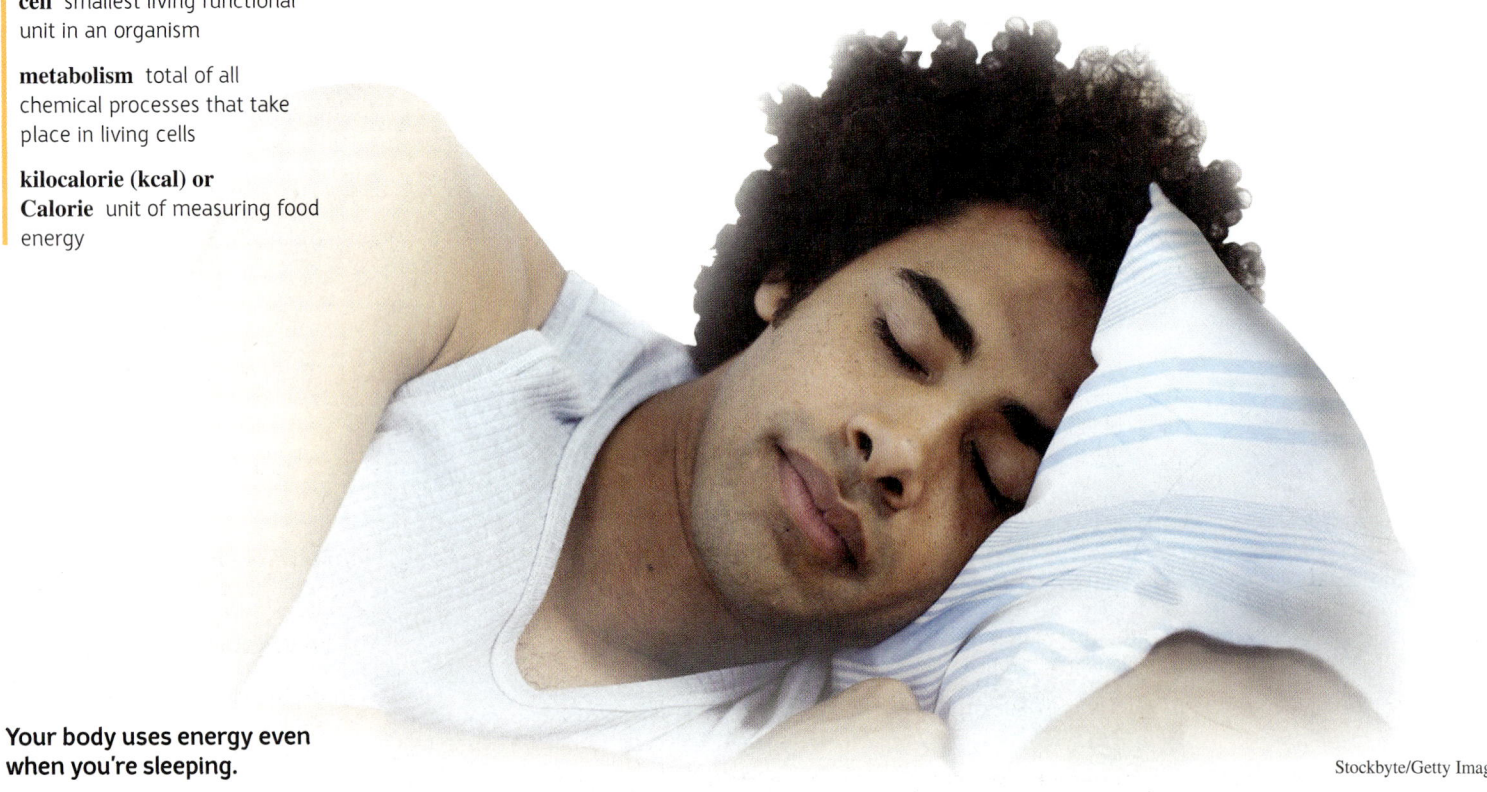

Your body uses energy even when you're sleeping.

Stockbyte/Getty Images

1.2c Macronutrients and Micronutrients

Carbohydrates, fats, and proteins are sometimes called **macronutrients** because the body needs relatively large amounts of these nutrients daily. Vitamins and minerals are **micronutrients** because the body needs very small amounts of them to function properly. Macronutrients supply energy (kcal) for cells, whereas micronutrients do not. Although your body requires large amounts of water, this nutrient provides no energy and isn't usually classified as a macronutrient.

Nutrition experts often use metric measurements, such as grams (g) and liters (l), instead of household measures, such as ounces and cups. An ounce of salt, for example, weighs about 28 g. **Table 1.2** provides the meaning of some commonly used metric prefixes, including *kilo-* and *milli-*. In general, a serving of food supplies grams of carbohydrate, fat, and protein and *milligram (mg)* or *microgram (mcg or µg)* quantities of vitamins and minerals. **Appendix A** provides information about common English-to-metric and metric-to-household unit conversions.

Table 1.2 Common Metric Prefixes for Nutrition

- kilo- (k) = one thousand (1000)
- deci- (d) = one-tenth (0.1)
- centi- (c) = one-hundredth (0.01)
- milli- (m) = one-thousandth (0.001)
- micro- (mc or µ) = one-millionth (0.000001)

A gram of carbohydrate and a gram of protein each supplies about 4 kcal; a gram of fat provides about 9 kcal **(Fig. 1.5)**. Although alcohol isn't a nutrient, it does provide energy; a gram of pure alcohol furnishes 7 kcal.

If you know how many grams of carbohydrate, protein, fat, and/or alcohol are in a food, you can estimate the number of kilocalories it provides. For example, if a serving of food contains 10 g of carbohydrate and 5 g of fat, multiply 10 by 4 (the number of kcal each gram of carbohydrate supplies). Then multiply 5 by 9 (the number of kcal each gram of fat supplies). By adding the two values (40 kcal from carbohydrate and 45 kcal from fat), you'll determine that this food provides 85 kcal/serving.

A serving of food contains 30 g of carbohydrate, 10 g of fat, 5 g of protein, 60 mg of vitamin C, and 5 mg of iron. How many calories are in the serving of food? First, determine the amount of energy in each of the food's components.

$$30 \text{ g of carbohydrate} \times 4 \text{ kcal/g} = 120 \text{ kcal from carbohydrate}$$
$$10 \text{ g of fat} \times 9 \text{ kcal/g} = 90 \text{ kcal from fat}$$
$$5 \text{ g of protein} \times 4 \text{ kcal/g} = 20 \text{ kcal from protein}$$

Now, add together the calories for the three sources of energy: 120 kcal + 90 kcal + 20 kcal = 230 kcal/serving.

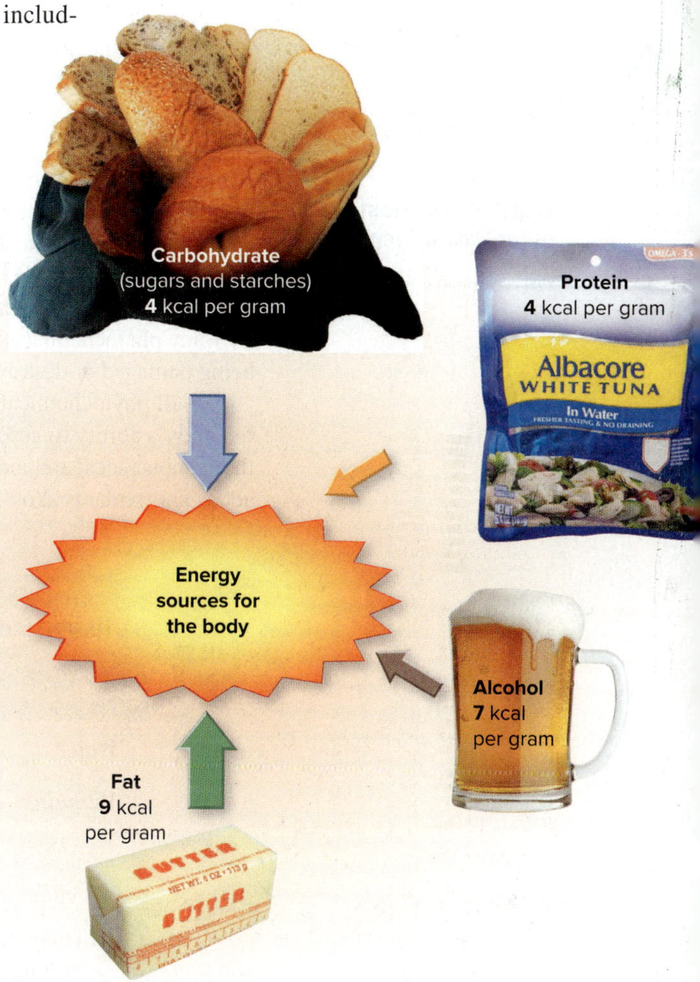

Figure 1.5 Energy sources for the body. Alcohol isn't a nutrient.

■ *How can you estimate the amount of calories in a serving of food?*

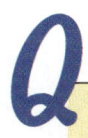

Answer This

Why don't you need to include vitamin C and iron in your calorie calculations? You'll find the answer on the last page of this unit.

macronutrients nutrients needed in gram amounts daily and that provide energy; carbohydrates, proteins, and fats

micronutrients nutrients needed in milligram or microgram amounts (vitamins and minerals)

Basket of bread: Wendy Schiff; Beer mug: dr3amer/iStock.com; Package of tuna: Holly Curry/McGraw-Hill Education; Stick of butter: D. Hurst/Alamy

1.2d What's an Essential Nutrient?

Your body can make many nutrients, such as fat and cholesterol (types of lipids), but about 50 nutrients must be supplied by food because the human body does not produce the nutrient or make enough to meet its needs. Such nutrients are **essential nutrients (Table 1.3).** Water is the most essential nutrient. You can live for months without iron or vitamin C but only a few days without water.

If an essential nutrient is missing from the diet, a **deficiency disease** occurs as a result. The deficiency disease is a state of health characterized by certain abnormal *physiological* (functional) changes that result in signs and symptoms of disease. Such signs and symptoms may include skin rashes, diarrhea, and loss of night vision. Treating a deficiency disease is usually simple: When the missing essential nutrient is added to the diet, the deficiency disease is cured.

1.2e What's a Nonnutrient?

Some foods, particularly those from plants, contain nonnutrients: substances that are not nutrients, yet may have healthful benefits. Alcohol is an energy-supplying nonnutrient that can have harmful as well as beneficial effects on your health. Plants make hundreds of **phytochemicals** *(fi'-toe-kem'-ih-kalz)*. Caffeine, for example, is a phytochemical naturally made by coffee plants that has a stimulating effect on the body. Later units of this text provide more information about caffeine and alcohol.

Many phytochemicals function as **antioxidants.** An antioxidant protects cells and their components from being damaged or destroyed by chemically unstable factors that are called **free radicals.**

Not all phytochemicals have beneficial effects on the body; some are *toxic* (poisonous) or can interfere with the body's ability to absorb nutrients. **Table 1.4** lists several phytochemicals, identifies rich food sources of these substances, and indicates their effects on the body, including possible health benefits. Certain vitamins act as antioxidants. You'll learn more about them in Unit 8, which focuses on vitamins.

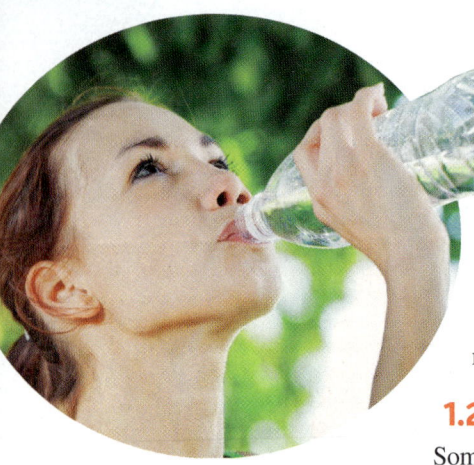

Water is the most essential nutrient.

vm/Getty Images

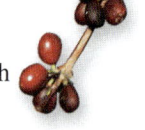

Coffee beans

Source: USDA Natural Resources

essential nutrient nutrient that must be supplied by food

deficiency disease state of health that occurs when a nutrient is missing from the diet

phytochemicals substances made by plants that are not nutrients but may be healthful

antioxidant substance that protects cells and their components from being damaged or destroyed by free radicals

free radicals chemically unstable factors that can damage or destroy cells

TABLE 1.3 ESSENTIAL NUTRIENTS FOR HUMANS

Water

Vitamins

A			C	
B vitamins			D*	
Thiamin	Pantothenic acid	B-6	E	
Riboflavin	Biotin	B-12	K	Choline**
Niacin	Folic acid (folate)			

Glucose (from carbohydrate-containing foods)†

Minerals

Calcium	Copper	Magnesium	Phosphorus	Sodium
Chloride	Iodine	Manganese	Potassium	Sulfur
Chromium	Iron	Molybdenum	Selenium	Zinc

The following components of proteins (amino acids) are generally recognized as essential:

Histidine	Lysine	Threonine
Isoleucine	Methionine	Tryptophan
Leucine	Phenylalanine	Valine

Fats that contain linoleic and alpha-linolenic acids

*The body makes vitamin D after exposure to sunlight, but a dietary source of the nutrient is often necessary.
**The body makes choline but may not make enough to meet needs. Often classified as a *vitamin-like* substance.
†A source of glucose is needed to supply the nervous system with energy and spare protein from being used for energy.

Table 1.4 Phytochemicals

Examples	Rich Food Sources	Biological Effects/ Possible Health Benefits
Alpha-carotene, beta-carotene, lutein, lycopene	Orange, red, yellow, dark green fruits and vegetables; egg yolks	Antioxidant activity, especially beta-carotene; may inhibit cancer growth. The body can convert alpha- and beta-carotene into vitamin A.
Quercetin	Apples, tea, red wine, onions, olives, raspberries, cocoa	Antioxidant activity, may inhibit cancer growth, may reduce risk of heart disease
Anthocyanins	Red, blue, or purple fruits and vegetables	Antioxidant activity, may inhibit cancer growth, may reduce risk of heart disease
Resveratrol	Red wine, purple grapes and grape juice, dark chocolate, cocoa	Antioxidant activity, may inhibit cancer growth, may reduce risk of heart disease
Isoflavonoids	Soybeans and other legumes	Antioxidant activity, may inhibit cancer growth, may reduce risk of heart disease
Sulfur compounds	Garlic, onions, leeks, broccoli, cauliflower, cabbage, kale, bok choy, collard and mustard greens	Antioxidant activity, may inhibit cancer growth, may reduce risk of heart disease
Caffeine	Coffee, tea, cocoa	Stimulant effects
Saponins	Chickpeas, beans, oats, grapes, olives, spinach, garlic, quinoa	May kill certain microbes, inhibit certain cancers, and reduce risk of heart disease
Capsaicin	Chili peppers	May provide some pain relief, when applied to skin

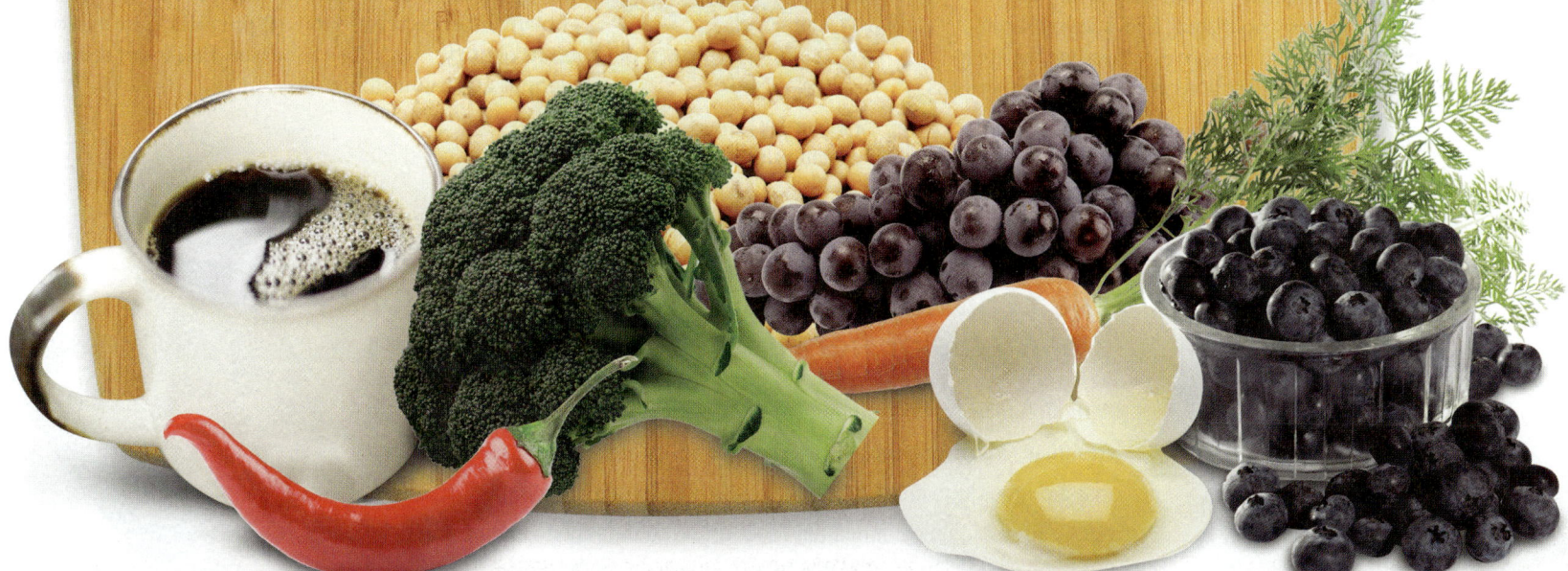

Cutting board: Mark A. Dierker/McGraw-Hill Education; Cup of coffee: Ingram Publishing/SuperStock; Broccoli: lynx/iconotec.com/Glow Images; Chili pepper: Maks Narodenko/Shutterstock; Soybeans: Fabrizio Troiani/Alamy Stock Photo; Carrot: Clover/SuperStock; Purple grapes: lynx/iconotec.com/Glow Images; Broken egg: Photodisc/Getty Images; Bowl of blueberries: Purestock/SuperStock

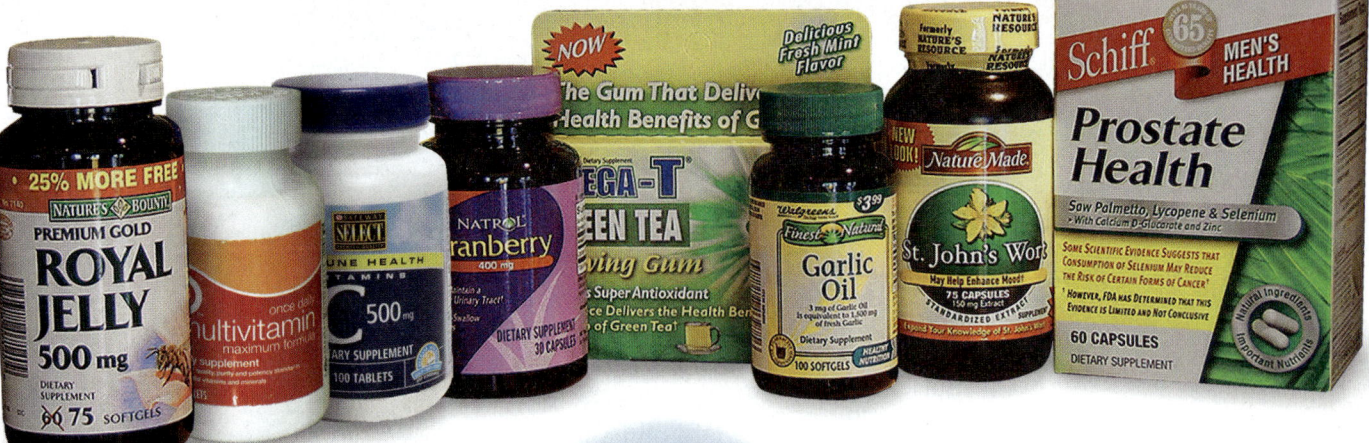

1.2f What Are Dietary Supplements?

Many Americans take dietary supplements such as vitamin pills and herbal extracts to improve their health. A **dietary supplement** is a product (excluding tobacco) that contains a vitamin, a mineral, an herb or other plant product, an amino acid, or a dietary substance that supplements the diet by increasing total intake.[3] According to scientific evidence, some dietary supplements, such as vitamins, minerals, and certain herbs, can have beneficial effects on health. However, results of scientific testing also indicate that many popular dietary supplements are not helpful and may even be harmful. Information about specific dietary supplements is in Unit 3 and woven into other units of this textbook where appropriate.

1.2g What's Malnutrition?

Malnutrition is a state of health that occurs when the body is improperly nourished. Everyone must consume food and water to stay alive, yet despite the abundance and variety of nutritious foods, many Americans consume nutritionally poor diets and suffer from malnutrition as a result. Some people select nutritionally inadequate diets because they lack knowledge about nutritious foods or the importance of nutrition to health. Low-income people, however, are at risk for malnutrition because they have limited financial resources for making wise food purchases. Other people who are at risk of malnutrition include those who are frail and living in long-term care facilities, have severe eating disorders, are addicted to drugs such as alcohol, or have certain serious diseases.

Many people associate malnutrition with *under*nutrition and starvation. *Over*nutrition, the long-term excess of energy or nutrient intake, is also a form of malnutrition. Overnutrition is often characterized by unhealthy amounts of body fat (*obesity*). You may be surprised to learn that overnutrition is more common in the United States than undernutrition. Obesity is widespread in countries where most people have the financial means to buy plenty of food, have an ample food supply, and obtain little exercise. Unit 10 provides information about obesity; Unit 11 discusses the international problem of undernutrition.

Obesity is a form of malnutrition.

dietary supplement product that contains a vitamin, a mineral, an herb or other plant product, an amino acid, or a dietary substance that supplements the diet

malnutrition state of health that occurs when the body is improperly nourished

Nutrition Fact or Fiction?

The typical college student gains 15 pounds during his or her freshman year.

Although many college students (more than 51%) gain weight during their freshman year in college, the average weight gain is 7.6 pounds.[4] Factors that are thought to contribute to the weight gain include feeling "stressed out," eating too much unhealthy food, drinking too much alcohol, and being less physically active than before they entered college.

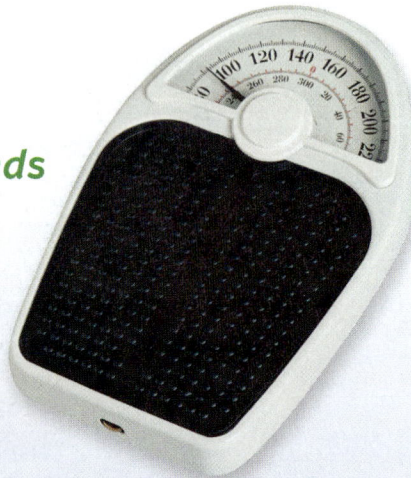

Supplements: Wendy Schiff; Obese woman: Lars A. Niki; Bathroom scale: Comstock Images/Getty Images USA, Inc.

Module 1.3

Key Nutrition Concepts

1.3 - Learning Outcomes

After reading Module 1.3, you should be able to

1. Define all of the **key terms** in this module.
2. Classify foods as nutrient dense, energy dense, or high in empty calories.
3. Identify key basic nutrition concepts, including the importance of eating a variety of foods and no naturally occurring food supplies all nutrients.

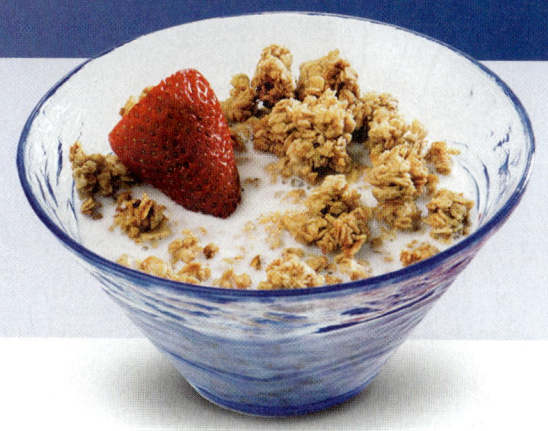

Design Pics Inc./Alamy

Before learning about nutrients and their roles in health, it's important to grasp some key basic nutrition concepts (**Table 1.5**). Each of the sections of this module focuses on one of these concepts. The content in the units that follow will build upon these key concepts and can help you make more informed choices concerning your dietary practices.

1.3a There Are No "Good" or "Bad" Foods

Do you refer to pizza, chips, candy, doughnuts, ice cream, and sugar-sweetened soft drinks as "bad foods" or "junk foods"? All foods have nutritional value, so no food deserves to be labeled "bad" or "junk." Although pies, doughnuts, and ice cream contain a lot of fat and sugar, these foods also supply small amounts of protein, vitamins, and minerals to diets. A chocolate doughnut, for example, provides 6 g protein, 2 mg niacin (a B vitamin), 4 mg iron, and 4 g fiber. (Most forms of fiber are classified as carbohydrates.) Even sugar-sweetened soft drinks provide two nutrients: water and the carbohydrate sugar, a source of energy. As you read this textbook, you'll learn why certain foods are healthier choices than others.

A food *is* bad for you if it contains toxic substances or is contaminated with bacteria, viruses, or microscopic animals that cause food-borne illness. You've probably suffered from a food-borne illness at least once. The abdominal cramps, nausea, vomiting, and diarrhea that usually accompany a food-borne illness occur within a few hours or days after a person eats the contaminated food. Unit 11 discusses food safety concerns, including major types of food-borne illnesses and how to prevent them.

Empty Calories

Some foods and beverages, such as candies, pastries, snack chips, sugar-sweetened drinks, and some alcoholic beverages, may be described as sources of "empty calories."[5] **Empty calories** are calories from unhealthy types of fat, added sugar, and/or alcohol. Thus, a food that contains a lot of empty calories usually isn't a good source of vitamins and minerals. Eating too many foods that are high in empty calories may displace more nutritious foods from your diet. In later units of this text, you'll learn more about empty calories, including alcohol.

What's a Nutrient-Dense Food?

Certain foods provide more "key beneficial nutrients" than others. Key beneficial nutrients are protein; fiber; vitamins A, C, and E; and the minerals iron, calcium, magnesium, and potassium.[6] A **nutrient-dense** food or beverage contains more key beneficial nutrients in relation to total calories, especially calories from unhealthy fats, added sugars, and/or alcohol. Broccoli, leafy greens, fat-free milk, orange juice, lean meats, eggs, and whole-grain cereals are examples of nutrient-dense foods.

> **empty calories** calories from unhealthy fats, added sugars, and/or alcohol
>
> **nutrient dense** describes foods or beverages that supply more key beneficial nutrients in relation to total calories

Table 1.5 Key Nutrition Concepts

1. There are no good or bad foods.
2. Variety, moderation, and balance are features of healthy diets.
3. Food is the best source of nutrients and phytochemicals.
4. There is no "one size fits all" approach to good nutrition.
5. Foods and nutrients are not cure-alls.

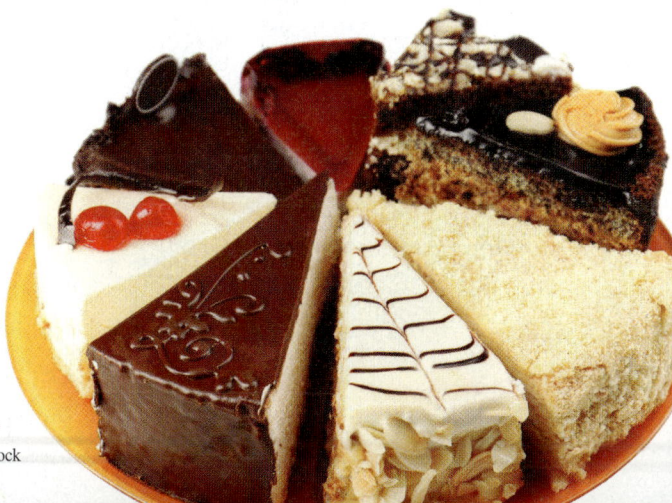

Foods that contain a lot of empty calories usually aren't nutrient dense.

Africa Studio/Shutterstock

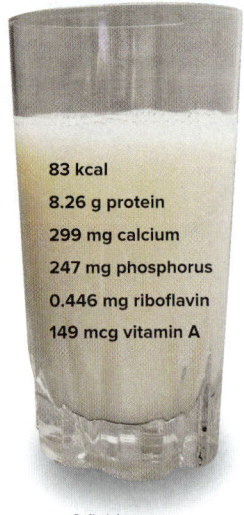
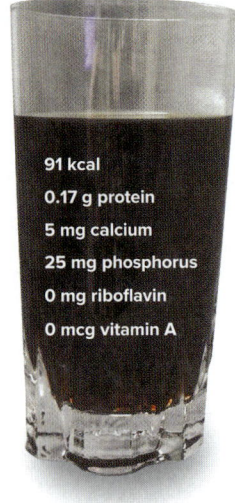

8 fluid ounces fat-free milk
83 kcal
8.26 g protein
299 mg calcium
247 mg phosphorus
0.446 mg riboflavin
149 mcg vitamin A

8 fluid ounces sugar-sweetened soft drink
91 kcal
0.17 g protein
5 mg calcium
25 mg phosphorus
0 mg riboflavin
0 mcg vitamin A

Figure 1.6 Nutrient density.

■ *What distinguishes a food that is a rich source of empty calories from a nutrient-dense one?*

Figure 1.6 compares amounts of energy and certain nutrients provided by 8-ounce servings of fat-free milk and a cola-type, sugar-sweetened ("regular") soft drink. Although the drinks supply similar amounts of calories, the milk provides far more protein and riboflavin (a B vitamin), and minerals calcium and phosphorus. A healthy diet contains a variety of nutrient-dense foods and limits empty calories.

Which Foods Are Energy Dense?

Energy density describes the energy value of a food in relation to the food's weight. For example, a chocolate, yeast-type frosted doughnut that weighs about 3.5 ounces and is about 4 inches in diameter provides about 400 kcal; eight medium strawberries also weigh about 3.5 ounces, but they provide only 32 kcal. You'd have to eat 100 of the strawberries to obtain the same amount of food energy that's in the chocolate doughnut (**Fig. 1.7**). Therefore, the doughnut is an energy-dense food in comparison to the berries. In general, high-fat foods such as doughnuts are energy dense because they're concentrated sources of energy. Most fruits aren't energy dense because they contain far more water than fat.

It's important to note that not all energy-dense foods are rich sources of empty calories. Nuts, for example, are high in fat and, therefore, energy dense. However, nuts are also nutrient dense because they contribute protein, vitamins, minerals, and fiber to diets. You can find information about the energy and nutrient contents of foods by using "What's in the Foods You Eat *Search Tool*" that's available at the U.S. Department of Agriculture's website: https://www.ars.usda.gov/.

| **energy density** energy value of a food in relation to the food's weight

TASTY Tidbits

Almonds and other nuts are nutrient and energy dense. For example, 1 ounce of plain, roasted almonds (about 23 whole nuts) supplies about 170 kcal, 6 g of protein, 15 g of fat, 6.5 mg of vitamin E, and small amounts of iron, calcium, and B vitamins. Snack on a handful of nuts or add them to your cereal.

Figure 1.7 Energy density.

■ *What distinguishes an "energy-dense" food from a food that's not energy dense?*

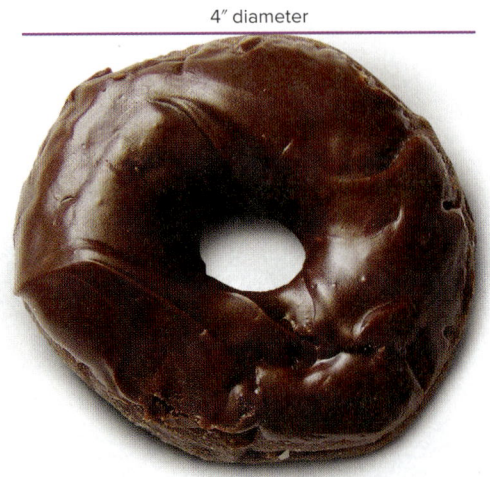

4" diameter

400 kcal

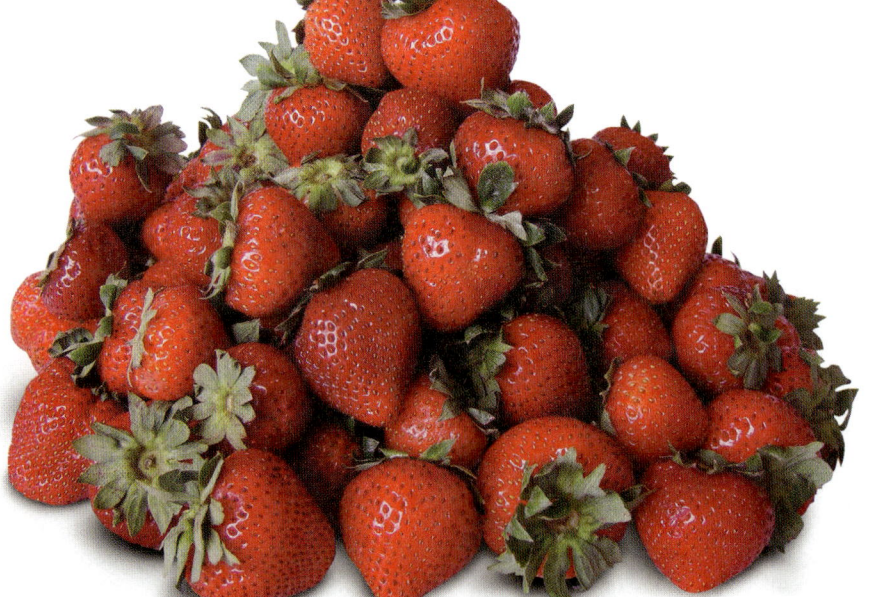

400 kcal

Milk, Soft drink, Doughnut, Strawberries: Wendy Schiff; Almonds: onair/Shutterstock

Key Nutrition Concepts   15

Culture & Cuisine

Traditional Mexican meals typically include some form of corn, such as tortillas made from cornmeal; beans; chili peppers; and rice. Meals may also feature eggs, pork, chicken, beef, and fish as well as a wide variety of fruits and vegetables. Main dishes, dips, sauces, and snacks often incorporate fresh avocados, tomatillos, papayas, pineapples, limes, mangoes, chayote, cherimoya, jicama, tomatoes, garlic, onions, plantains, and the fruit (*tuna*) and young stems (*nopales* or pads) of the prickly pear cactus. Cilantro; oregano; cumin; parsley; and various dried peppers, such as chile de árbol, chipotle, cascabel, and pasilla, are used to add distinctive flavors to Mexican cuisine. The traditional Mexican diet is high in fiber, vitamins C and A, potassium, magnesium, and beneficial phytochemicals.

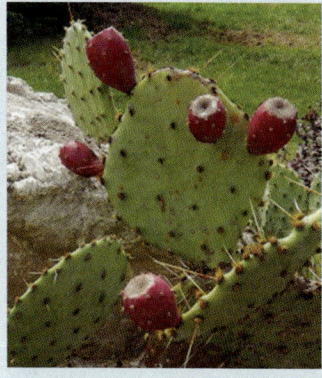
Prickly pear cactus with fruit (tuna) and green stems (pads or nopales)

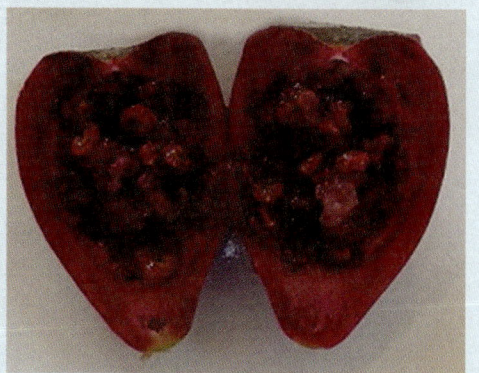
Prickly pear fruit (tuna), sliced in half to show seeds and pulp

1.3b Variety, Moderation, and Balance Are Features of Healthy Diets

Most foods are mixtures of nutrients, but no natural food is "perfect" in that it contains all nutrients in amounts that your body needs. To help ensure that your diet provides all the essential nutrients as well as beneficial phytochemicals, choose a **variety** of nutrient-dense foods and consume them in reasonable amounts (**moderation**). Furthermore, **balance** (match) your caloric intake with enough physical activity to maintain a healthy weight. Unit 3 provides more information about healthy diets, including recommendations for serving sizes.

1.3c Food Is the Best Source of Nutrients and Phytochemicals

The most natural, reliable, and economical way to obtain nutrients and beneficial phytochemicals is to base your diet on a variety of "whole" and minimally processed foods. For most Americans, eating 100% raw foods isn't practical and, in some instances, it's unsafe. Many foods undergo some form of processing, such as peeling, refining, and heating, before they're eaten. Such treatments can make food safer and more convenient to eat.

Plant foods naturally contain a variety of nutrients and phytochemicals, but processing the foods often removes some of the most healthful parts. For example, a wheat kernel is stripped of its germ and outer hull (*bran*) during refinement into white flour **(Fig. 1.8)**. Wheat germ is a rich source of vitamin E and beneficial ("healthy") fats. Wheat bran contains fiber and certain phytochemicals, and it's a concentrated source of several micronutrients. The endosperm is primarily starch (a form of carbohydrate) with some protein and very small amounts of micronutrients and fiber. A "whole grain" includes the bran and germ portions of the kernel along with the endosperm. By replacing refined grain products, such as white bread, with 100% whole-grain products, you can increase the likelihood of obtaining a wide variety of nutrients and phytochemicals.

> **variety** including many different nutrient-dense foods in your diet
>
> **moderation** consuming foods in reasonable amounts
>
> **balance** matching calorie intake with enough physical activity to maintain a healthy weight

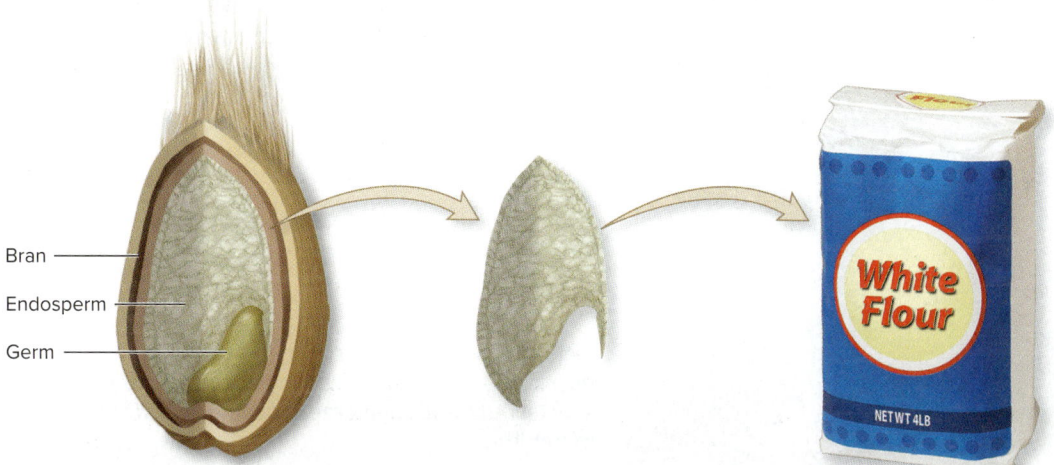

Figure 1.8 What is white flour? During refinement, a wheat kernel is stripped of its nutrient-rich germ and bran. The endosperm (white flour) that remains is mostly starch.

■ *Why is it important to choose a variety of foods, especially those that are whole or minimally processed?*

Cactus, Cactus fruit: Wendy Schiff; White flour: Michael Scott/McGraw-Hill Education

Should You Take Nutrient Supplements?

Your body is designed to obtain nutrients from foods, not supplements. In some instances, nutrients from food are more available—that is, more easily digested and absorbed than those in supplements.

It's important to understand that nutrient supplements don't contain everything you need for optimal nutrition. For example, they don't contain the wide variety of phytochemicals found in plant foods. Although supplements that contain phytochemicals are available, they may not provide the same healthful benefits as those obtained by consuming the plants that contain these substances. Why? Nutrients and phytochemicals may need to be consumed together to provide desirable effects in the body. Food naturally contains combinations of these chemicals in very small amounts and certain proportions. There's nothing "natural" about gulping down handfuls of supplements.

For each micronutrient, there's a range of safe intake. In their natural states, most commonly eaten foods contain safe levels of micronutrients. However, you can develop health problems by taking high doses of dietary supplements that contain vitamins and/or minerals.

For each nutrient, there is a range of safe intake.

1.3d There's No "One Size Fits All" Approach to Good Nutrition

By using food guides presented in Unit 3, you can individualize your diet so that it's nutritionally adequate and suits your food likes and dislikes, budget, and lifestyle. Individualizing a diet doesn't mean only eating foods that "match" your blood type, hair color, personality, or shoe size. If someone promotes a diet based on such personal traits, steer clear of the diet and the promoter. Consider this: Human beings wouldn't have survived as a species for thousands of years if their diets had to be matched to physical characteristics or personalities.

It's important to note that nutritional needs of healthy people vary during different stages of their lives. Thus, infants, children, pregnant women, and older adults often need nutrient supplements to boost their nutrient intakes. Additionally, physicians often prescribe nutrient supplements or special diets for chronically ill people.

1.3e Foods and Nutrients Aren't Cure-Alls

Although specific nutrient deficiency diseases can be cured if you eat foods that contain the nutrient that's missing or is in short supply, nutrients don't "cure" other ailments. Diet is only one aspect of yourself that influences your health. Other lifestyle factors as well as genetics and environment also play major roles in determining your health status.

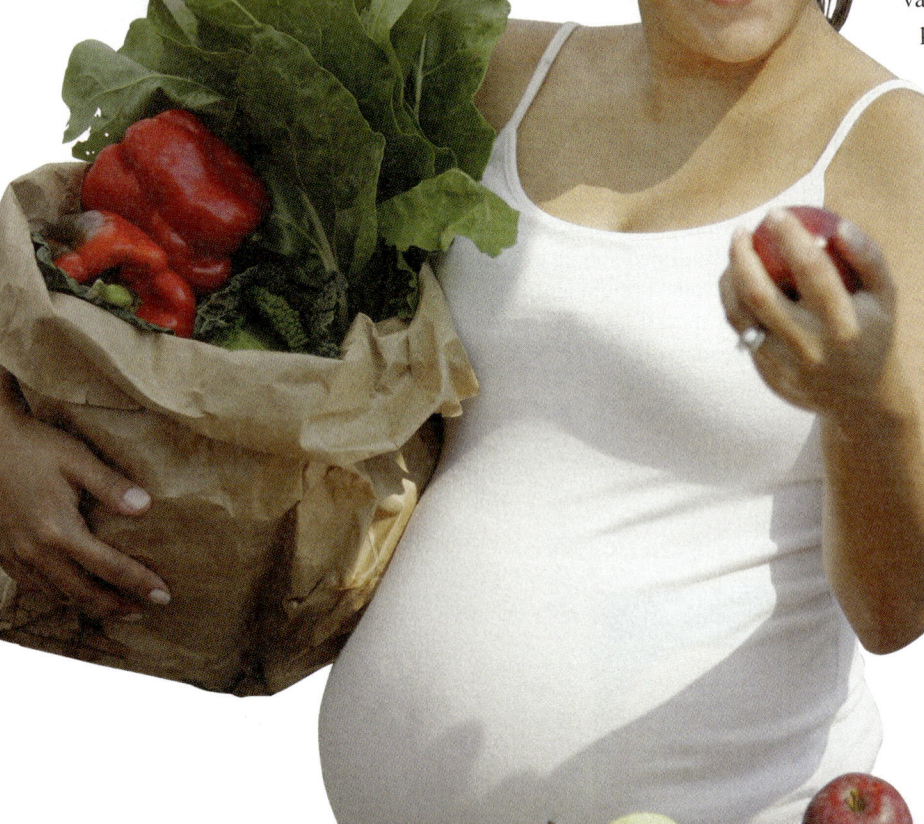

Although a pregnant woman may choose nutritious foods, she still may need to take a special nutrient supplement during this stage of her life.

Vladimir Pcholkin/Getty Images USA, Inc.

What *IS* That?

Pitaya (or pitahaya) is the fruit of a night-blooming cactus that's also called "dragon fruit." Although some farmers in Florida and California grow species of cactus that produce sweet pitaya (usually *H. undatus*), most of the pitayas that are available in grocery stores have been imported from Vietnam, a country in Southeast Asia.

Depending on the variety of cactus, pitayas can have white, red, or purplish-pink pulp that's dotted with numerous tiny, black seeds. Although the seeds are edible, they're not digested by the intestinal tract, and, as a result, can have a mild laxative effect.

Before eating a fresh pitaya, wash the skin. Then, slice the fruit in half, remove the peel, and cut the pulp into bite-size pieces. Because sweet pitaya can have a bland taste (especially the fruit with white pulp), it's often blended with more flavorful fruits to make juice.

A 3.5-ounce serving of bite-size pitaya cubes supplies 60 kcal, mostly from natural sugars. Fresh pitaya isn't a nutrient-dense food, but the fruit is low in sodium and fat, and a serving adds about 3 grams of fiber and a small amount of vitamin C to diets. Varieties of pitaya that have red pulp are a rich source of plant pigments called *betalains*, which may act as antioxidants in the body. Nevertheless, there's a lack of scientific evidence that pitayas have healthful benefits for humans. If you occasionally eat large amounts of pitayas with red pulp, expect your urine and stools to become red temporarily.[7]

What Are Functional Foods?

Many foods and beverages are manufactured for specific health-related functions. Although there's no legal definition for *functional foods*, such products have health-related purposes.[8] Functional foods are often made to boost nutrient intakes or help manage specific health problems. For example, you can increase your calcium intake by purchasing orange juice that has the mineral added to it. Certain margarine substitutes contain beneficial fats and phytochemicals that may lower the risk of heart disease. Many yogurt products contain specific forms of bacteria that may relieve diarrhea. These bacteria are *probiotics*—that is, living microorganisms that can benefit human health (see Unit 4). Although some functional foods can help people improve their health in other ways, more research is needed to determine their benefits as well as possible harmful effects.

1.3f Some Closing Thoughts

By applying what you learn about nutrition and the role of diet in health, you may be able to live longer and healthier as a result. Furthermore, you may become a more careful consumer of nutrition-related information by studying the content of this textbook. You must eat to live, so you'll have plenty of opportunities to use the information and, in some instances, develop new food-related attitudes and habits. Enjoy!

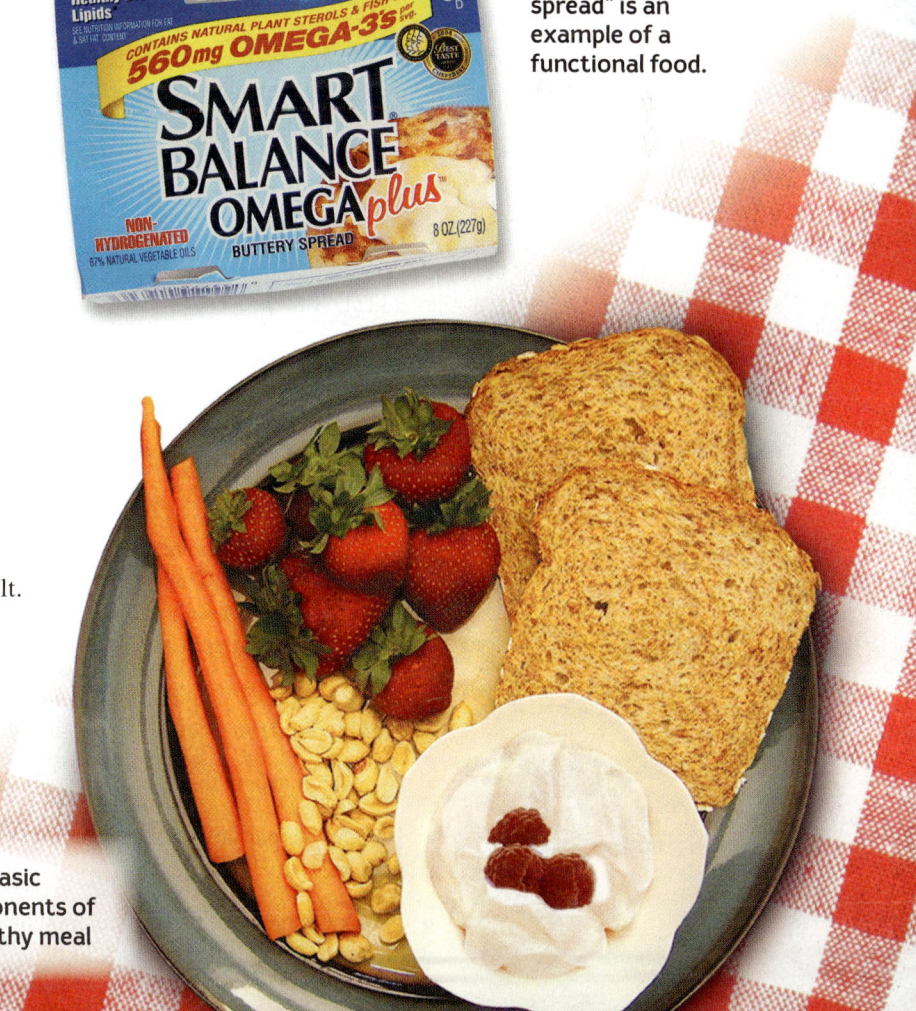

This "buttery spread" is an example of a functional food.

Basic components of a healthy meal

Dragon fruit, Smart Balance, Plate of bread, fruit, vegetables: Wendy Schiff; Tablecloth: cheminsnumeriques/Getty Images USA, Inc.

In a Nutshell

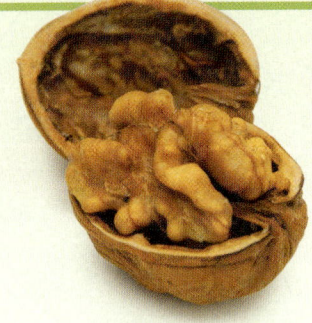

Module 1.1 Why Learn About Nutrition?
- Many factors, including friends, income, and cultural/ethnic background, influence personal food choices.

- Lifestyle choices, including poor eating habits and lack of physical activity, contribute to the development of many of the leading causes of premature deaths for American adults, including heart disease, cancer, stroke, and diabetes. You may be able to live longer and be healthier by applying what you learn about nutrition and the role of diet and health.

- Chronic diseases, such as heart disease and cancer, are long-term health problems that generally have multiple risk factors. A risk factor is a personal characteristic such as family history and lifestyle practices that increases your chances of developing such diseases. There are ways you may be able to reduce your risk of developing a chronic disease, especially one that's among the leading causes of death in the United States. Such actions include modifying your diet, increasing your physical activity, and improving other aspects of your lifestyle.

Module 1.2 Nutrition Basics
- Nutrients are chemicals in foods that the body needs for proper functioning. Nutrition is the scientific study of nutrients and how the body uses them. There are six classes of nutrients: carbohydrates, lipids, proteins, vitamins, minerals, and water.

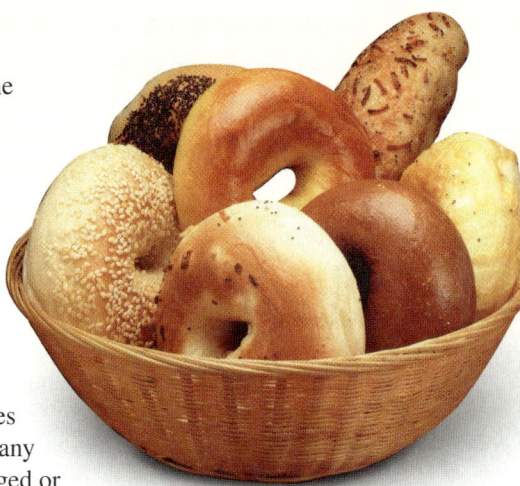
Stan Sholik/Alamy

- The body needs certain nutrients for energy, growth and development, and regulation of processes, including the repair and maintenance of cells. The human body can make many nutrients, but about 50 of these chemicals are dietary essentials that must be supplied by food because the body doesn't produce them or make enough to meet its needs.

- Plant foods naturally contain a variety of phytochemicals, substances that aren't classified as nutrients yet may have healthful benefits. Many phytochemicals are antioxidants that protect cells from being damaged or destroyed by exposure to certain environmental factors. However, some phytochemicals are toxic.

xefstock/Getty Images USA, Inc.

- Every cell needs energy. Calories or kilocalories (kcal) are used to indicate the energy value in food. A gram of carbohydrate and a gram of protein each supplies about 4 kcal; a gram of fat provides about 9 kcal. Although alcohol isn't a nutrient, a gram of pure alcohol furnishes 7 kcal.

- Carbohydrates, fats, and proteins are referred to as macronutrients because the body needs relatively large amounts of these nutrients daily. Vitamins and minerals are micronutrients because each day, the body needs very small amounts. Although the body requires large amounts of water, this nutrient provides no energy and isn't usually classified as a macronutrient.

Module 1.3 Key Nutrition Concepts
- Most naturally occurring foods are mixtures of nutrients, but no food contains all the nutrients needed for optimal health. Thus, nutritionally adequate diets include a variety of nutrient-dense foods that are consumed in moderation. It's also important to balance calorie intake with physical activity to avoid unwanted weight gain.

- Instead of classifying foods as "good" or "bad," you can focus on eating all foods in moderation and limiting foods and beverages that are sources of empty calories.

- For each nutrient, there's a range of safe intake.

- Healthy people should rely on eating a variety of foods to meet their nutrient needs instead of taking nutrient supplements.

- Although nutrients are vital to good health, foods and the nutrients they contain are not cure-alls. There's no "one size fits all" approach to planning a nutritionally adequate diet.

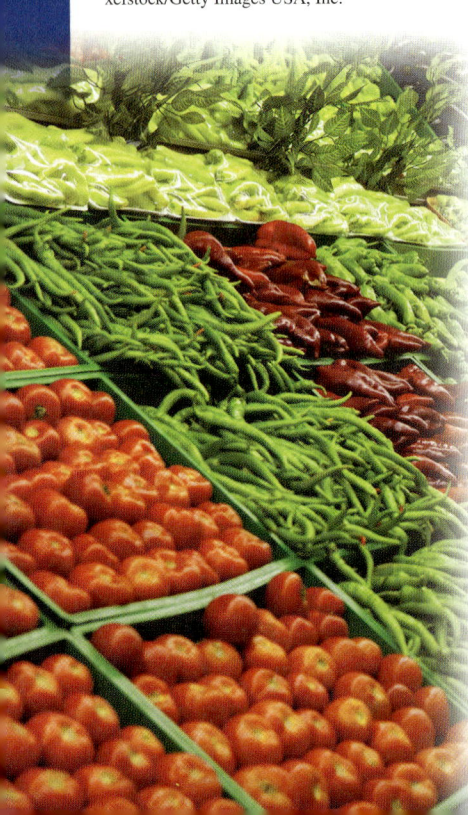

What's in Your Diet?!

1. If you purchase food regularly, keep your grocery store receipts for a week.

   a. How much money did you spend on the foods you purchased at these markets?

   b. Which foods were the most expensive?

   c. How much do you spend on food and beverages that supply a lot of empty calories, such as salty snacks, cookies, soft drinks, and candy?

   d. What percentage of your food dollars was spent on foods that were high in empty calories? _____ (Divide the amount of money you spent on such foods by the total cost of food for the week. Move the decimal point over 2 places to the right and place a percent sign after the number.)

   e. How much money did you spend on nutrient-dense foods, such as whole-grain products, peanut butter, eggs, fruits, and vegetables?

   f. What percentage of your food dollars was spent on nutrient-dense foods? _____ (Divide the amount of money you spent on nutrient-dense foods by the total cost of food for the week. Move the decimal point over 2 places to the right and place a percent sign after the number.)

2. For one week, keep a detailed log of your usual convenience store purchases, including the item(s) purchased and amount of money you spent for each purchase.

   a. What types of foods and beverages did you buy from the stores?

   b. How many soft drinks did you consume each day that were purchased at convenience stores?

   c. How much money did you spend on foods and beverages that were purchased at convenience stores?

   d. Based on this week's convenience store food and beverage expenditures, estimate how much money you spend on such purchases in a year.

3. For one week, keep a detailed log of the foods and beverages that you bought from fast-food restaurants and food trucks. Record when you made the purchases and the amount of money you spent on them.

   a. According to your weekly record, how often do you buy food from fast-food places?

   b. What types of foods did you usually buy?

   c. How much money did you spend on fast foods?

   d. Based on this week's expenditures, estimate how much money you spend on fast-food purchases in a year.

4. Over the past month, did you purchase dietary supplements? If your response is "Yes," which product or products did you purchase? _____

   _____

   How much did you spend on such products? _____

5. Over the past month, did you buy coffee at commercial coffee outlets? If your response is "Yes," which kinds of coffee did you purchase and how were they prepared? _____

   How much did you spend on such products? _____

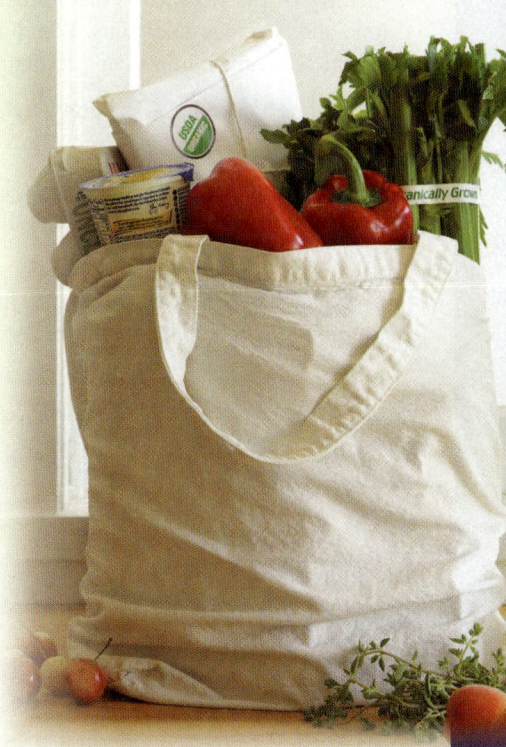

Annabelle Breakey/Getty Images USA, Inc.

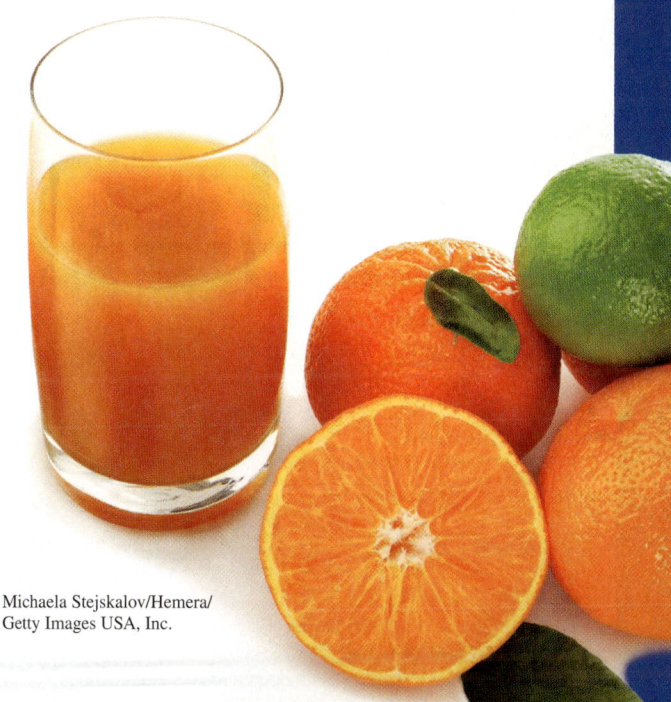

Michaela Stejskalov/Hemera/ Getty Images USA, Inc.

Consider This...

1. Identify at least six factors that influence your food and beverage selections. Which of these factors is the most important? Explain why.

2. "Everyone's on a diet." Explain why this statement is true.

3. Consider your current eating habits. Explain why you think your diet is or isn't nutritionally adequate.

4. If you were at risk of developing a chronic health condition that could be prevented by changing your diet, would you make the necessary changes? Explain why or why not.

5. "Everything in moderation." Explain what this statement means in terms of your diet.

6. Recall everything that you ate or drank in the past 24 hours. Identify the foods that were energy dense, nutrient dense, or high in empty calories. Are you interested in changing your intake of such foods? Explain why or why not.

Test Yourself

Select the best answer.

1. Diet is a
   a. practice of restricting energy intake.
   b. pattern of food choices.
   c. method of reducing portion sizes.
   d. technique to reduce carbohydrate intake.

2. Which of the following health conditions isn't one of the 10 leading causes of death in the United States?
   a. Cancer
   b. Diabetes
   c. Arthritis
   d. Stroke

3. Which of the following substances is a nutrient that provides energy?
   a. Glucose
   b. Water
   c. Alcohol
   d. Vitamin C

4. _____ refers to all chemical processes that occur in living cells.
   a. Physiology
   b. Catabolism
   c. Anatomy
   d. Metabolism

5. Phytochemicals
   a. are essential nutrients.
   b. generally have no effects on health.
   c. should be avoided.
   d. are in plant sources of food.

6. Which of the following foods is energy and nutrient dense?
   a. Strawberries
   b. Peanuts
   c. Fat-free milk
   d. Iceberg lettuce

7. Which of the following foods is a rich source of phytochemicals?
   a. Egg whites
   b. Blueberries
   c. Canned salmon
   d. Chicken

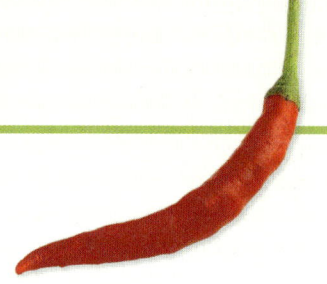
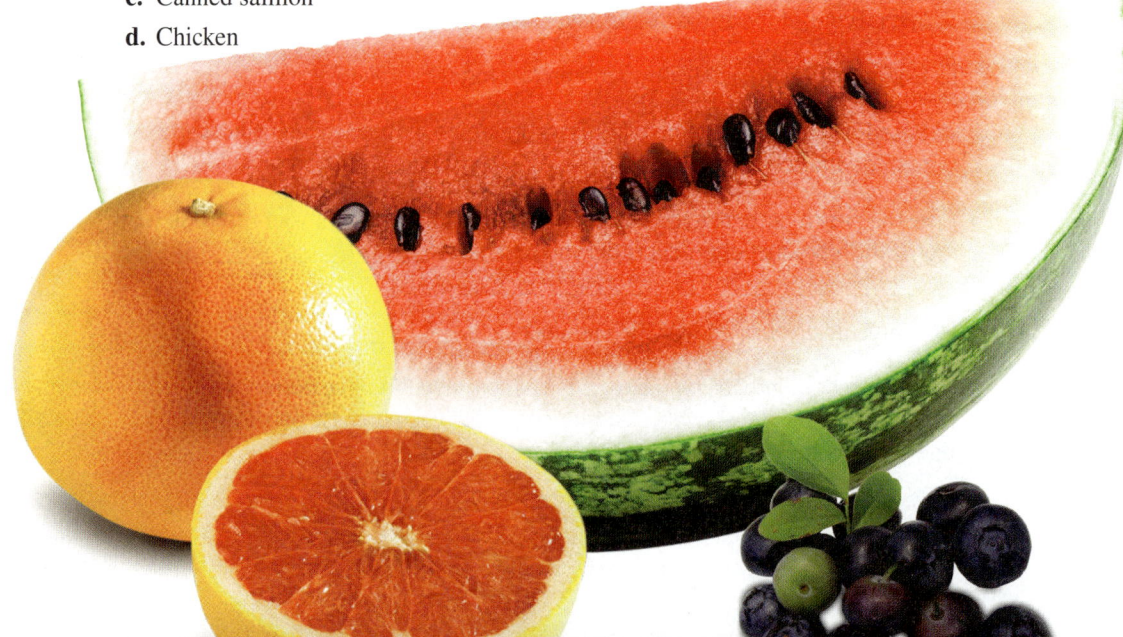

Watermelon: Digital Vision/Getty Images; Pink grapefruit: Purestock/SuperStock; Blueberries: Wendy Schiff

8. Which of the following conditions is a chronic disease?
   a. Heart disease
   b. Upset stomach
   c. Broken rib
   d. Common cold

9. In the United States, the primary cause of preventable deaths is
   a. tobacco use.
   b. auto accidents.
   c. high-fat diet.
   d. excessive alcohol intake.

10. A serving of food contains 20 g carbohydrate, 6 g protein, and 9 g fat. Based on this information, a serving of this food supplies ____ kcal.
    a. 64
    b. 124
    c. 162
    d. 185

11. Which of the following items is high in empty calories?
    a. Cottage cheese
    b. Chocolate chip cookie
    c. Green grapes
    d. Egg yolk

12. Which of the following foods is the most nutrient dense?
    a. 15 French fries
    b. 1 celery stalk
    c. 1 tablespoon butter
    d. 1/2 cup raspberries

13. Which of the following substances isn't a dietary supplement?
    a. Iron
    b. Alcohol
    c. Vitamin A
    d. Calcium

14. Which of the following foods supplies all of the essential nutrients for human beings?
    a. Whole milk
    b. Lean meat
    c. Whole eggs
    d. None of these is correct.

15. Which of the following statements is false?
    a. A healthy diet can be individualized to suit a person's budget and lifestyle.
    b. For each nutrient, there is a range of safe intakes.
    c. Vitamin and mineral supplements contain every substance needed for optimal nutrition.
    d. Food processing can make raw foods safer to eat.

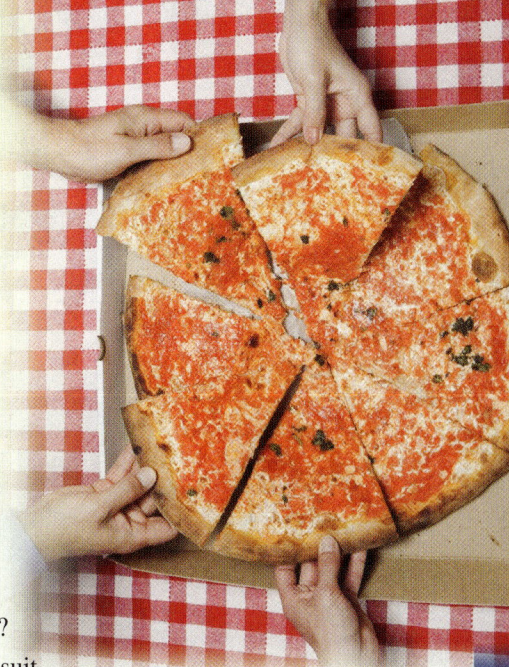

Fuse/Getty Images

Answers: 1. b 2. c 3. a 4. d 5. d 6. b 7. b 8. a 9. a 10. d 11. b 12. d 13. b 14. d 15. c

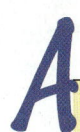 **Answer This (Module 1.2c)**

Iron and vitamin C are micronutrients; they provide no calories.

References → See Appendix D.

Design Elements: Spiral notebook paper background, Stacked paper with clip background, Marginal note clip, and Culture & Cuisine globe icon: ©McGraw-Hill Education; In a Nutshell walnut: ©McGraw-Hill Education/Mark A. Dierker, photographer; Test Yourself red pepper: Iconotec/Glow Images

Unit 2

Nutrition Information
FACT OR FICTION?

What's on the Menu?

Module 2.1
Nutrition: Science for Consumers

Module 2.2
Spreading Nutrition Misinformation

Module 2.3
Becoming a More Critical Consumer of Nutrition Information

Module 2.4
Seeking Reliable Nutrition Information

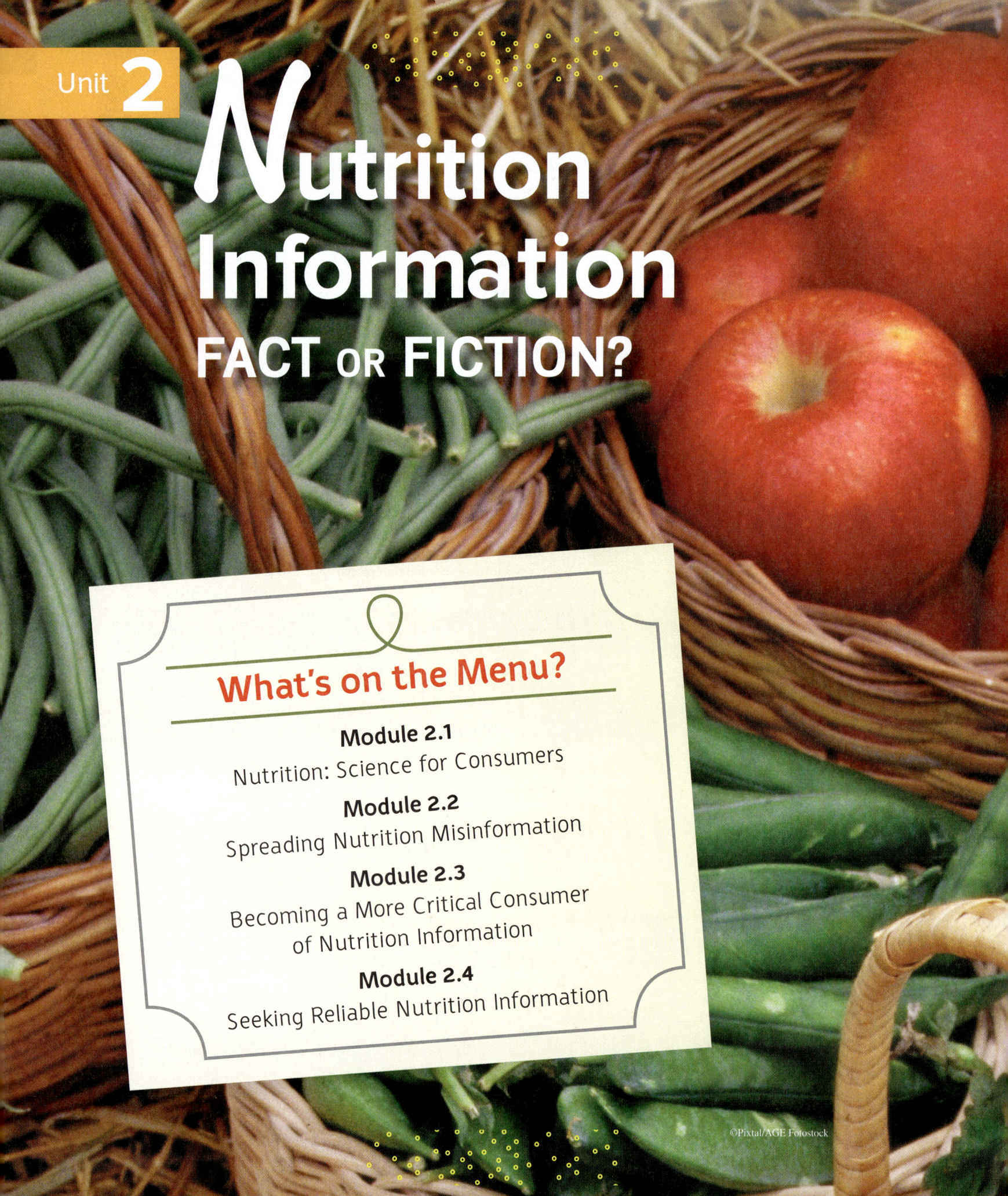
©Pixtal/AGE Fotostock

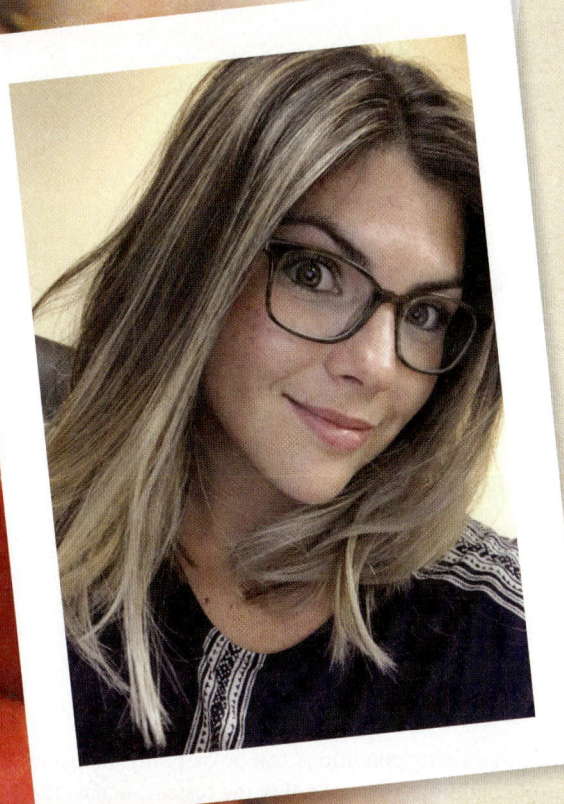

Mary Wester

"I believe in taking care of myself, because I want to be as healthy as possible and live a long life. My diet is healthy . . . I eat mostly whole foods, including lean meats, fruits, and vegetables, but I also take a supplement. It's not a pill; it's a green 'superfood' supplement powder that has the nutritional benefits of several fruits and vegetables. Sometimes I mix the powder with flavored water to hide the taste. You honestly have to plug your nose and chug the stuff."

"Drinking a serving of the green superfood supplement is equal to eating servings of 11 different fruits and vegetables. I really think it helps me, especially my skin. Before I used the supplement, I had a lot of skin blemishes. Since I've been taking it, my skin is clearer, and I have more energy and feel better."

Mary Wester

Mary Wester is a senior majoring in nursing at the University of South Dakota. As a nursing major, she's learned about foods and the importance of following a healthy diet, but she sometimes finds it's difficult to take the time to prepare and eat nutrient-dense foods. She's busy taking college classes, training and participating in competitive athletics (track and field), and working part time. To help maintain her good health, she uses the green superfood supplement as dietary "insurance."

Mary's positive experience with the green superfood supplement is intriguing, but it's an anecdote. Anecdotes are reports of one's personal experiences. Although they can be interesting, anecdotes aren't scientific evidence. Would you buy the green superfood supplement and regularly consume the unpleasant-tasting beverage made with it because Mary thinks it improves her health? How can you find out whether the product is safe to use and actually provides health benefits?

We consume food, and we consume nutrition information. Magazines, books, ads, the Internet, and even family members and friends contribute to the "flood" of nutrition information. Unfortunately, much of this information isn't supported by scientific evidence. The challenge is learning how to be a skeptical consumer who questions the reliability of nutrition-related information, including anecdotes and manufacturers' health claims. This unit takes a closer look at how scientists collect information that relates to nutrition. The unit also provides practical tips for judging the honesty and reliability of popular sources of nutrition information, such as Internet sites and magazine articles.

Wendy Schiff

Module 2.1

Nutrition: Science for Consumers

2.1- Learning Outcomes

After reading Module 2.1, you should be able to

1. Define all of the **key terms** in this module.
2. List the basic steps of the scientific method as it relates to nutrition research in general.
3. Discuss ways that scientists conduct nutrition-related research that involves human subjects.
4. Explain why results of similar studies can provide different findings.

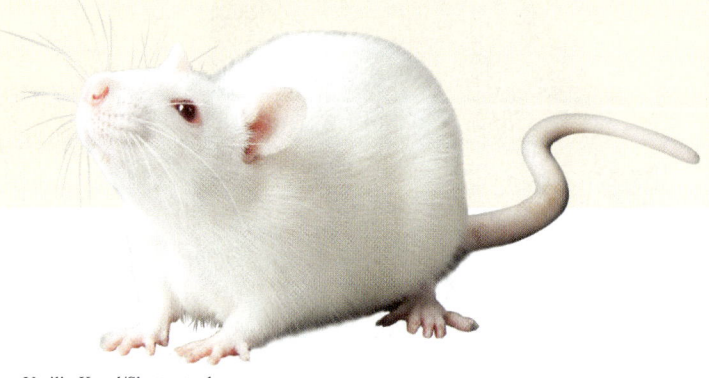

Vasiliy Koval/Shutterstock

In the past, nutrition facts and recommended dietary practices were often based on intuition, common sense, "conventional wisdom" (tradition), or **anecdotes** (reports of personal experiences). Today, registered dietitians and other nutrition experts discard conventional beliefs, explanations, and practices when the evidence obtained by current scientific research no longer supports them.

2.1a Collecting Science-Based Evidence

Scientists generally use the *scientific method* to answer questions about natural and physical observations. Scientists, for example, have answered questions such as: "How does the stomach break down food proteins?" "Why do babies need the mineral iron to develop normally?" and "Why is vitamin C necessary to maintain good health?"

An **experiment** is a way of testing a scientific question. Because of safety and ethical concerns, nutrition scientists often conduct experiments on small mammals before performing similar research on humans. Certain kinds of mice and rats are raised for experimentation purposes. The rodents are inexpensive to house in laboratories, and their food and other living conditions can be carefully controlled. Researchers control conditions that are not being tested, such as the ways the animals are handled and the kinds of physical activity the animals receive. Otherwise, their findings are likely to be unclear or inaccurate.

Essential Concept 2.1 describes the basic steps of the scientific method as applied to a nutrition-related experiment involving laboratory mice.

Essential Concept

2.1 Applying the Scientific Method

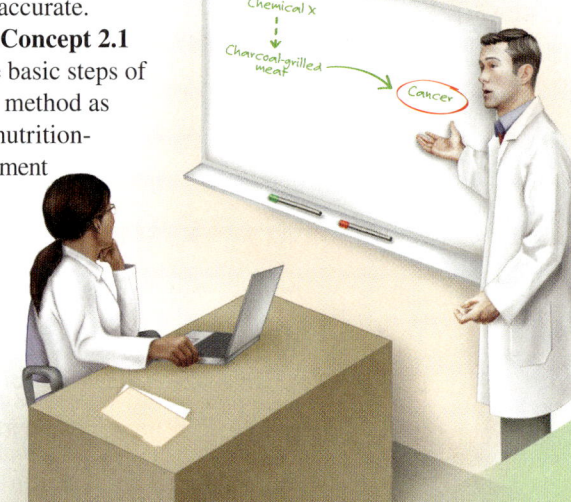

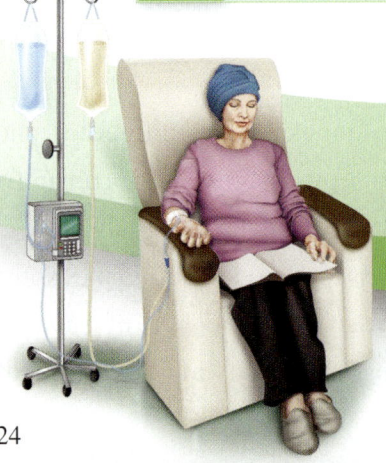

1 Observe
Scientists observe a group of hospitalized patients who have stomach cancer. After obtaining dietary information from all the patients, the researchers determine that the patients with stomach cancer eat more charcoal-grilled meat than other people who are the same age but don't have stomach cancer.

2 Develop a question
The researchers think eating charcoal-grilled meat increases the risk of stomach cancer. They develop a question: "Chemical X is only in meat that has been charcoal grilled. If chemical X is given to a group of laboratory mice for 6 months, will they develop more cases of stomach cancer than mice that have not eaten chemical X?"

anecdotes reports of personal experiences

experiment a way of testing a scientific question

peer review expert critical analysis of a research article before it's published

Nutrition: Science for Consumers

5 Analyze the findings
At the end of the 6-month study, the scientists review all the data and use statistical tests to analyze the findings. The researchers are particularly interested in comparing the health of the two groups of mice, especially whether any of the mice developed stomach cancer.

4 Collect information
Every month the researchers collect information (*data*) about each mouse.

3 Test
The scientists test the question by dividing a group of 100 3-week-old laboratory mice into two groups that have 50 mice in each group. One group of mice in the study (subjects) is the treatment (or experimental) group. Each of these mice is fed ½ teaspoon of charcoal-grilled meat along with their ration of regular mouse chow every day. The other group of mice is called the control group. Instead of receiving ½ teaspoon of charred meat, mice in the control group only eat the mouse chow.

FINDINGS
Mice that ate charred meat were 3x as likely to develop stomach cancer than mice that didn't eat the meat.

6 Form conclusions
After analyzing the data, the researchers form conclusions based on their findings. Now, the scientists can answer their original question. According to the results of their study, the mice that consumed the charred meat were more likely to develop stomach cancer, compared to the mice that didn't eat the charred meat.

Purestock/SuperStock

7 Share the results
The team shares the results of their findings, usually by preparing an article that describes the study and its findings. The team submits the article to the editor of a scientific journal. The article undergoes **peer review**—that is, the editor sends copies of the article to a group of peer reviewers—scientists who are qualified to judge the findings presented in the article. The researchers don't know the identities of the peer reviewers. If the peer reviewers accept the study's findings as being scientifically reliable, the journal's editor agrees to publish the article.

8 Conduct more research
After reading the article in the journal, other researchers conduct more research to examine the original question. Scientists do not accept the results of the study until the findings are supported by evidence from more studies, especially those conducted by different researchers.

TASTY Tidbits

Placebos can produce beneficial results, particularly in subjects who have conditions that involve pain.[1] Because participants in the control group believe they are receiving a real treatment, their faith in the "treatment" can stimulate the release of chemicals in the brain that alter pain perception, reducing their discomfort. Therefore, when people report that a treatment was helpful, they may not have been imagining the positive response, even when they were taking a placebo. This is because the chemicals released in the brain actually relieved the pain.

double-blind study experimental design in which neither the participants nor the researchers are aware of each participant's group assignment

treatment group group being studied that receives a treatment

Human Intervention Studies

Researchers must be careful when applying the results of laboratory experiments involving animals to people because of the many differences between people and "lab" animals. Nutrition scientists, however, do conduct experimental (intervention) studies using humans to obtain information about health conditions (outcomes) that can result from specific dietary practices. In such instances, scientists often design a double-blind study. In a **double-blind study,** the researchers and subjects don't know which participants are assigned to the **treatment** and **control groups.** Maintaining such secrecy is important during the course of a study because researchers and subjects may try to predict their group assignments. If the investigators who interview the participants are aware of their individual group assignments during the study (a single-blind study), they may convey clues to each subject. For example, a researcher's tone of voice or body language could influence a subject's belief about being in the experimental or control group. Subjects who think they're in the control group may report no changes in their condition. Ideally, subjects shouldn't be able to figure out their group assignment during the study.

When conducting double-blind studies, researchers provide all study participants with the same instructions and a "treatment," such as a dietary supplement or experimental food. However, only members of the treatment group actually receive the treatment. Subjects in the control group are given a placebo.

Placebos are not simply "sugar pills"; they are a fake treatment, such as a sham pill, injection, or medical procedure. If the treatment is a pill, the placebo pill looks, tastes, and smells like the pill that contains the active ingredient that is given to the subjects in the treatment group. The placebo pill, however, contains substances that don't produce any measurable physical changes. Providing placebos to members of the control group enables scientists to compare the extent of the treatment's response with that of the placebo.

What Is the Placebo Effect?

People often report positive or negative reactions to a treatment even though they received the fake treatment. If a patient believes a medical treatment will improve his or her health, the patient is more likely to report positive results for the therapy. Such wishful thinking is called the **placebo effect.**

At the present time, there is little scientific evidence to support claims that dietary supplements are "superfoods" with exceptional health benefits. For example, people who drink a "green" superfood dietary supplement may believe their health has improved as a result. Such positive beliefs may be the result of the placebo effect. On the other hand, the people who use the green supplement might be experiencing positive effects that have not been considered or measured by researchers. As more people consume green superfood dietary supplements, scientists are likely to conduct studies to determine whether the products actually have any effects on health, including negative ones.

Nutrition Fact or Fiction?

Medical researchers can make important discoveries without following the scientific method.

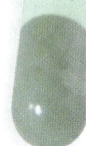
H. pylori

Yes! In 1982, Dr. Barry Marshall and Dr. Robin Warren proposed that a type of bacterium (*Helicobacter pylori* [*H. pylori*]) causes gastritis, inflammation of the stomach lining.[2] Gastritis can lead to stomach ulcers. Initially, other physicians were skeptical about this notion because it challenged traditional medical beliefs. To provide support for his idea, Marshall experimented on himself, which is very risky and not a common practice among scientists. He actually swallowed some of the bacteria and developed severe stomach inflammation as a result. Because of Dr. Marshall's daring experiment, physicians now accept the notion that *H. pylori* is a primary cause of gastritis and stomach ulcers. Today, people who have ulcers and *H. pylori* in their stomachs are treated with antibiotics that kill the bacterium. Unit 4 has more information about stomach ulcers.

Single purple pill, Pill and bottle: Wendy Schiff; *Helicobacter pylori* bacterium: Heather Davies/Science Source

What IS That?

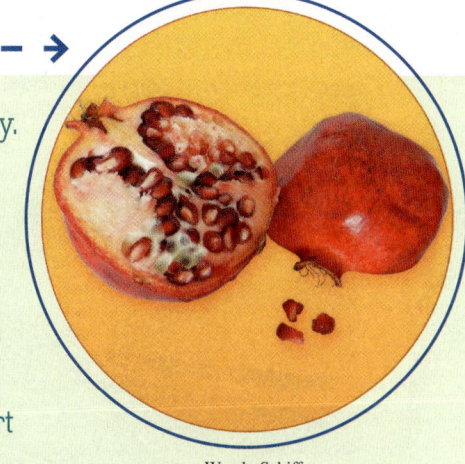
Wendy Schiff

Pomegranate (*Punica granatum*) is a leathery-skinned fruit that is filled with pockets of edible, juicy seeds that have a sweet, tangy taste. In the United States, pomegranates are grown mostly in California, but the plant is native to northern India, the Mediterranean region, and certain Middle Eastern countries. Pomegranate seeds are often crushed and strained to collect their juice. People from countries that have grown and eaten pomegranates for centuries may use a syrup (pomegranate "molasses") made from the fruit to flavor meat marinades and add to desserts. You may be able to find pomegranate syrup in markets that specialize in selling global food products.

When compared to other fruits, pomegranate juice has very high contents of phytochemicals with antioxidant activity. Nevertheless, results of scientific studies fail to provide good evidence that the juice is useful for reducing the risk of serious health problems such as heart disease. Pomegranate juice, however, may help prevent infections and reduce inflammation in people who have kidney disease.[3]

Although pomegranate is high in phytochemicals, it's not a good source of most vitamins and minerals. A ½-cup serving of 100% pomegranate juice supplies 67 kcal and 265 mg of potassium.

Population Studies

For decades, nutrition scientists have noted differences in rates of chronic diseases and causes of death among various populations. To understand why these differences exist, researchers rely on physical examinations, such as height and weight measurements, of large numbers of people to obtain health data. Additionally, they may collect information about a specific population's health and food-related practices by conducting surveys. Such surveys often question people about their personal and family medical histories, environmental exposures, and dietary practices.

The Framingham Heart Study
The Framingham Heart Study, which began in 1949 in Massachusetts, is one of the most well-known population studies that relates to nutrition. At the beginning of the study, the over 5000 healthy participants underwent physical examinations and were questioned about their family and personal medical histories as well as their dietary and other lifestyle practices. Over the following years, a group of medical researchers periodically collected information concerning each participant's health and, if the person died, the cause of death. The scientists analyzed this information and found relationships among a variety of personal characteristics and health outcomes. Findings from the Framingham Heart Study identified numerous risk factors for heart disease, including poor diet and cigarette smoking. Today, medical researchers are still collecting information from original Framingham Heart Study participants as well as their descendants.

control group group being studied that does not receive a treatment

placebo fake treatment, such as a sham pill, injection, or medical procedure

placebo effect response to a placebo

Tom Mareschal/Alamy

2.1b Confusion and Conflict

One day, the news media highlight research about the health benefits of eating garlic, dark chocolate, brown rice, or cherries. A few weeks later, the media report the results of new scientific investigations that don't support the earlier findings. Consumers often become confused and disappointed when they learn about conflicting results generated by nutrition studies. As a result, some people think nutrition scientists don't know what they are doing. Why can't scientists agree and provide proof that eating specific foods benefits health?

Conflicting findings often result from differences in the ways that various studies are designed. Even when investigating the same question, different groups of scientists often conduct their studies and analyze the results differently. For example, the numbers, ages, and physical conditions of people who participate in each study (*subjects*), the type and length of the study, the amount of the treatment provided, and the methods used to analyze results typically vary among studies. Furthermore, situational, genetic, behavioral, and environmental differences among individuals account for much of the variation in the ways they respond to a treatment. Not only are people genetically different, they also have different lifestyles, and they typically recall or report dietary information and follow instructions concerning health care practices differently. These and other factors can influence the results of nutrition research involving human subjects. This is why dietary recommendations shouldn't be made from the results of a single study. The popular media, however, often report the findings of a study if they're sensational, that is, they grab your attention.

Getty Images

What's Research Bias?

Scientists expect other researchers to avoid relying on their personal attitudes and biases ("points of view") when collecting and analyzing data, and to evaluate and report their results objectively and honestly. However, the funding sources of scientific research may have certain expectations or biases about research outcomes. As a result, such groups are more likely to finance studies of scientists whose research efforts support their interests. The beef industry, for example, might not fund scientific investigations to find connections between high intakes of beef and the risk of certain cancers. On the other hand, the beef industry might be interested in supporting a team of scientists whose research indicates that a high-protein diet that contains plenty of beef is beneficial for people who are trying to lose weight.

Peer-reviewed journals usually require authors of articles to *disclose* (mention) their affiliations and sources of financial support. (Peer review is discussed in Essential Concept 2.1.) Such disclosures might appear either on the first page or at the end of the article. By having this information, readers can decide whether research bias may have influenced the researchers. For example, you read an article in what appears to be a scientific journal that describes a study about the numerous health benefits of drinking apple cider vinegar. The article provides the names of the researchers who authored the article and their disclosure statement. According to the disclosure, all of the authors work for the same company. While searching for information about the company, you discover it manufactures apple cider vinegar. How reliable or biased would you rate the researchers' findings? Although peer review helps ensure that the scientists are as ethical and objective as possible, it's impossible to eliminate all research bias.

What kinds of nutrition-related research are likely to be funded by the beef industry?

Carson Ganci/Design Pics

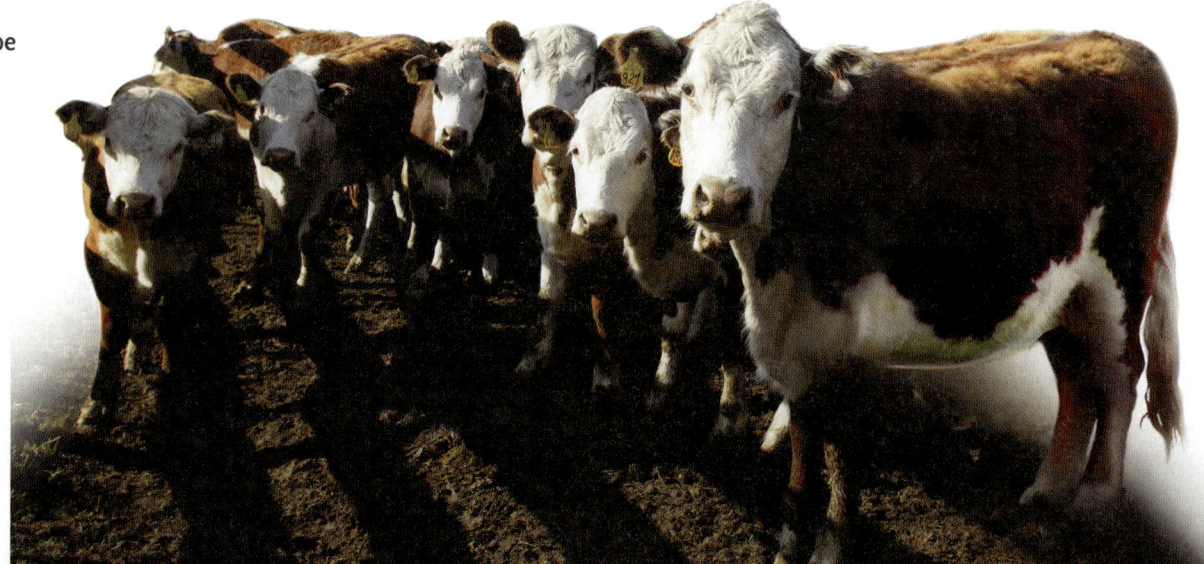

Cause and Effect

Population studies involving people and their eating practices generally cannot establish *cause and effect*—that is, whether a practice is responsible for an outcome. When two different natural events occur simultaneously within a population, it doesn't necessarily mean they're related to each other. For example, when a population's intake of sugar-sweetened soft drinks increases, the percentage of overweight people in the population also increases. Does this prove that drinking sugary soft drinks causes weight gain? Not necessarily. What appears to be a relationship between a dietary practice and a physical outcome could be a coincidence—that is, a chance happening.

In cases involving chronic diseases such as heart disease and cancer, it is difficult to prove that a single factor is responsible for the development of the condition. Multiple risk factors, including your *genetic susceptibility* (inherited proneness) to develop the disease, usually influence whether you'll develop a chronic disease. Other factors that play a role in the development of heart disease include high blood pressure, age, tobacco use, and intake of certain fats. Unit 6 provides more information about heart disease.

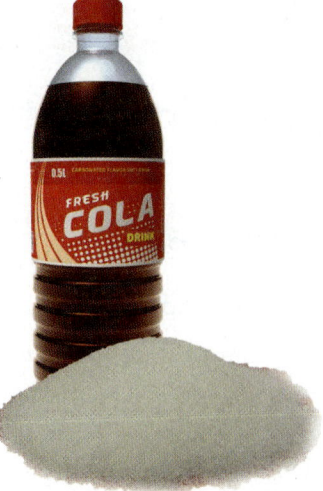

Q Answer This

Lemonade consumption increases in the summer, and drowning deaths also increase in the summer. Does this prove that drinking lemonade increases the risk of drowning? This answer is on the last page of this unit.

What IS That?

For centuries, people in Asia have used the *rhizomes* (rye'-zhomes), fleshy underground stems, of the tropical plant ginger (*Zingiber officinale*) to treat stomach pain, nausea, and diarrhea.[4] Popular forms of ginger include fresh or candied rhizomes, ginger extracts, and the dried, powdered seasoning that many Americans enjoy in pies and cakes.

Eating small amounts of ginger for a short time may be a safe way to relieve "morning sickness"—the nausea and vomiting that often accompany early pregnancy. However, pregnant women should always check with their physicians before taking dietary supplements. If you consume ginger, particularly the powdered form of the herb, you may experience side effects, including intestinal gas and heartburn.

Wendy Schiff

Culture & Cuisine

During the first 350 years after the discovery of the New World, most of the people who immigrated to North America (excluding African slaves) were from western European countries. Western European immigrants generally followed a "meat-and-potatoes" diet. Main meals typically included a large portion of fatty red meat (beef, pork, or mutton [flesh of adult sheep]) served with boiled or mashed white potatoes, gravy, white breads, and butter. Salt was used as a seasoning and preservative. Today, the mainstream American diet, which is sometimes referred to as the "Western" diet, still provides large amounts of fatty red meat (primarily beef or pork) and white potatoes (usually peeled and fried), but the diet also contains generous amounts of processed meats, such as sausage, ham, and bacon; salt; sugar; and refined (white) flour products. The mainstream American diet lacks fruit, whole grains, nuts, and a variety of vegetables. Populations that follow this food pattern generally have high rates of certain chronic diseases, particularly heart disease, cancer of the large intestine, and type 2 diabetes, which are discussed in later units of this textbook.

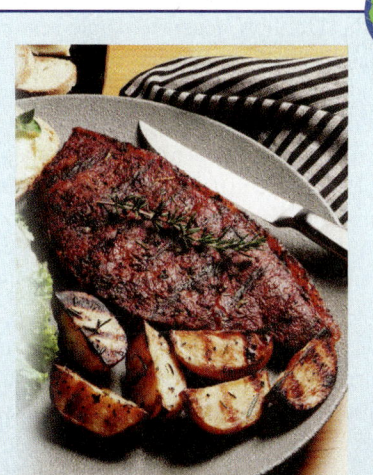

Ernie Friedlander/Cole Group/Getty Images

Bottle of soft drink: scanrail/Getty Images; Sugar: Wendy Schiff

Module 2.2
Spreading Nutrition Misinformation

2.2 - Learning Outcomes
After reading Module 2.2, you should be able to
1. Define all of the **key terms** in this module.
2. Explain the difference between an anecdote and a testimonial.
3. Explain why there is so much nutrition misinformation.

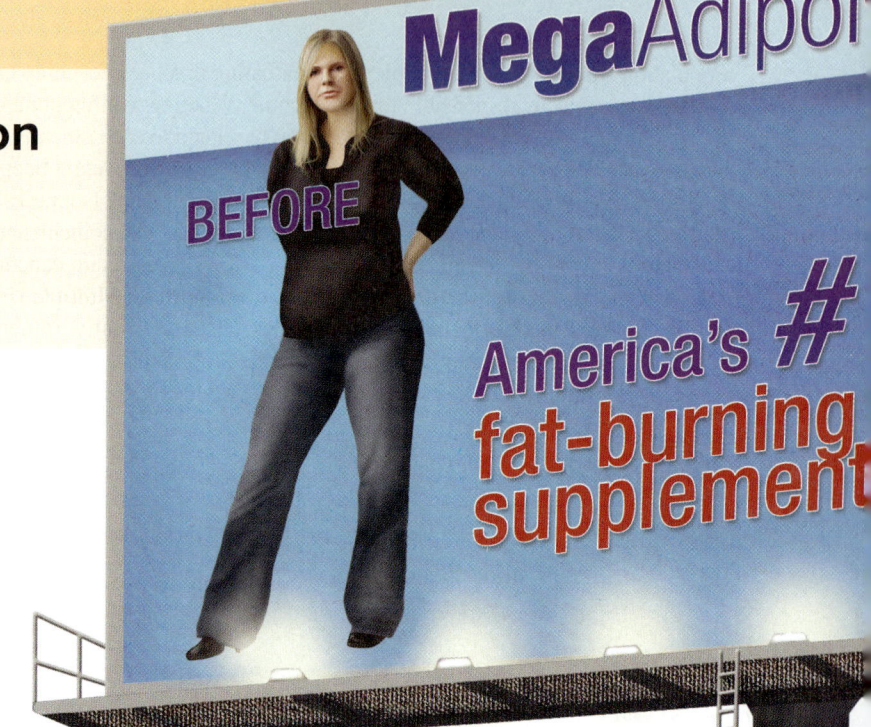

If you think you already know a lot of nutrition facts, what were your sources of the information? Did you rely on magazines or the Internet? Why did you think these sources were trustworthy? In many instances, such popular sources of nutrition information are not reliable. Let's take a closer look at why you need to be careful when seeking nutrition information and advice.

2.2a Anecdotes and Testimonials

The host of a popular TV program interviews an attractive, young actress who claims to have lost a lot of weight after she started taking weight-loss pills made from a rare type of cactus. A few days later, a friend mentions that she's lost 3 pounds since she began taking this product a week ago. You'd like to lose a few pounds without restricting your food intake or exercising. Should you take this dietary supplement? It's promoted by the TV show host and helped the actress and your friend. Perhaps it will help you.

Although the TV show host is a likable person who seems to be honest and the personal experiences of the actress and your friend seem to provide evidence that the weight-loss supplement is effective, can you trust their judgment?

The actress's information is a **testimonial,** a personal endorsement of a product. People are usually paid to provide their testimonials for advertisements; therefore, their remarks might be biased in favor of the product. Your friend's experience with the weight-loss product is an anecdote, as is Mary's experience with a green superfood dietary supplement (see this unit's opener). When your source of nutrition information is a testimonial or an anecdote, it's not scientific. If the nutrition information is in an advertisement, you cannot be sure that the information is based on scientific facts. Thus, testimonials, anecdotes, and ads aren't reliable sources of nutrition information.

| **testimonial** personal endorsement of a product

2.2b A Matter of Mistrust

Although people's lives have improved as a result of scientific advancements in medicine, many Americans mistrust the motives of scientists, dietitians, and other medical professionals. Promoters of nutrition misinformation use this mistrust to sell their products. For example, they may claim that physicians are more interested in making money than doing what's best for their patients, such as recommending dietary supplements. Are physicians driven by the desire to make money from their patients' illnesses? Do they hide information about natural cures from them?

It's true that physicians need incomes to support themselves and their families. However, people who tell you that the "medical/scientific establishment is hiding information about natural cures from you just to make money from your misery" are using *scare tactics* to build your mistrust in the medical establishment. Consider this: If your physician makes a mistake, you can sue him or her for malpractice. If you purchase a nutrition-related product or service, then your money enters the promoter's pockets. If the product or service doesn't live up to the promoter's claims or is harmful, what can you do?

As a group, physicians strive to diagnose and treat diseases using techniques that are scientifically tested for safety and effectiveness. Physicians have nothing to gain from concealing a cure from the public, but they have much to gain from treating their patients kindly and effectively. If you follow a physician's advice and have positive results, how likely are you to be that doctor's patient for a long time and recommend the practitioner to others?

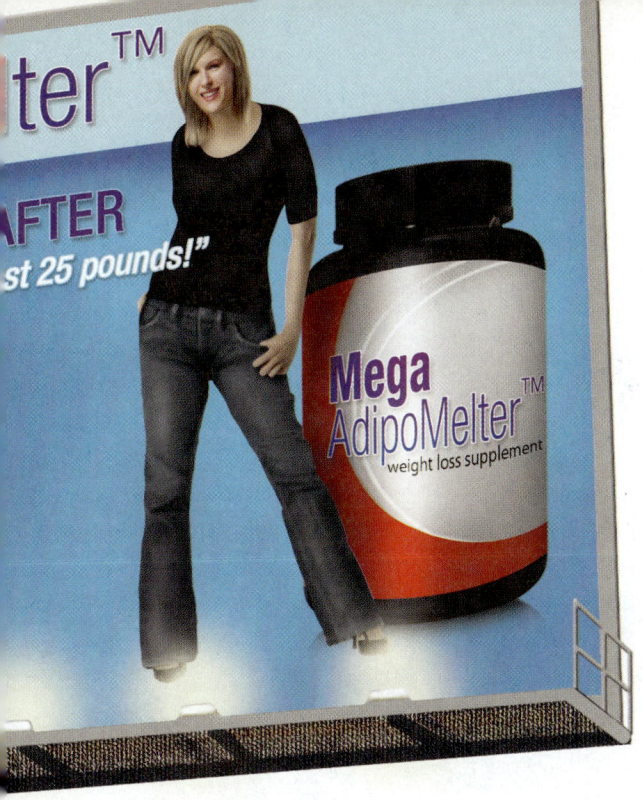

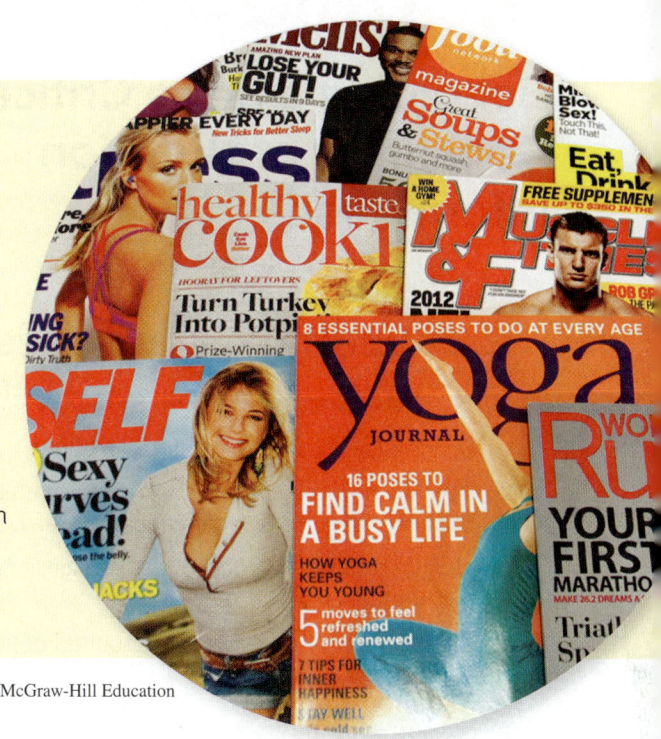

TASTY Tidbits

You can often distinguish a peer-reviewed scientific journal from a popular magazine simply by looking at their covers and skimming their pages. Compared to scientific journals, popular magazines typically have

- More colorful, attractive covers and photographs;
- Articles that are shorter and easier for the average person to read; and
- Advertisements for products mentioned in articles.

Mark Dierker/McGraw-Hill Education

If your car breaks down, you probably would want people who have the best training, tools, and equipment to determine the problem and repair it. If you think something is wrong with your body, it's wise to seek information and opinions from medical professionals who have the best scientific training and experience to diagnose and treat health disorders.

2.2c Why Is There So Much Nutrition Misinformation?

People may think they've learned facts about nutrition by reading popular magazine articles or best-selling books, by visiting Internet websites, or by watching television news, commercials, infomercials, or home shopping network programs. In many instances, however, they've been misinformed. To be a careful consumer, you shouldn't assume that all nutrition information presented in the popular media is reliable. Why?

First Amendment Freedoms

The First Amendment to the U.S. Constitution guarantees freedom of the press and freedom of speech. As a result, people can provide nutrition information that's not true. Thus, the First Amendment doesn't protect consumers with freedom from nutrition misinformation or false nutrition claims.

The **U.S. Food and Drug Administration (FDA)** can regulate nutrition- and health-related claims on product labels, but the agency cannot prevent the spread of health and nutrition misinformation published in books or pamphlets or presented in television or radio programs. People who promote nutrition misinformation often profit from these freedoms. As a consumer, you are responsible for questioning and researching the accuracy of nutrition information as well as the credentials of the people making nutrition-related claims.

U.S. Food and Drug Administration (FDA) federal agency that regulates claims on product labels

larry1235/Shutterstock

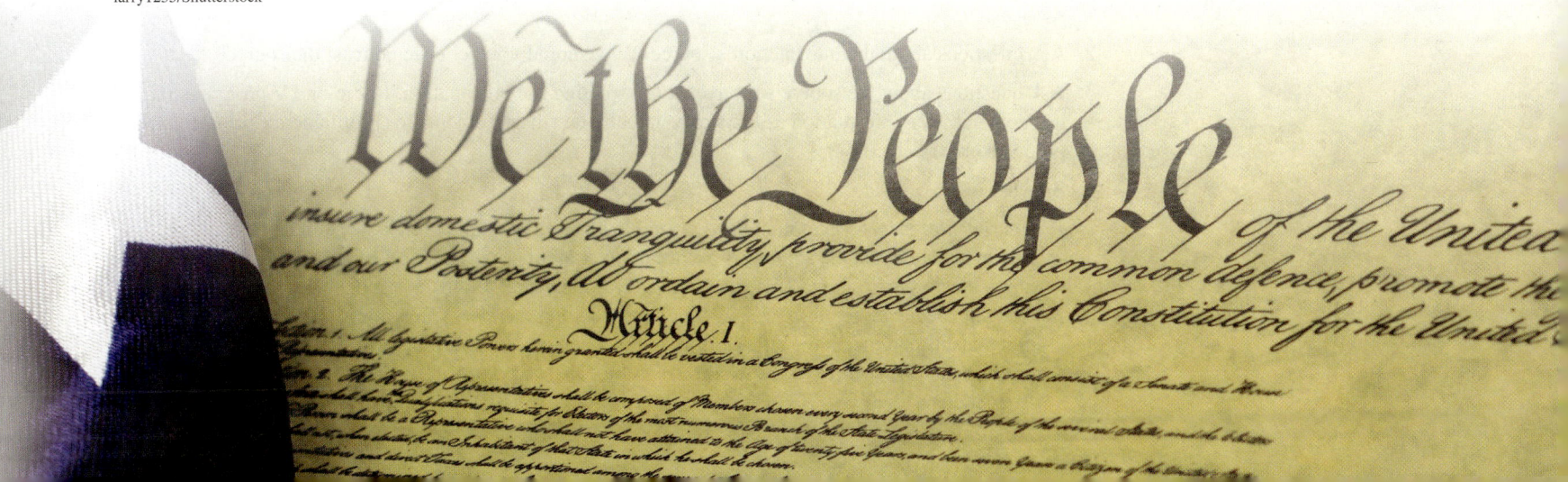

Module 2.3
Becoming a More Critical Consumer of Nutrition Information

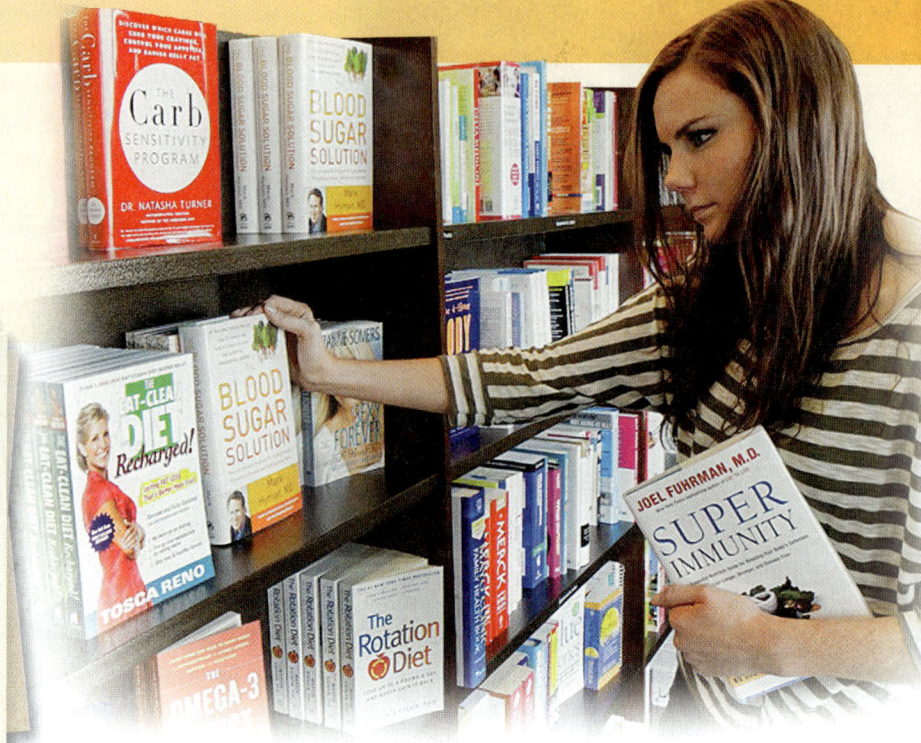

2.3 - Learning Outcomes

After reading Module 2.3, you should be able to

1. Define all of the **key terms** in this module.
2. Describe how you can become a more careful and critical consumer of nutrition information.
3. Identify common "red flags" that are signs of nutrition misinformation.
4. Describe how to identify reliable sources of nutrition information.

Mark Dierker/McGraw-Hill Education

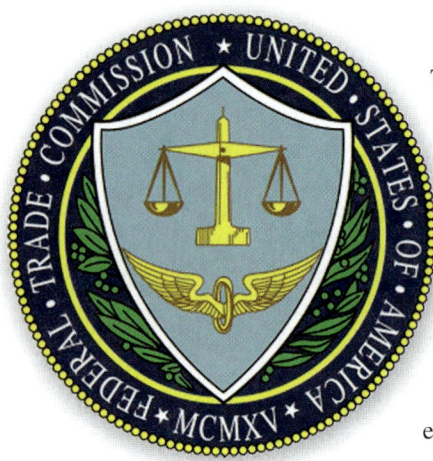

Source: Federal Trade Commission

The **Federal Trade Commission (FTC)** enforces U.S. consumer protection laws and investigates complaints about false or misleading health claims that are used in advertising. According to the FTC, Americans spend billions of dollars annually on fraudulently marketed and unproven health-related products and treatments that are often useless.[5] Claims for such products often promise cures for common and serious medical conditions, including obesity and cancer. When the products prove to be ineffective, the people who believed the claims and bought the products are cheated out of their money and, in some instances, their health declines as a result of wasting time using the worthless product.

If you're like most people, you don't want to waste your money on things you don't need or that are useless or potentially harmful. Promoters of worthless nutrition products often use clever marketing methods, including sensational claims about the products' effectiveness, to attract people to make unnecessary purchases. Skeptical people don't believe the claims without checking into them.

2.3a Becoming a More Skeptical Consumer

How can you become a more careful, critical consumer of nutrition-related information, products, or services? By being more *skeptical*.

1. Don't believe everything you hear or read about nutrition, including nutrition-related products or services.
2. Ask questions about the information's source. Why should you believe and trust the source?
3. Ask questions about the source's motives for promoting the information. Radio or TV programs that promote nutrition information as facts may actually be advertisements for profitable nutrition-related products or services.
4. Be wary of
    - *Salespeople.* Salespeople often have favorable biases toward the things they sell and, therefore, they may not be reliable sources of information about these products. Clerks in a dietary supplements store, for example, may wear a white lab coat to look as though they have a science or medical educational background. Keep in mind that the clerks were hired to sell dietary supplements and may have little or no scientific training. Furthermore, the clerks may receive commission for what they sell, so they might not inform you about the negative aspects of using a product or service.

Federal Trade Commission (FTC) federal agency that enforces U.S. consumer protection laws and investigates health claims

- *Nutrition "experts."* Anyone can call him- or herself a "nutritionalist" to appear to be a "nutrition expert." What is the person's educational background? Are his or her nutrition degrees from accredited institutions? What is the person's professional experience? Is it limited to the industry that's marketing nutrition-related products?

- *Claims that the product was "scientifically tested" or "clinically tested at a major university."* Where can you read the article about the study? Which university was involved in the clinical tests? Is it an accredited university? How was the testing done?

- *Citations to what appear to be scientific journal articles.* Promoters often make up journal citations or cite "journals" that were created by the products' manufacturers to provide the appearance of scientific credibility.

- *Scientific-sounding terms,* such as "enzymatic therapy," "nutritionals," or "colloidal chelated extract." Promoters typically use such vague or meaningless terms when presenting false or misleading information as factual and obtained by scientific methods. Such terms are designed to convince people without science backgrounds that the nutrition-related information is true.

- *Popular sources of nutrition information,* such as magazines and the Internet, because such sources generally don't subject articles or blogs to expert review before publishing the information. A reliable source has information about research that supports claims of a product's effectiveness as well as scientific studies that don't support its usefulness. Furthermore, reliable sources of information will alert consumers to possible health risks linked to using the products.

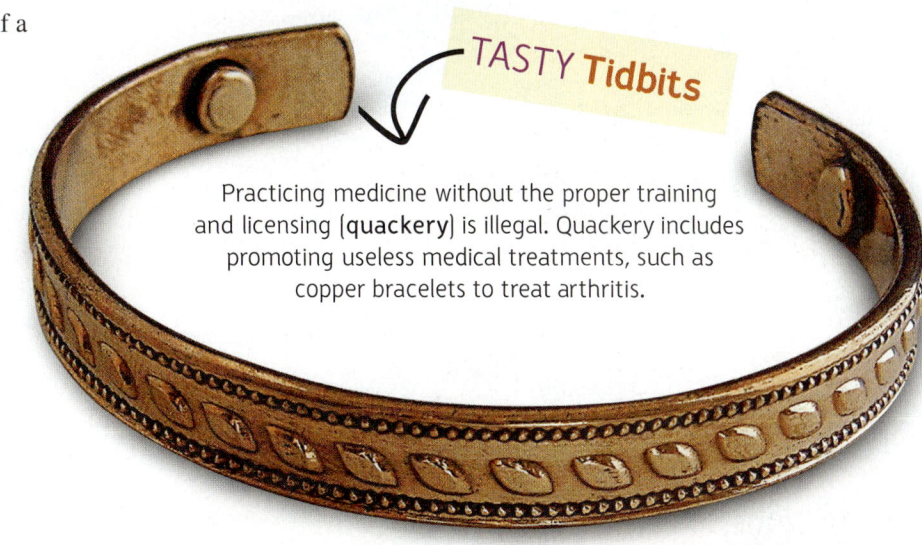

TASTY Tidbits

Practicing medicine without the proper training and licensing (**quackery**) is illegal. Quackery includes promoting useless medical treatments, such as copper bracelets to treat arthritis.

Wendy Schiff

quackery practicing medicine without the proper training and licensing

2.3b Look for "Red Flags" of Misinformation

A *red flag* is a term or expression that draws your attention. For consumers of nutrition information, red flags are clues or signals of misinformation in media, advertising, and personal communications. Common red flags include

1. **Promises of quick and easy health remedies,** such as: "Our product helps you lose weight fast, *without* exercising or dieting."

2. **Claims that sound too good to be true,** such as: "You can eat everything you like and still lose weight" and "Garlic pills cure heart disease." These claims are rarely true. Remember, if the claim sounds too good to be true, it probably isn't true.

3. **Scare tactics,** such as: "Your liver is loaded with toxins and needs cleansing" and "There are chemicals in your food!" Such statements are meant to frighten people. The truth: Your liver can't be "cleansed," and everything in your environment is chemical in nature.

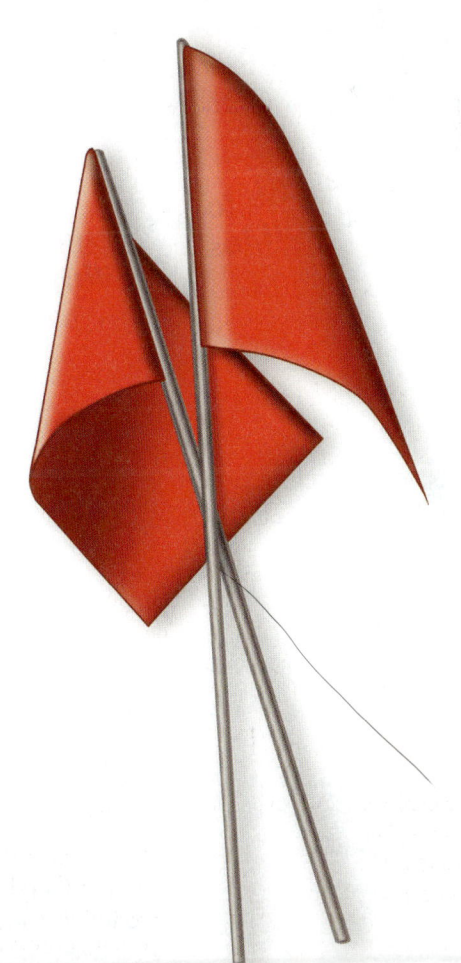

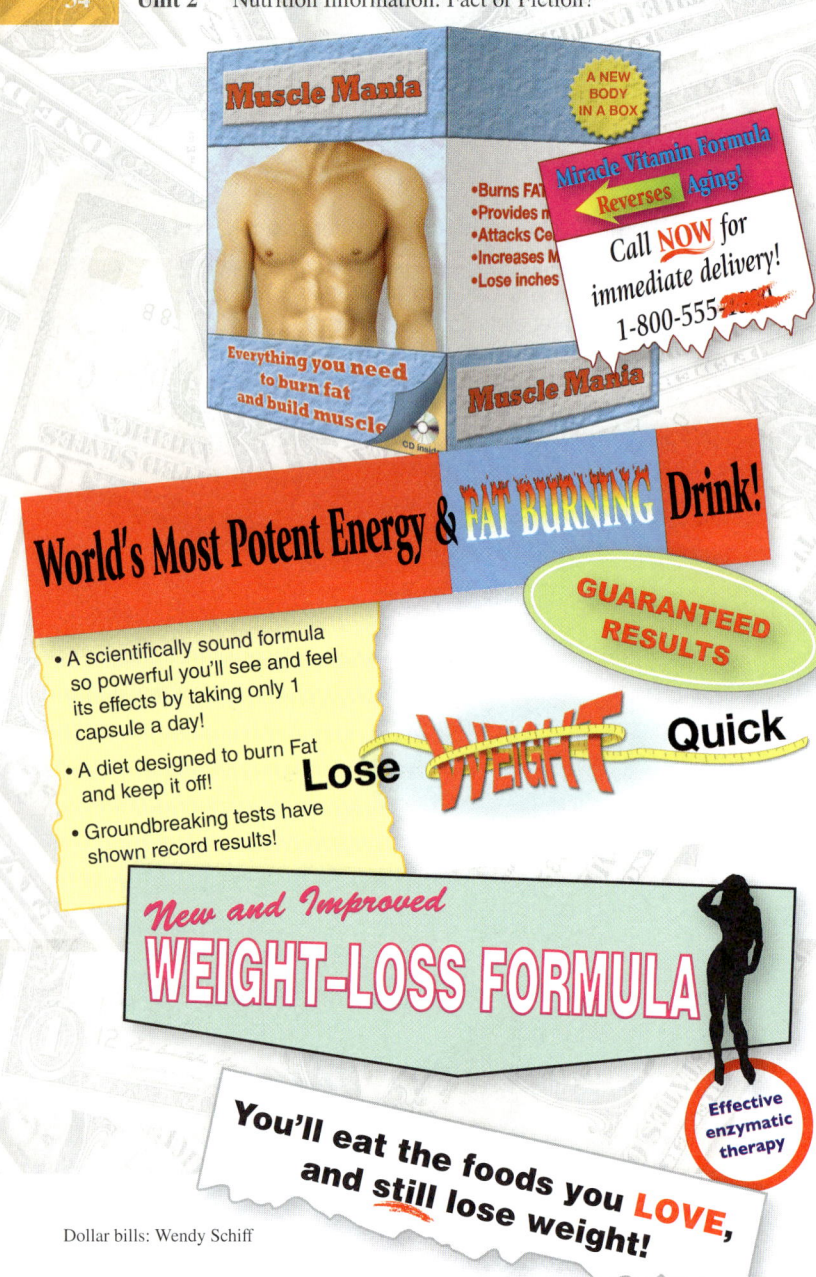

4. **"Money back" guarantees,** such as: "No risk. Just return the partially empty container and pay only shipping and handling." Or "You have nothing to lose!" You *lose* money on worthless, ineffective, and potentially unsafe dietary supplements. Furthermore, you may lose valuable time trying to diagnose and treat a serious health problem on your own, rather than seeking more conventional and, usually, more effective medical care.

5. **Statements about the superiority of unconventional medical practices,** such as: "Russian scientists have discovered the countless health benefits of taking Siberian ginseng" or "Herbal tea is the only cure for intestinal cancer."

6. **Testimonials and anecdotes as evidence of effectiveness,** such as: "I lost 50 pounds in 30 days using this product" or "I rubbed this vitamin E–containing lotion on my scar and it disappeared in days." As mentioned earlier, testimonials and anecdotes are not scientific.

7. **Information that promotes a product's benefits while overlooking its risks:** "Our all-natural supplement boosts your metabolism naturally so it won't harm your body." Beware of any source of information that fails to mention the possible side effects of using a dietary supplement or nutrition-related treatment. Anything you consume, even natural substances such as water and minerals, can be toxic in high doses.

8. **Recommendations based on a single study:** "Research conducted at our private health facility proves coffee enemas can cure cancer." Results of such research are likely to be biased.

9. **Information concerning nutrients or the human body that's not supported by reliable scientific evidence:** "This book explains how to combine certain foods based on your blood type" or "Most diseases are caused by undigested food that gets stuck in your guts" or "People with alkaline bodies don't develop cancer."

10. **Disclaimers, usually in small or difficult-to-read print:** "Results may vary," "Results not typical," or "This product is not intended to diagnose, cure, or prevent any disease." Disclaimers are often clues that the product probably won't live up to your expectations or the manufacturer's claims.

2.3c The Internet

You can find abundant sources of information about nutrition and the benefits of dietary supplements on the Internet. Before trusting the information, you must be careful and consider the sources. The same critical consumer tools for evaluating nutrition information from other sources can be applied to judging the reliability of information on the Internet (see Modules 2.3a and 2.3b).

A careful consumer of nutrition information

- Uses multiple sites, especially government agency sites (*.gov), such as the Centers for Disease Control and Prevention (www.cdc.gov) and the Food and Drug Administration (www.fda.gov).

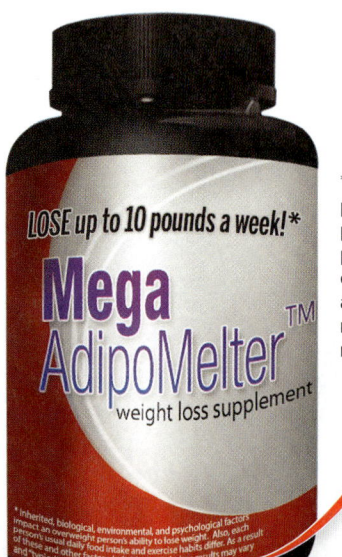

* Inherited, biological, environmental, and psychological factors impact an overweight person's ability to lose weight. Also, each person's usual daily food intake and exercise habits differ. As a result of these and other factors, individual weight loss results may vary and "typical" results are not possible to determine.

This disclaimer may be a red flag that this product has little or no effectiveness.

Dollar bills: Wendy Schiff

TASTY Tidbits

The Health on the Net is a nonprofit, international organization that promotes the HONcode, a set of principles for standardizing the reliability of health information on the Internet. When you are searching for reliable nutrition or health information on the Internet, look for the HONcode symbol on the main page of the website. For more information about HONcode, visit Health on the Net's website (www.hon.ch/).

Source: https://www.hon.ch/en/

- Is skeptical of information in blogs. Blogs might be interesting to read, but they aren't necessarily reliable.
- Is wary of websites that promote or sell products for profit (*.com) because such sources of information may be biased. Be wary if an *.org site sells dietary supplements online and/or includes articles that promote a product's benefits without mentioning its risks.
- Is wary of sites that include disclaimers. Examples of disclaimers include "The FDA has not evaluated this website" or "The author and owner of this site are not liable for personal actions taken as a result of the site's contents."

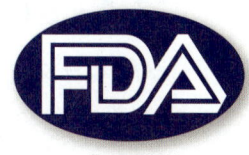

Source: FDA

- Doesn't trust sites that include attacks on the trustworthiness of the medical or scientific establishment.
- Avoids sites that provide online diagnoses and treatments.
- Avoids giving personal information at the site because its confidentiality may not be protected.

- Relies primarily on sites that are sponsored by groups of qualified health professionals. In general, websites sponsored by nationally recognized health organizations (*.org) such as the Academy of Nutrition and Dietetics (www.eatright.org) and nonprofit organizations such as the American Cancer Society (www.cancer.org) and National Osteoporosis Foundation (www.nof.org) are reliable sources of nutrition information. Nationally accredited colleges and universities (*.edu) are excellent sources of credible nutrition information.

The FTC enforces consumer protection laws and investigates complaints about false or misleading health claims that appear on the Internet. To obtain more information to help you evaluate nutrition and health-related claims, visit the agency's website. To complain about a product, you can complete and submit the FTC's complaint form at the agency's website: www.ftc.gov/faq/consumer-protection/submit-consumer-complaint-ftc or call the agency's toll-free line (1-877-382-4357).

TASTY Tidbits

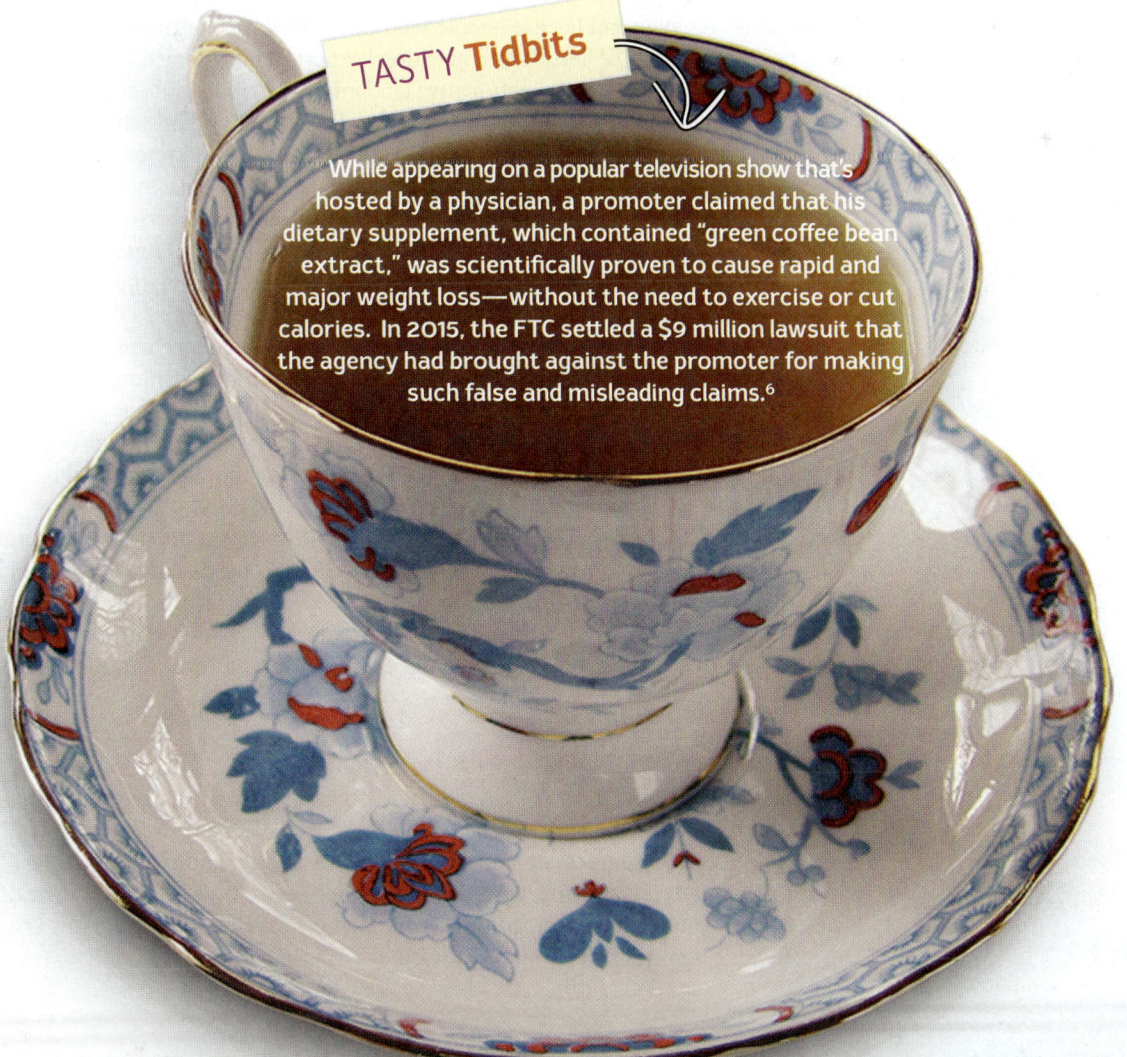

While appearing on a popular television show that's hosted by a physician, a promoter claimed that his dietary supplement, which contained "green coffee bean extract," was scientifically proven to cause rapid and major weight loss—without the need to exercise or cut calories. In 2015, the FTC settled a $9 million lawsuit that the agency had brought against the promoter for making such false and misleading claims.[6]

Wendy Schiff

Module 2.4
Seeking Reliable Nutrition Information

2.4 - Learning Outcome

After reading Module 2.4, you should be able to
1. Explain how to identify reliable nutrition experts.

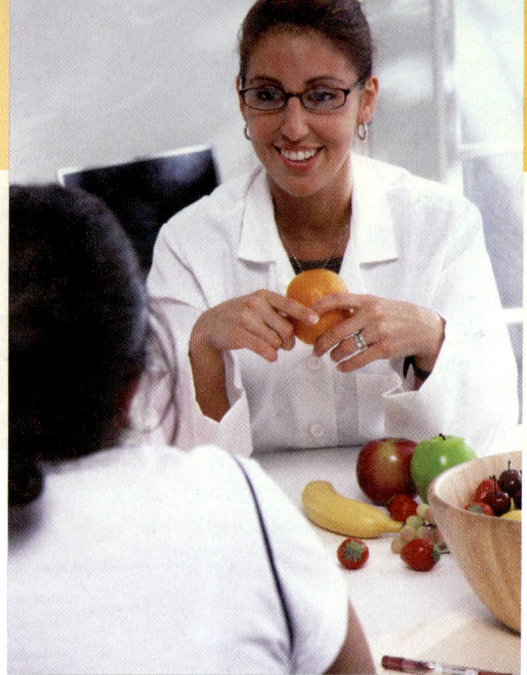
liquidlibrary/PictureQuest

Pick up a fitness, food, or health magazine, and you're likely to find something about nutrition. An article in a popular men's fitness magazine, for example, refers to an herbal tea recipe developed by a "physical fitness guru and nutrition expert." It seems that anyone who eats food can describe him- or herself as a nutritionist and provide nutrition- and food-related advice.

If you have questions about food or nutrition, where do you find factual answers? Should you ask your friends, dentists, doctors, or coaches? Who can be trusted to provide the facts?

2.4a Identifying Nutrition Experts

Although many states regulate and license people who call themselves nutritionists, you cannot always rely on someone who refers to him- or herself as a nutrition "expert," "nutritionist," or "nutritionalist" for reliable nutrition information. There are no nationally standardized legal definitions for these descriptors.

"Doctors" may not be physicians or nutrition scientists. Most physicians aren't nutrition experts because they didn't have extensive training in human nutrition while they were in medical school. Furthermore, a so-called nutrition expert who's referred to as "Doctor" may not have a doctorate degree (Ph.D.) in human nutrition from an accredited university. Such persons may have obtained their degrees simply by purchasing them on the Internet or through a mail-order outlet, without having taken appropriate coursework or graduated from an accredited university or college.

To obtain information about an author's or nutritionist's credentials, enter the person's name at an Internet search engine and evaluate the results. For example, is the person a nutrition scientist or registered dietitian nutritionist associated with an accredited school of higher education, such as a state or private university, or a government agency such as the U.S. Department of Agriculture? You can also visit www.quackwatch.org and submit an "Ask a Question" e-mail requesting information about a person's credentials.

If your university or college has a nutrition or dietetics department, you are likely to find qualified nutrition experts, including nutrition professors and registered dietitians, who are faculty members. Nutrition professors generally have doctorate degrees in human nutrition from accredited universities and extensive educational

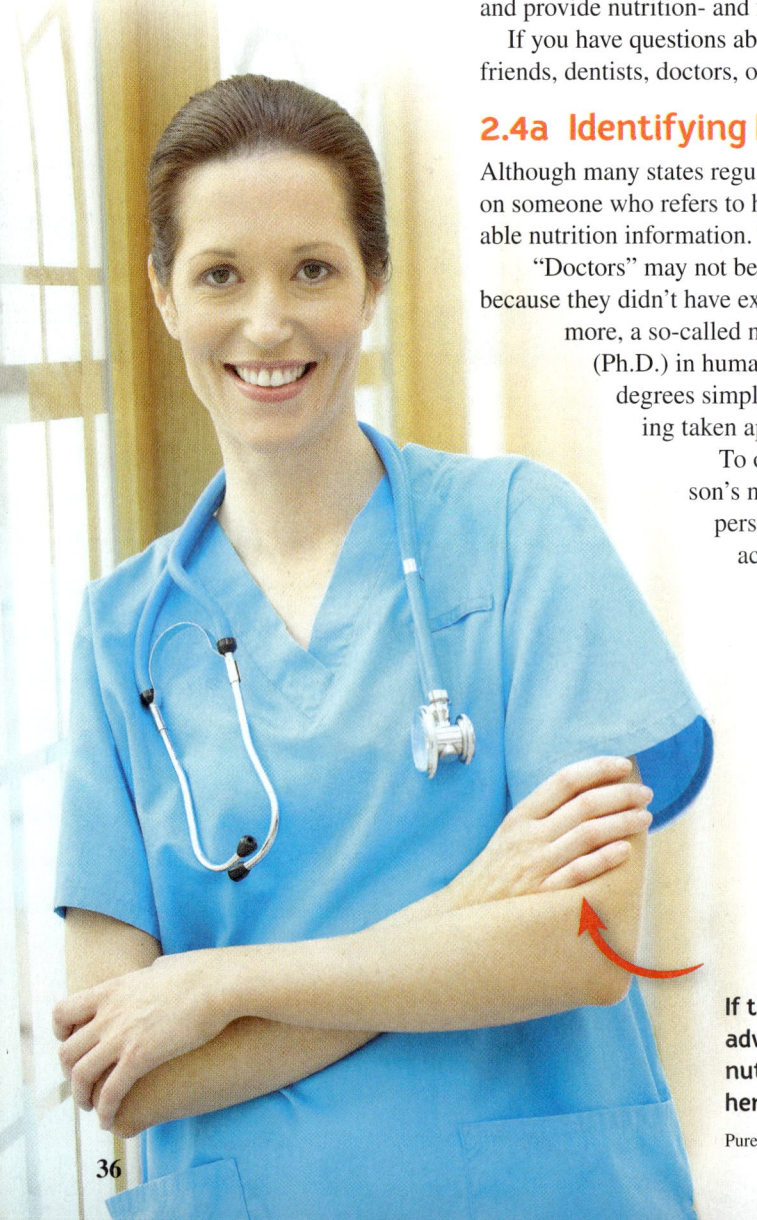

If this person appeared on a television show or in a magazine advertisement, would you consider her to be a reliable source of nutrition information? Explain why you would or would not trust her nutrition-related advice.

Purestock/SuperStock

backgrounds that emphasize coursework in human nutrition. Such instructors teach nutrition courses, conduct nutrition research, or do both.

A registered dietitian (RD) or a registered dietitian nutritionist (RDN) is a college-trained health care professional who has extensive knowledge of foods, nutrition, and dietetics. Dietetics is the application of nutrition and food information to treat many health-related conditions. Registered dietitian nutritionists are certified and must maintain their certification regularly by meeting nationally established standards. The titles "registered dietitian" and "registered dietitian nutritionist" are legally protected, so people cannot refer to themselves as RDs or RDNs without having the proper certification. You can also locate registered dietitians by contacting your local dietetic association or visiting the Academy of Nutrition and Dietetics website (www.eatright.org) or the dietitians of Canada's website (www.dietitians.ca).

In a Nutshell

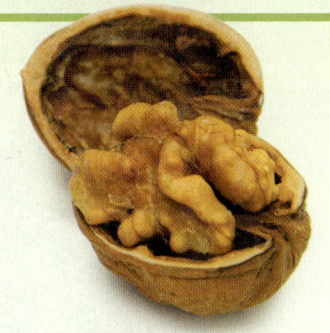

Module 2.1 Nutrition: Science for Consumers

- Scientists generally use the scientific method to answer questions about natural and physical observations.

- Nutrition research relies on scientific methods that generally involve making observations, asking questions, performing tests, collecting and analyzing data, drawing conclusions from data, and reporting on the findings. Other scientists can test the findings to confirm or reject them.

- Experimental studies using humans often involve double-blind studies and placebos. In studies that don't involve experiments, nutrition scientists may collect information about a specific population's health and food-related practices by conducting surveys.

- Scientists expect other researchers to avoid relying on their personal attitudes and biases when collecting and analyzing data, and to evaluate and report their results objectively and honestly.

- Scientists share results of their findings, usually in an article that describes the study and its findings. Before publishing the article, the editor of a scientific journal sends copies of it to peer reviewers. If peer reviewers accept the study's findings as being scientifically reliable, the journal's editor agrees to publish the article.

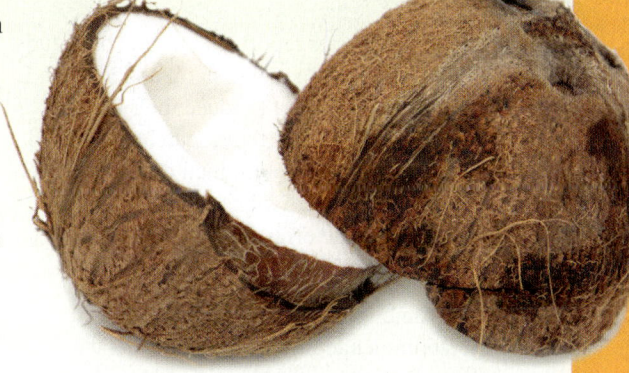

Bernatskaya Oxana/Shutterstock

- Conflicting research findings often result because different teams of researchers use different study designs, populations, and ways of analyzing results. Other factors, such as individual genetic and lifestyle differences, can also influence the results of nutrition research involving human subjects.

- Studies involving people and their food-related practices generally cannot establish cause and effect. When two different natural events occur simultaneously within a population, it doesn't necessarily mean they're related to each other. What appears to be a relationship between a dietary practice and a physical outcome could be a coincidence.

Module 2.2 Spreading Nutrition Misinformation

- Although testimonials and anecdotes are often used to promote nutrition-related products, you cannot be sure that this information is reliable or based on scientific facts. Personal observations are not evidence of cause-and-effect relationships because many factors, such as lifestyle and environment, can influence outcomes.

- Popular magazine articles, best-selling popular books, Internet websites, television news reports, and other forms of media are often unreliable sources of nutrition information.

- The First Amendment to the U.S. Constitution guarantees freedom of the press and freedom of speech. The FDA can regulate nutrition- and health-related claims on product labels, but the agency cannot prevent the spread of health and nutrition misinformation presented in the media.

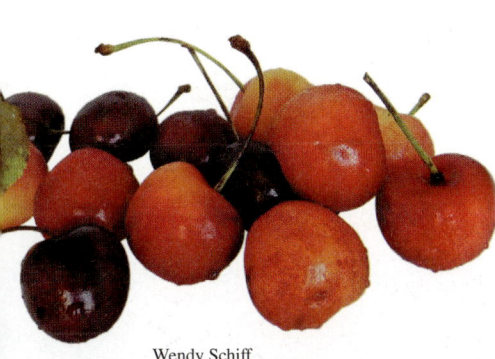

Wendy Schiff

Module 2.3 Becoming a More Critical Consumer of Nutrition Information

- To become a more critical consumer of nutrition information, consider being more skeptical about the reliability of the nutrition information that's readily available from family, friends, and the media. To determine whether a source of information is reliable, ask questions to determine the source's reasons for promoting the information. You can also look for red flags that indicate misinformation, such as claims that sound too good to be true and scare tactics.

- Much of the nutrition information that's on the Internet is unreliable and intended to promote sales. Websites sponsored by nonprofit organizations, nationally recognized health associations, government agencies, and nationally accredited colleges and universities are generally reliable sources of information.

- The FTC enforces consumer protection laws and investigates complaints about false or misleading health claims that appear on the Internet.

Module 2.4 Seeking Reliable Nutrition Information

- Many states regulate and license nutritionists, but there's no standard legal definition for "nutrition expert" or "nutritionist" in the United States.

- For reliable food, nutrition, and dietary information, consult persons with degrees in human nutrition from accredited institutions of higher learning, such as nutrition instructors, RDs, and RDNs. To locate registered dietitians, contact local dietetic associations or visit the Academy of Nutrition and Dietetics website (www.eatright.org).

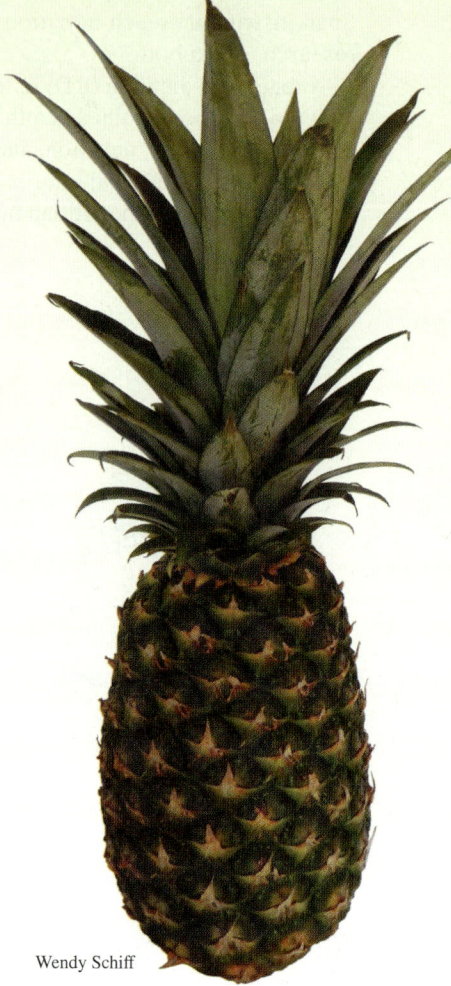
Wendy Schiff

Consider This...

1. A news broadcaster reports the results of a study in which people who took fish oil and vitamin E supplements daily didn't reduce their risk of heart attack. Moreover, the researchers stopped the study when they determined the supplements increased the subjects' risk of stroke! Explain how you would determine whether this information is reliable.

2. Recall someone, maybe a parent or friend, who recommended that you take a dietary supplement or eat an unusual food because it provided health benefits. Describe the recommendation and explain why you did or didn't follow the advice.

3. Search the Internet for a website that promotes and sells dietary supplements. Record the URL for the site. Use the information in Module 2.3 to judge the reliability of the nutrition information provided by the site.

4. Browse through popular magazines to find an article or advertisement that relates to nutrition, and make a copy of the article or advertisement. Analyze each sentence or line of the article or advertisement for signs of unreliability. Is the article or advertisement a reliable source of information? Explain why it is or why it isn't.

5. In the opening of this unit, a young woman reported that drinking a beverage made with a superfood dietary supplement improved her skin. Design a scientific study that would test the effectiveness of this product as a treatment for skin blemishes.

Test Yourself

Select the best answer.

1. The first step of the scientific method usually involves
   a. making observations.
   b. developing a question.
   c. identifying relationships between personal characteristics.
   d. gathering data.

2. The government agency that enforces consumer protection laws by investigating false or misleading health-related claims is the
   a. Federal Bureau of Investigation (FBI).
   b. Environmental Protection Agency (EPA).
   c. Federal Trade Commission (FTC).
   d. Centers for Disease Control and Prevention (CDC).

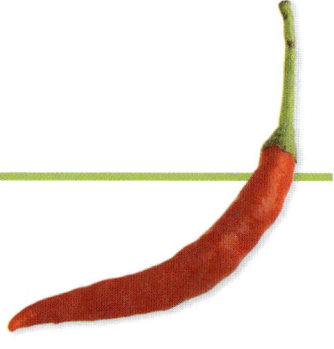

3. A testimonial is a(an)
   a. unbiased report about a product's value.
   b. scientifically valid claim.
   c. form of scientific evidence.
   d. personal endorsement of a product.

4. Which of the following websites is most likely to provide biased and unreliable nutrition information?
   a. A site that sells dietary supplements (*.com)
   b. The site of a nationally recognized, nonprofit health association (*.org)
   c. A U.S. government agency's site (*.gov)
   d. The site of an accredited college or university (*.edu)

5. A(An) _____ is a fake treatment that may be used in nutrition-related studies that have human subjects.
   a. anecdote   c. control
   b. placebo   d. double blind

6. The federal agency that can regulate nutrition claims on food labels is the
   a. FSIS.   c. EPA.
   b. FTC.   d. FDA.

7. You read an article about vegetables grown in the United States. According to the article's author, Americans need to take dietary supplements because the vegetables lack essential nutrients. This claim is an example of a(an)
   a. scare tactic.
   b. scientific fact.
   c. anecdote.
   d. evidence-based report.

8. A nutrition scientist designs a study in which he assigns 100 people to the treatment group and 100 people to the control group. Although the scientist knows each person's group assignment, the subjects aren't aware of their group placement. This is an example of a(an)
   a. double-blind study.
   b. uncontrolled study.
   c. single-blind study.
   d. biased study.

9. Each day, one of your relatives drinks a smoothie made from wheatgrass. He claims it helps keep his immune system "energized and balanced." His claim is an example of
   a. an anecdote.
   b. a direct observation.
   c. an indirect correlation.
   d. a validated bias.

10. A person claiming to be a doctor recommends coffee enemas as the treatment for cancer of the large intestine. This recommendation is an example of
    a. professional bias.
    b. controlled experimentation.
    c. the placebo effect.
    d. quackery.

11. Someone who has _____ credentials after his or her name is most likely a reliable source of food and nutrition information.
    a. RDN   c. LED
    b. MD   d. PE

Answers: 1. a 2. c 3. d 4. a 5. b 6. d 7. a 8. c 9. a 10. d 11. a

A Answer This (Module 2.1b)

There is no relationship between drinking lemonade and drowning. This observation is a coincidence and not a case of cause and effect. Why? During warm weather, people are more likely to drink lemonade, and people are also more likely to go swimming. Although these two events tend to occur at the same time of year, they're not related to each other.

Wheatgrass

References → See Appendix D.

Design Elements: Spiral notebook paper background, Stacked paper with clip background, Marginal note clip, and Culture & Cuisine globe icon: ©McGraw-Hill Education; In a Nutshell walnut: ©McGraw-Hill Education/Mark A. Dierker, photographer; Test Yourself red pepper: Iconotec/Glow Images

Wendy Schiff

Unit 3
Making More Nutritious Choices

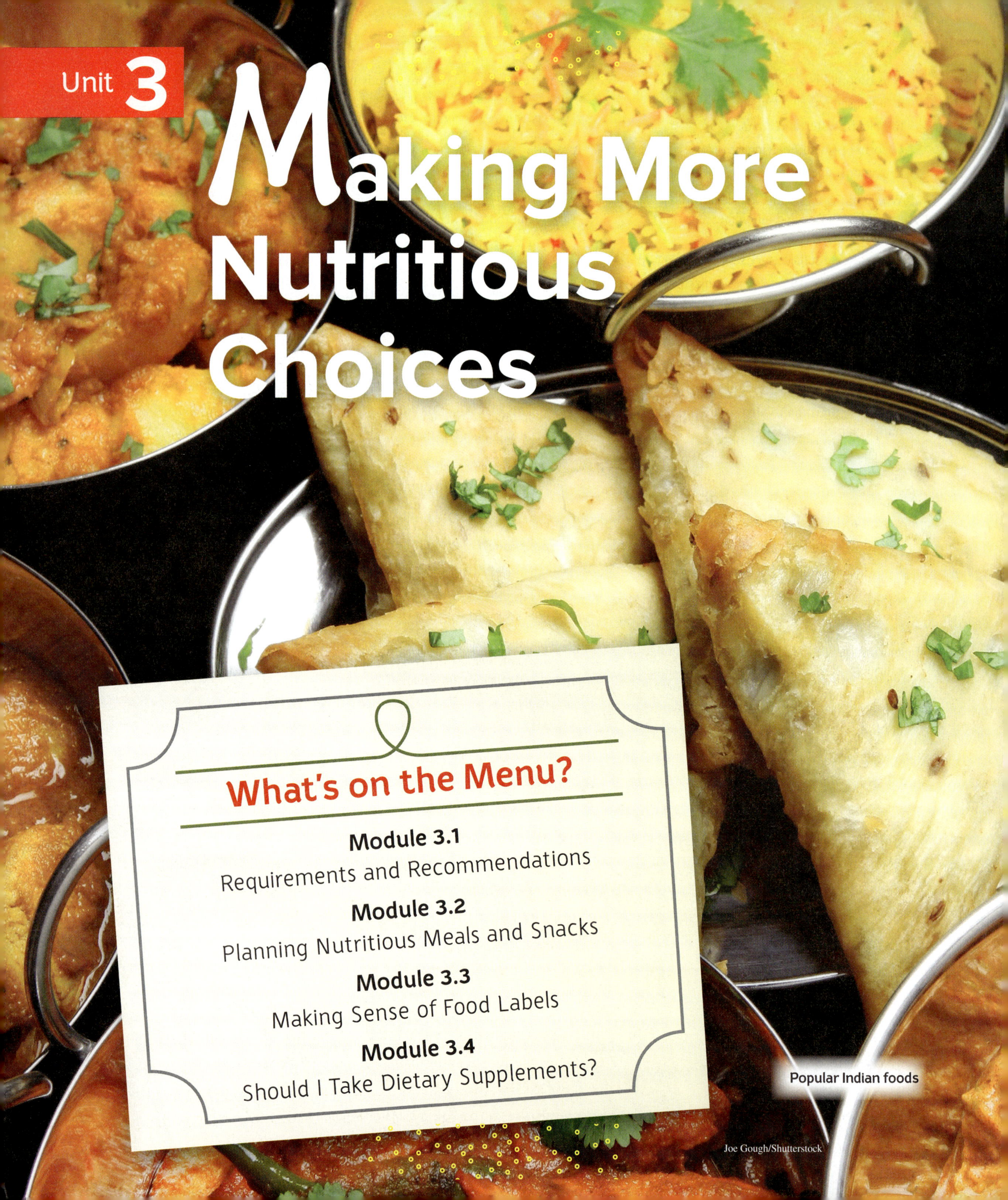

What's on the Menu?

Module 3.1
Requirements and Recommendations

Module 3.2
Planning Nutritious Meals and Snacks

Module 3.3
Making Sense of Food Labels

Module 3.4
Should I Take Dietary Supplements?

Popular Indian foods

Joe Gough/Shutterstock

"I was born in Madras (Chennai), India... I moved to the United States with my family when I was nine years old. I love Indian food. When I visit India, my diet is very different than what I eat here. You can buy a variety of spicy foods, such as peppery corn-on-the-cob and vazhakkai bajji (banana slices that are fried after being dipped in besan flour mixed with chili powder), that are cooked in stalls that line city streets. The variety of fresh, tropical fruits is amazing. I love fresh jackfruit! I can't find fresh jackfruit where I now live."

"My mom makes naan (nahn) and roti from scratch. Naan and roti are flatbreads that are often served with a spicy lentil and/or curry gravy. I like sticky white rice with meals, and I eat all types of vegetables, beans, and lentils. I'll also eat poultry, eggs, dairy foods, and seafood, but I don't eat red meat because I think it's unhealthy. My parents don't eat foods from animals."

Sachin Raghothaman

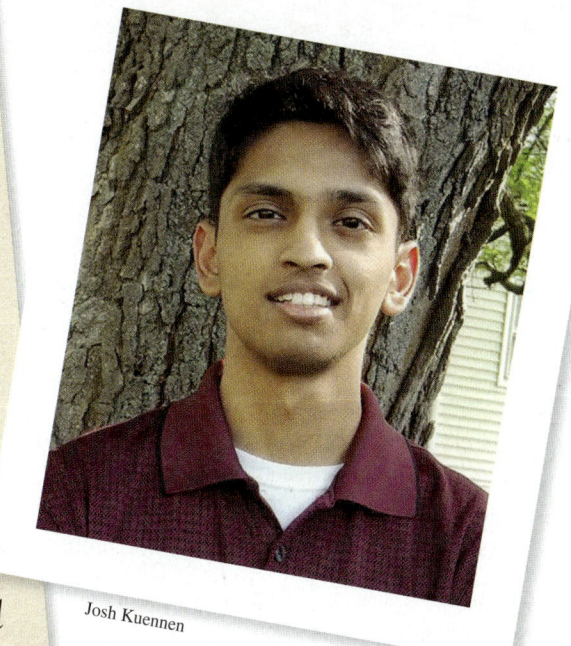

Josh Kuennen

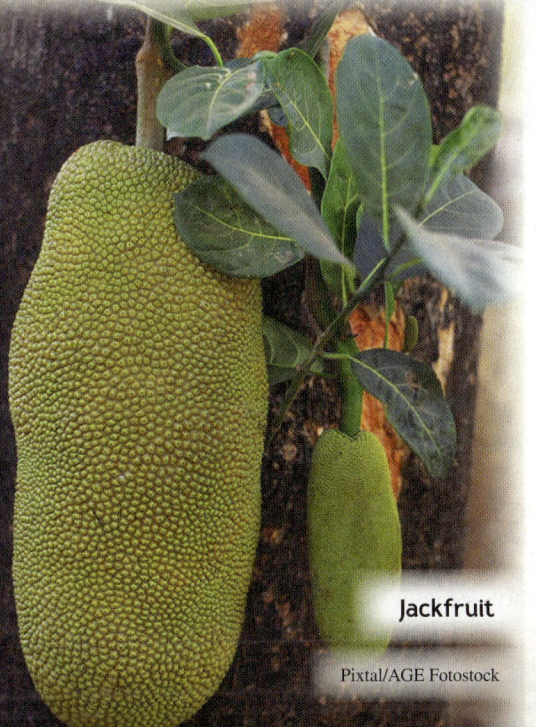

Jackfruit

Pixtal/AGE Fotostock

Aparajith ("Sachin") Raghothaman is a senior majoring in mechanical engineering at Iowa State University. As he described, his diet is quite different than the typical American college student's. Traditional Asian diets, such as Sachin's, often contain small amounts of animal foods and larger amounts of locally grown fresh fruits, vegetables, and rice or noodles. Registered dietitian nutritionists generally recommend that Americans increase their consumption of plant foods, such as beans and lentils, and reduce their intakes of red meats, and, especially, processed meat. Such meat includes sausage, bacon, hot dogs, and "deli meats." Making these dietary changes might improve the long-term health status of many Americans.

How can you plan nutritious meals and snacks that don't rely on red meats, processed meat, fried potatoes, canned applesauce, and iceberg lettuce? Unit 3 discusses dietary standards; practical ways for you to plan a nutritionally adequate, well-balanced diet; and how you can interpret and use nutrition-related information that appears on food and dietary supplement labels.

Module 3.1

Requirements and Recommendations

3.1 - Learning Outcomes

After reading Module 3.1, you should be able to

1. Define all of the **key terms** in this module.
2. Differentiate among the various dietary standards of the Dietary Reference Intakes.
3. Identify and apply the Acceptable Macronutrient Distribution Ranges for carbohydrate, protein, and fat intakes for adults.

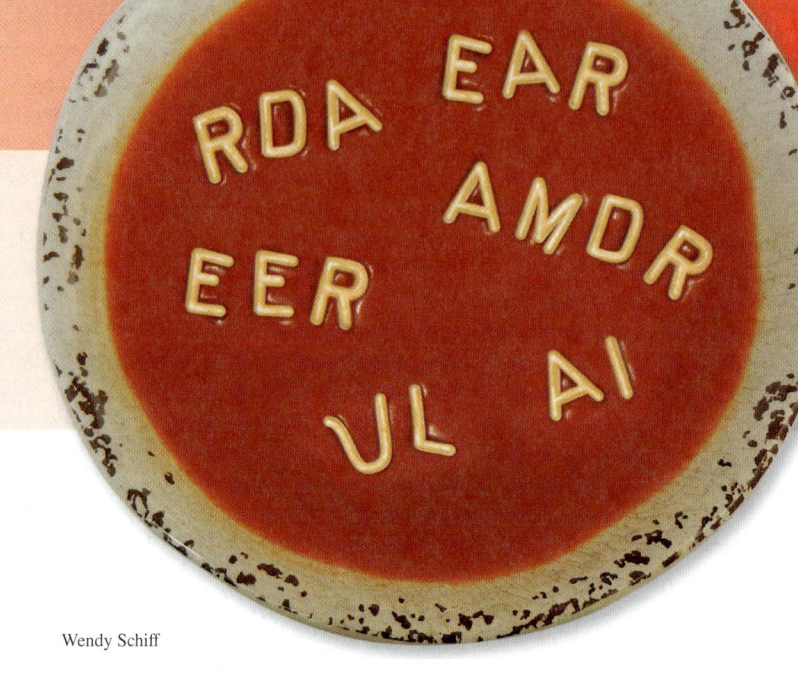

Wendy Schiff

By using research methods discussed in Unit 2, scientists have been able to estimate required amounts of many essential nutrients. A **requirement** can be defined as the smallest amount of a nutrient that maintains a defined level of nutritional health.[1] This amount, when consumed daily, prevents the development of the nutrient's deficiency disease. For example, the requirement for vitamin C (generally, 10 mg/day) prevents scurvy, the vitamin's deficiency disease.[2] The requirement (need) for a particular nutrient varies to some degree from person to person. Your age, sex, general health status, physical activity level, and life cycle stage (pregnancy, for example) are among factors that influence your nutrient requirements.

Your body stores many nutrients, including vitamin D and the minerals iron and calcium. Major storage sites are your liver, body fat, and/or bones. Other nutrients, however, such as vitamin C and most B vitamins, aren't stored by your body. For optimal nutrition, you need to consume enough of these nutrients each day to maintain adequate levels of them in your body.

Your body uses its nutrient stores much like you can use a savings account to help manage your money. When you have some extra cash, it's wise to place the money in a savings account, so you can withdraw some of the reserves to meet future needs without going into debt. When your intake of certain nutrients is more than enough to meet your needs, the body stores the excess. During a serious illness or recovery from such an illness, your body's needs for many nutrients are likely to be greater than normal. However, you may not feel like eating. When this situation happens, your body can withdraw some nutrients from storage. As a result of having optimal levels of stored nutrients, you may recover more quickly.

3.1a Introducing the DRIs

Dietary Reference Intakes (DRIs) encompass a variety of energy and nutrient intake standards that can be used to help people reduce their risk of nutrient deficiencies and excesses, prevent disease, and achieve optimal health **(Fig. 3.1)**.[3] Registered dietitians refer to DRIs when planning nutritious diets for groups of people and evaluating

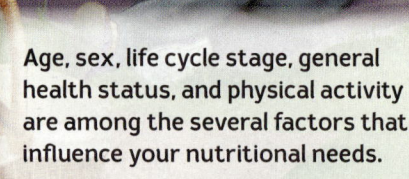

Age, sex, life cycle stage, general health status, and physical activity are among the several factors that influence your nutritional needs.

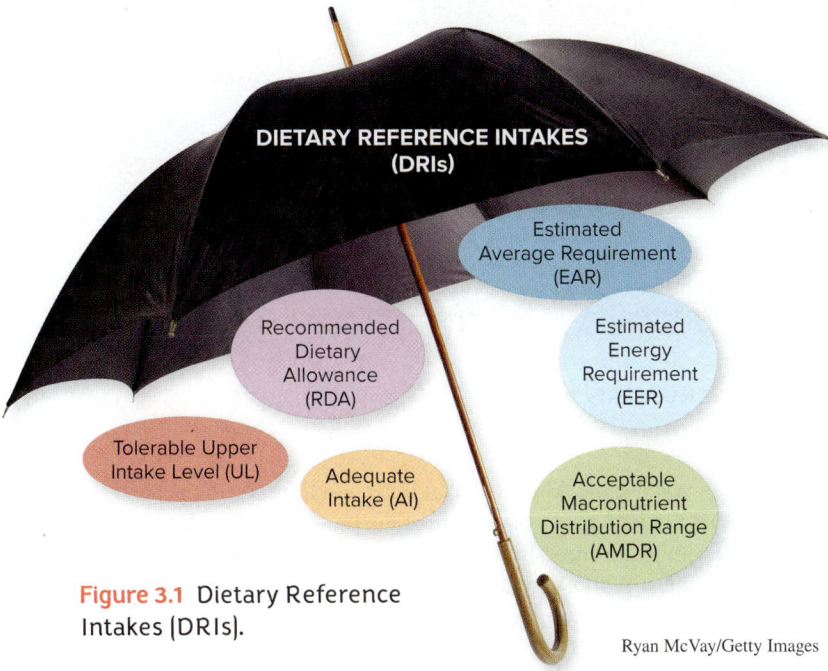

Figure 3.1 Dietary Reference Intakes (DRIs).

Ryan McVay/Getty Images

the nutritional adequacy of a population's diet. However, you can use DRIs to evaluate the nutritional quality of your diet (see **Appendix E**).[4]

Estimated Average Requirement (EAR)

An **Estimated Average Requirement (EAR)** is the amount of the nutrient that meets the needs of 50% of healthy people who are in a particular life stage/sex group (**Fig. 3.2**). Life stage/sex groups classify people according to age, sex, and whether females are pregnant or breastfeeding. Because the EAR for a nutrient meets the requirements of only 50% of the population, you shouldn't use the standard to judge whether your daily intake is adequate. Scientists, however, use EARs for setting nutrient recommendations.

Estimated Energy Requirement (EER)

The **Estimated Energy Requirement (EER)** is the average daily energy (calorie) intake that meets the needs of a healthy person who is maintaining his or her weight. The EER takes into account the person's physical activity level, height, and weight, as well as sex and life stage. Because the EER is an average figure, you may have energy needs that are higher or lower.

Recommended Dietary Allowance (RDA)

Simply consuming required amounts of nutrients doesn't always result in optimal nutritional status. Some people may naturally have higher requirements. What if your requirement for a particular nutrient is higher than average? If that's the case, your body is likely to develop the nutrient's deficiency disease, unless you consume more than the typical person's required amount.

The **Recommended Dietary Allowances (RDAs)** are standards for recommending daily intakes of several nutrients. RDAs meet the nutrient needs of nearly all healthy individuals (97 to 98%) in a particular life stage/sex group (see Figure 3.2).

To establish an RDA for a nutrient, nutrition scientists add a "margin of safety" amount to the EAR that allows for individual variations in nutrient

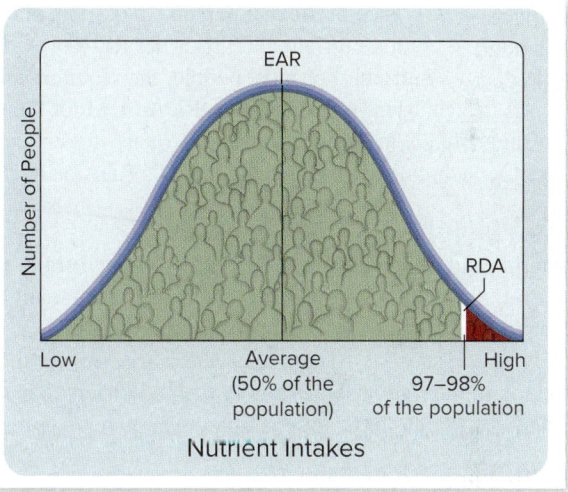

Figure 3.2 The EAR. This graph shows the distribution of nutrient intakes within a population. Note the positions of the EAR and RDA.

■ *What is an EAR?*

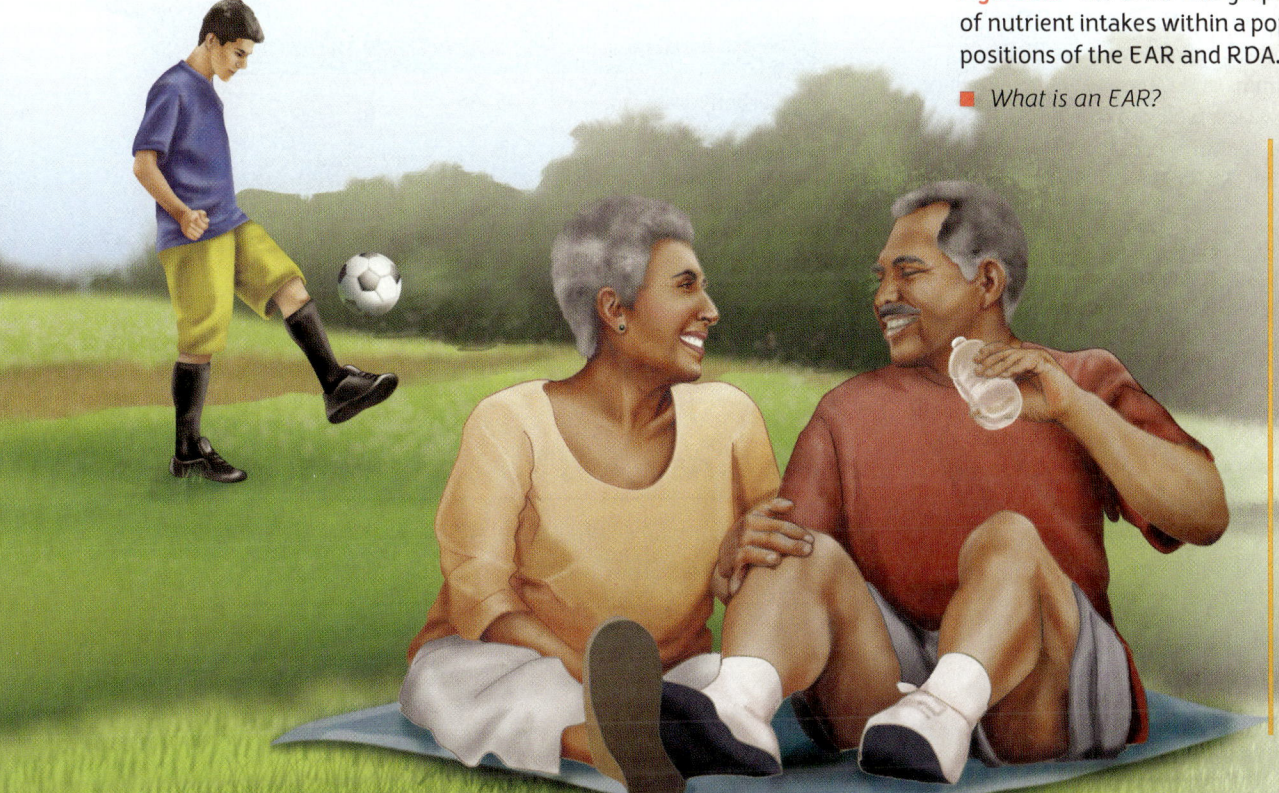

requirement smallest amount of a nutrient that maintains a defined level of nutritional health

Dietary Reference Intakes (DRIs) various energy and nutrient intake standards for Americans

Estimated Average Requirement (EAR) amount of a nutrient that meets the needs of 50% of healthy people in a life stage/sex group

Estimated Energy Requirement (EER) average daily energy intake that meets the needs of a healthy person maintaining his or her weight

Recommended Dietary Allowances (RDAs) daily nutrient recommendations that meet the needs of 97–98% of healthy people in a life stage/sex group

needs and helps maintain tissue stores. For example, the adult RDA for vitamin C (nonsmokers) is 15 mg higher than the EAR—75 mg for women who aren't pregnant or breastfeeding and 90 mg for men.[3]

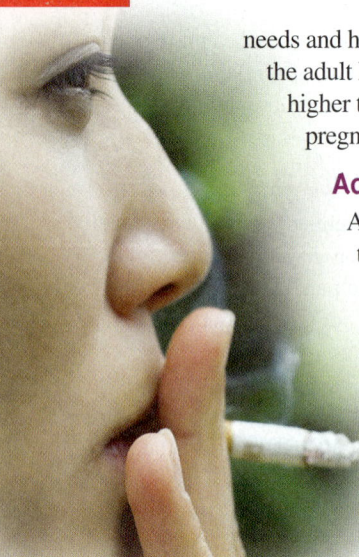

Smoking increases the body's need for vitamin C.

Adequate Intakes (AIs)

A few nutrients don't have RDAs because there's not enough information about them to determine human needs. Scientists set **Adequate Intakes (AIs)** for these particular nutrients. To establish an AI, scientists record eating patterns of a group of healthy people and estimate the group's average daily intake of the nutrient. If the group of people under observation shows no evidence of the nutrient's deficiency disorder, the average level of intake must be adequate and that amount becomes the AI (**Fig. 3.3**).

It is important to understand the difference between a person's requirement ("need") for a nutrient and his or her RDA or AI for that nutrient. For most people, the requirement for a nutrient is less than the RDA or AI for the nutrient. Thus, your diet is likely to be nutritionally adequate if your average daily intake for each nutrient meets the nutrient's RDA or AI value.

Tolerable Upper Intake Level (UL)

Many vitamins and minerals have a **Tolerable Upper Intake Level (Upper Level, or UL)**. The UL is the highest average amount of a nutrient that's unlikely to harm most people when the amount is consumed daily (see Figure 3.3). The risk of a *toxicity disorder* increases when a person regularly consumes amounts of a nutrient that exceed its UL. The UL for vitamin C, for example, is 2000 mg/day for adults.

Acceptable Macronutrient Distribution Ranges (AMDRs)

Acceptable Macronutrient Distribution Ranges (**AMDRs**) indicate ranges of carbohydrate, fat, and protein intakes that are likely to provide adequate amounts of vitamins and minerals and may reduce the risk of diet-related chronic diseases. You can use the AMDRs to determine whether your diet has a healthful balance of macronutrients. **Table 3.1** lists adult AMDRs.

Adequate Intakes (AIs) dietary recommendations that assume a population's average daily nutrient intakes are adequate because no deficiency diseases are present

Tolerable Upper Intake Level (Upper Level or UL) standard representing the highest average amount of a nutrient that's unlikely to be harmful when consumed daily

Acceptable Macronutrient Distribution Ranges (AMDRs) macronutrient intake ranges that are nutritionally adequate and may reduce the risk of diet-related chronic diseases

---

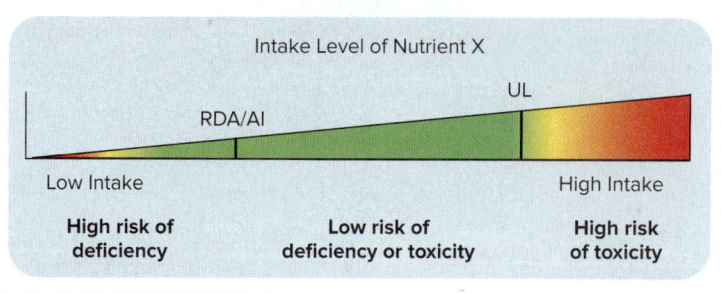

Figure 3.3 RDAs, AIs, and ULs.

■ *What is a UL?*

How can you use the AMDRs? You'll need to translate the percentages of AMDRs into grams of carbohydrate, protein, and fat. Let's say you generally consume 1800 kcal/day to maintain your weight. You want to meet AMDR guidelines for carbohydrate and protein by making 50% (0.50) of your total kcal from "carbs" and 25% (0.25) of your kcal from protein. Let's start with carbohydrates. Multiply 0.50 × 1800 kcal, which equals 900 kcal. To figure out how many grams of carbohydrates this represents, divide 900 g by 4 kcal (each gram of carbohydrate supplies 4 kcal). Thus, you can consume 225 g of carbohydrates daily. To make 25% of your calorie intake from protein, multiply 0.25 × 1800 kcal, which equals 450 kcal. Divide 450 kcal by 4 kcal (each gram of protein provides 4 kcal). Your daily intake of protein is 112.5 g. Now, you've accounted for all but 25% of your daily calories. To figure out how many grams of fat you can eat each day, multiply 0.25 × 1800 kcal, which equals 450 kcal. Each gram of fat supplies 9 kcal, so divide 450 kcal by 9 kcal to get 50 g of fat. Now, you've accounted for 100% of your daily energy intake.

TABLE 3.1 ACCEPTABLE MACRONUTRIENT DISTRIBUTION RANGES: ADULTS

Macronutrient	AMDR (% of total energy intake)
Carbohydrate	45–65
Protein	10–35
Fat*	20–35

*Fat intake should include essential fatty acids (see Unit 6).

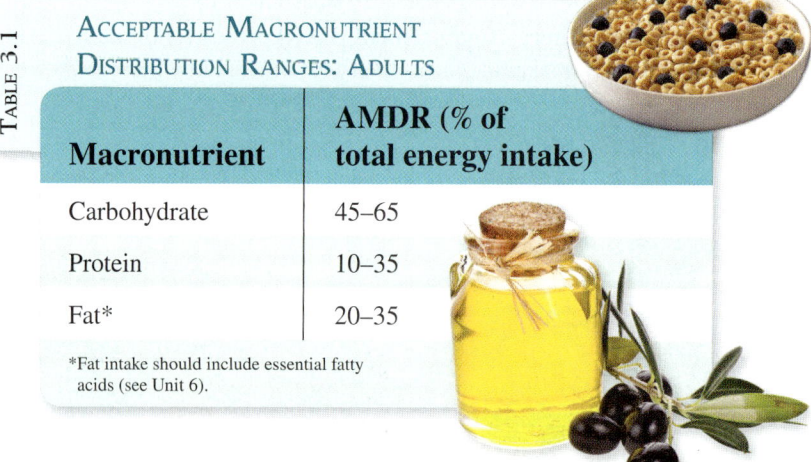

Q Answer This

If your total calorie intake is 2400 kcal per day and fat provides 30% of your calories, how many grams of fat do you consume? You'll find the answer on the last page of this unit.

Woman smoking: ZenShui/Frederic Cirou/Getty Images; Olive oil, Small twig with black olives: ANCH/Shutterstock; Bowl of toasted oat cereal: Robert Santos/Getty Images

Module 3.2

Planning Nutritious Meals and Snacks

3.2 - Learning Outcomes

After reading Module 3.2, you should be able to

1. Define all of the **key terms** in this module.
2. List major food groups, identify foods that are typically classified in each group, and indicate nutritional equivalents of foods in each group.
3. Discuss recommendations of the *2015–2020 Dietary Guidelines for Americans* and describe features of a healthy dietary pattern (according to these guidelines).
4. Use MyPlate and other dietary tools to develop nutritionally adequate daily menus.

3.2a Introducing the Food Groups

The DRIs aren't easy to use for planning menus, so nutrition experts develop more consumer-friendly food (dietary) guides. In general, food guides classify foods into major groups according to their natural origins and key nutrients. Most commonly consumed dairy foods, for example, are made from cow's milk, which is a good source of calcium. Food guides usually recommend amounts of foods from each group that should be eaten daily. You can use such guides to plan what to eat each day as well as add variety and nutritional balance and adequacy to your diet.

The serving equivalents charts on the following pages of Section 3.2a show amounts of commonly eaten foods from each group that are considered nutritionally equal to each other. These food standards have been set by the U.S. Department of Agriculture (USDA).[5]

Grains

Grains include products made from wheat, rice, and oats. Pasta, noodles, crackers, and flour tortillas are members of this group. Cornmeal and popcorn are usually grouped with grain products. Although corn is a type of grain, it's often used as a vegetable in meals.

Carbohydrate (starch) and protein are the primary macronutrients that are naturally in grains. Dietary guides generally recommend that you choose foods made with *whole grains*. **Whole grains** are the entire, ground, cracked, or flaked seeds of cereal grains, such as wheat, buckwheat, oats, corn, rice, wild rice, rye, and barley.[6] In general, the grains that are used to make whole-grain foods haven't undergone as much processing (*minimally processed*) as a refined-grain food, such as white bread or plain buns. Whole-grain foods, such as whole-grain breads and whole-grain cereals, are good sources of micronutrients and fiber.

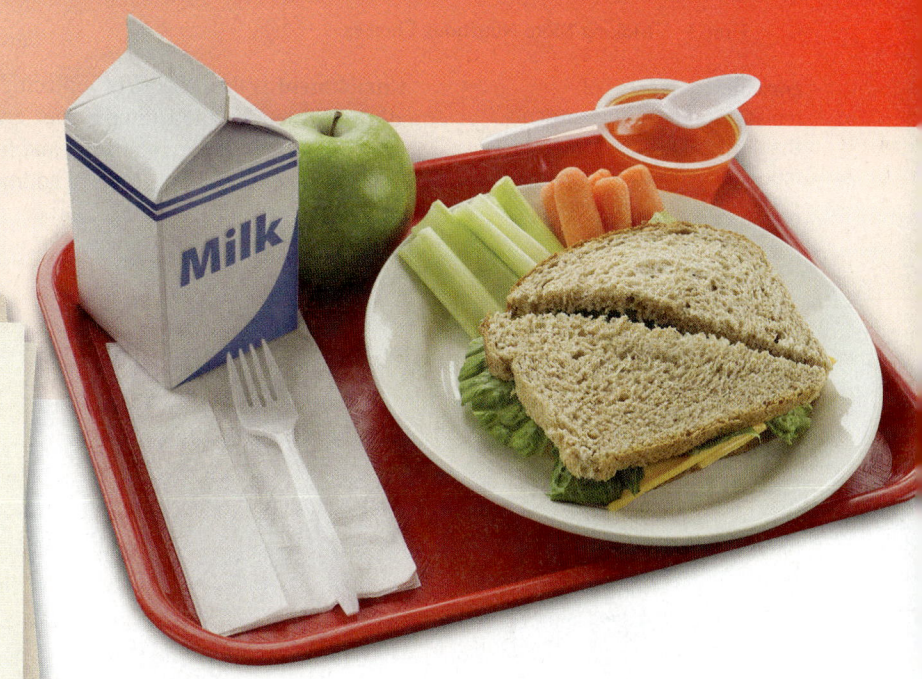

TASTY Tidbits

Compared to refined-grain products, foods made with whole grains naturally contain more fiber. Be careful of products that have the claim "Made with 18 grams of whole grains" on the label. Such claims can be misleading because whole grains aren't nutrients. You need to be concerned about amounts of fiber and other nutrients in a serving of the product. For that information, read the nutrition information on the product's label.

A serving of this cereal has 18 g "whole grains," but how much fiber does it provide?

whole grains the entire, ground, cracked, or flaked seeds of cereal grains, such as wheat, buckwheat, oats, corn, rice, wild rice, rye, and barley

Lunch on tray: Tetra Images/SuperStock; Whole-grain serving label: Wendy Schiff; Magnifying glass: Siede Preis/Getty Images

46 Unit 3 Making More Nutritious Choices

enrichment process of replacing some of the nutrients that were lost during a raw food's refinement

fortification addition of any nutrient to food

Enrichment is the process of replacing some, but not all, of the nutrients that were lost during a raw food's refinement. In the United States, enriched-grain products have specific amounts of iron and the B vitamins thiamin, riboflavin, niacin, and folic acid added to refined cereal grain products, such as enriched breads and rice. **Fortification** is the addition of any nutrient to foods. Nutrient fortification may restore nutrients in foods that were lost during processing or provide specific health benefits. Examples of fortification include the addition of vitamins and/or minerals to ready-to-eat cereals and granola bars, calcium to orange juice, and vitamins A and D to milk.

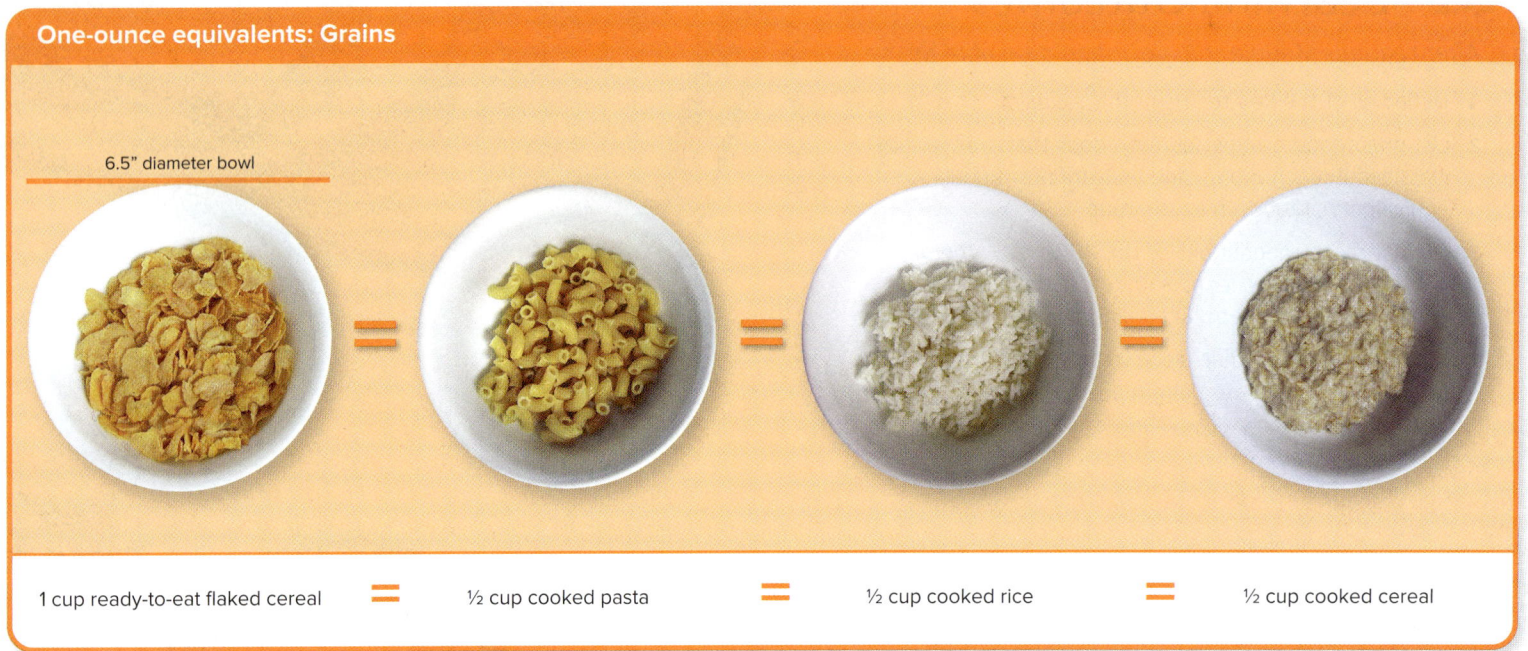

One-ounce equivalents: Grains

6.5" diameter bowl

1 cup ready-to-eat flaked cereal = ½ cup cooked pasta = ½ cup cooked rice = ½ cup cooked cereal

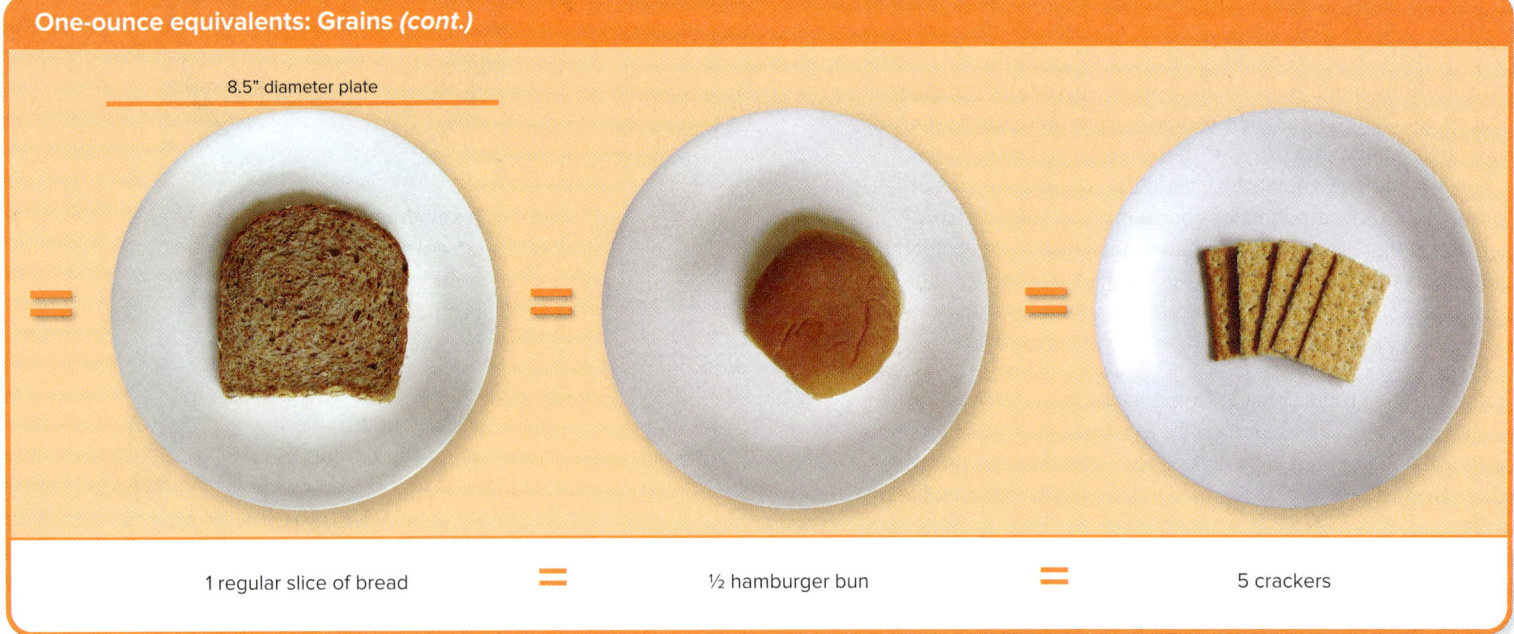

One-ounce equivalents: Grains *(cont.)*

8.5" diameter plate

1 regular slice of bread = ½ hamburger bun = 5 crackers

All images: Wendy Schiff

Planning Nutritious Meals and Snacks 47

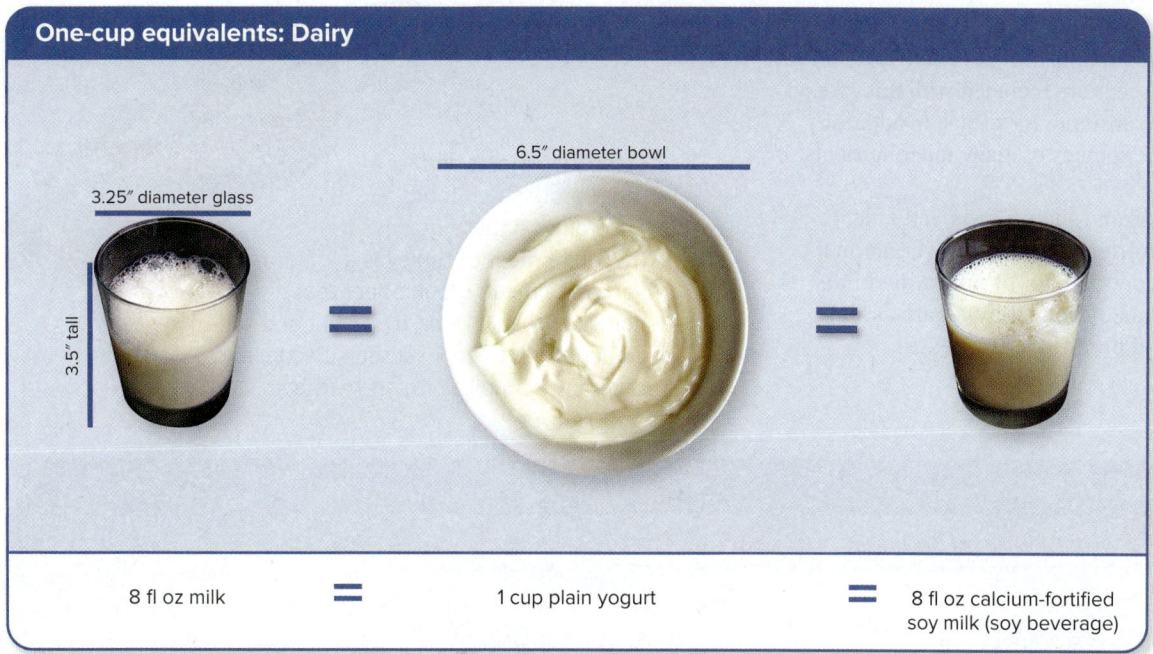

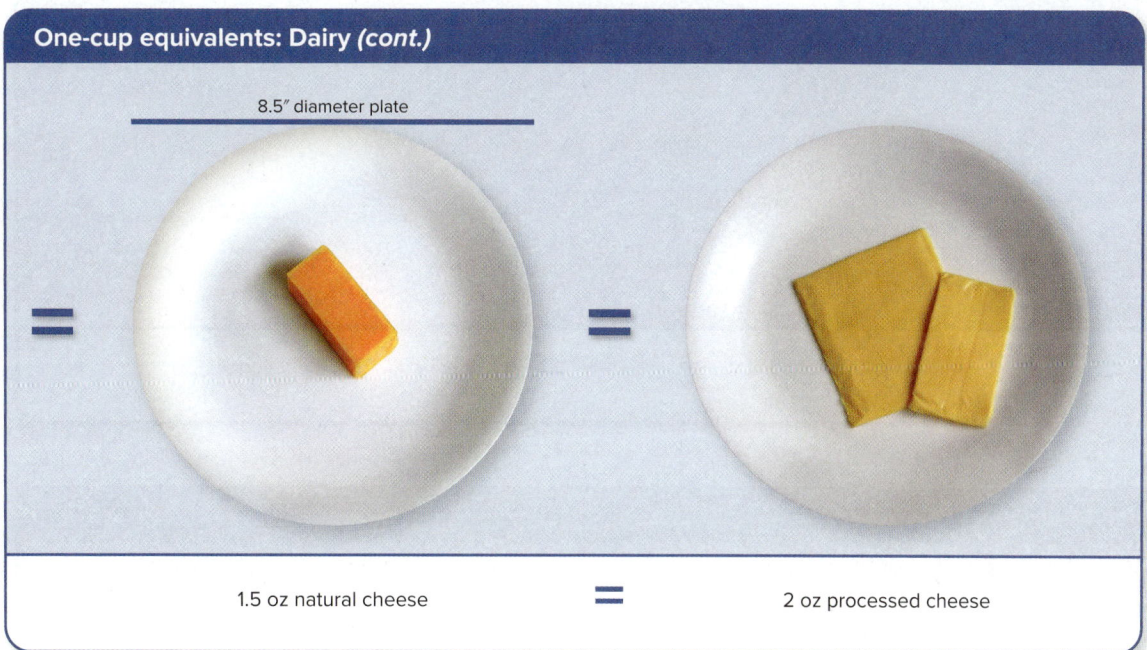

All images: Wendy Schiff

Dairy Foods

Dairy foods include milk and products made from milk that retain some or most of their calcium content after processing. In addition to calcium, many dairy foods are excellent sources of protein, phosphorus and potassium (minerals), and the vitamins A and D (if fortified), and riboflavin. Foods made from soybeans (for example, soy "milks") can substitute for cow's milk, if they are fortified with calcium and other micronutrients.

Ice cream, pudding, and frozen yogurt are often grouped with dairy foods, even though they often have high added-sugar and fat contents. Although cream cheese, cream, and butter are made from milk, they aren't included in this group because they have high amounts of fat and little or no calcium.

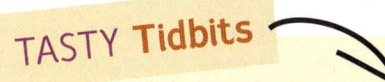
TASTY Tidbits

A serving of whole milk is about 3.25% fat by weight. Obviously, "2% milk" is 2% fat by weight. Low-fat milk contains only 1% fat by weight and is often called "1% milk." Most dietary guides recommend choosing dairy products that have most of the fat removed, such as low-fat milk or *fat-free* (nonfat or skim milk), which has less than 0.5% fat.

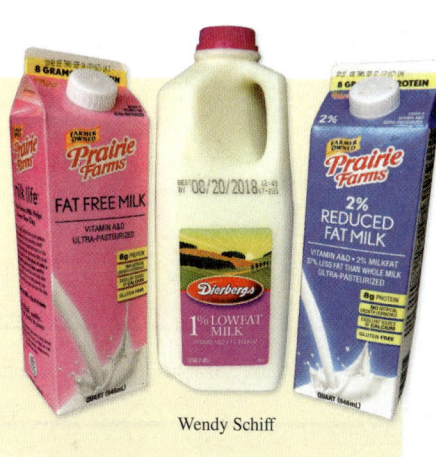
Wendy Schiff

Protein Foods

Protein-rich foods include beef, pork, lamb, fish, shellfish, liver, and poultry. Beans, eggs, nuts, tofu, and seeds are included with this group because these protein-rich foods can substitute for meats. In addition to protein, foods in this group are rich sources of many micronutrients, especially iron, zinc, and B vitamins.

In general, the body absorbs minerals, such as iron and zinc, more easily from animal foods than from plants. However, animal foods, especially red meats, often contain a lot of unhealthy kinds of fat. Diets that supply high amounts of unhealthy fat are associated with increased risk of heart and blood vessel diseases.

TASTY Tidbits

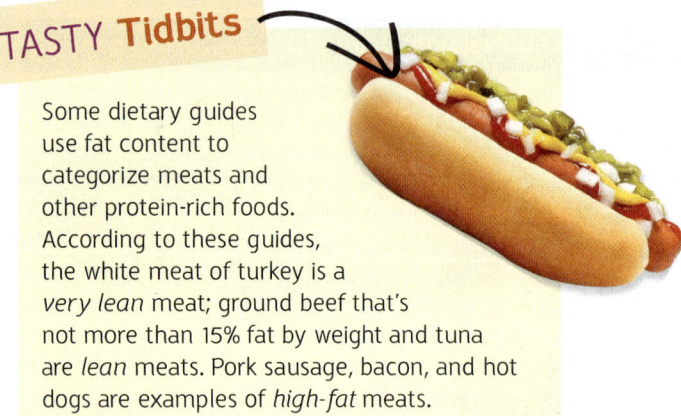

Some dietary guides use fat content to categorize meats and other protein-rich foods. According to these guides, the white meat of turkey is a *very lean* meat; ground beef that's not more than 15% fat by weight and tuna are *lean* meats. Pork sausage, bacon, and hot dogs are examples of *high-fat* meats.

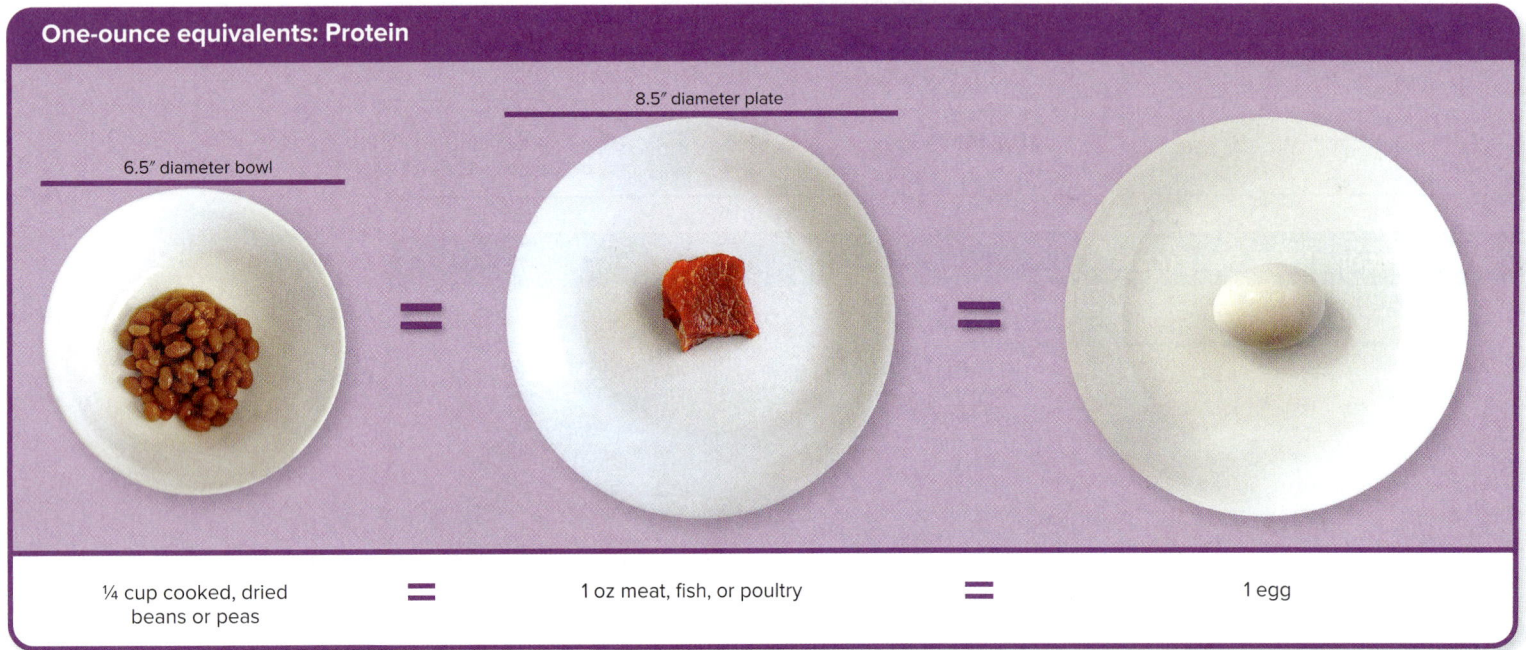

One-ounce equivalents: Protein

¼ cup cooked, dried beans or peas = 1 oz meat, fish, or poultry = 1 egg

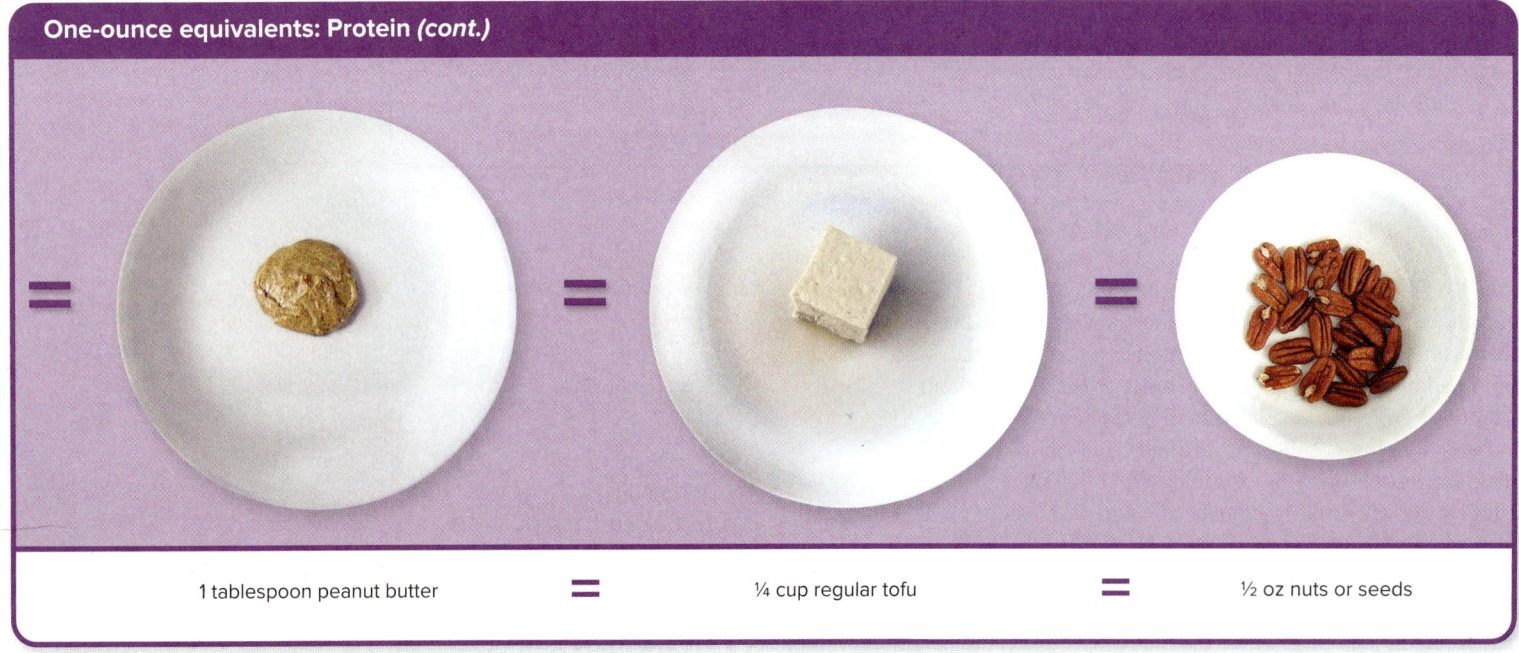

One-ounce equivalents: Protein *(cont.)*

= 1 tablespoon peanut butter = ¼ cup regular tofu = ½ oz nuts or seeds

Hot dog: Lauri Patterson/E+/Getty Images; Protein foods: Wendy Schiff

Fruits

Fruits include fresh, dried, frozen, sauced, and canned fruit, as well as 100% fruit juice.[7] Although fruits aren't good sources of protein, most fruits are low in fat and good sources of phytochemicals and micronutrients, especially the mineral potassium and vitamins C and folate. Although 100% juice can count toward your fruit intake, the majority of your choices from this group should be whole or cut-up fruits.[8] Why? Whole or cut-up fruits are healthier options than juices because they contain more fiber.

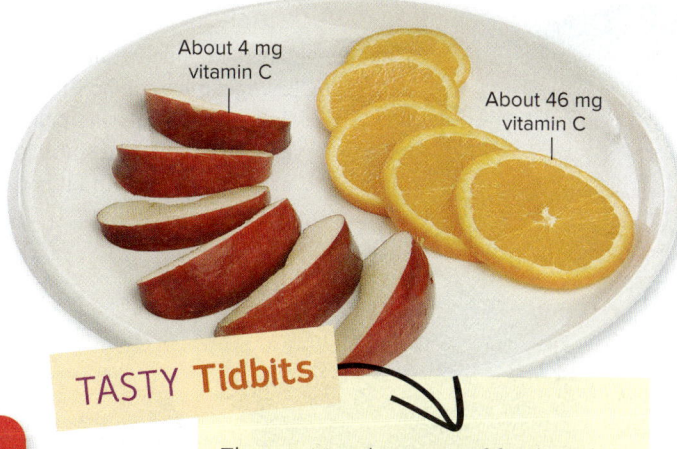

TASTY Tidbits

The nutritional content of foods within each group often varies widely. For example, 3.5 ounces of fresh sliced apples and 3.5 ounces of fresh orange slices each supplies about 50 kcal. However, the apples contribute about 4 mg of vitamin C, whereas oranges supply about 46 mg of the vitamin to diets. That's why you should eat a variety of foods from each food group.

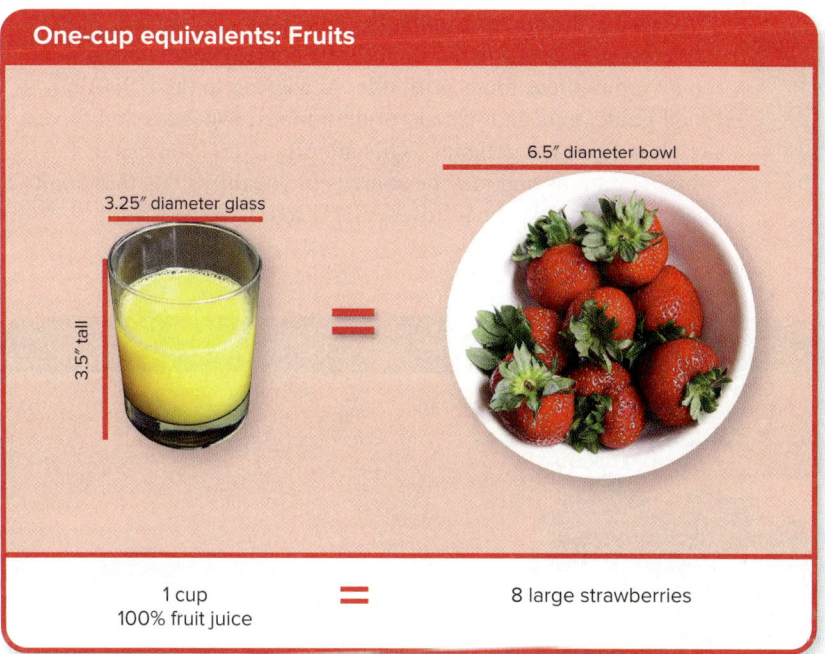

One-cup equivalents: Fruits

1 cup 100% fruit juice = 8 large strawberries

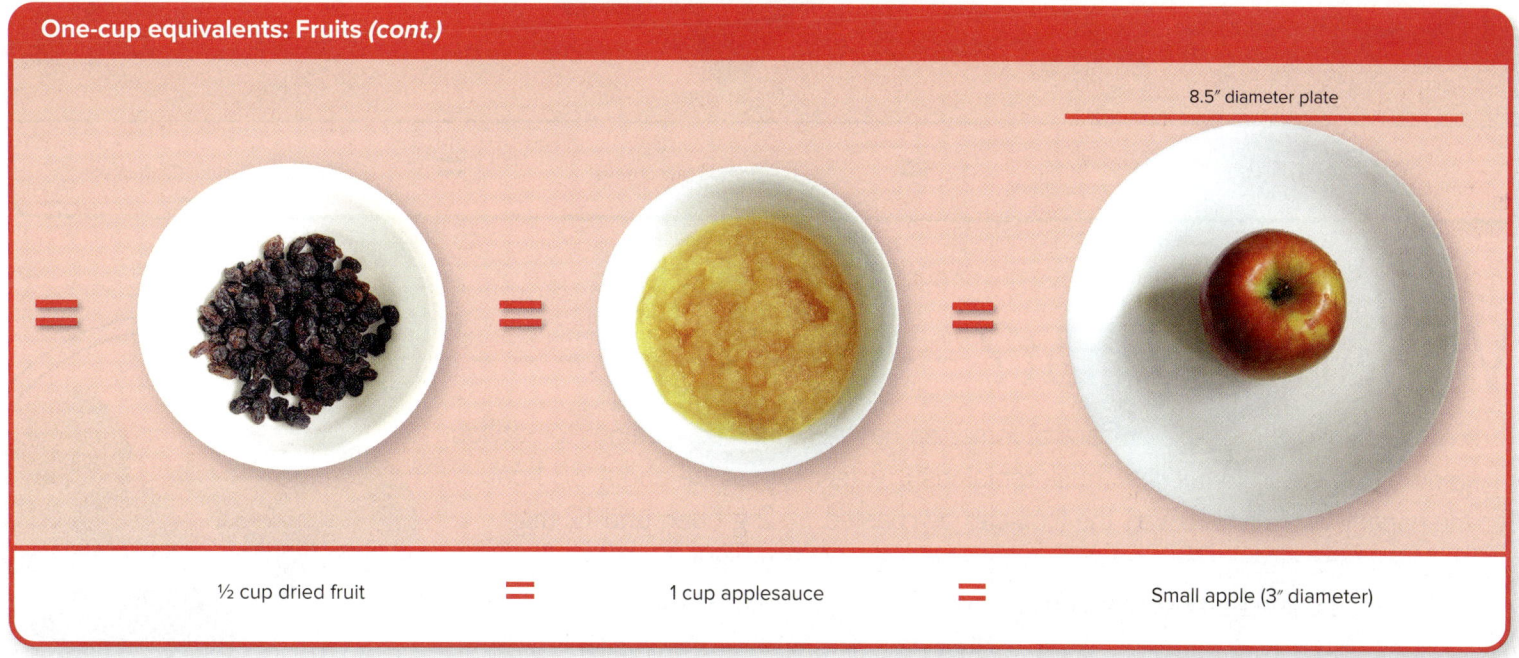

One-cup equivalents: Fruits *(cont.)*

= ½ cup dried fruit = 1 cup applesauce = Small apple (3" diameter)

Fruit plate: Christopher Kerrigan/McGraw-Hill Education; Fruits: Wendy Schiff

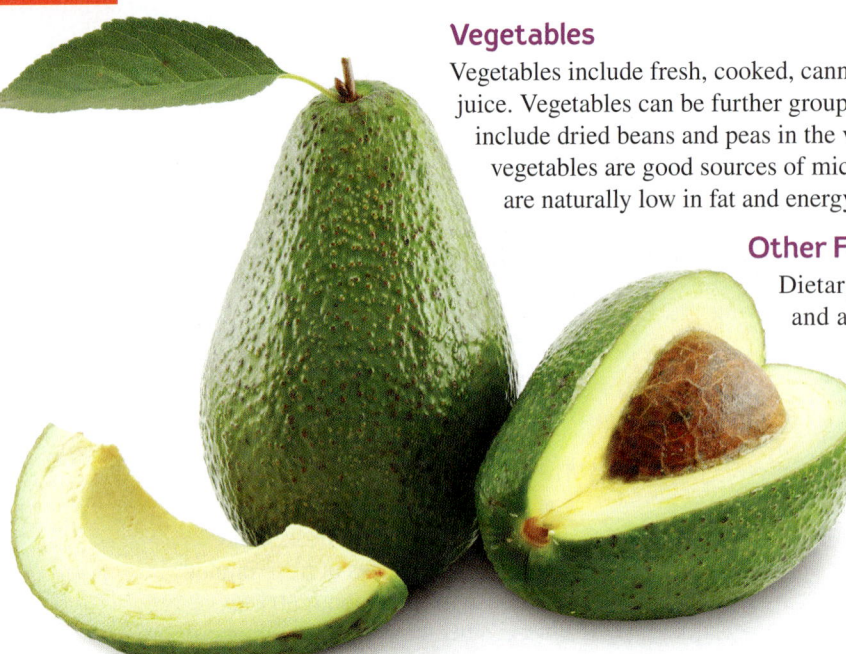

Vegetables

Vegetables include fresh, cooked, canned, frozen, and dried/dehydrated vegetables, and 100% vegetable juice. Vegetables can be further grouped into dark green, orange, and starchy categories. Some guides include dried beans and peas in the vegetable group as well as in the protein foods group. Many vegetables are good sources of micronutrients, fiber, and phytochemicals. Furthermore, most vegetables are naturally low in fat and energy.

Other Foods

Dietary guides, other than the USDA's guide, may include an oils group and a group for sugary foods and alcoholic beverages. Oils include canola, corn, and olive oils, as well as other fats that are liquid at room temperature. Certain spreadable foods made from vegetable oils, such as mayonnaise, margarine, and salad dressing, are also rich sources of oils. Because nuts, olives, avocados, and some types of fish have high fat contents, a dietary guide may group these foods with oils. According to the USDA's food guide, nuts and fish are protein foods; avocados and olives are classified as vegetables.[9] Oils are often good sources of fat-soluble vitamins and may be sources of "healthy" fats that don't increase your risk of cardiovascular disease.

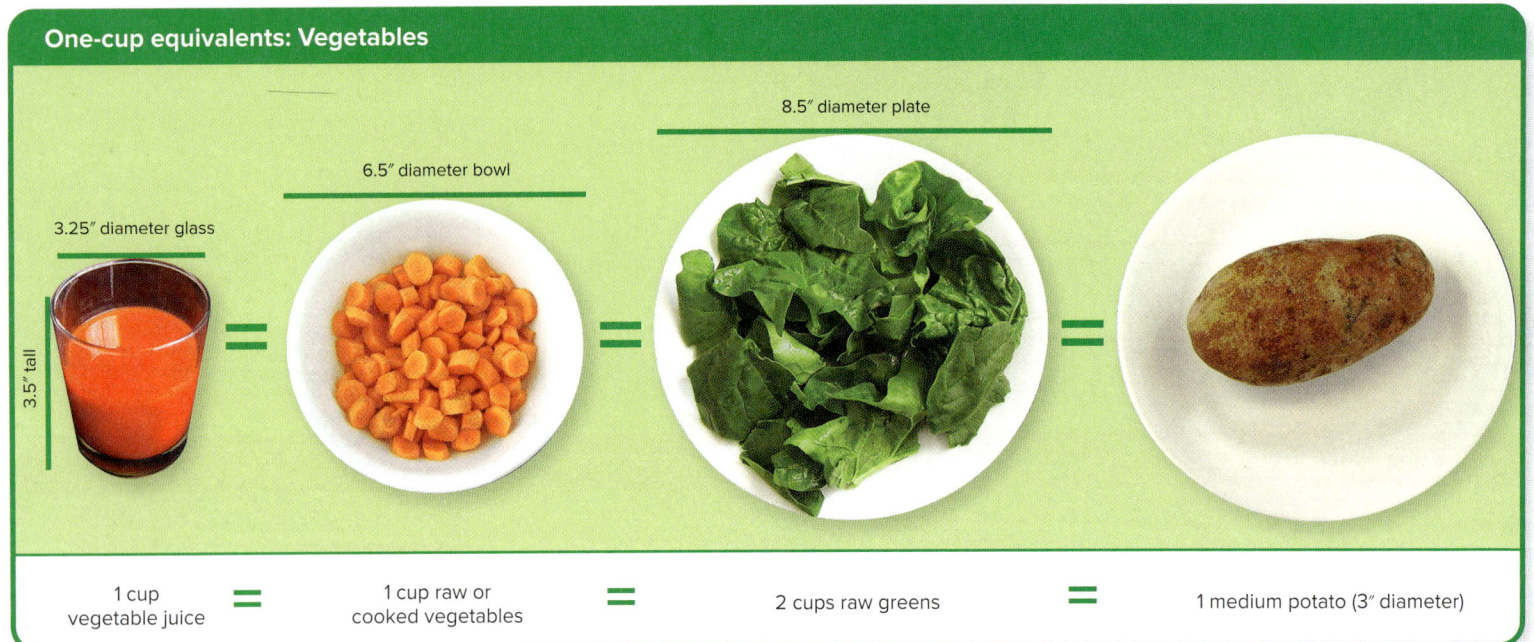

One-cup equivalents: Vegetables

1 cup vegetable juice = 1 cup raw or cooked vegetables = 2 cups raw greens = 1 medium potato (3" diameter)

What IS That?

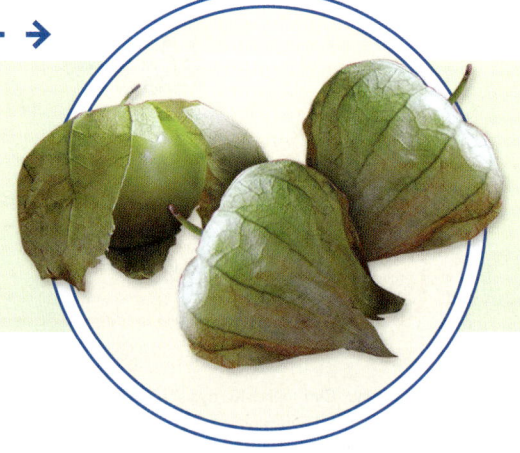

For centuries, the people of Central America have grown and eaten *tomatillos* ("husk-tomatoes"). After the papery husk is removed, the fruit can be roasted, chopped, and mixed with ground chili peppers to form sauces, such as *salsa verde* (green sauce).

Three medium tomatillos provide about 33 kcal, 2 g fiber, and 12 mg vitamin C.

Avocado: ZoonarShullye Serhi/age fotostock; Vegetables, Tomatillos: Wendy Schiff

Nutrition Fact or Fiction?

Organic foods are more nutritious than conventional foods.

The production of **organic foods** involves "environmentally friendly" (sustainable) farming methods that don't rely on the use of antibiotics, hormones (*chemical messengers*), synthetic fertilizers and pesticides, genetic improvements, or ionizing radiation.[10] Results of scientific studies generally don't indicate that organic food crops are more nutritious than conventionally grown food crops.[11] However, eating organic food may reduce your exposure to pesticide residues and antibiotic-resistant bacteria.[11] To learn about organic farming methods and organic food standards, visit the USDA's website (www.usda.gov) and under "Topics," search for "Organic."

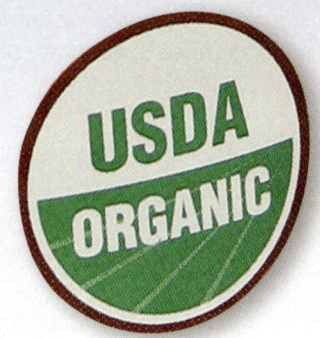

Solid fats, such as beef fat, butter, lard (pork fat), and shortening, are fairly hard at room temperature. Solid fats contain unhealthy types of fats that may increase your risk of cardiovascular disease. Cream, cream cheese, and sour cream are liquid or soft at room temperature, but these foods are usually classified as solid fats. Unit 6 discusses how dietary fats can affect health.

Sugary foods ("sweets") contain high amounts of sugar added during processing. Sugary foods and alcoholic beverages are sources of empty calories that supply few or no micronutrients in relation to their energy content.[12, 13]

Rich Sources of Empty Calories Many commonly eaten foods and beverages contain lots of empty calories. Such foods and beverages include

- candy, cakes, cookies, pastries, and doughnuts;
- sugar-sweetened soft drinks and sports, energy, and fruit drinks;
- cheese (source of solid fat);
- pizza (source of solid fat); and
- ice cream.

3.2b How Do I Classify Combination Foods?

How do you classify menu items that combine small amounts of foods from more than one food group, such as pizza, sandwiches, and casseroles? The first step is to determine the ingredients and classify each into an appropriate food group. A slice of pizza, for example, has a crust made with wheat flour (grains), which is topped with tomato sauce (vegetable) and cheese (dairy). Estimate the number of cups or ounces of each ingredient and record the amounts contributed from a particular food group. The slice of pizza may provide ¼ cup of a vegetable, 2 ounces of grains, and ¼ cup of dairy. The familiar items in **Figure 3.4** can help you judge serving sizes without keeping handy a set of measuring cups and a scale for weighing foods.

— Grain group
— Vegetable group
— Dairy group

Wendy Schiff

organic foods foods produced without the use of antibiotics, hormones, synthetic fertilizers and pesticides, genetic improvements, or ionizing radiation

Figure 3.4 You can use familiar items such as these to estimate serving sizes.

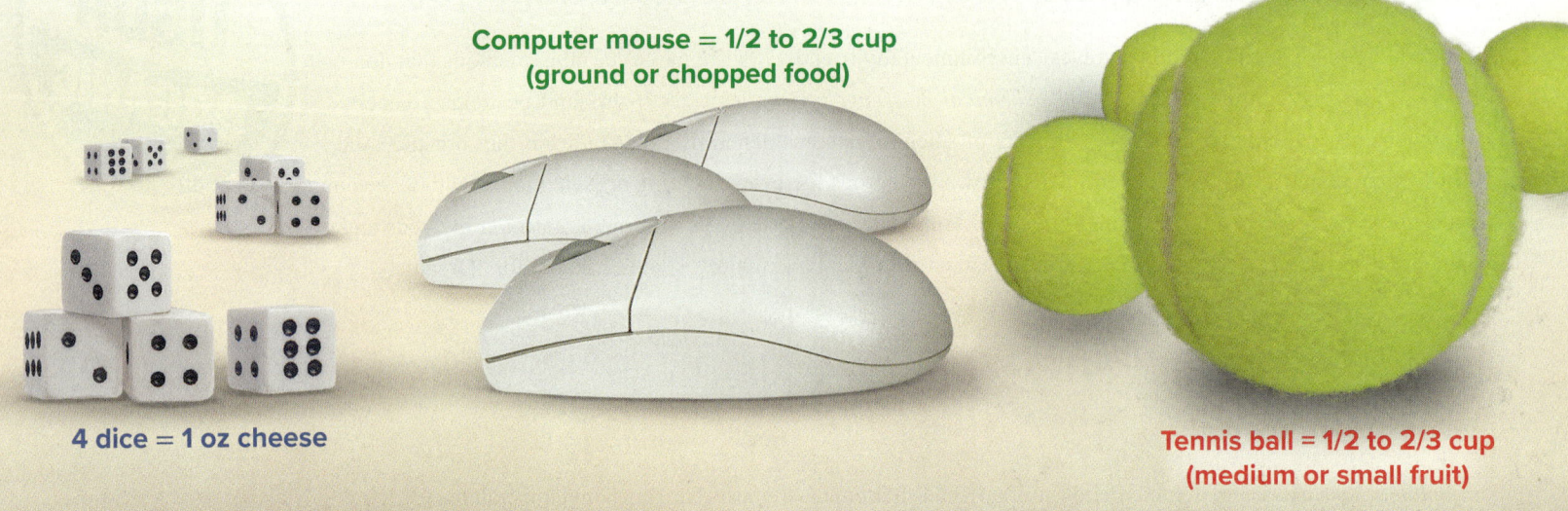

Computer mouse = 1/2 to 2/3 cup (ground or chopped food)

4 dice = 1 oz cheese

Tennis ball = 1/2 to 2/3 cup (medium or small fruit)

3.2c Dietary Guidelines

About 75% of Americans have unhealthy diets. In general, Americans don't eat the recommended amounts of fruits, vegetables, dairy products, and healthy oils. On the other hand, we tend to eat a lot of foods that contain too much added sugars, saturated (unhealthy) fats, and sodium.[14] Such unhealthy food choices can lead to obesity and high blood pressure (hypertension), which are major public health problems among Americans.

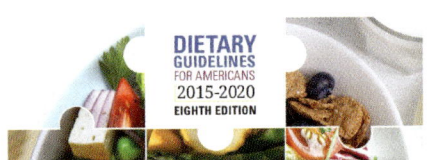

The U.S. Department of Health and Human Services (HHS) and the USDA publish the *Dietary Guidelines for Americans* (Dietary Guidelines), a set of general nutrition-related lifestyle recommendations that are intended for healthy people over 2 years of age.[14] The Dietary Guidelines are designed to promote adequate nutritional status and good health, and to reduce the risk of major nutrition-related, chronic health conditions, such as obesity, high blood pressure (hypertension), and cardiovascular disease.

The most recent version of the guidelines, the *2015–2020 Dietary Guidelines for Americans*, promotes a "healthy eating pattern" and has five overarching general guidelines:

1. Follow a healthy eating pattern across the life span;
2. Focus on variety, nutrient density, and amount;
3. Limit calories from added sugars and saturated fats, and reduce sodium intake;
4. Shift to healthier food and beverage choices; and
5. Support healthy eating patterns for all.

The features of a healthy eating pattern (diet) are listed in **Table 3.2**. The following section provides more specific advice from the 2015–2020 Dietary Guidelines. These guidelines are updated about every 5 years, so a new version should be available by 2021.

TABLE 3.2 HEALTHY EATING PATTERNS

According to the Dietary Guidelines, a healthy eating pattern provides

- A variety of vegetables;
- A variety of fruit, especially whole fruit;
- Grains, especially whole grains;
- Fat-free or low-fat dairy products;
- Various protein foods; and
- Oils.

According to the Dietary Guidelines, a healthy eating pattern limits

- Unhealthy fats, added sugars, and sodium.

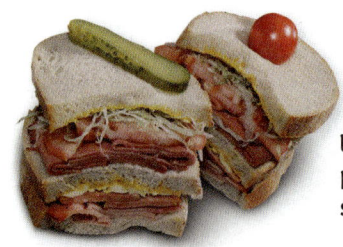

Deli meats and dill pickles are high in sodium.

Dice: Christopher Kerrigan/McGraw-Hill Education; Computer mice: Amos Morgan/Getty Images; Tennis balls: Wendy Schiff; Cover of Dietary Guidelines: Source: U.S. Dept. of Agriculture; Sandwich: Purestock/SuperStock

Planning Nutritious Meals and Snacks   53

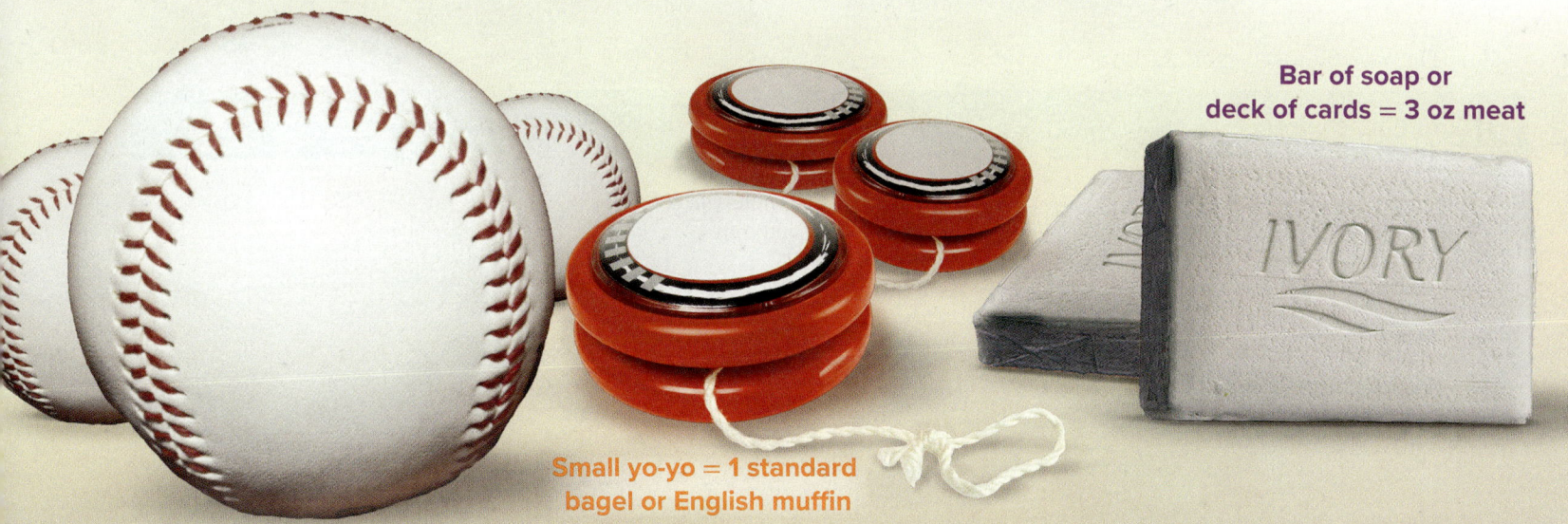

Baseball or human fist = 1 cup (large apple or orange, or 1-cup serving of ready-to-eat cereal)

Bar of soap or deck of cards = 3 oz meat

Small yo-yo = 1 standard bagel or English muffin

Key Recommendations of the 2015–2020 Dietary Guidelines

- Increase the variety of protein foods you consume, and each week, incorporate about 8 ounces of various seafood into your meals. Avoid eating tile fish, shark, swordfish, and king mackerel because they may contain high amounts of the toxic substance methylmercury.
- Increase your intake of nutrient-dense vegetables.
- Eat more nutrient-dense fruits for snacks, for desserts, or in side dishes.
- Choose enriched grain products and make at least half of your grains whole grains.
- Consume fat-free or lower-fat versions of milk, yogurt, and cheese.
- Consume less than 10% of daily calories from added sugars. Added sugars contribute calories to foods and beverages, but they lack essential nutrients. For people consuming 2000 kcal per day, the upper limit of 10% of total calories is 200 kcal, the amount of energy in about 12 teaspoons of sugar.
- Consume less than 10% of daily calories from saturated fats. Solid fats, fatty red meats, and whole-fat dairy products are generally rich sources of saturated fat.
- Consume less than 2300 mg of sodium per day. Eating too much sodium may increase your risk of high blood pressure (hypertension) and heart disease. Sodium is a mineral that's in table salt. Processed foods and fast foods (chips and French fries, for example) supply most of the salt in Americans' diets.
- Choose foods that provide potassium, dietary fiber, calcium, and vitamin D, which are "nutrients of public health concern" because Americans tend to consume them in limited amounts. Iron is an additional nutrient of public health concern for pregnant women.
- Achieve or maintain a healthy body weight. Increasing your physical activity level can help support this recommendation.
- Use vegetable oils when preparing foods. Consume as little trans fat and cholesterol as possible while following a healthy diet.
- If you consume alcohol, the beverage should be consumed in moderation and only if you are of legal drinking age. "Moderation" is up to one drink per day for women and up to two drinks per day for men. If you don't drink alcohol, you shouldn't start drinking for any reason. Furthermore, certain individuals, including pregnant women, should not consume any alcohol.

TASTY Tidbits

Many kinds of fruit make quick and easy snacks that can be carried in knapsacks, purses, and briefcases. Fresh fruit such as apples, oranges, tangerines, kiwifruit, and grapes can be kept for a few days at room temperature in a fruit bowl. You can store fresh fruits for longer periods by placing them in the refrigerator. Banana peels, however, turn dark brown when the fruit's refrigerated, but the fruit is still good to eat.

Baseballs: Ryan McVay/Getty Images; Yo-yos: Stockdisc/Getty Images; Ivory soap: Christopher Kerrigan/McGraw-Hill Education; Salt shaker: C Squared Studios/Getty Images; Bowl of fruit: Wendy Schiff

Unit 3 Making More Nutritious Choices

Applying the Dietary Guidelines

Table 3.3 provides some ways to incorporate the Dietary Guidelines into your diet.

TABLE 3.3 THE DIETARY GUIDELINES IN ACTION

If You Usually Eat:	Consider Replacing with:
White bread and buns	Whole-wheat bread and rolls
Sugary ready-to-eat cereals	High-fiber cereal sweetened with fruit
Cheeseburger, French fries, and a regular soft drink	Roasted chicken or turkey sandwich, baked beans, and fat-free milk or soy milk
Potato salad or coleslaw	Leafy greens salad
Sweet rolls, doughnuts, and salty snacks	Small bran muffin, bagel topped with peanut butter and raisins, or unsalted sweet potato chips
Regular soft drinks, whole milk	Water, fat-free or low-fat milk, or 100% fruit juice
Fatty meats such as bacon, sausage, and hot dogs	Chicken, turkey, or fish; lean meats such as ground round
Chocolate chip, iced, or cream-filled cookies	Oatmeal cookies or fresh fruit

Hamburger bun: Alamy Stock Photo; Sugary cereal: Sean Justice/Corbis; Cheeseburger, French fries, soft drink: Boarding1Now/Getty Images; Potato salad, Cole slaw, Doughnut, Chips in bowl, Whole milk in large glass, Fatty meats, Iced cookie, Cereal with berries, Leafy greens salad, Bran muffin, Bagel topped with peanut butter, Sweet potato chips, Fat-free milk, Roast chicken, Oatmeal cookie: Wendy Schiff; Cinnamon bun: Brian Hagiwar/Getty Images; Soft drink: M. Unal Ozmen/Shutterstock; Chocolate chip cookie: Purestock/Getty Images; Slice of bread: Ingram Publishing; Turkey panini: Ingram Publishing/SuperStock; Water: 81a/age fotostock; Orange juice: Stockbyte/Getty Images; Apples: Purestock/SuperStock

3.2d MyPlate

In 2011, the USDA introduced **MyPlate.** MyPlate is an online dietary and menu planning guide that has some interactive features. MyPlate focuses on five different food groups: fruits, vegetables, protein foods, grains, and dairy (**Fig. 3.5**).[5] According to the USDA, "oils" isn't a food group, even though they provide some essential nutrients.[9] The government agency, however, notes the need for some fat in the diet, especially oils.

To learn more about MyPlate's five food groups, visit the "ChooseMyPlate.gov" website (www.choosemyplate.gov/). Under "Eat Healthy" on the menu bar, click on "What is MyPlate?" to obtain a list of food groups. Then click on each food group for practical information about foods in the group, including dietary patterns (how much of the food should be eaten), major nutrients, scientifically supported health benefits of the food, and helpful food-related tips. ChooseMyPlate.gov also includes a variety of other food and nutrition resources for consumers, such as recipes and quizzes. Furthermore, the website has nutrition information that applies to teens and pregnant women.

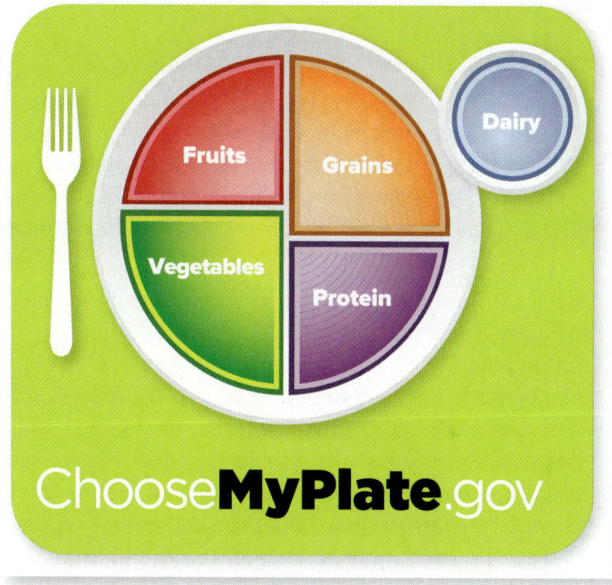

Figure 3.5 MyPlate is the USDA's planning guide.

■ *Which MyPlate food groups are represented in a taco that contains black beans, shredded lettuce, salsa, and cheddar cheese?*

Source: USDA

Using MyPlate

MyPlate has 12 different nutritionally adequate daily food patterns that supply from 1000 to 3200 kcal/day (www.choosemyplate.gov/MyPlatePlan). Each pattern is individualized to meet some of your characteristics, including age, sex, and physical activity level. You can also individualize a daily food pattern so it considers your food likes and dislikes. The dietary patterns generally emphasize nutrient-dense foods and beverages that contain little or no empty calories. The MyPlate Plans also provide upper limits for intakes of sodium, unhealthy fats, and added sugars.

MyPlate can be helpful for planning menus because it promotes food variety, nutritional adequacy, and moderation. You can also use MyPlate to evaluate the nutritional quality of your daily diet by recording your food and beverage choices, classifying your choices into food groups, and estimating your intake of servings from each food group. **Table 3.4** shows suggested amounts of foods for average, healthy, 20-year-old women and men.

MyPlate USDA's dietary and menu planning guide

Other Dietary Guides

Before introducing MyPlate, the USDA promoted a food guide called the "MyPyramid Plan." The MyPyramid Plan inspired the development of other dietary pyramids for people who follow cultural and ethnic food traditions that differ from the mainstream American ("Western") diet. Examples of such guides include the Mediterranean Diet Pyramid (**Fig. 3.6**) and the Asian Diet Pyramid (**Fig. 3.7**).

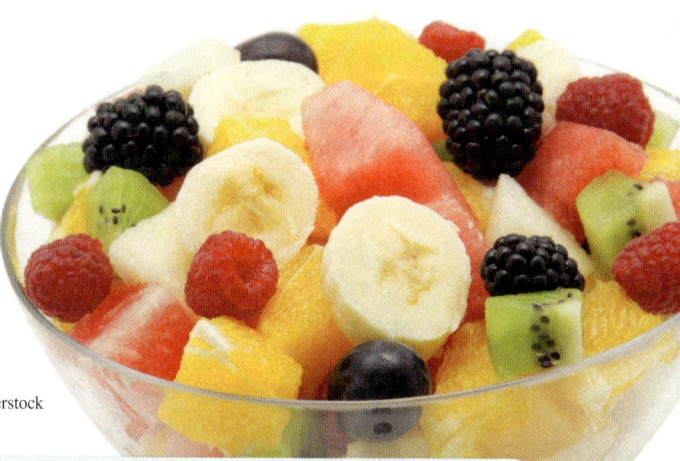

Nataliia K/Shutterstock

"I think my diet is healthier than other college students', because I generally avoid fast foods and cook most of my meals using fresh ingredients. There are several Indian grocery stores in town, so I can buy most of the spices and raw foods that I need. I also enjoy playing sports, especially soccer, so I stay in shape and have fun, too!"

Sachin

Table 3.4 MyPlate: Recommendations for Average, Healthy, 20-Year-Old Women and Men

MyPlate Guidelines (Daily)	Women	Men
Kilocalories	2000–2400	2600–3200
Fruits	2 cups	2–2.5 cups
Vegetables	2.5–3 cups	3.5–4.0 cups
Grains	6–8 oz	9–10 oz
Protein	5.5–6.5 oz	6.5–7 oz
Dairy	3 cups	3 cups

Culture & Cuisine

If you like foods that incorporate a variety of spices, you'll love Indian cuisine. Popular Indian dishes are often seasoned with ginger, cloves, cardamom, fresh curry leaves, cumin, coriander, turmeric, and garlic. The outcome is an amazing array of flavorful food combinations.

India is a huge country made up of various regions and cultures. Each region is known for particular foods and food preparation methods. Main meals, however, generally feature a spicy sauce (*curry*) made with vegetables, such as potatoes, chickpeas, lentils, and beans. Curry may be served on rice or used as a dip for flatbread. Main meals often include a starchy food such as basmati rice or flatbreads (naan or roti, for example); vegetables; and *chutney*. Chutney is a type of condiment that's made with fresh, chopped cilantro or mint with green chilies and a little lemon.

The majority of Indians are followers of the Hindu religion, which regards cattle as sacred, so the animal cannot be eaten. Many Indians are vegetarians, but some members of the population eat chicken, goat, and lamb. Dairy foods are widely consumed; Indian food preparation typically uses *ghee*, a type of butter, to cook onions and garlic. Plain yogurt may be added to sauces. The most popular dessert is *gulab jamun*, sweet round dumplings that are fried and then soaked in rose- or jasmine-flavored syrup. Milk-based puddings, such as carrot pudding, are also popular.

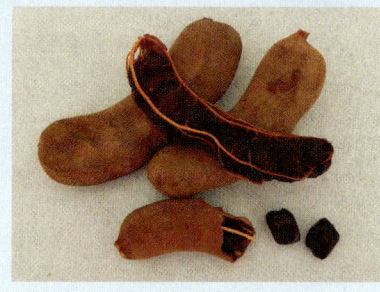

Tamarind pods with some pulp exposed. Note the two hard seeds that were removed from the pulp.

Wendy Schiff

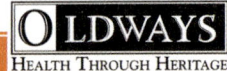
Mediterranean Diet Pyramid

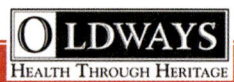
Asian Diet Pyramid

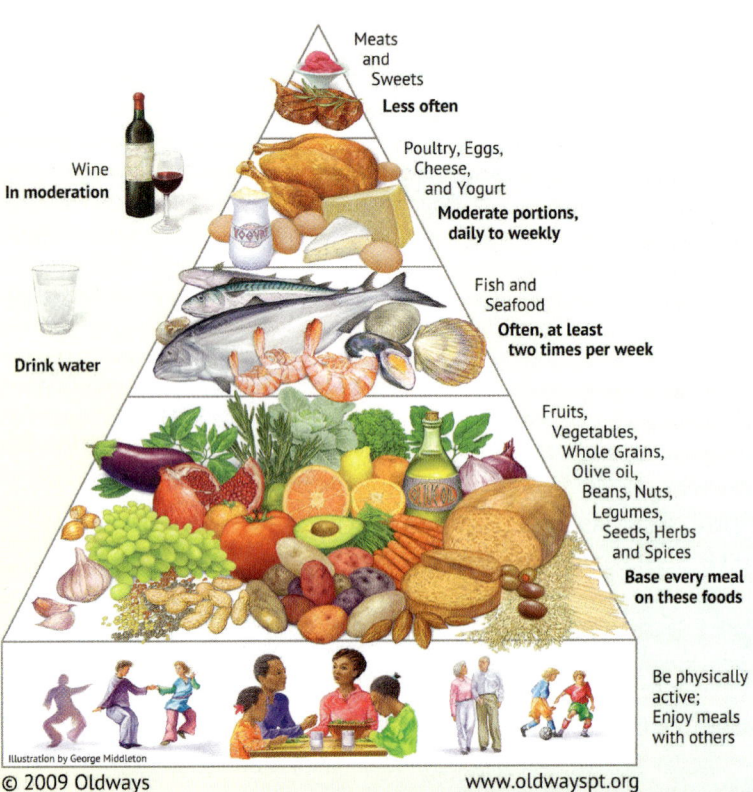

Figure 3.6 The traditional Mediterranean Diet Pyramid.

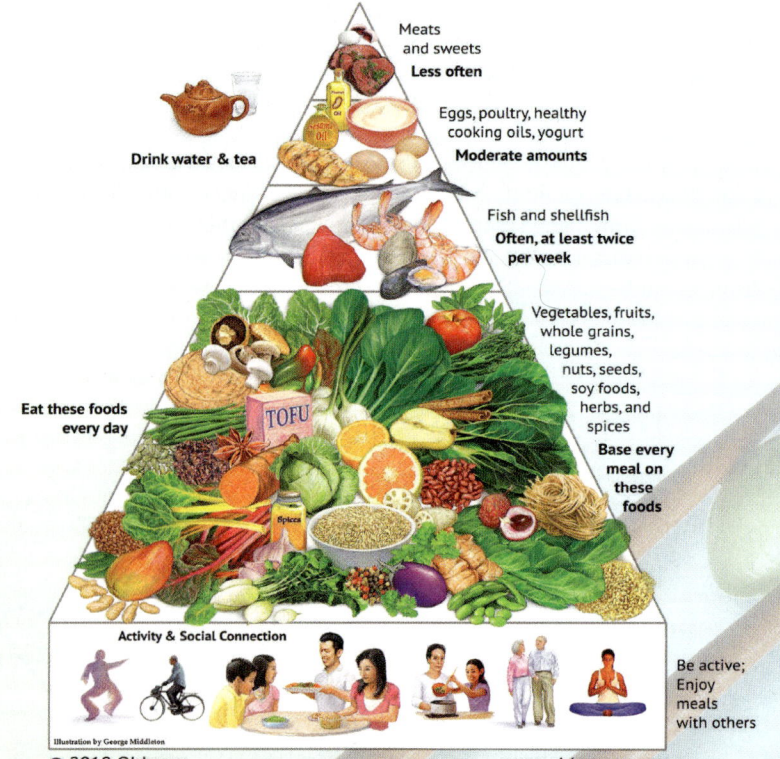

Figure 3.7 The traditional Asian Diet Pyramid.

■ *Which foods form the foundation of the traditional Asian Diet Pyramid?*

Mediterranean Diet Pyramid: 2009 Oldways Preservation & Exchange Trust, oldwayspt.org; Asian Diet Pyramid: 2018 Oldways Preservation & Exchange Trust, oldwayspt.org; Chopsticks with soybean: D. Hurst/Alamy

Module 3.3
Making Sense of Food Labels

3.3 - Learning Outcomes

After reading Module 3.3, you should be able to

1. Define all of the **key terms** in this module.
2. Use the Nutrition Facts panel to make more nutritious food choices.
3. Discuss the FDA's role in regulating food product labels.
4. Identify the types of nutrition-related claims that may be on food labels.

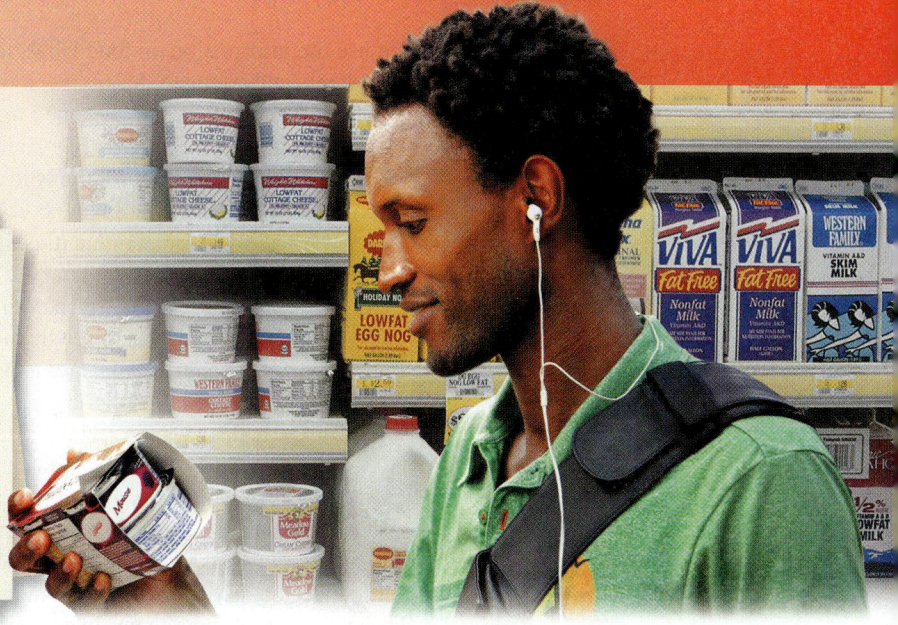

Fuse/Getty Images

3.3a Nutrition Facts

Today, nearly all packaged foods and beverages must have labels that provide the product's name to identify the food. The label should also have the manufacturer's name and address, and the amount of product in the package (**Fig. 3.8a**). In addition to this information, the Food and Drug Administration (FDA) requires food manufacturers to use a special labeling format, the **Nutrition Facts panel,** to display information about the energy and nutrient contents of most packaged foods (**Fig 3.8b**).[15] You

> **Nutrition Facts panel** information on food packaging that indicates nutrition information per serving of the food

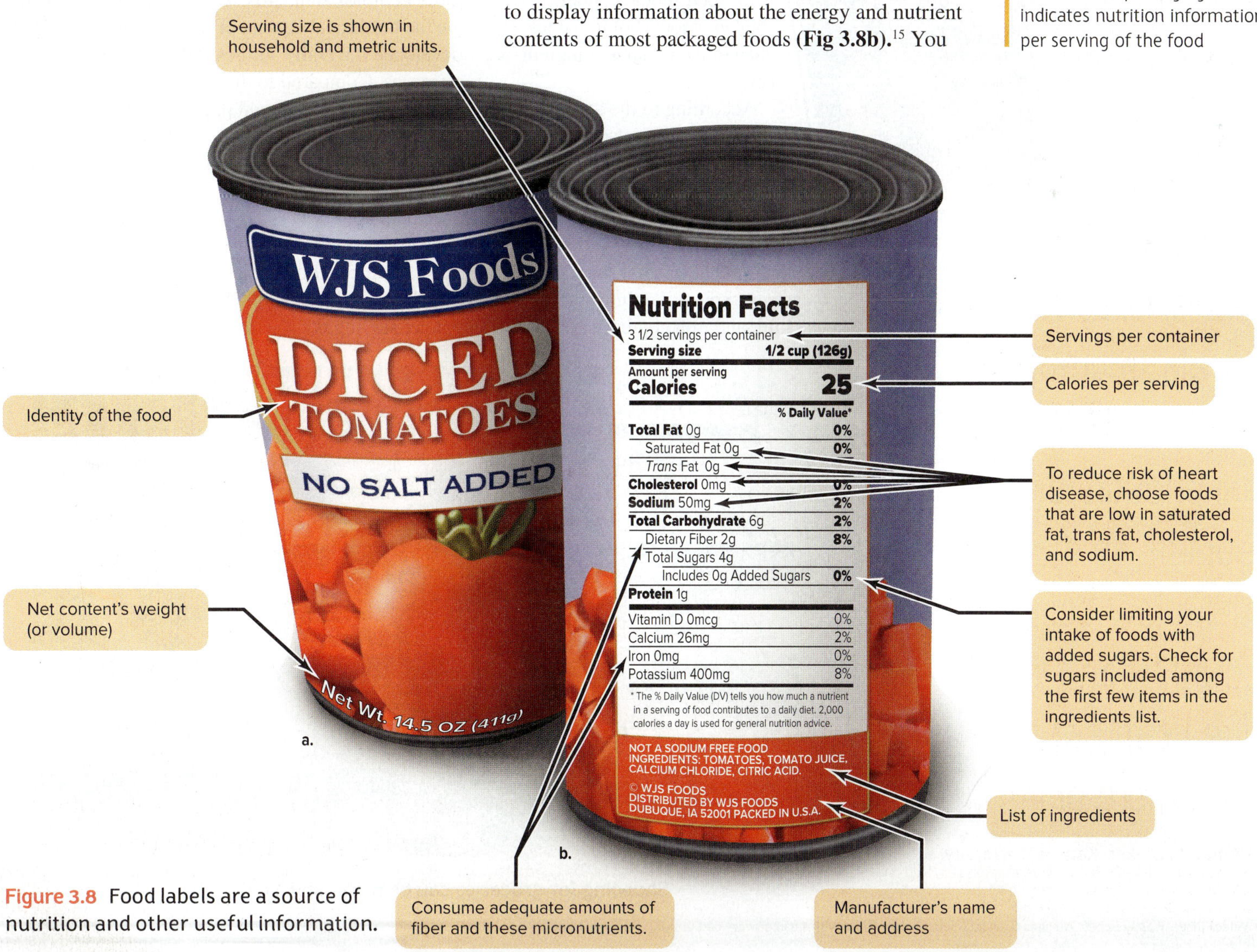

Serving size is shown in household and metric units.

Identity of the food

Net content's weight (or volume)

Servings per container

Calories per serving

To reduce risk of heart disease, choose foods that are low in saturated fat, trans fat, cholesterol, and sodium.

Consider limiting your intake of foods with added sugars. Check for sugars included among the first few items in the ingredients list.

List of ingredients

Consume adequate amounts of fiber and these micronutrients.

Manufacturer's name and address

Figure 3.8 Food labels are a source of nutrition and other useful information.

TASTY Tidbits

Fresh and frozen fruits and vegetables; fresh poultry, fish, and shellfish; and some other food items must declare the product's *country of origin* either on the packaging or where the product is located in stores.

Daily Values (DVs) set of nutrient intake standards developed for labeling purposes

"What is my main source of nutrition information? Food labels. I use food labels to compare products. I need to eat enough food to feel full, so if a food has a low calorie count, then I feel like I can eat a little more of it."

—Amanda Croker, Kansas Univeristy

can use the information on food labels to determine ingredients and compare the energy and nutrient contents of similar packaged food products.

In 2016, the FDA introduced a new format for the Nutrition Facts panel (see Figure 3.8b). Most food manufacturers must use the new format by January 2020.

Until then, you will continue to see the original Nutrition Facts panel on packaged foods. The top of the panel displays the serving size and total amount of energy, indicated as numbers of calories in a serving. The panel uses grams (g) and milligrams (mg) to indicate amounts of nutrients in a serving of food.

Products that have more than one ingredient must display a list of the ingredients in descending order according to weight. Note the list of ingredients displayed under the Nutrition Facts panel on the can of diced tomatoes shown in Figure 3.8b. This particular product has tomatoes as the first ingredient. Thus, this food should contain higher amounts of tomatoes than of the remaining ingredients listed.

According to the new labeling format, the Nutrition Facts panel must provide information about the food's total fat, specific fats (saturated fat and trans fat), cholesterol, sodium, total carbohydrate, fiber, total sugars, added sugars, protein, vitamin D, potassium, calcium, and iron contents. Keep in mind, "total fat" includes amounts of saturated, monounsaturated, polyunsaturated, and trans fats. "Total carbohydrates" includes amounts of fiber, naturally occurring sugars, and added sugars. Recall that fiber, vitamin D, potassium, calcium, and iron are "nutrients of public health concern," according to the Dietary Guidelines for Americans. Food manufacturers can also indicate amounts of other nutrients in their products.

Be careful when using the Nutrition Facts panel; don't assume the information applies to the entire package. For example, the Nutrition Facts panel on a package of food indicates there are four servings in the container. If you eat all the container's contents, you must multiply the information concerning calories, fat, and other food components by four. Why? Because you ate four servings and the nutritional information on the Nutrition Facts panel applies to only *one* serving.

Understanding Daily Values (DVs)

The RDAs and AIs are sex-, age-, and life stage–specific. Therefore, it's not practical to provide nutrient information on food labels that refers to these complex standards. To help consumers evaluate the nutritional content of food products, the FDA developed the **Daily Values (DVs)** for labeling purposes. Compared to the RDAs/AIs, the DVs are a more simplified and practical set of nutrient standards. The adult DV for a nutrient is based on a diet that supplies 2000 kcal/day. Not all nutrients have DVs. For a list of DVs, see **Appendix B.**

Percentages of DVs are designed to help consumers compare nutrient contents of packaged foods to make more healthful choices. The general rule of thumb: A food that supplies 5%DV or less of a nutrient per serving is a *low source* of the nutrient; a food

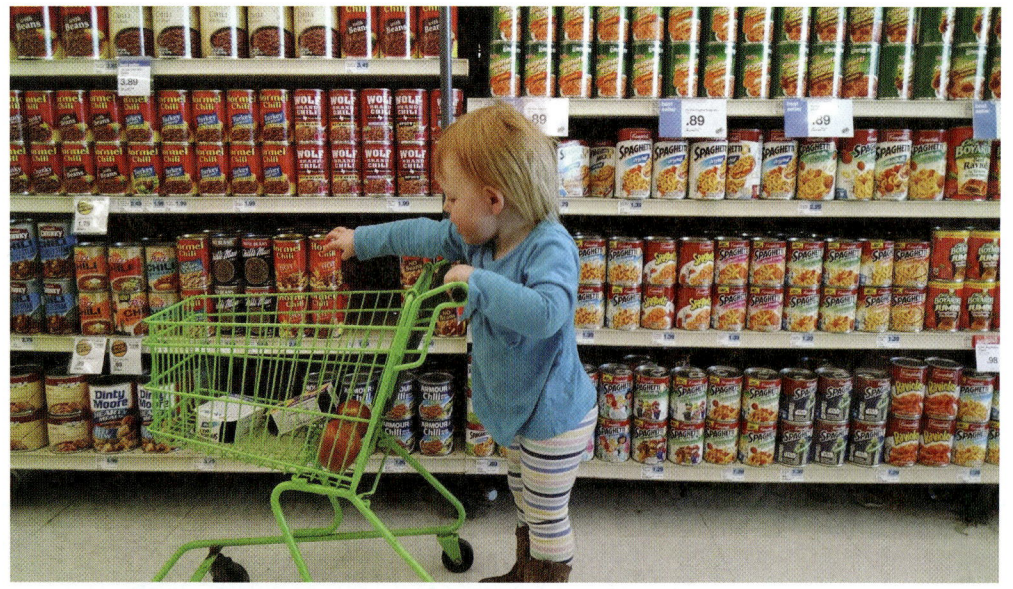

Shopping for groceries can be fun at any age!

Daily Values label: Wendy Schiff; Amanda Croker: Alicia Croker; Child with small grocery cart in store: Darlene Schueller

that provides 20%DV or more per serving is a *high source* of the nutrient.[15]

When evaluating or planning nutritious menus, your goal is to obtain at least 100% of the DVs for fiber, vitamins, and most minerals each day. High intakes of saturated fat, added sugars, and sodium may have negative effects on your health. Thus, you may need to consume *less* than 100% of the DV for these nutrients each day.

Claims on Food Labels To make their foods more appealing to consumers, manufacturers often promote products as having certain health benefits or high amounts of nutrients. In the United States, the FDA regulates much of the information that is on food labels. The FDA permits food manufacturers to include certain *health, structure/function,* and *nutrient content claims* on labels **(Fig. 3.9)**.

- A **health claim** describes the relationship between a food or food ingredient and the reduced risk of a nutrition-related condition. The FDA, for example, allows this health claim: "Adequate calcium as part of a healthful diet, along with physical activity, may reduce the risk of osteoporosis in later life."

- A **structure/function claim** describes the role a nutrient plays in maintaining a structure, such as bone, or promoting a normal function, such as digestion. "Calcium builds strong bones" and "Fiber maintains bowel regularity" are examples of structure/function claims that the FDA allows on food labels.

- A **nutrient content claim** describes levels of nutrients in packaged foods. Such claims can use terms such as "free," "high," or "low" to describe how much of a nutrient is in the product. Additionally, nutrient content claims can use terms such as "more" or "reduced" to compare amounts of nutrients in a product to those in a similar product (*reference food*).

A *light* or lite food has
- at least one-third fewer kilocalories OR half the fat of the reference food.

A reduced-fat food contains
- at least 25% less fat per serving than the reference food.

A low-fat food contains
- 3 g or less fat per serving.

A low-calorie food contains
- 40 kcal or less per serving.

Lean meat or poultry provides
- less than 10 g of fat, 4.5 g or less of saturated fat, and less than 95 mg of cholesterol per serving.

The FDA regulates the use of terms such as "health" and "healthy" on food labels. In general, a serving of food that contains more than 13 g of fat, 4 g of saturated fat, 60 mg of cholesterol, or 480 mg of sodium can't have a health claim on the label.[16] As of July 2018, the FDA was reviewing its definition of a "healthy food."

As of July 2018, the FDA had not developed a standard definition for "natural food." In the past, the agency allowed manufacturers to include the term "natural" on the label if the food didn't contain food coloring agents, synthetic flavors, or other manufactured substances. For the latest information about claims that can be used for labeling purposes, visit the FDA's website at www.fda.gov.

health claim statement that describes relationship between a food or food ingredient and reduced risk of a nutrition-related condition

structure/function claim statement that describes the role a nutrient plays in maintaining a structure of the body or promoting a normal body function

nutrient content claim statement that describes levels of nutrients in a packaged food

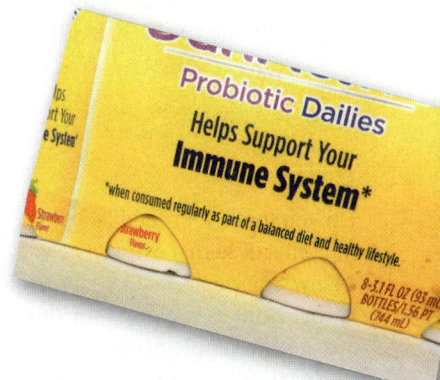

Note the health claim on this food package.

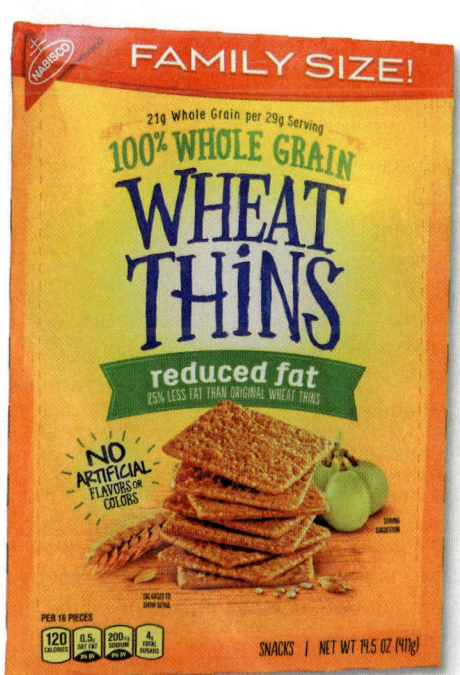

Figure 3.9 Note the claims on this food package.

■ *What kinds of claims are allowed on food labels?*

All: Wendy Schiff

TASTY Tidbits

Often, the only difference between a creamy salad dressing, such as ranch or blue cheese, and the "light" version of the dressing is the amount of water they contain. Instead of paying more for calorie-reduced bottled salad dressings, make your own light salad dressing by adding about ¼ cup water to a jar of regular creamy salad dressing, then stir or shake the mixture.

Module 3.4

Should I Take Dietary Supplements?

3.4 - Learning Outcomes

After reading Module 3.4, you should be able to

1. Define all of the **key terms** in this module.
2. Identify popular dietary supplements and discuss the benefits and risks of taking such products.
3. Identify people who should take specific dietary supplements.

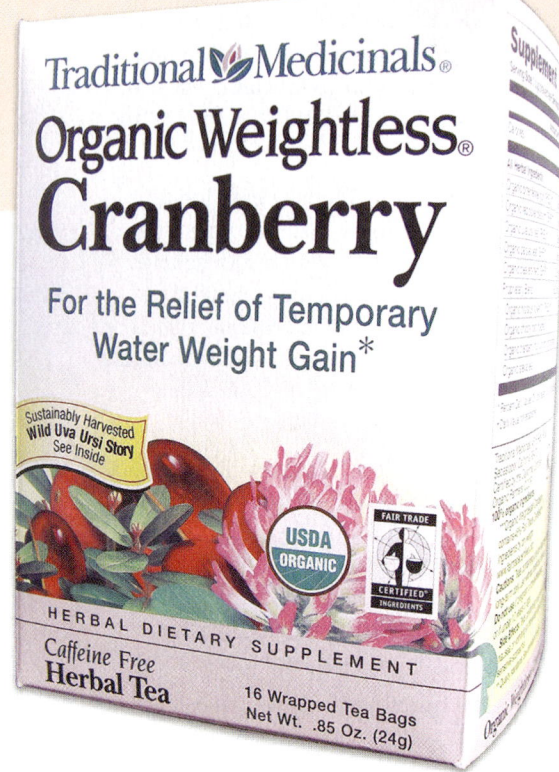

Do you think your food lacks vitamins and minerals? Do you take vitamin pills or herbal extracts because you want to improve your health? Many Americans take dietary supplements such as vitamin pills and herbal extracts because they think they are necessary or helpful. What are dietary supplements?

Recall from Unit 1 that a dietary supplement is a product (excluding tobacco) that's taken by mouth and supplements the diet by increasing total intake.

A dietary supplement can contain

- a vitamin,
- a mineral,
- an herb or other plant product, or
- an amino acid (component of proteins), enzyme, or other dietary ingredient.

The Dietary Supplement Health and Education Act (DSHEA) of 1994 allows manufacturers to classify dietary supplements as a special category of foods. As a result, manufacturers of dietary supplements don't need to test their products for safety and effectiveness. Some dietary supplements, such as vitamins and certain herbs, can have beneficial effects on health. In many instances, there's no scientific evidence that supports the usefulness as well as the safety of nonnutrient dietary supplements, including plant-based products.[17]

The FDA doesn't regulate the production of dietary supplements as strictly as it regulates the manufacturing of over-the-counter and prescription medications. As a result, you can't always be certain of the product's ingredients. Herbal products, for example, have been found to be missing the main ingredient that was listed on the label or contain ingredients that weren't listed on the label. In some instances, the extra ingredients were toxic (poisonous) or caused allergic reactions.

3.4a Popular Dietary Supplements

In the United States, the most commonly used dietary supplements are multivitamin/multimineral (MV/M) products that typically contain several vitamins and minerals.[18] Among American adults, the most popular dietary supplements that don't contain vitamins or minerals are

- fish oil or "omega 3,"
- glucosamine and/or chondroitin,
- probiotics and prebiotics, and
- coenzyme Q_{10} and melatonin.[19]

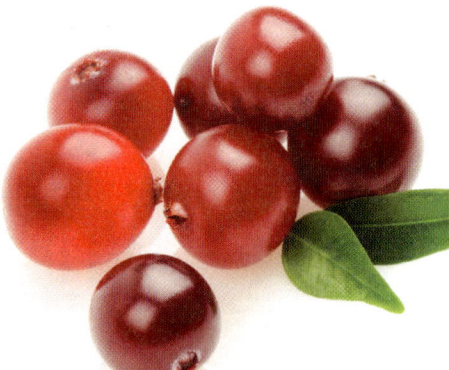

Ripe cranberries

When researchers asked a group of people why they used nonnutrient dietary supplements, the majority of the subjects (85%) reported they used the products to promote wellness; about 40% used the supplements to treat health conditions.[20]

Cranberry tea box: Wendy Schiff; Cranberries: azure1/Shutterstock

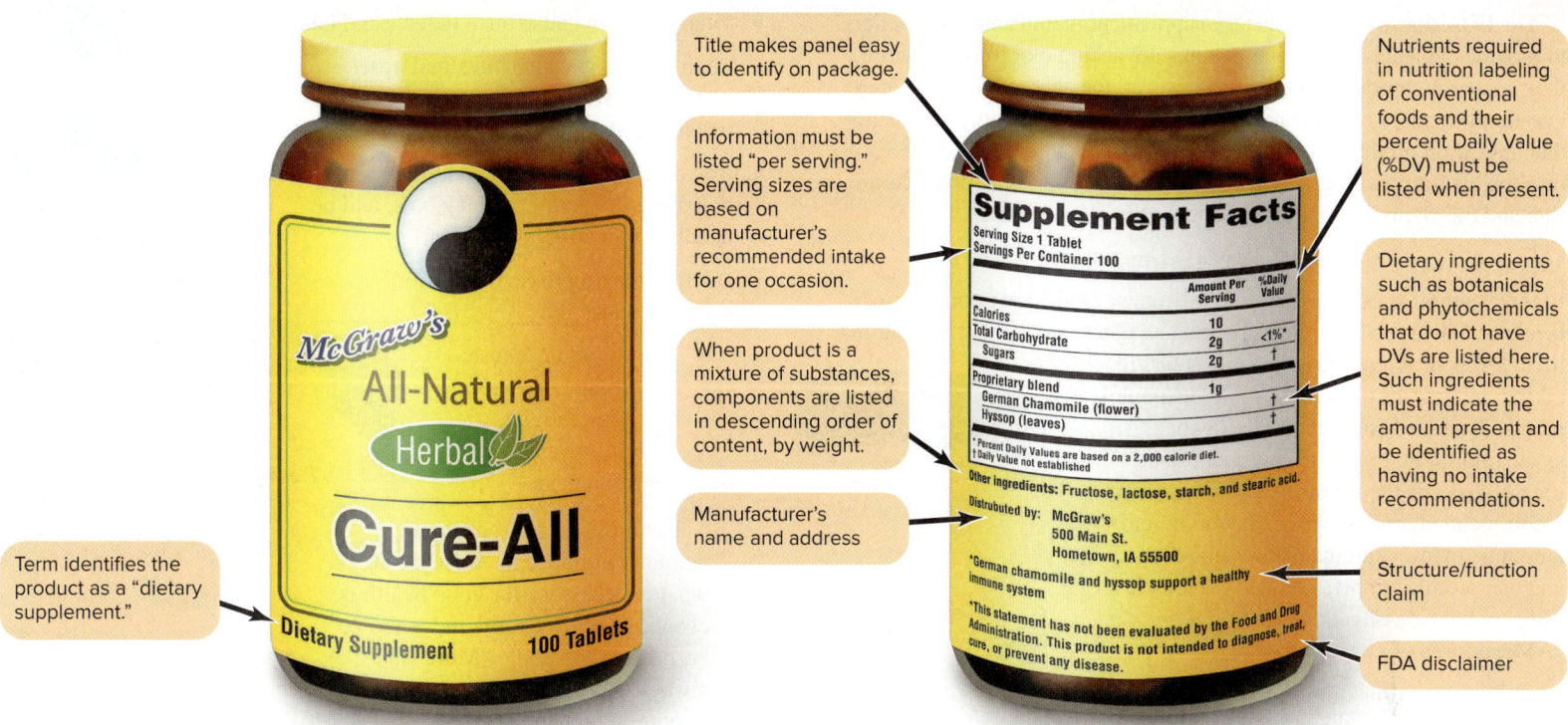

Figure 3.10 Dietary supplement labels must provide information in a specific format.

Dietary Supplement Labels

Every dietary supplement container must be properly labeled (**Fig. 3.10**). The label must include the term "dietary supplement" or a similar term that describes the product's particular ingredient, such as "herbal supplement" or "vitamin C supplement." Furthermore, the label must include facts about the product's contents in a special format—the "Supplement Facts" panel (see Figure 3.10). The panel provides information about the serving size, amount per serving, and percent Daily Value (%DV) for ingredients, if one has been established. Although Daily Values (DVs) are standard desirable or maximum intakes for several nutrients, DVs have not been established for nonnutrient products, such as melatonin and cranberry fruit concentrate.

According to the FDA, dietary supplements aren't intended to treat, diagnose, cure, or alleviate the effects of diseases. Therefore, the agency doesn't permit manufacturers to market a dietary supplement product as a treatment or cure for a disease or to relieve signs or symptoms of a disease. Although such products generally cannot prevent diseases, some can improve health or reduce the risk of certain diseases or conditions. Therefore, the FDA allows supplement manufacturers to display structure/function claims on labels. Manufacturers of iron supplements, for example, may have a claim on the label that states: "Iron is necessary for healthy red blood cell formation." If the FDA has not reviewed a claim, the label must include the FDA's disclaimer indicating that the claim has not been evaluated by the agency (**Fig. 3.11**).

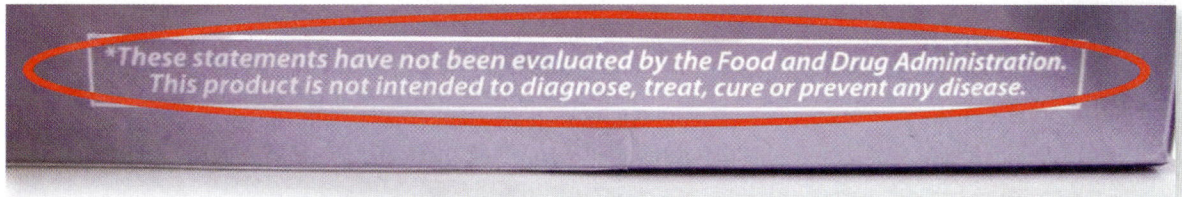

Figure 3.11 Disclaimers can be difficult to read on labels.

■ *Why does the FDA require disclaimers on certain food and dietary supplement package labels?*

Wendy Schiff

The FDA doesn't require dietary supplement manufacturers or sellers to provide evidence that labeling claims are accurate or truthful before they appear on product containers. However, the agency's officials may question the safety of a dietary supplement or the truthfulness of claims that appear on product labels. In such cases, the manufacturers are responsible for providing the FDA with evidence that their products are safe and the claims on labels are honest and not misleading.

Vitamin and Mineral Supplements: Safety

In their natural states, most commonly eaten foods don't contain toxic levels of nutrients. You probably don't need to worry about consuming toxic levels of micronutrients, unless you're taking *megadoses* of vitamin/mineral supplements. A **megadose** is generally defined as an amount of a vitamin or mineral that greatly exceeds the scientifically determined recommended amount. When taken in high amounts, many vitamins behave like drugs and can produce unpleasant and even toxic (poisonous) side effects.

Megadoses of

- B-vitamin niacin may cause facial flushing, itchy skin, and liver damage;
- vitamin B6 can cause nausea, heartburn, and severe nerve damage;
- vitamin C can cause intestinal upset and diarrhea;

megadose generally defined as an amount of a vitamin or mineral that greatly exceeds the recommended amount

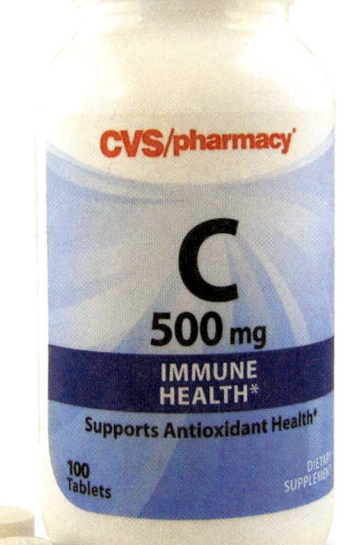

Each of these vitamin C pills provides over 5 times the new DV for the vitamin, which is 90 mg for adults.

- vitamin A can cause birth defects and be deadly;
- vitamin D may cause intestinal upset, weakness, confusion, disorientation, heart rhythm irregularities, and kidney damage;
- iron may cause nausea, vomiting, constipation, diarrhea, and dark-colored stools, and be deadly, especially for children;
- calcium may increase the risk of kidney stones; and
- selenium may cause gastrointestinal upsets, hair loss, fatigue, irritability, and mild nerve damage.

Pennyroyal

For most people, consuming amounts of nutrients that exceed what is necessary for good health is economically wasteful and could be harmful to the body. "More isn't always better," when it relates to optimal nutrition.

Herbal Supplements: Safety

Herbal supplements may be made from plants that have toxic parts. Comfrey, pennyroyal, sassafras, kava, lobelia, and ma huang are among the plants known to be highly toxic or cancer-causing. Products containing material from these plants should be avoided. Herbal teas may contain pollens and other parts of plants that can cause allergies, particularly in people who are sensitive to the herbs or their related species. Some people who take supplements that contain echinacea develop allergic responses that can be severe.[21] Therefore, people who have asthma or allergies should be very careful when using plant-based supplements.

Consumers also need to be aware that medicinal herbs may contain substances that interact with prescription or over-the-counter medications as well as other herbs. Such responses can produce unwanted and even dangerous side effects (see **Table 3.5**). Ginkgo biloba, for example, can interact with aspirin, increasing the risk of bleeding. Garlic and vitamin E supplements can also increase bleeding. Kava and valerian act as sedatives (calming agents) and can amplify the effects of anesthetics used during surgery. Therefore, consult a physician or pharmacist before using any dietary supplement or giving such products to your children. Additionally, treat dietary supplements as drugs: Store them away from children and provide your physicians and other health care professionals with a list of the ones you're taking.

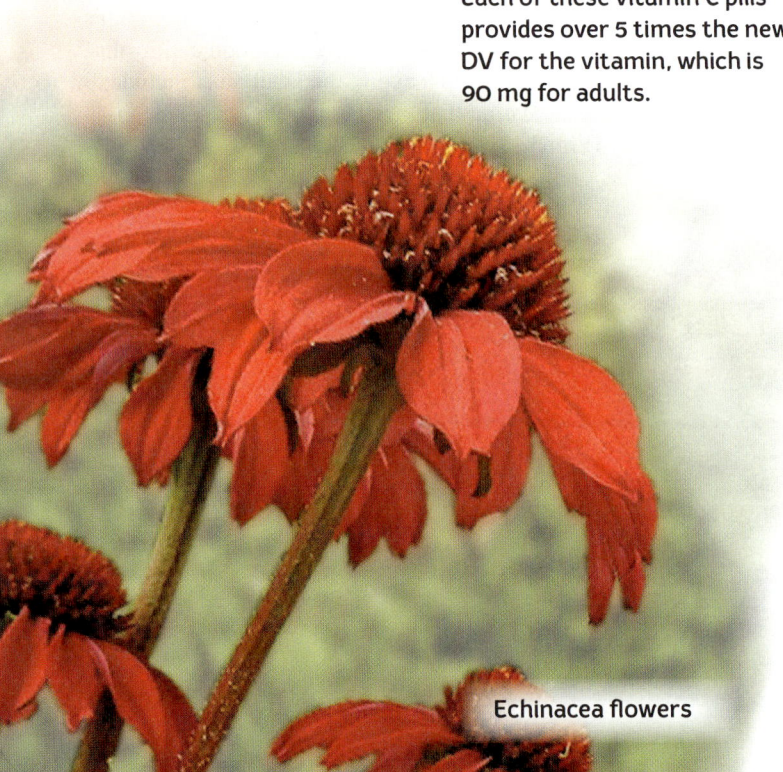

Echinacea flowers

Pennyroyal leaves: Pixtal/AGE Fotostock; Vitamin C bottle, Flowers: Wendy Schiff

3.4b Should You Take Dietary Supplements?

In 2018, sales of dietary supplements were estimated to be $31 billion in the United States.[22] In many instances, however, people don't need dietary supplements, and they are wasting their money by purchasing them—money that could be better spent on natural sources of nutrients and phytochemicals, particularly fruits, vegetables, and whole-grain cereals.

The human body is designed to obtain nutrients and phytochemicals from foods, not supplements. It's important to understand that nutrient supplements don't contain everything you need for optimal health. For example, they don't contain the wide variety of phytochemicals found in plant foods. Furthermore, supplements that contain phytochemicals may not provide the same healthful benefits as those obtained when you consume the plants that contain these substances. Why? Nutrients and phytochemicals may need to be consumed together to provide desirable effects in the body. Food naturally contains combinations of these chemicals in very small amounts and certain proportions. There's nothing "natural" about gulping down handfuls of supplements.

Some people take dietary supplements, particularly those containing nutrients, because the products are recommended by their physicians or registered dietitians. When compared to nonpregnant women, pregnant women require higher amounts of many nutrients. Thus, physicians usually recommend a special MV/M supplement for their pregnant patients. In rare cases, people are born with inherited conditions that increase their requirements for micronutrients. Older adults and people with chronic diseases may also need supplemental vitamins because their bodies don't absorb or use the nutrients normally.

Most dietary supplements are available without the need for prescriptions, so people can take them without their doctors' knowledge and approval. In general, there appears to be little danger in taking an MV/M supplement that provides 100% of recommended amounts of micronutrients daily.[23] However, healthy adults should consider taking such supplements as an "insurance policy" and not a substitute for eating a variety of nutritious foods.

If you use or are thinking about using one or more dietary supplements:

- Discuss your need for the supplement with your physician or a dietitian before you purchase or use the product. This action is particularly important if you're pregnant, are breastfeeding a baby, or have a chronic medical condition such as diabetes or heart disease.

- Consult a physician as soon as you develop signs and symptoms of a serious illness. Using supplements to treat serious diseases instead of seeking conventional medical care that has proven effectiveness is a risky practice. In these instances, delaying or forgoing useful medical treatment may result in the worsening of the condition or even be life threatening.

- Be wary of claims made about a supplement's benefits and investigate the claims used to promote the product. Seek websites that provide reliable information about dietary supplements and aren't in the business of selling the products.

- Determine hazards associated with taking the supplement.

You can find information about the risks and benefits of various dietary supplements at the Office of Dietary Supplements' website: http://ods.od.nih.gov. "Herbs at a Glance," another government-sponsored website, provides a series of fact sheets with information about popular plant-based dietary supplements. These fact sheets can be accessed at: https://nccih.nih.gov/health/herbsataglance.htm. If you experience negative side effects after using a particular dietary supplement, it's a good idea to be examined by a physician immediately. Furthermore, you, as well as your physician, should report the problem to the FDA's MedWatch program by calling (800) FDA-1088 or visiting the agency's website at: www.fda.gov/safety/medwatch/.

TABLE 3.5   Some Popular Dietary Supplements

Dietary Supplement	Major Claims	Known Health Effects* Benefits	Known Health Effects* Risks
Acidophilus (Lactobacillus)	Live bacterial culture (a probiotic) reduces risk of diarrhea and other intestinal problems	May improve health by restoring the balance of beneficial bacteria in the intestinal tract	Likely safe for most healthy people, when taken in appropriate amounts and by mouth
Beta-carotene	Antioxidant; Reduces risk of cancer and heart disease	Source of vitamin A; Antioxidant	High doses can turn skin an orange color and may increase the risk of death from all causes
Chondroitin sulfate	Relieves joint damage associated with arthritis	Conflicting scientific evidence to support health benefit claims; more research is needed; Often combined with glucosamine	When taken by mouth, may cause mild intestinal discomfort, including gas, bloating, and cramps
Coenzyme Q_{10}	Increases exercise tolerance; Prevents heart disease and cancer; Reverses signs of aging and disease	Antioxidant made by the body and involved in energy metabolism; may improve immune system function; Insufficient scientific evidence to support most claims	No serious side effects reported; May interact with certain medications, particularly medications that lower blood cholesterol levels
Echinacea	Boosts immune system; Prevents the common cold and reduces cold symptoms	Mixed scientific evidence to support common cold prevention claims, but research is ongoing	Generally safe but may provoke allergic response or intestinal upset
Evening primrose oil	Treats eczema (a common skin condition); Relieves arthritis and postmenopausal symptoms	Insufficient scientific evidence to support claims	May cause mild intestinal upset; Safety of long-term use has not been determined
Fish oil	Prevents heart disease and stroke; Cures rheumatoid arthritis; Reduces depression and risk of Alzheimer's disease	Source of omega-3 fatty acids; May provide some mild relief for symptoms of rheumatoid arthritis; Lack of evidence that fish oil is beneficial for other health conditions	May interfere with blood clotting, increasing the risk of hemorrhagic stroke; Cod liver oil contains vitamin A, which is toxic when taken in large doses
Flaxseed and flaxseed oil	Acts as a laxative (flaxseed); Reduces blood cholesterol levels	Nonanimal source of omega-3 fatty acids; Seeds have laxative effects; May benefit people with high blood cholesterol levels, but more research is needed	Raw or unripe seeds are toxic; Can cause diarrhea
Garlic	Lowers blood cholesterol levels	Doesn't lower cholesterol consistently; May reduce elevated blood pressure	Can cause allergic reaction and unpleasant body odor; may increase risk of bleeding
Ginger	Treats "morning sickness" and other forms of nausea; Relieves stomach upsets	May help relieve morning sickness and other forms of nausea; Lack of scientific evidence to support other health benefit claims	Mild intestinal discomfort, including heartburn, gas, and diarrhea

Glucosamine: Jill Braaten/McGraw-Hill Education; Pink flower: Wendy Schiff; Yellow evening primrose: Carol Wolfe; Garlic: Photodisc/Getty Images; Flax flowers: Pixtal/SuperStock; Ginger: Stockbyte

Dietary Supplement	Major Claims	Known Health Effects* Benefits	Risks
Ginkgo biloba	Improves memory. Reduces the risk of Alzheimer's disease and other forms of dementia	Lack of scientific evidence to support health benefit claims	May increase the risk of bleeding and cause allergic reactions, headaches, and intestinal upsets. Raw or roasted gingko seeds are toxic
Ginseng (Asian)	Boosts overall health. Treats erectile dysfunction (male impotence) and hepatitis C	Lack of scientific evidence to support health benefit claims	May cause headaches, sleep disturbances, allergic responses, and gastrointestinal upsets. May interfere with regulation of blood glucose and pressure levels, which can be dangerous
Glucosamine hydrochloride	Relieves joint damage associated with arthritis	Some scientific evidence supports health benefit claims, but more research is needed (frequently used with chondroitin)	May interfere with a certain blood-clotting medication
Green tea	Prevents or treats cancer. Promotes weight loss. Reduces blood cholesterol levels	Extracts are not helpful for weight loss. May reduce heart disease risk, but more research is needed. Lack of reliable evidence to support other health benefit claims	Green tea extracts may damage the liver. Caffeine content may cause sleep disturbances, irritability, and digestive upset
Kava	Reduces stress	Potential harm of using kava outweighs any benefit	Toxic—can damage the liver and cause death. May cause heart problems, yellowed skin, and eye irritation
Lavender	Reduces anxiety, treats sleep disorders	Lack of scientific evidence that supports health benefit claims	May be unsafe when used for aromatherapy; lavender oil may be poisonous if consumed
Melatonin	Treats some sleep disorders. Prevents jet lag	May be effective for treating certain sleep disorders and preventing jet lag	Questions about long-term safety
St. John's wort	Reduces depression	Evidence to support claims is inconsistent	May weaken certain medications, including prescription antidepressants and oral contraceptives
Valerian	Promotes relaxation. Treats sleep disorders	Evidence to support claims is inconsistent	Dizziness, headache, stomach upset. Questions about long-term safety

*Sources: www.cancer.gov/about-cancer/treatment/cam/hp/coenzyme-q10-pdq; https://ods.od.nih.gov/factsheets/list-all/; https://nccih.nih.gov/health/glucosaminechondroitin; https://nccih.nih.gov/health/melatonin; https://nccih.nih.gov/health/herbsataglance.htm. Accessed: July 23, 2018.
Ginkgo biloba: Jill Braaten; Chinese herbs, Bottles of herbal medicine: Corbis RF/Alamy Stock Photo; Tea and saucer: Wendy Schiff; Kava kava bottle, Melatonin: Jill Braaten/McGraw-Hill Education; St John's wort: Pixtal/SuperStock; Valerian: Pixtal/AGE Fotostock

In a Nutshell

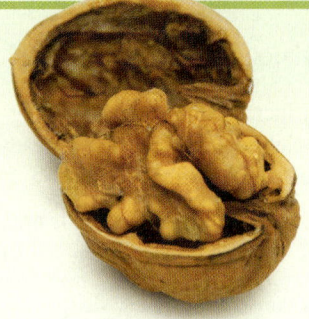

Module 3.1 Requirements and Recommendations

- A requirement is the smallest amount of a nutrient that maintains a defined level of nutritional health. Numerous factors influence your nutrient requirements, including age and state of health. Scientists use information about nutrient requirements and the body's storage capabilities to establish specific dietary recommendations.

- Dietary Reference Intakes (DRIs) encompass a variety of energy and nutrient intake standards that can be used to help people reduce their risk of nutrient deficiencies and excesses, prevent disease, and achieve optimal health. An Estimated Average Requirement (EAR) is the amount of the nutrient that meets the needs of 50% of healthy people in a particular life stage/sex group. The Estimated Energy Requirement (EER) is used to evaluate a person's energy intake. The Recommended Dietary Allowances (RDAs) meet the needs of nearly all healthy individuals (97 to 98%) in a particular life stage/sex group. The RDA or AI for a nutrient is not the same as the requirement for that nutrient.

- When nutrition scientists are unable to determine an RDA for a nutrient, they establish an Adequate Intake (AI) value. The Tolerable Upper Intake Level (UL) is the highest average amount of a nutrient that's unlikely to harm most people when the amount is consumed daily.

- Acceptable Macronutrient Distribution Ranges (AMDRs) indicate ranges of carbohydrate, fat, and protein intakes that provide adequate amounts of vitamins and minerals and may reduce the risk of diet-related chronic diseases.

Module 3.2 Planning Nutritious Meals and Snacks

- Dietary guides generally classify foods into groups according to their natural origins and key nutrients. Such guides usually feature major food groups, including grains, dairy foods, and vegetables. Some dietary guides also include a group for oils.

- The Dietary Guidelines are a set of general nutrition-related lifestyle recommendations designed to promote adequate nutritional status and good health, and to reduce the risk of major chronic health conditions. These guidelines are updated every 5 years.

- The *Dietary Guidelines for Americans* (2015–2020 version) has five overarching concepts. These concepts are follow a healthy eating pattern across the life span; focus on variety, nutrient density, and amount; limit calories from added sugars and saturated fats, and reduce sodium intake; shift to healthier food and beverage choices; and support healthy eating patterns for all.

- ChooseMyPlate.gov is the USDA's online source of food, nutrition, and physical activity information. The MyPlate website can be helpful for planning menus because it promotes food variety, nutritional adequacy, and moderation.

Module 3.3 Making Sense of Food Labels

- Consumers can use information on food labels to determine ingredients and compare nutrient contents of packaged foods and beverages.

- Nearly all foods and beverages sold in supermarkets must be labeled with the product's name, manufacturer's name and address, amount of product in the package, ingredients listed in descending order by weight, and country of origin. Food labels must use a special format for listing specific information on the Nutrition Facts panel.

- The Daily Values (DVs) are a practical set of nutrient standards for labeling purposes. The nutrient content in a serving of food is listed on the label as a percentage of the DV (%DV). Not all nutrients have DVs. A dietary goal is to obtain at least 100% of the DVs for fiber, vitamins, and minerals (except sodium) each day.

- The FDA regulates much of the information that can be placed on food labels. The FDA permits food manufacturers to include certain health, structure/function, and nutrient content claims on food labels.

Wendy Schiff

Module 3.4 Should I Take Dietary Supplements?

- According to the DSHEA, a dietary supplement is a product (excluding tobacco) that is taken by mouth and contains a vitamin, a mineral, an herb or other plant product, an amino acid, or a dietary ingredient that supplements the diet by increasing total intake.

- The FDA regulates the labeling of dietary supplements. According to the FDA, dietary supplements aren't intended to treat, diagnose, cure, or alleviate the effects of diseases. Therefore, the agency doesn't permit manufacturers to market a dietary supplement product as a treatment or cure for a disease, or to relieve signs or symptoms of a disease.

- According to scientific evidence, some dietary supplements can have beneficial effects on health. However, results of scientific testing also indicate that many popular dietary supplements aren't helpful and may even be harmful.

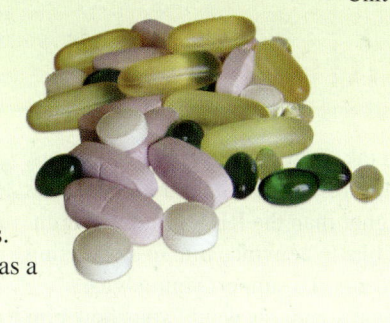

What's in Your Diet?!

I. Record Keeping
   A. 24-Hour Dietary Recall
   1. Recall every food and beverage that you have eaten over the past 24 hours. Recall how much you consumed and how it was prepared.
      a. How easy or difficult was it to recall your food intake?
      b. Recall your intake of nutrient supplements such as vitamin C.
   B. Three-Day Diet Record
   1. Without changing your usual diet, keep a detailed log of your food and beverage intake for 3 days; one of the days should be Friday or Saturday. Use a separate log for each day. Remember to include your daily intake of nutrient supplements in your record.

II. Analysis
Using nutritional analysis software, analyze your daily food and nutrient supplement intakes and answer questions in Part III of this activity. Keep the record on file for future applications.

   A. Computer-Generated Dietary Analysis, such as Nutrition CalcPlus
   1. Load the software into the computer, or log on to the software website.
   2. Choose the DRIs or related nutrient standard from **Appendix E**, based on your life stage, sex, height, and weight.
   3. Enter the information from the 3-day food intake record. Be sure to enter each food and drink and the specific amounts. Enter your intake of nutrient supplements.
   4. The software program will give you the following results:
      a. The appropriate RDA (or related standard) for each nutrient
      b. The total amount of each nutrient and the kilocalories consumed for each day
      c. The percentage intake compared with the standard amount for each nutrient that you consumed each day
   5. Keep this assessment for activities in other units.

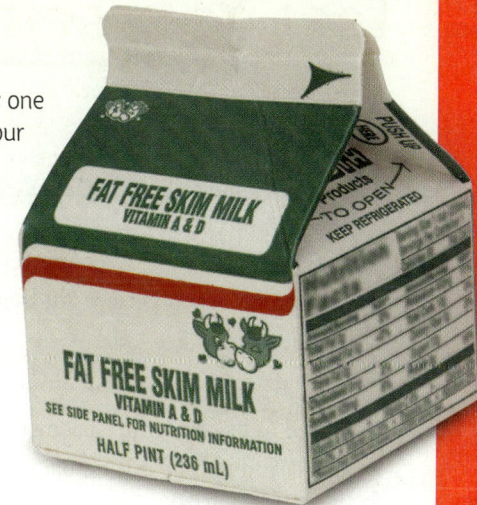

III. Evaluation of Nutrient Intakes
Remember, it is not necessary to consume the maximum of your nutrient recommendations every day. A general standard is meeting at least 70% of the standards averaged over several days. It is best not to exceed the Upper Level (if set) over the long term to avoid potential toxic effects of some nutrients.

   A. For which nutrients did your average intake fall below the recommended amounts—that is, to less than 70% of the RDA/AI?
   B. For which nutrients did your average intake exceed the Upper Level (if a UL has been set)?

IV. MyPlate
This activity determines how your diet stacks up when compared to the amounts of foods from each food group that are recommended in the USDA's www.choosemyplate.gov.

   A. Refer to your 3-day food intake record. Classify each food item in the appropriate food group of MyPlate. For each food group, indicate whether you ate the recommended amount daily for your sex, age, height, weight, and physical activity level. Note that some of your food choices—pizza, for example—may contribute to more than one food group. Enter a minus sign (−) if your total falls below the MyPlate recommendation or a plus sign (+) if it equals or exceeds the daily recommendation for each food group.

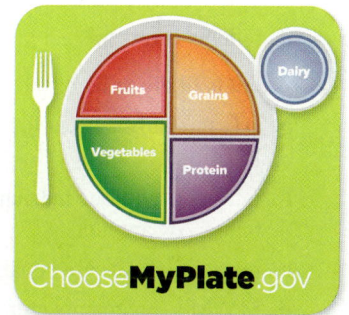

Pills: Wendy Schiff; Milk carton: Mark Steinmetz/McGraw-Hill Education; ChooseMyPlate: Source: USDA

Consider This...

1. Your friend takes several dietary supplements daily and, as a result, his vitamin B-6 intake is 50 times higher than the RDA for the vitamin. You would like to convince him to stop taking the supplements. To support your advice, which nutrient standards would you show him? Explain why.

2. Why should you use MyPlate to plan menus instead of the DRIs?

3. How do your sodium, saturated fat, and added sugar intakes compare to the recommendations of the latest U.S. Dietary Guidelines?

4. How can you determine whether the wheat crackers that are made by a company in England have animal or vegetable fat in them?

5. Visit the USDA's website to access "What's in the Foods You Eat *Search Tool*," a database for searching the nutritional content of foods. To practice using this search tool, find the number of kilocalories and the amounts of fiber, potassium, iron, sodium, and calcium in 1 cup of raw jicama, 1 cup of 2% milk with added vitamin A, and ¼ cup of dry roasted, salt-added sunflower seed kernels (no hulls).

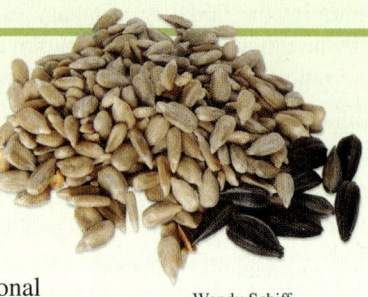
Wendy Schiff

Test Yourself

Select the best answer.

1. The amount of a nutrient that should meet the needs of almost all of the healthy people in a particular group is the
    a. Estimated Average Requirement (EAR).
    b. Recommended Dietary Allowance (RDA).
    c. Adequate Intake (AI).
    d. Tolerable Upper Intake Level (UL).

2. Which of the following statements is false?
    a. RDAs are standards for daily intakes of certain nutrients.
    b. RDAs meet the nutrient needs of nearly all healthy people.
    c. RDAs contain a margin of safety.
    d. RDAs are requirements for nutrients.

3. The Estimated Energy Requirement (EER)
    a. has a margin of safety.
    b. doesn't account for a person's height, weight, or physical activity level.
    c. is based on the average daily energy needs of a healthy person.
    d. reflects a person's actual daily energy needs.

4. A diet is likely to be unsafe if
    a. average daily intakes for nutrients meet RDA or AI values.
    b. intakes of various nutrients are slightly less than EAR amounts.
    c. nutrient intakes are consistently above ULs.
    d. MV/M supplements aren't included.

5. According to MyPlate, which of the following foods is grouped with dairy products?
    a. Eggs
    b. Yogurt
    c. Butter
    d. Sour cream

6. Protein-rich food sources that also contain saturated fat and cholesterol include
    a. cheese.
    b. split peas.
    c. nuts.
    d. ripe bananas.

7. In general, whole fruits are a good source of all of the following substances, except
    a. fiber.
    b. vitamin C.
    c. phytochemicals.
    d. protein.

8. The Nutrition Facts panel on a package of food must display amounts of ___ in a serving of the food.
    a. vitamin D
    b. fluoride
    c. magnesium
    d. vitamin E

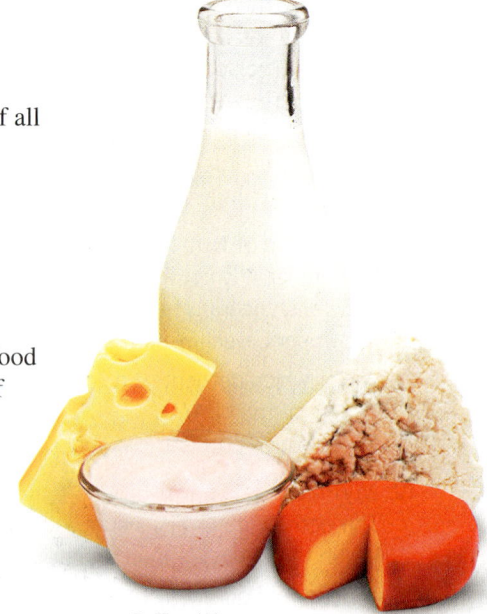
D. Hurst/Alamy

9. Which of the following statements is true?
   a. According to MyPlate, vegetable oils are grouped into the "Fats and Oils" food group.
   b. The MyPlate menu planning guide cannot be individualized to meet a person's food preferences.
   c. A person can use www.choosemyplate.gov to evaluate his or her diet's nutritional adequacy.
   d. MyPlate was the first food guide developed for Americans.

10. Which of the following information isn't provided by the Nutrition Facts panel?
    a. Percentage of calories from fat
    b. Amount of carbohydrate per serving
    c. Serving size
    d. Amount of protein per serving

11. Daily Values are
    a. for people who consume 1200 to 1500 kilocalorie diets.
    b. based on the lowest RDA or AI for each nutrient.
    c. dietary standards developed for food-labeling purposes.
    d. used to evaluate the nutritional adequacy of a population's diet.

12. When consumed, which of the following dietary supplements isn't likely to cause serious side effects?
    a. Pennyroyal
    b. Acidophilus
    c. Lobelia
    d. Ma huang

Answers: 1. b 2. d 3. c 4. c 5. b 6. a 7. d 8. a 9. c 10. a 11. c 12. b

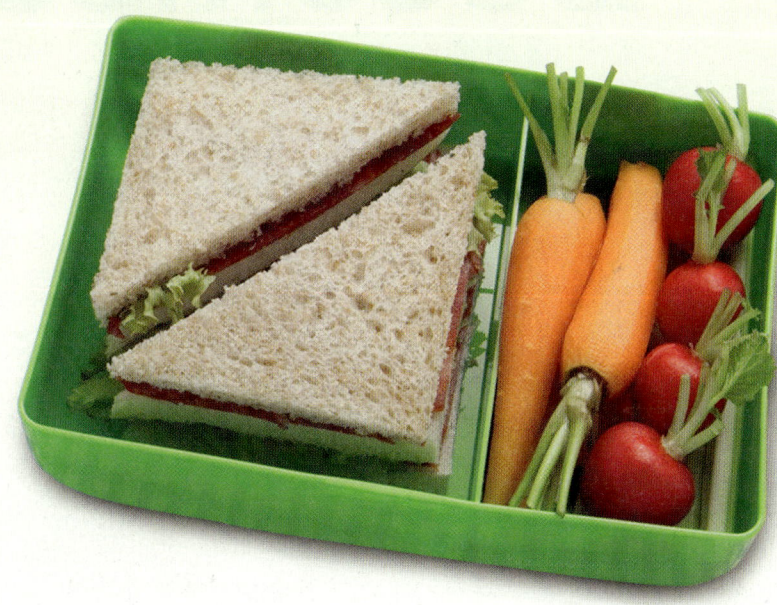

A. Huber/U. Starke/Corbis

Answer This (Module 3.1b)
80 g

References → See Appendix D.

Design elements: Spiral notebook paper background, Stacked paper with clip background, Marginal note clip, and Culture & Cuisine globe icon: ©McGraw-Hill Education; In a Nutshell walnut: ©McGraw-Hill Education/Mark A. Dierker, photographer; Test Yourself red pepper: Iconotec/Glow Images

Unit 4
How Food Becomes You

What's on the Menu?

Module 4.1
From Cells to Systems

Module 4.2
Digestive System

Module 4.3
Common Digestive System Disorders

Module 4.4
Metabolism Basics

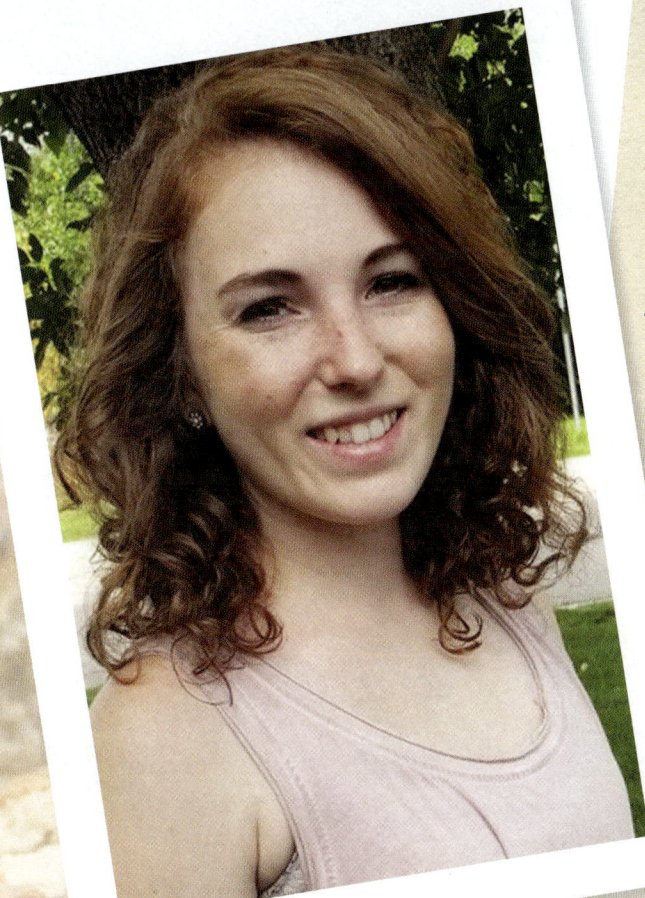

"I have celiac disease, so I can't eat anything that contains gluten. I make my own meals and snacks . . . when I shop for food, I always check labels to see if the food is gluten free. Eating things that I haven't prepared can cause problems for me, so I don't go out to eat that often. I even bring my own foods to parties . . . it's just not worth getting sick. When I was in college, I had to live off campus because I couldn't eat dorm food. . . . If you or someone you know has celiac disease, don't take the disease lightly. Continuing to eat gluten can lead to worse health problems, so eat the right foods!"

Karlin West

Karlin West recently graduated from the University of Northern Iowa with a business degree. During her sophomore year in high school, she developed abdominal pain and vomiting after eating. Because she was unable to "keep food down," her weight began to drop. She soon learned that she could follow a diet of "protein shakes" without getting sick, but she felt hungry and tired all of the time. According to Karlin, "doctors didn't know what was wrong with me, even after they performed lots of tests on my digestive tract." Alarmed, Karlin's parents took their ailing daughter to a major medical center in Iowa City, hoping that its specialists could diagnose her mysterious illness. It didn't take much time for the physicians to identify Karlin's disorder—*celiac disease*. A person with celiac disease can't eat anything that contains *gluten,* a protein in wheat, buckwheat, and rye. When gluten enters the person's intestinal tract, it sparks an immune response by the small intestine that damages the structure's lining. Such damage makes it difficult for the body to obtain nutrients from foods and beverages. Over time, the condition results in malnutrition, particularly vitamin and mineral nutrient deficiencies, and weight loss. Many popular foods, including breads, doughnuts, and other baked goods, are made with wheat flour, which contains gluten. By following a gluten-free diet, people with celiac disease generally can enable their digestive tract to heal. Unit 7 provides more information about celiac disease, including risk factors for the condition.

Unit 4 focuses primarily on the digestive system, including how your body obtains and delivers nutrients to where it needs them. Module 4.3 provides general information about some common intestinal problems, including constipation, heartburn, and cancer.

Module 4.1
From Cells to Systems

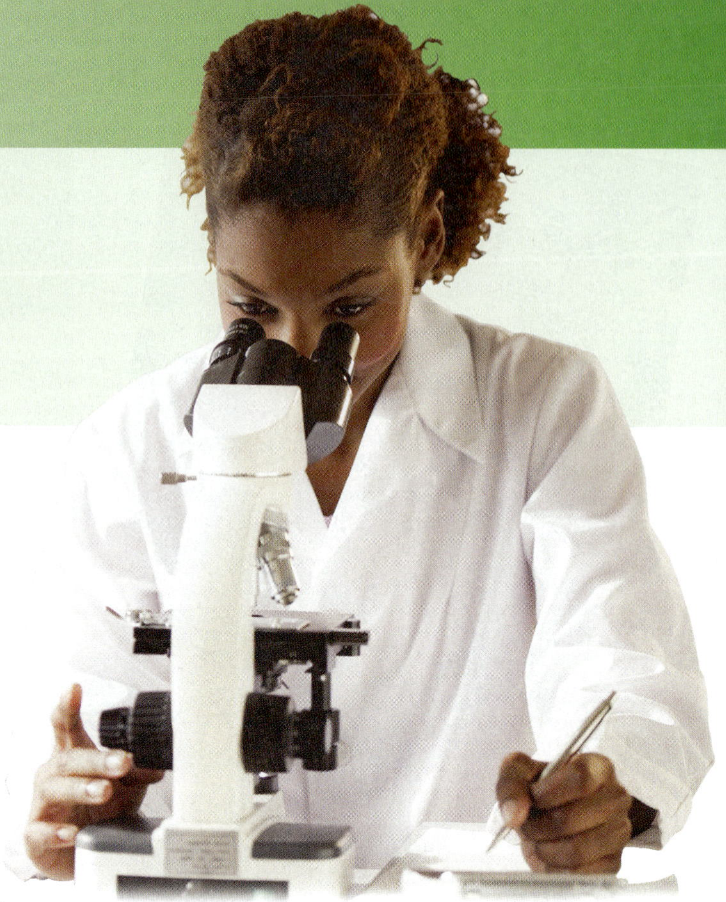

4.1 - Learning Outcomes

After reading Module 4.1, you should be able to

1. Define all of the **key terms** in this module.
2. Explain how the body is organized into cells, tissues, organs, and organ systems.
3. Identify the primary organs in each organ system.
4. Discuss at least one major function of each organ system.

4.1a The Organization of Your Body

By learning about your body, you may appreciate its complexity and be amazed at the variety of metabolic activities that keep you alive, physically active, mentally alert, and healthy. As mentioned in Unit 1, a cell is the smallest living functional unit in your body. Your body has about 100 *trillion* cells that can be classified into numerous cell types. Each type of cell has a specific function. For example, muscle cells are necessary for movement; nerve cells send messages; red blood cells transport oxygen; and certain white blood cells protect your body from disease-causing bacteria and viruses. Each human cell has a membrane that surrounds it and controls the passage of nutrients and other substances into and out of the cell.

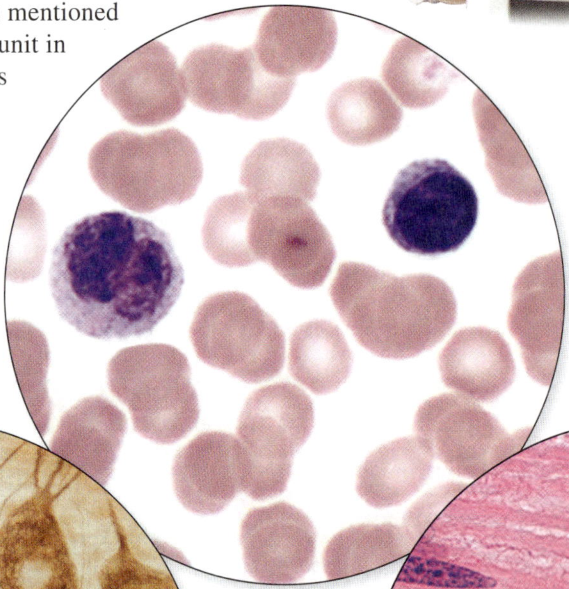

Blood cells

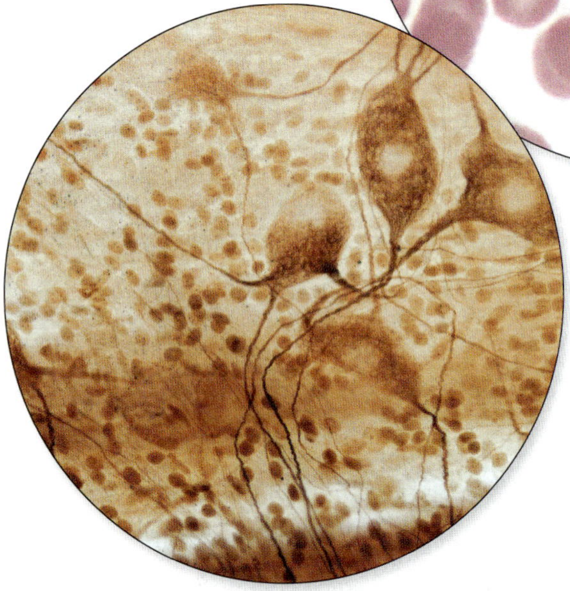

Nerve cells

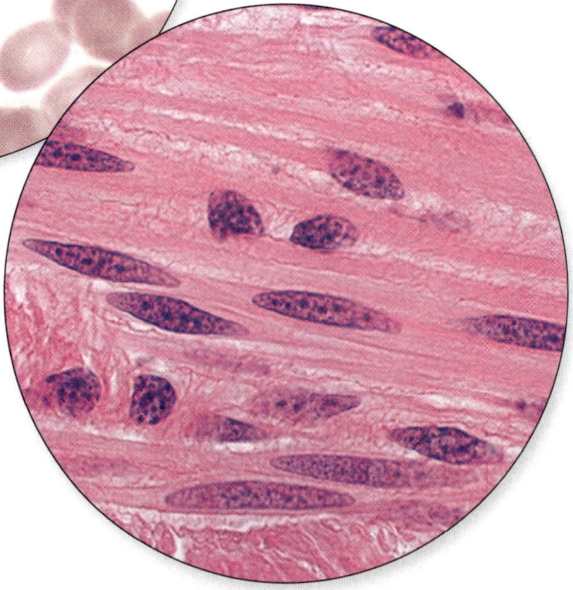

Smooth muscle cells

Woman looking into microscope: JGI/Daniel Grill/Blend Images/Getty Images; Micrograph of blood cells: Al Telser/McGraw-Hill Education; Micrograph of nerve cells: xia yuan/Getty Images; Micrograph of smooth muscle cells: McGraw-Hill Education/Dennis Strete

Essential Concept

4.1 Your Body's Organization

tissues masses of cells that have similar characteristics and functions

organ collection of tissues that function in a related fashion

organ system group of organs that work together for a similar purpose

1 Cell
For example, muscle cells are necessary for movement.

2 Tissue
Cells that have similar characteristics and functions are usually joined together into larger masses called **tissues**.

3 Organ
An **organ** is composed of various tissues that function in a related fashion. The stomach, for example, is an organ because it contains different kinds of tissue that work together to churn food and break down the food's components.

4 Organ system
An **organ system** is a group of organs that work together for a similar purpose. The digestive system, for example, includes several organs, including the stomach and intestines.

5 Organism
A healthy person is composed of organ systems that function together properly.

4.1b Your Body's Organ Systems

The organ systems are dependent on each other. If your liver, for example, isn't functioning properly, the rest of your body won't be able to function properly. By following a nutritionally adequate diet, you may be able to achieve better health. **Table 4.1** lists each system's major organs or tissues and summarizes their primary functions.

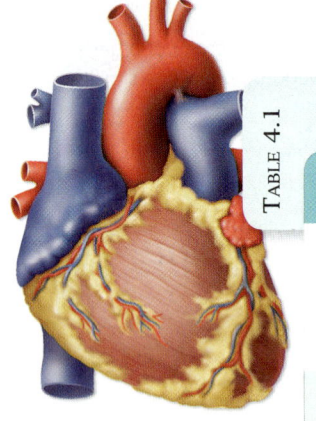

TABLE 4.1 THE ORGAN SYSTEMS OF YOUR BODY

System	Major Organs or Tissues	Primary Functions
Digestive	Mouth, salivary glands, esophagus, stomach, intestines, pancreas, liver, gallbladder	Digestion and absorption of nutrients
Cardiovascular	Heart, blood vessels, blood	Circulation of blood throughout the body
Respiratory	Nose, pharynx, larynx, trachea, bronchi, lungs	Exchange of oxygen and carbon dioxide
Lymphatic and Immune	Lymphatic fluid, white blood cells, lymph vessels and nodes, spleen, thymus	Defense and immunity against infectious agents, fluid balance, white blood cell production, and absorption of fat-soluble nutrients from intestinal tract
Urinary	Kidneys, bladder	Elimination of salts, water, and wastes; and maintenance of fluid balance
Muscular	Muscles	Movement and stability of the body
Skeletal	Bones, tendons, ligaments	Support, movement, protection, and production of blood cells
Nervous	Brain, spinal cord, nerves, sensory receptors	Thought processes, regulation and coordination of many body activities, and detection of changes in external and internal environments
Endocrine	Glands or organs that secrete hormones (chemical messengers), including fat tissue	Regulation and coordination of many body activities, including growth, nutrient balance, and reproduction
Integumentary	Skin, hair, nails	Protection and immunity, regulation of body temperature, and vitamin D synthesis
Reproductive	Gonads, genitals	Procreation (creating children)

Source: Adapted from: Widmaier EP, and others: *Vander's human physiology*, 12th ed. Boston: McGraw-Hill Publishing Company, 2011.

Module 4.2
Digestive System

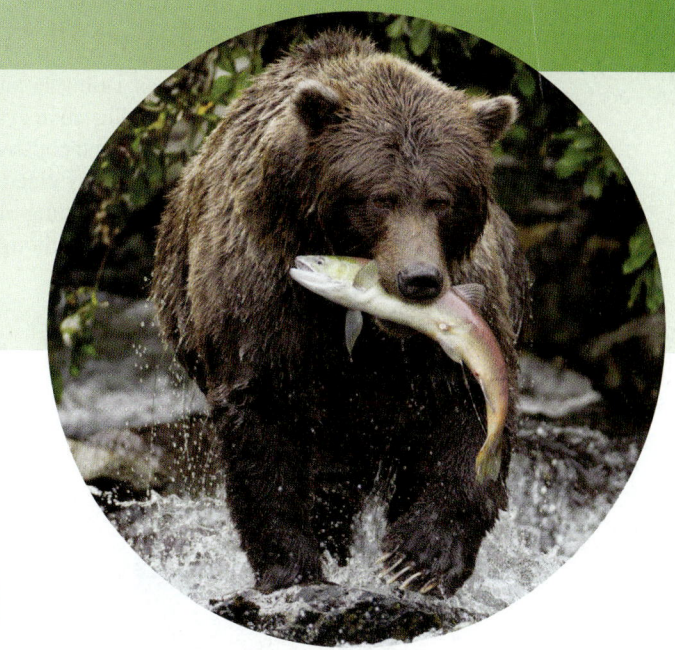

4.2 - Learning Outcomes
After reading Module 4.2, you should be able to

1. Define all of the **key terms** in this module.
2. Explain the difference between mechanical and chemical digestion and provide an example of each.
3. Identify organs and structures of the digestive system, including accessory organs, and describe their primary functions.
4. Discuss the overall process of digestion and absorption.

4.2a Overview of Digestion

Grizzly bears are omnivores. In addition to salmon, they eat other animals, but fruit, nuts, leaves, and roots form the foundation of their diet. You're an **omnivore,** an organism that can digest and absorb nutrients from plants; animals; fungi, which include mushrooms; and even bacteria. The human digestive system is designed to receive food from all of these sources, process it into nutrients, transport the nutrients into the bloodstream, and eliminate the waste products. Your body doesn't need food—your cells need the nutrients that are in food to carry out their work.

Digestion is the process of breaking down large food components into smaller chemical units (**molecules**), including individual nutrients. This process involves mechanical and chemical digestion.

- **Mechanical digestion** involves the physical breakdown of foods, including the biting action of teeth and mixing movements of the stomach.
- **Chemical digestion** refers to the chemical breakdown of foods by substances secreted into the **digestive tract,** which is sometimes called the "GI" (gastrointestinal) tract.

Absorption is the process by which nutrients and other substances are taken up by the digestive tract and enter the bloodstream or lymphatic system (see Table 4.1). This module focuses on the functions of your digestive system.

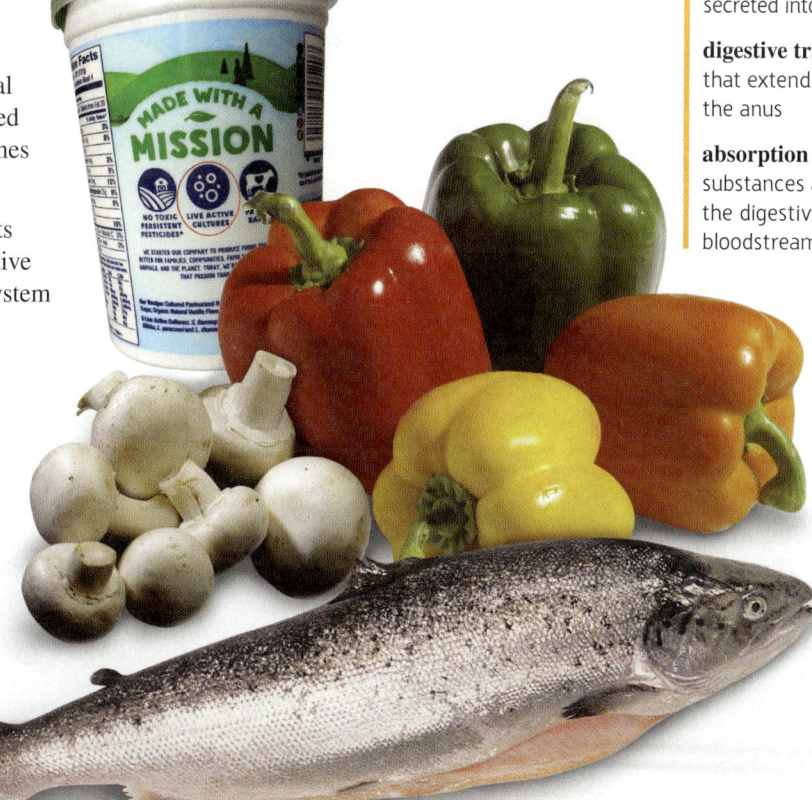

An omnivore's food includes plants, animals, fungi, and bacteria, such as certain live bacteria in the yogurt.

omnivore organism that can digest and absorb nutrients from plants, animals, fungi, and bacteria

digestion process by which large food components are mechanically and chemically broken down

molecules basic chemical units that make up substances

mechanical digestion physical breakdown of foods

chemical digestion chemical breakdown of foods by substances secreted into the digestive tract

digestive tract muscular tube that extends from the mouth to the anus

absorption process by which substances are taken up from the digestive tract and enter the bloodstream or the lymph

Bear, Fish: Justinreznick/Getty Images;
Container of yogurt: Wendy Schiff;
Mushrooms, Peppers: Purestock/SuperStock;
Salmon: Getty Images/Digital Vision

accessory organs organs of the digestive system that assist digestive tract function

4.2b Your Digestive Tract

The mouth, esophagus, stomach, and small and large intestines are the major organs of the digestive tract and components of the digestive system (**Fig. 4.1a**). The digestive tract forms a continuous muscular tube that begins at the mouth and ends with the anus.

The teeth, tongue, salivary glands, liver, gallbladder, and pancreas are **accessory organs** of the digestive system that assist the functioning of the digestive tract (**Fig. 4.1b**). The liver, gallbladder, and pancreas play major roles in digestion, even though food doesn't move through them.

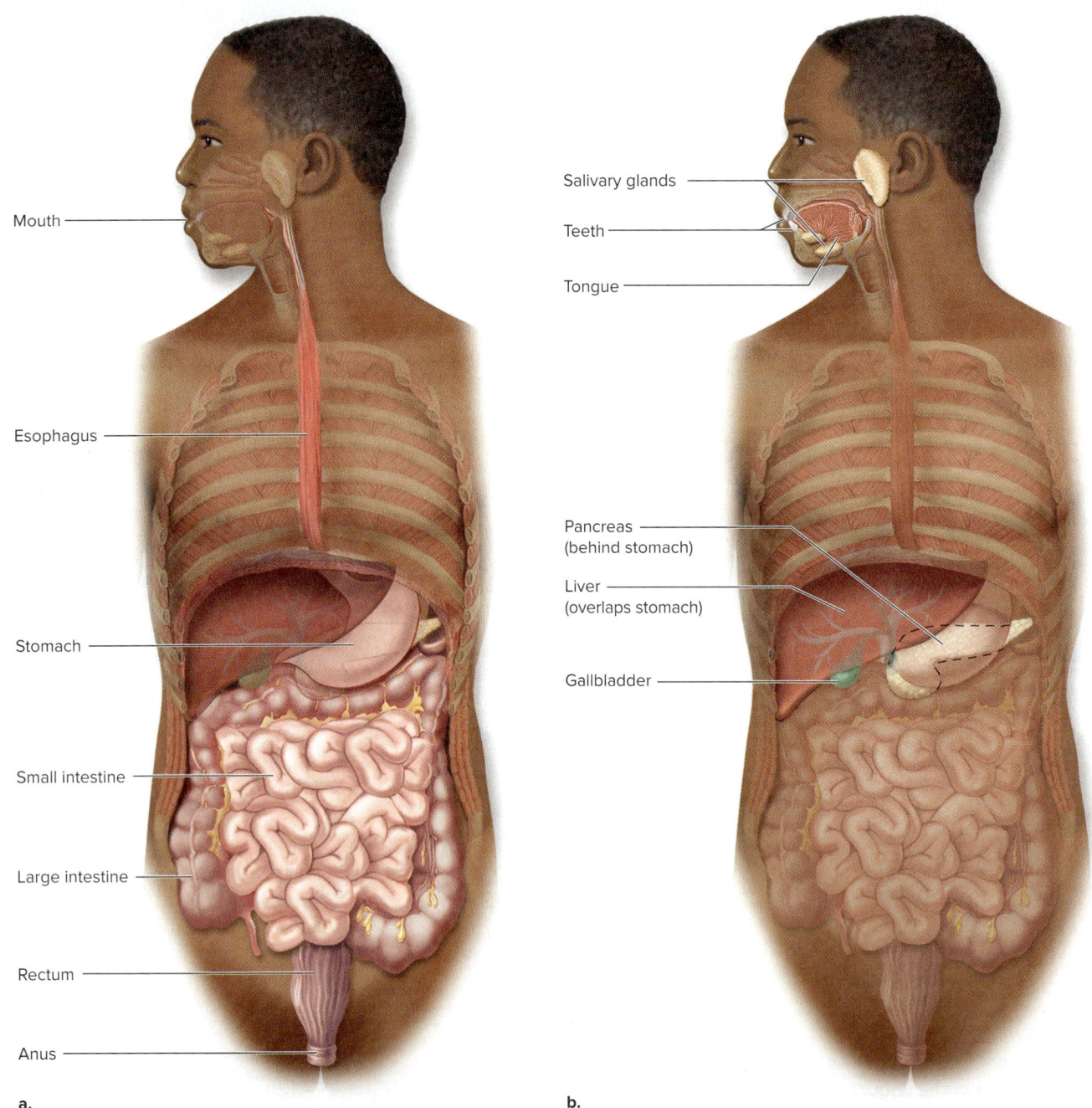

Figure 4.1 Your digestive tract. (a) The major organs of the digestive system. **(b)** Accessory organs of the digestive system.

Mouth

Digestion actually starts in the mouth:

- Teeth begin the mechanical digestion of food by biting, tearing, and grinding chunks of food into smaller pieces that are easier to swallow.
- Salivary glands secrete **saliva,** a watery fluid that mixes with food and makes it easier to swallow. Saliva contains an enzyme that enables a minor amount of starch to undergo chemical digestion. **Enzymes** are proteins that help certain chemical changes occur, such as the breakdown of large substances.
- The tongue senses the taste and texture of foods and directs food to the back of the mouth where it can be swallowed.

A Matter of Taste Taste buds that are located primarily on the tongue have specialized cells that help you distinguish sweet, sour, salty, bitter, and umami (*ew-mom´-ē*) tastes. Umami is often described as a meaty taste. Taste buds are also able to sense fat in foods.[1]

The entire tongue can detect the different kinds of tastes, but the areas close to the sides and tip of the tongue have the most taste buds. The middle of the tongue isn't as sensitive to taste as other parts of the organ.

- Foods that taste sweet, such as ripe fruit, usually contain simple sugars that can provide energy for your cells.
- Foods that taste sour may be good sources of vitamin C, such as citrus fruit.
- The rear portion of the tongue is more likely to detect bitter substances than are other regions of the organ. Bitter-tasting substances are often poisonous. Thus, having a lot of taste buds on the back of the tongue that detect the bitter taste can give you a chance to spit out a bitter substance before you swallow it.

The sense of smell also contributes to your ability to taste. As you chew food, it releases chemicals that become airborne and stimulate nerves inside your nose. Your brain receives this information and combines it with information about taste sensations from your mouth to identify foods' flavors. Thus, favorite foods may seem tasteless and unappealing when you have an upper respiratory tract infection and the inside of your nose is congested.

saliva watery fluid secreted by the salivary glands that mixes with food in the mouth

enzymes proteins that help chemical reactions occur

TASTY Tidbits

Children have more taste buds than do adults, which may explain why they often reject strong-flavored foods such as liver, cooked broccoli, and raw onion. As you age, the number of taste buds in your mouth declines, and as an older adult, you might find yourself adding more seasoning to food to improve its taste.

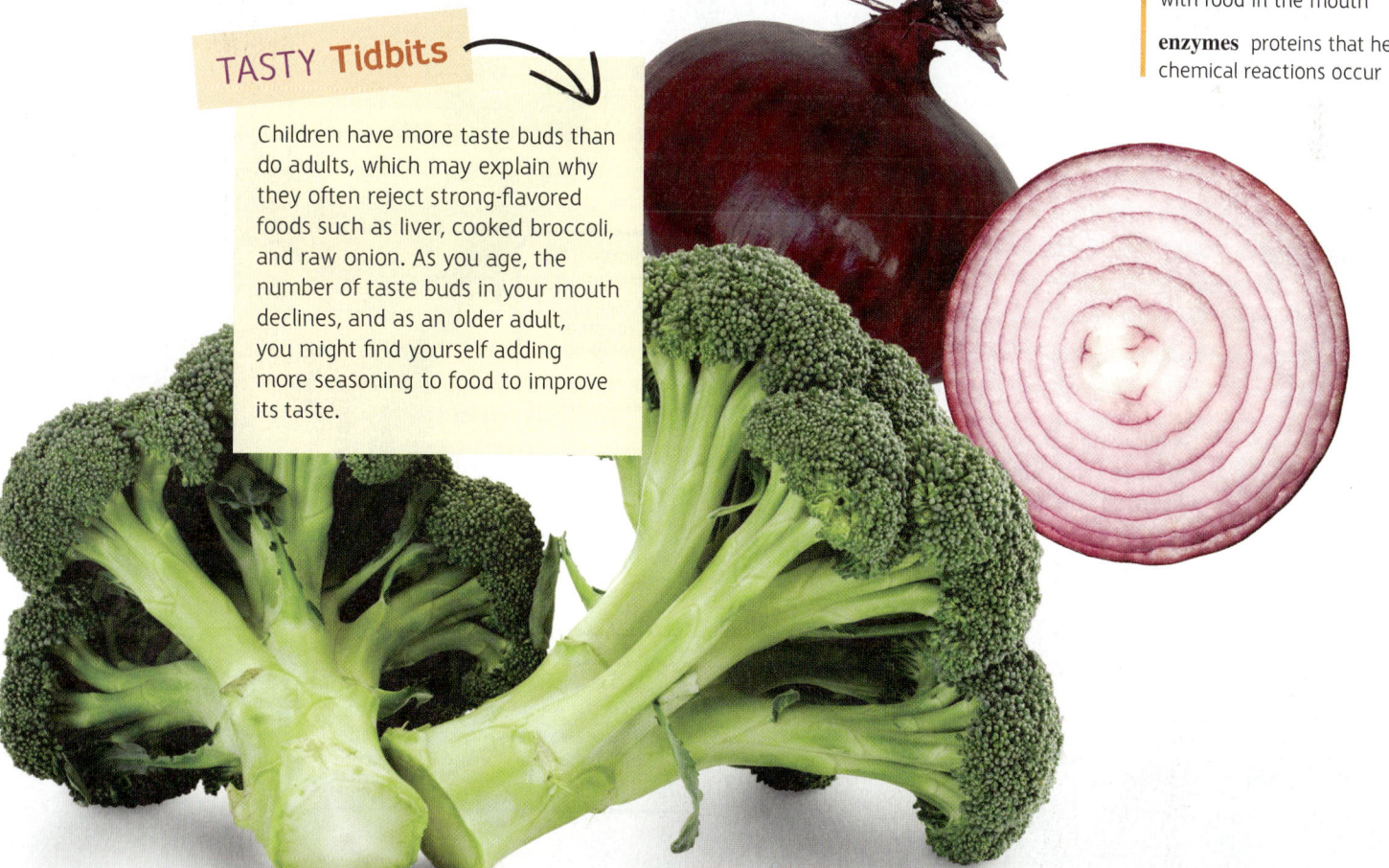

Child: Ingram Publishing; Broccoli: Creative Studio Heinemann/Getty Images; Whole red onion: Wendy Schiff; Red onion (cut): Mtsaride/Shutterstock

Unit 4 How Food Becomes You

Essential Concept

4.2 What Happens When You Swallow?

Esophagus

The **esophagus** (*eh-sof´-ah-gus*) is a muscular tube that extends about 10 inches from the back of the mouth to the top of the stomach. **Essential Concept 4.2** illustrates what happens to the material that's in your mouth when you swallow.

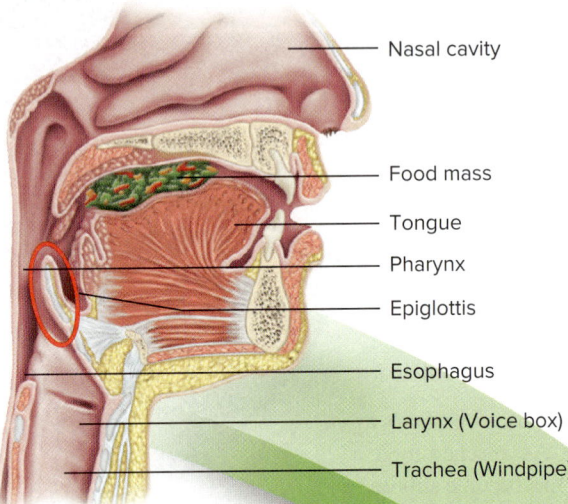

- Nasal cavity
- Food mass
- Tongue
- Pharynx
- Epiglottis
- Esophagus
- Larynx (Voice box)
- Trachea (Windpipe)

1 The esophagus transfers a mass of swallowed food into the stomach. The entrance to the esophagus is near the larynx and the opening of the trachea (windpipe). The **epiglottis** (*ep-eh-glot´-tis*) is a flap of tissue that can cover the trachea.

esophagus tubular organ of the digestive tract that connects the back of the mouth with the stomach

epiglottis flap of tissue that covers the entrance to the trachea (windpipe) to keep food from entering the lungs during swallowing

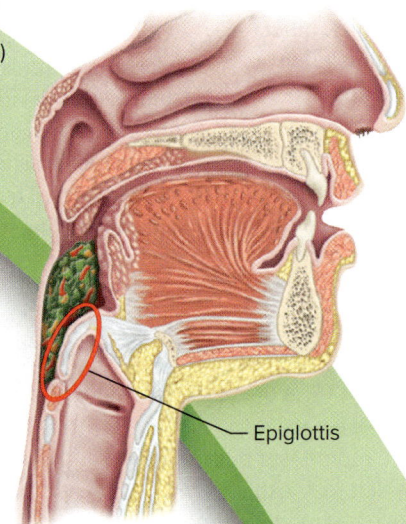

- Epiglottis

2 When you swallow, the epiglottis covers the entrance to the trachea. This prevents the food from "going down the wrong pipe" (entering the larynx and trachea), which can cause choking.

- Epiglottis

3 After swallowing the mass of food, the epiglottis returns to its usual position. Now, you can talk and breathe again because the larynx and trachea are able to obtain air.

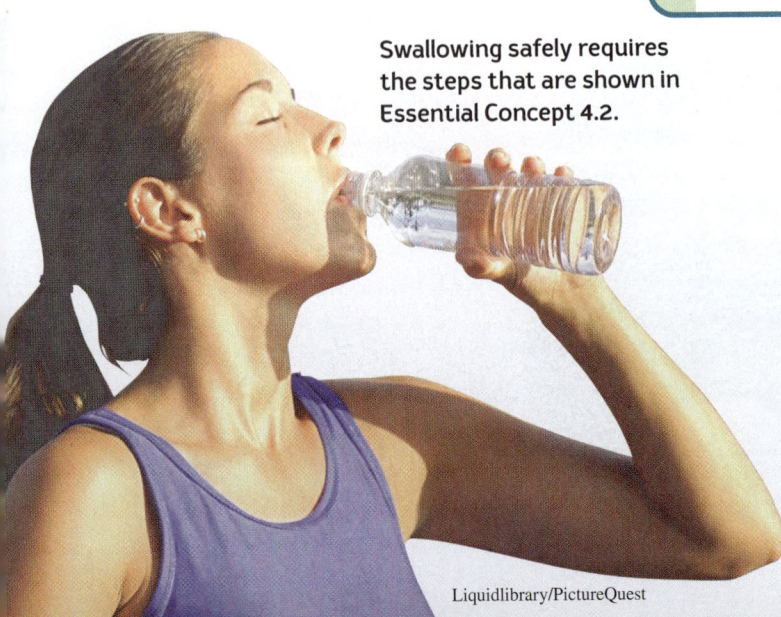

Swallowing safely requires the steps that are shown in Essential Concept 4.2.

Liquidlibrary/PictureQuest

Swallowing food stimulates **peristalsis** (*per-uh-stall´-sis*), waves of muscular activity along the digestive tract that help propel food material through the tract. **Figure 4.2** shows how peristalsis moves a mass of food through the esophagus and to the stomach. Peristalsis also occurs in the stomach and intestines.

Peristalsis is an involuntary response, which means the muscular movements happen without the need to think about them.

Lifesaving Lesson Accidental choking is a major cause of preventable deaths. A common distress sign of choking is grabbing the throat with one or both hands. Choking danger signs include bluish skin color; difficulty breathing; inability to speak; weak, ineffective coughing; and loss of consciousness ("passing out").[2] The **Heimlich maneuver** (also called "abdominal thrusts") is a first aid technique that can help clear the blocked airway of a choking person. By learning the simple Heimlich maneuver, you can save a life, perhaps even your own.

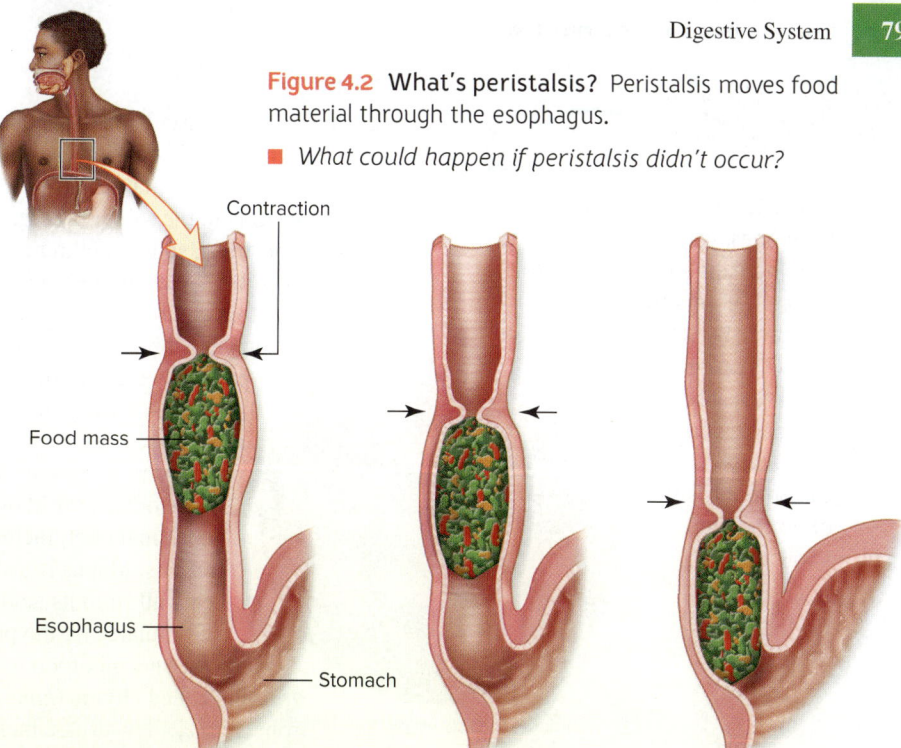

Figure 4.2 What's peristalsis? Peristalsis moves food material through the esophagus.

■ *What could happen if peristalsis didn't occur?*

Essential Concept

4.3 First Aid for Choking: The Heimlich Maneuver

peristalsis type of muscular contraction of the digestive tract

Heimlich maneuver life-saving technique for people who are choking

1 A hand or hands wrapped around the throat is a common sign of choking.

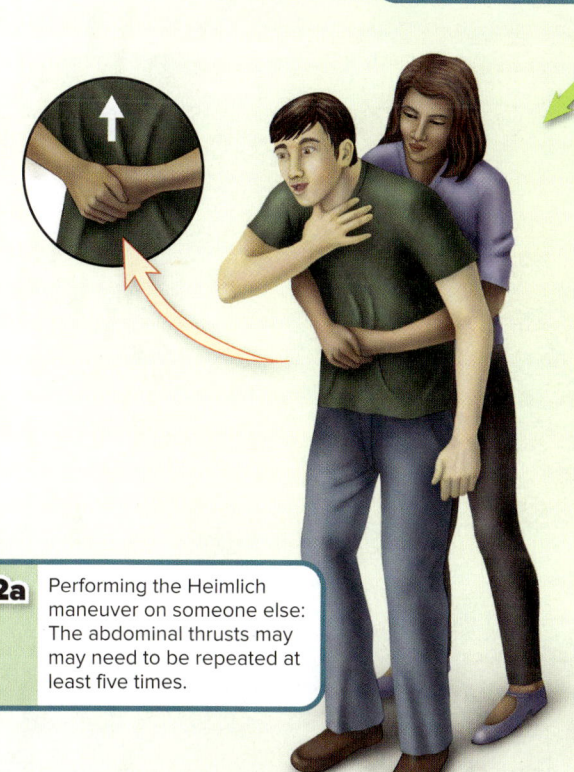

2a Performing the Heimlich maneuver on someone else: The abdominal thrusts may may need to be repeated at least five times.

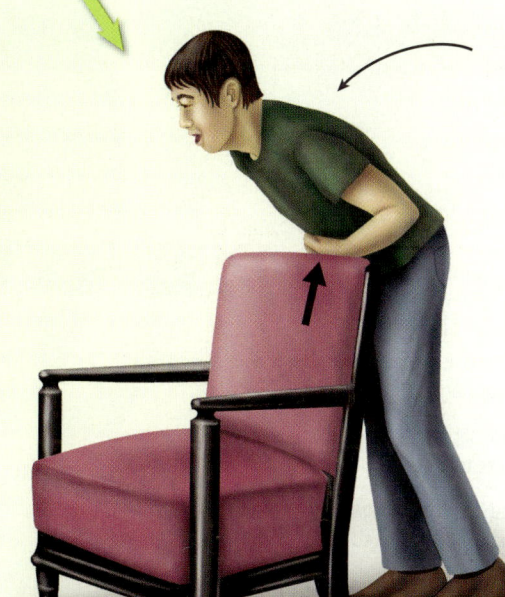

2b Performing the Heimlich maneuver on yourself: This procedure may need to be repeated at least five times.

TASTY Tidbits

When you eat foods or drink beverages, you swallow some air. Burping expels most of this air before it enters the stomach. By slowing down the rate at which you eat and drink, you can reduce the amount of air that you swallow.

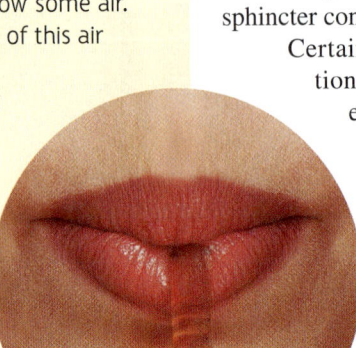

Nick Koudis/Getty Images

Stomach

The stomach is a muscular sac that can expand and hold about 4 to 6 cups of food after a typical meal. The **lower esophageal sphincter** (*eh-sof-ah-jee´-al sfink´-ter*) is the ring of muscular tissue at the lower end of the esophagus that controls the opening to the stomach (**Fig. 4.3**). After food enters the stomach, this sphincter constricts, so the food remains in the organ.

Certain cells within the stomach secrete gastric juice, a watery solution that contains hydrochloric acid (HCl) and enzymes. The enzymes break down some protein and fat. HCl helps make proteins easier to digest. The acid also kills many dangerous, disease-causing microorganisms that may be in food.

As you can see in Figure 4.3, the stomach's walls consist of layers of muscle. Muscle contains protein—so how does the stomach avoid digesting itself? Special cells that line the intestinal tract, including the inside of the stomach, produce **mucus.** Mucus is a slippery substance that protects the stomach wall from its acid and enzymes.

Stimulated by the presence of food, the stomach's churning movements mix food with gastric juice. At this point, the food is a semisolid liquid called **chyme** (*kime*). Although the stomach absorbs very few nutrients from chyme, a few drugs, including some alcohol, can pass through the organ's walls and enter the bloodstream.

The **pyloric** (*pie-lor´-ic*) **sphincter** is the ring of muscular tissue at the base of the stomach. When this sphincter relaxes, small amounts of chyme leave the stomach and enter the small intestine (see Figure 4.3).

Following a meal, the stomach empties in about 3 to 4 hours, depending on the contents and size of the meal. Carbohydrate-rich meals or snacks spend less time in the stomach; protein-rich or fatty meals spend more time there. As you'd expect, larger meals take longer to empty from the stomach than smaller meals.

McGraw-Hill Education/matt meadows

lower esophageal sphincter ring of muscle in the lower part of the esophagus; controls the opening between the esophagus and stomach

mucus slippery fluid that protects certain cells

chyme mixture of gastric juice and partially digested food

pyloric sphincter ring of muscle at the base of the stomach that controls the rate at which chyme leaves the stomach

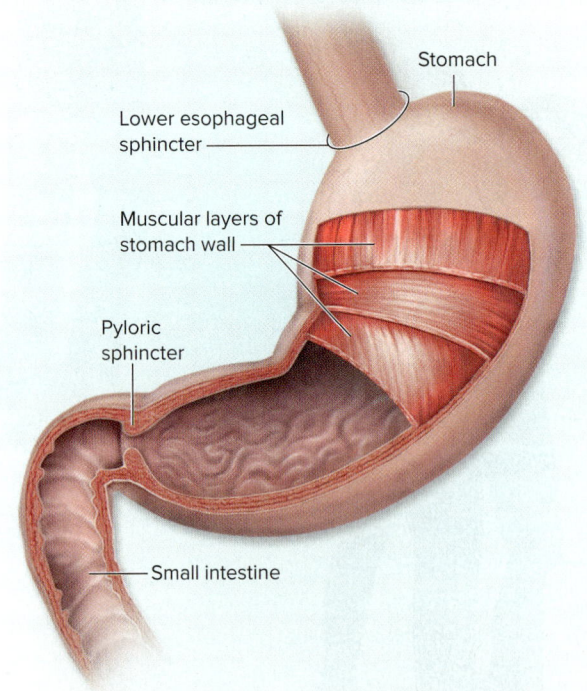

Figure 4.3 The stomach.

- *What structure controls the entrance to the stomach?*
- *What is the function of the pyloric sphincter?*

Small Intestine

The small intestine is a highly coiled tube that extends from the stomach to the large intestine. Most nutrient digestion and absorption occurs in the small intestine. The small intestine has three sections (**Fig. 4.4**):

- **duodenum** (*do-wah-dee´-num*)
- **jejunum** (*jeh-ju´-num*)
- **ileum** (*il´-lee-um*)

The pancreas and gallbladder release fluids into the duodenum that neutralize the acidic chyme from the stomach. As a result, enzymes that don't function in acidic conditions are able to digest chyme in the small intestine.

What Are Villi?

The lining of the small intestine is covered by tiny, fingerlike projections called **villi** (singular, **villus**) (**Fig. 4.5a**). A villus has an outer layer of special cells called **absorptive cells** (**Fig. 4.5b**). Absorptive cells have tiny structures called microvilli that are exposed to chyme. Villi and microvilli increase the surface area of the small intestine, which increases your body's ability to digest and absorb nutrients.

Microvilli have enzymes that help complete digestion. As a result of enzyme action, macronutrients are broken down into their basic components. Proteins break down into amino acids, fats into fatty acids and glycerol, and most dietary carbohydrates into glucose. You will learn more about the digestion of these nutrients in Units 5, 6, and 7.

Absorptive cells remove (*absorb*) the breakdown products of digestion from chyme. Within each villus are tiny blood vessels that form a capillary network and a **lacteal**, a lymphatic system vessel that carries fluid called **lymph**. Essential Concepts 4.4 and 4.5 illustrate the absorption of water- and fat-soluble nutrients in the small intestine.

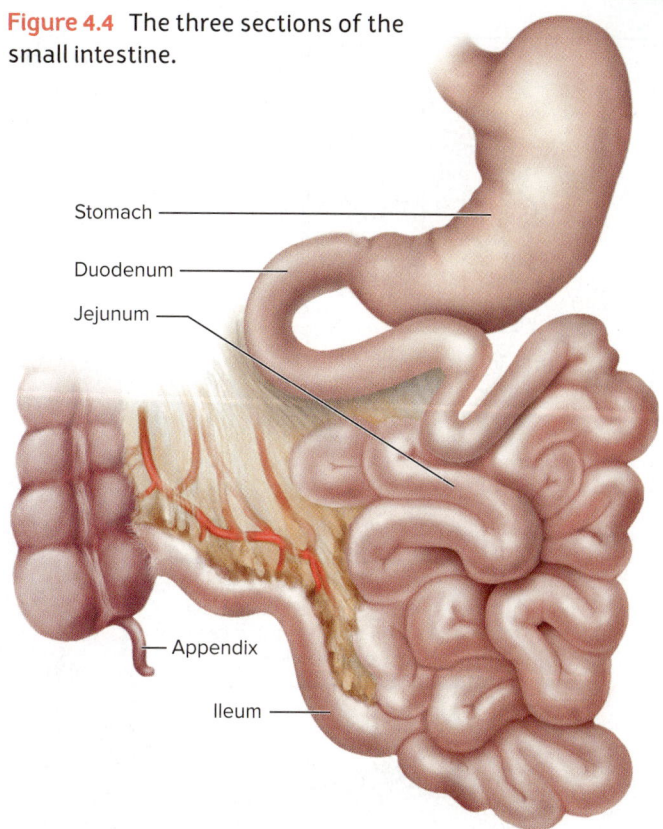

Figure 4.4 The three sections of the small intestine.

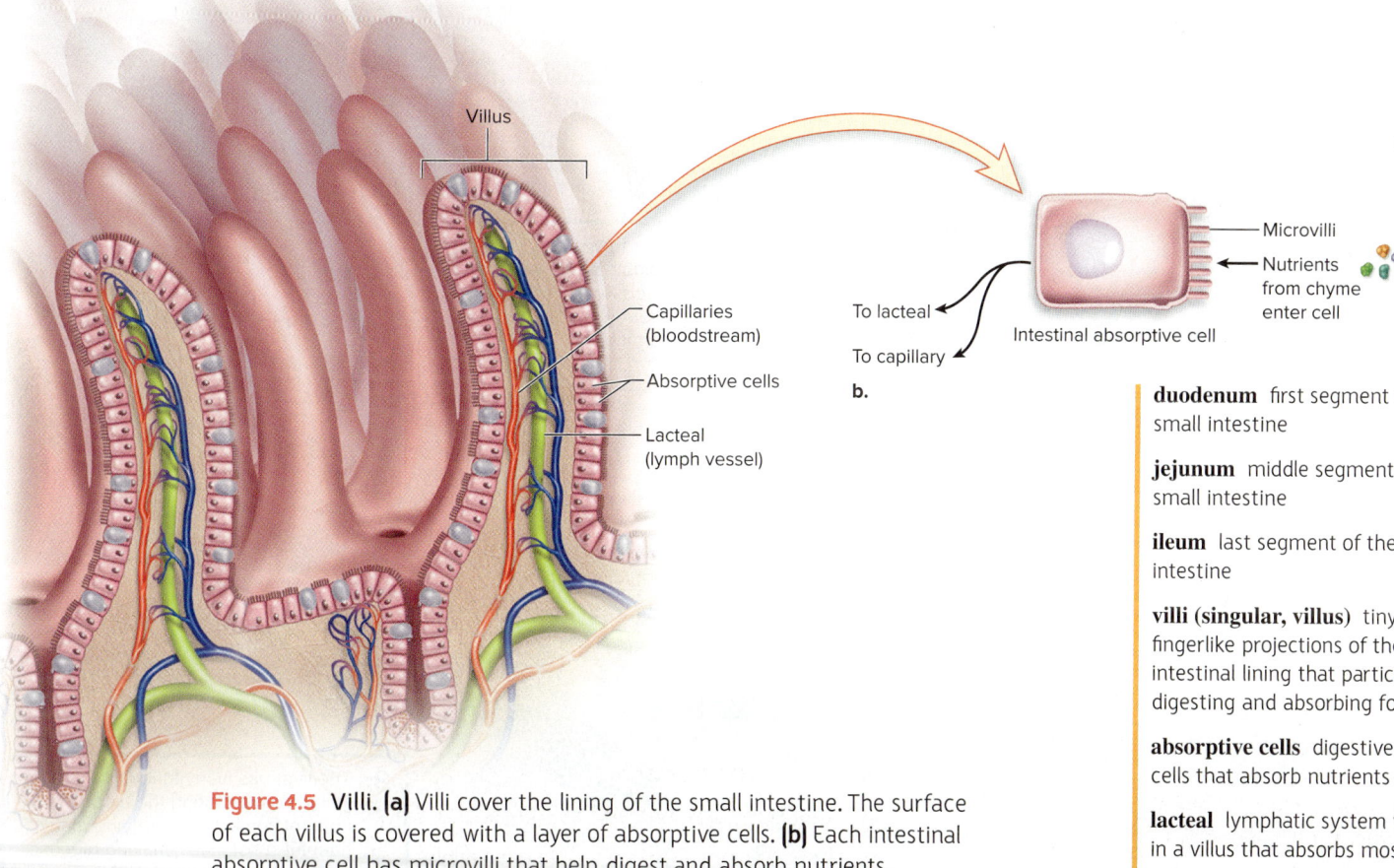

Figure 4.5 Villi. (a) Villi cover the lining of the small intestine. The surface of each villus is covered with a layer of absorptive cells. (b) Each intestinal absorptive cell has microvilli that help digest and absorb nutrients.

■ *What would happen if your small intestine didn't have villi?*

duodenum first segment of the small intestine

jejunum middle segment of the small intestine

ileum last segment of the small intestine

villi (singular, villus) tiny, fingerlike projections of the small intestinal lining that participate in digesting and absorbing food

absorptive cells digestive tract cells that absorb nutrients

lacteal lymphatic system vessel in a villus that absorbs most lipids

lymph fluid in the lymphatic system

Essential Concept

4.4 What Happens to Water-Soluble Nutrients?

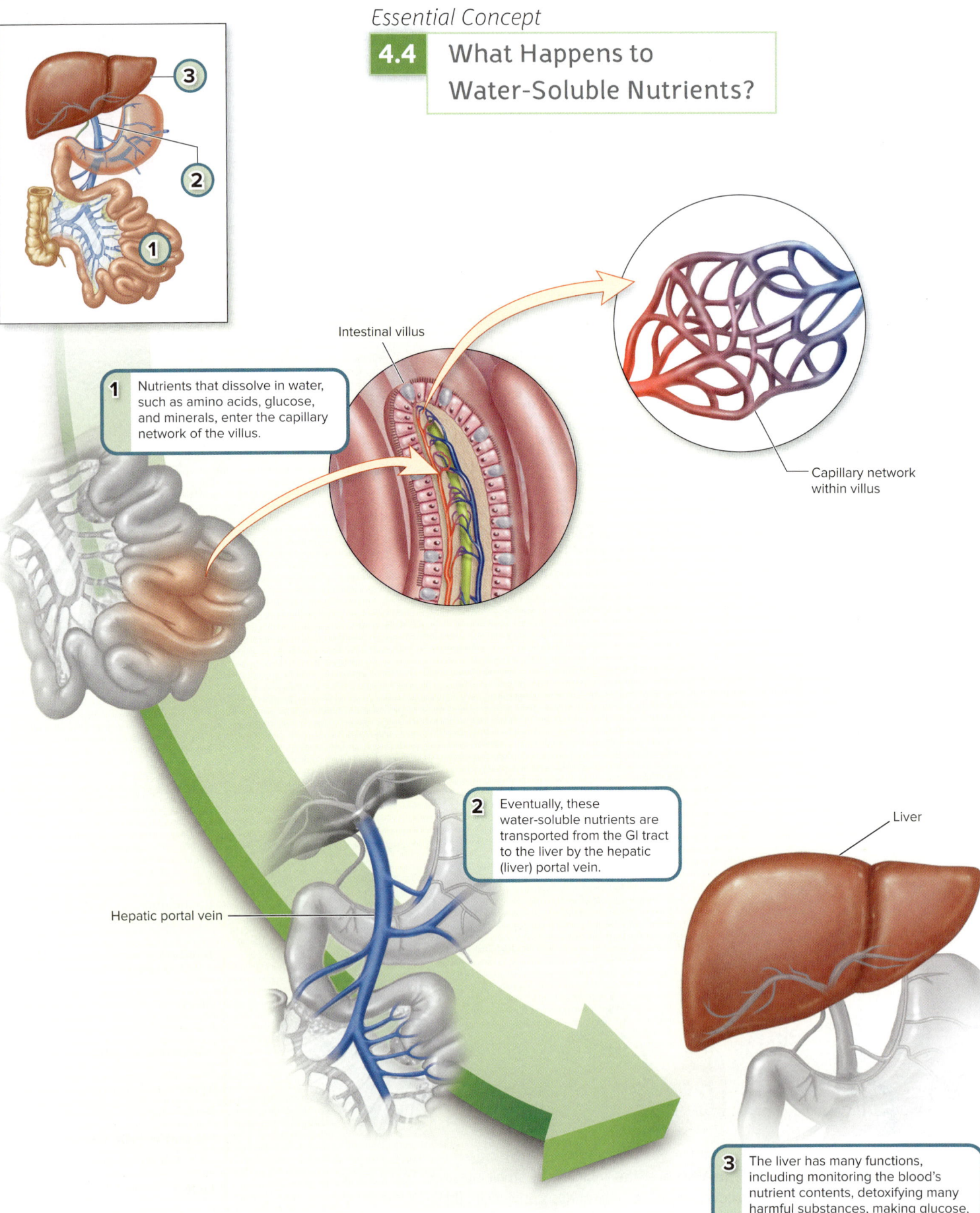

1. Nutrients that dissolve in water, such as amino acids, glucose, and minerals, enter the capillary network of the villus.

2. Eventually, these water-soluble nutrients are transported from the GI tract to the liver by the hepatic (liver) portal vein.

3. The liver has many functions, including monitoring the blood's nutrient contents, detoxifying many harmful substances, making glucose, and storing various nutrients.

Intestinal villus

Capillary network within villus

Hepatic portal vein

Liver

Essential Concept

4.5 What Happens to Fat-Soluble Nutrients?

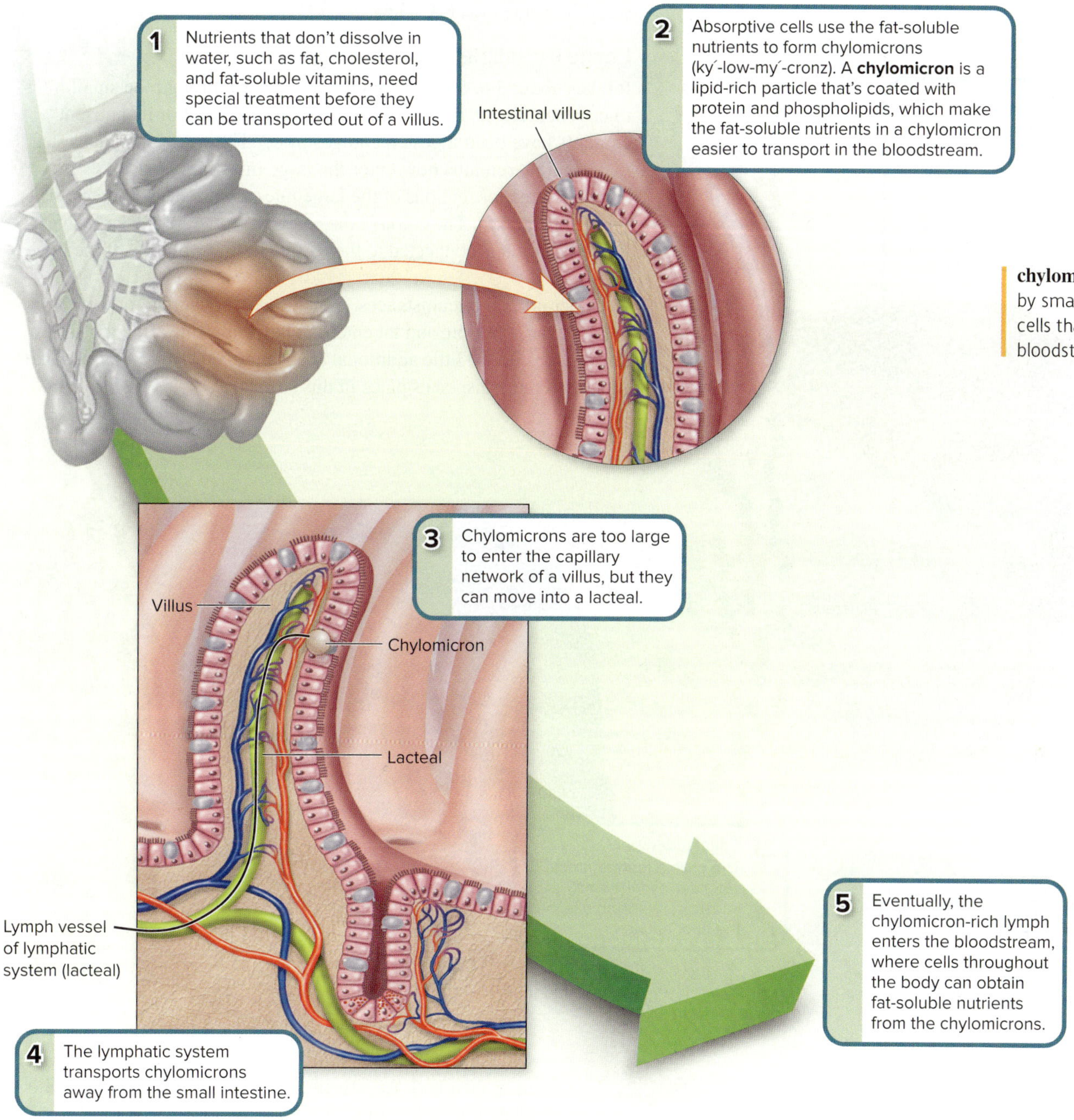

1 Nutrients that don't dissolve in water, such as fat, cholesterol, and fat-soluble vitamins, need special treatment before they can be transported out of a villus.

2 Absorptive cells use the fat-soluble nutrients to form chylomicrons (ky´-low-my´-cronz). A **chylomicron** is a lipid-rich particle that's coated with protein and phospholipids, which make the fat-soluble nutrients in a chylomicron easier to transport in the bloodstream.

Intestinal villus

chylomicron particle formed by small intestinal absorptive cells that transports lipids in the bloodstream

3 Chylomicrons are too large to enter the capillary network of a villus, but they can move into a lacteal.

Villus

Chylomicron

Lacteal

Lymph vessel of lymphatic system (lacteal)

4 The lymphatic system transports chylomicrons away from the small intestine.

5 Eventually, the chylomicron-rich lymph enters the bloodstream, where cells throughout the body can obtain fat-soluble nutrients from the chylomicrons.

What if you had a peanut butter sandwich and a glass of milk for lunch? Within a few hours, your intestinal tract has digested this food and absorbed its nutrients. Now, these nutrients are available for your cells to use. The calcium that was in the milk can be added to your bones. The amino acids that were in the peanut butter, milk, and bread can be used for making proteins that you need. The fat and carbohydrates that were in these foods can be burned for energy. Thus, you are what you eat!

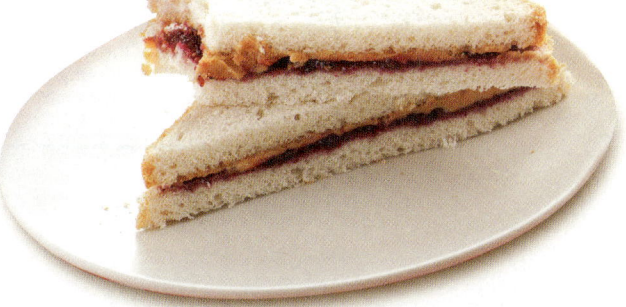

Hera Food/Alamy

Essential Concept

4.6 The Liver, Gallbladder, and Pancreas

1 Liver
The liver processes and stores many nutrients. The liver releases nutrients from storage when they are needed for various functions, including the production of new cells and repair of damaged cells.
- This organ makes cholesterol and uses the lipid to make **bile**, a substance that aids fat digestion and prepares fat and fat-soluble vitamins for absorption.
- Bile flows from the liver into the gallbladder, where it's stored until needed.

2 Gallbladder
The gallbladder contracts when fat is in the small intestine, releasing bile into the duodenum.

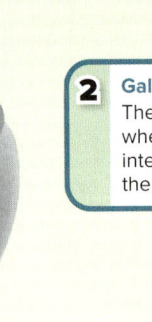

3 Pancreas
The pancreas produces and secretes most of the enzymes that break down carbohydrates, protein, and fat in the small intestine.

Accessory Organs Although chyme doesn't pass through the liver, gallbladder, and pancreas, these accessory organs help digestion in the small intestine (see **E.C. 4.6**).

Large Intestine

It takes about 3 to 5 hours for chyme to move through the small intestine. When chyme reaches the large intestine, most of its nutrient contents have been digested and absorbed. The water and undigested material that remains now enter the large intestine.

The two major sections of the large intestine are the **colon** and the **rectum** (Fig. 4.6). The colon is the primary section of the large intestine. The colon is connected to the rectum, a lower section of the large intestine.

Under normal circumstances, very little carbohydrate (other than dietary fiber), protein, and fat enter the large intestine. The large intestine has no villi, so little additional absorption, other than that of some water and minerals, takes place in this structure.

As chyme passes through the large intestine, most of its water content is absorbed. As a result, the residue becomes semisolid and is called *feces* or stools. Feces consist primarily of bacteria that normally live in the large intestine. Feces also contain undigested fiber from plant foods; some protein, water, and mucus; a small amount of fat; and cells that have been shed from the walls of the intestinal tract. Feces remain in the rectum until muscular contractions move the material into the anal canal and then out of the body through the anus.

bile substance needed for proper fat digestion

colon major structure of the large intestine

rectum lower section of the large intestine

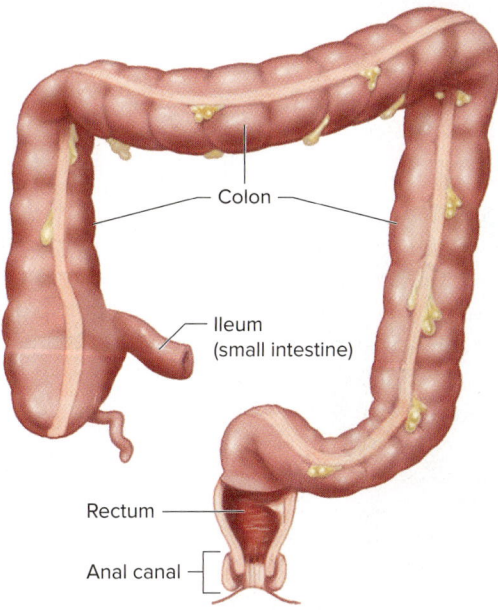

Figure 4.6 Large intestine.

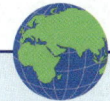

Culture & Cuisine

Kimchi (*kim-chee'*) is a traditional Korean food made with vegetables such as cabbage, cucumbers, or Korean radishes. A very popular kimchi uses leaves from fresh napa cabbages. The leaves are first carefully washed and then salted. The salt kills harmful bacteria and draws water out of the leaves so they become soft and limp. Next, the leaves are rinsed to remove the salt, and then each leaf is completely smeared with a paste-like mixture that is made with hot red chili pepper flakes, garlic, ginger, brown sugar, fish or shrimp sauce, and chopped Korean radishes, green onions, and *buchu* (Asian chives). The seasoned cabbage leaves are folded and stuffed into a sealed container, and the mixture is allowed to ferment for 1 to 5 days.

Fermentation is a natural process in which bacteria or yeast break down certain nutrients, producing acids, gases, and alcohol as a result. Many foods and beverages, including pickles, sauerkraut, yogurt, wine, and beer, are produced by fermentation.

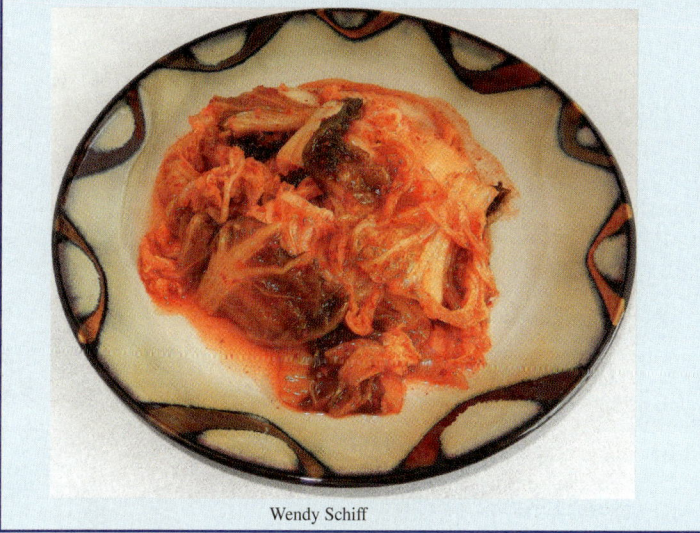

Wendy Schiff

Intestinal Bacteria A healthy person's large intestine is home to vast numbers and many types of bacteria, the "gut microbiome." These bacteria use *fermentation,* a chemical process that converts undigested food material to substances the bacteria can use for their nutrient needs. Intestinal bacteria make vitamins K and biotin, which you can absorb. These bacteria also make vitamin B-12, but it's not absorbed. Intestinal bacteria produce substances that your colon cells and, possibly, the rest of your body can use for energy. As a result of their metabolic activity, the bacteria contribute to *flatulence*—the release of intestinal gases that are expelled through your anus.

The gut microbiome plays a role in your immunity to infectious diseases. Furthermore, your risk of developing obesity, cancer, heart disease, and certain intestinal diseases may be linked to the diversity of your gut bacteria.[3,4]

Under normal conditions, the different bacterial populations that live in your gut maintain a balance that benefits your body. Starvation, antibiotic use, and excessive emotional stress can upset the normal balance of intestinal bacteria and result in intestinal infections. When you take an antibiotic for a bacterial infection, you kill the harmful bacteria that are making you sick as well as the beneficial bacteria in your large intestine. As a result, the harmful bacteria may flourish in the colon and limit the growth of the "good" bacteria.

To make yogurt, certain kinds of live bacteria (*cultures*) are added to milk. Warming the milk encourages the growth of the bacteria, which ferment the milk. Such bacteria are

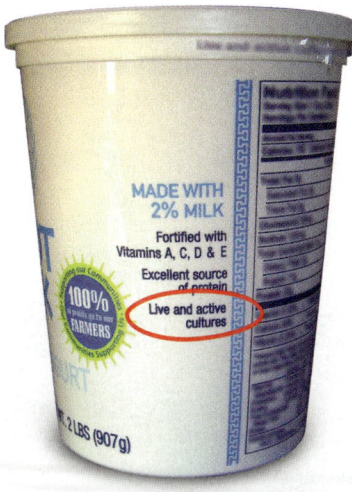

Wendy Schiff

probiotics, beneficial microbes that may help maintain or reestablish the normal balance of bacterial populations in your colon. When you buy yogurt, check the label to learn whether the product contains "live and active" cultures. You can take functional foods or dietary supplements that contain probiotics, but information about their long-term safety is unknown.[5,6] It's a good idea to check with your physician before taking such supplements.

Some kinds of intestinal bacteria can be quite harmful, and even deadly, if they enter other parts of your body or contaminate food. People should wash their hands after having bowel movements to reduce the likelihood of spreading dangerous microbes from their intestinal tract. Unit 11 discusses microorganisms that cause common food-borne infections and ways to limit your exposure to them.

probiotics live and active cultures of beneficial bacteria

4.2c Digestive System Summary

Your digestive system breaks down food into nutrients that can be absorbed and used by your body. **Figure 4.7** summarizes major functions of the organs and structures of the digestive system, including the accessory organs.

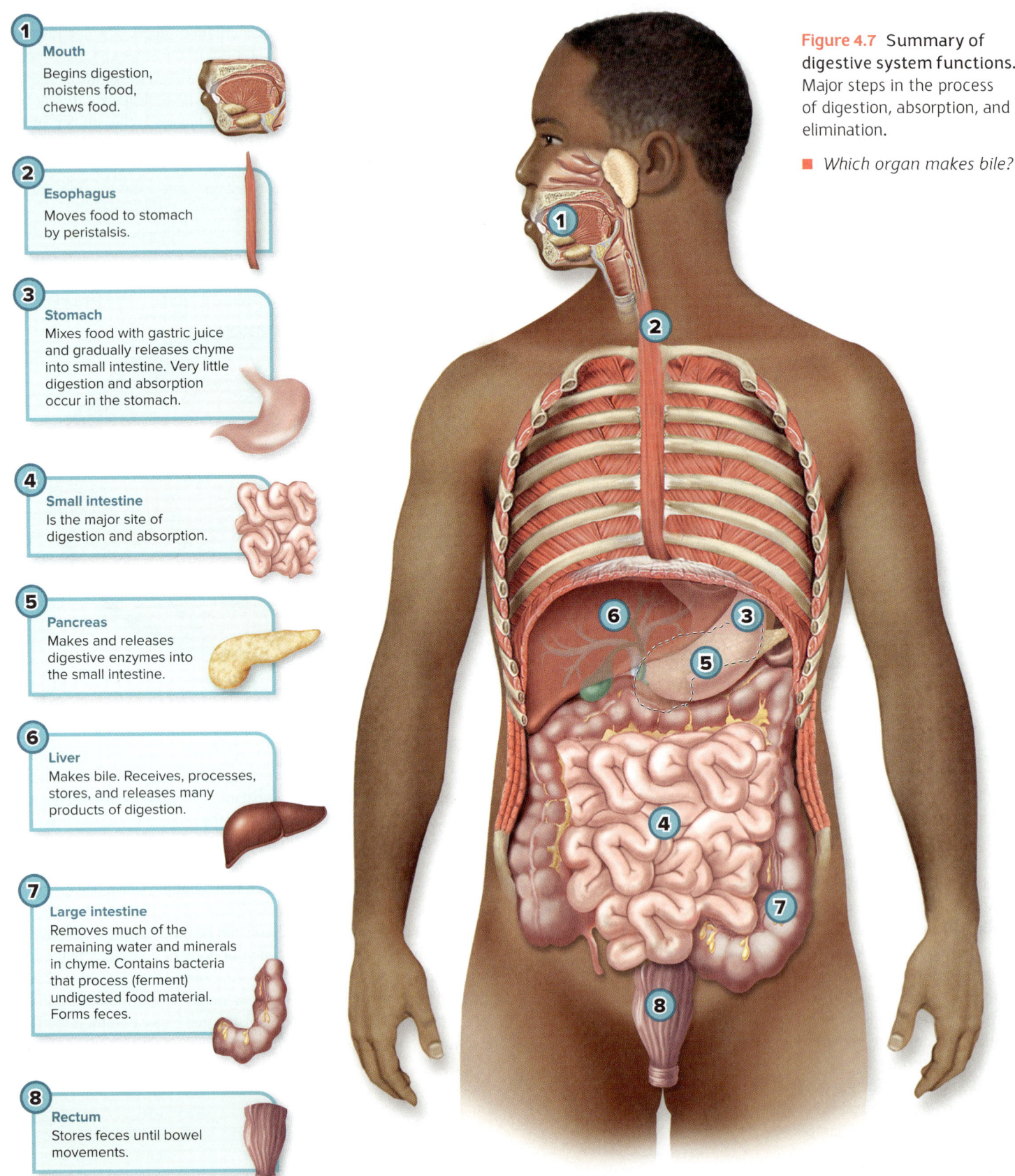

1 Mouth
Begins digestion, moistens food, chews food.

2 Esophagus
Moves food to stomach by peristalsis.

3 Stomach
Mixes food with gastric juice and gradually releases chyme into small intestine. Very little digestion and absorption occur in the stomach.

4 Small intestine
Is the major site of digestion and absorption.

5 Pancreas
Makes and releases digestive enzymes into the small intestine.

6 Liver
Makes bile. Receives, processes, stores, and releases many products of digestion.

7 Large intestine
Removes much of the remaining water and minerals in chyme. Contains bacteria that process (ferment) undigested food material. Forms feces.

8 Rectum
Stores feces until bowel movements.

Figure 4.7 Summary of digestive system functions. Major steps in the process of digestion, absorption, and elimination.

■ Which organ makes bile?

Module 4.3

Common Digestive System Disorders

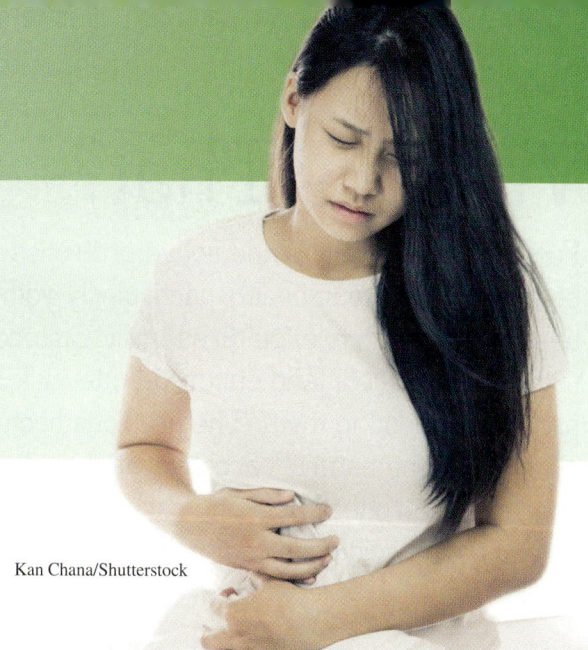

4.3 - Learning Outcomes

After reading Module 4.3, you should be able to

1. Define all of the **key terms** in this module.
2. Identify some common as well as serious digestive system problems; and discuss risk factors, preventive measures, and typical treatments for these conditions.

Kan Chana/Shutterstock

This module discusses some common disorders of the digestive system, including constipation, diarrhea, and vomiting. Information about chronic diseases of the intestinal tract, such as ulcerative colitis and colorectal cancer, is also provided.

4.3a Constipation

Although the normal frequency of bowel movements varies individually, a healthy person has at least three normal bowel movements per week.[7] When bowel movements occur less frequently and/or feces are dry and difficult or painful to eliminate, the person has **constipation**.

Many factors can reduce your frequency of bowel movements, including

- lack of dietary fiber,
- low water intake,
- lack of exercise, and
- changes in your typical routine, such as taking a long trip or having major surgery.

Furthermore, constipation can result if you regularly ignore your normal bowel urges and avoid making a trip to the bathroom when it's not convenient.

Chronic constipation can cause discomfort and may contribute to the development of swollen hemorrhoids and diverticula. **Hemorrhoids** are clusters of small veins in the anal canal that can become inflamed and swollen, causing itching and bleeding **(Fig. 4.8)**. **Diverticula** are small pouches that can form in the lining of the intestines, especially the large intestine **(Fig. 4.9)**. Diverticula can trap bacteria and feces, causing painful inflammation or infection. If diverticula become inflamed or infected, antibiotics are used, but sometimes surgery may be necessary to treat the condition (diverticulitis).

Scientists don't know what causes diverticula to form, but constipation, lack of physical activity, and excess body fat (obesity) may be risk factors.[8]

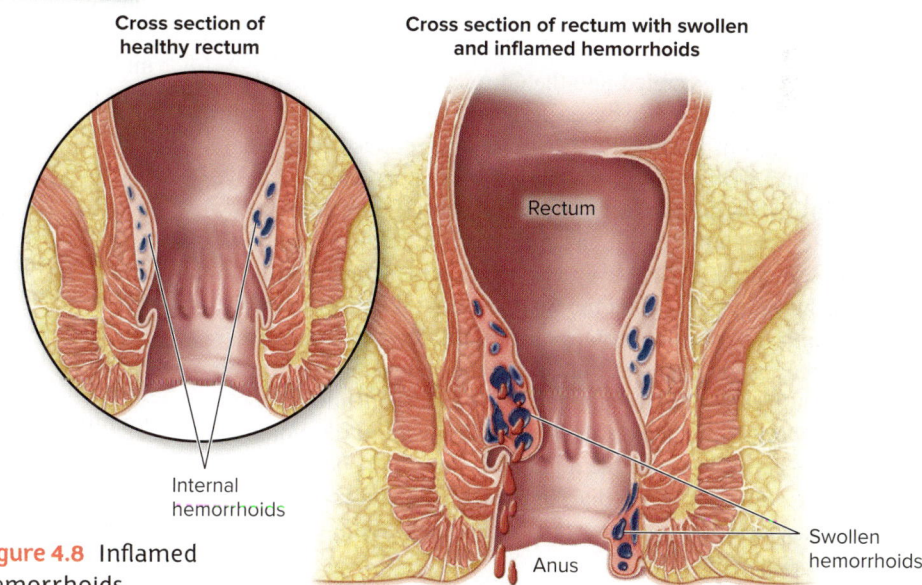

Figure 4.8 Inflamed hemorrhoids.

■ *What are inflamed hemorrhoids?*

If you're often constipated, discuss the matter with your physician. In many instances, exercising regularly and adding more fiber-rich foods to your diet is the first step to bowel "regularity." Unit 5 provides information about fiber, including rich food sources.

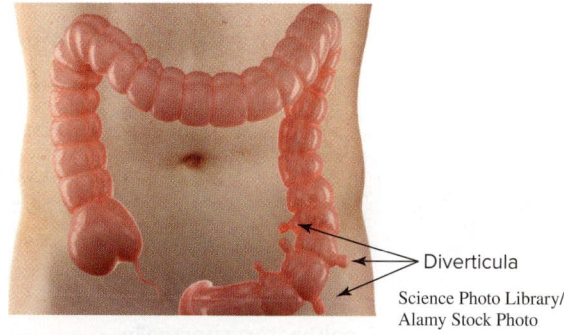

Science Photo Library/Alamy Stock Photo

Figure 4.9 Diverticula.

■ *What are diverticula?*

constipation bowel movements that occur less frequently than normal and/or are difficult to eliminate

hemorrhoids clusters of small veins in the anal canal that can become inflamed and swollen

diverticula small pouches that can form in the intestinal lining, especially the large intestine

What IS That?

Foods that contain live and active probiotics may be beneficial to your health, particularly your intestinal health. Kefir is a "cultured" milk. Cultured milks, such as kefir and cultured buttermilk, have probiotics added to them. The probiotic bacteria ferment the natural carbohydrate in milk for energy, and produce acid and carbon dioxide as a result. The acid curdles the milk and gives it a distinctive taste; the carbon dioxide provides some "fizz," like a carbonated soft drink. A 1-cup serving of kefir that's made from 2% milk supplies about the same energy and nutrient contents as 1 cup of 2% milk.

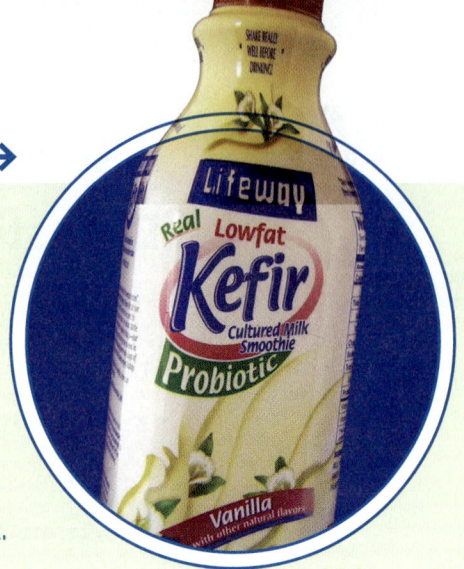
Wendy Schiff

4.3b Diarrhea

Diarrhea is a condition characterized by loose and watery stools that occur three or more times a day.[9] Diarrhea occurs when more water than normal is secreted into the GI tract or the tract absorbs less water than normal. Most cases of diarrhea result from bacterial or viral infections of the intestinal tract. The infectious bacteria or viruses produce irritating or toxic substances that increase the movements (motility) of the GI tract. As a result, the GI tract propels chyme more rapidly through it, absorbing less water than normal in the process. Increased GI motility also enables the large intestine to eliminate the watery feces and the toxic material it contains rapidly.

Loperamide, an over-the-counter medication, can be helpful for relieving an occasional bout of mild diarrhea in adults. Cases of severe diarrhea, however, require more immediate medical attention. Frequent watery stools can deplete the body's fluid volume (dehydration) and cause excessive losses of the minerals sodium and potassium. Therefore, treatment of severe diarrhea generally includes drinking watery replacement fluids that contain sodium, potassium, and simple sugars such as glucose.

Prompt treatment of severe diarrhea—within 24 to 48 hours—is especially crucial for infants and elderly people because they can become dehydrated quickly. In adults, diarrhea that's accompanied by bloody stools or lasts more than 7 days may be a sign of a serious intestinal disease, and a physician should be consulted.

Foods that contain probiotics, such as certain brands of cultured milk and yogurt, may help restore the normal bacterial population of your large intestine. More research, however, is needed to determine the most effective forms and doses of probiotics.

4.3c Vomiting

Not long after eating something toxic or drinking too much alcohol, you begin to feel queasy, or "sick to your stomach." Soon you become well aware that your body has an effective way of removing the harmful food or beverage—vomiting. Although vomiting is an unpleasant experience, it prevents toxic substances from entering your small intestine, where they can do more harm or be absorbed. Vomiting can also be a response to a food allergy, intense pain, "motion sickness," seasickness, migraine headaches, and hormonal changes in pregnancy (morning sickness).[10]

Treatment includes avoiding solid food until the vomiting resolves. Sipping small amounts of water or clear liquids, including noncarbonated soft drinks such as sports drinks, can help maintain body water. If you're able to drink small amounts of fluid without vomiting, you can try to drink increasing amounts of fluid until the vomiting subsides completely.

Vomiting generally doesn't last more than 24 hours. Repeated vomiting, however, can result in dehydration, especially if it's accompanied by diarrhea. Contact a physician when vomiting lasts longer than 2 days (adults) or is accompanied by

- dehydration (signs include dry mouth, extreme thirst, weakness, and dark-colored urine),
- severe headache or fever and stiff neck,
- abdominal pain, and/or
- rectal bleeding.[10]

Call 911 or have someone take you to an emergency room if you think you've been poisoned, there's blood in your vomit, or the vomit is green, or it looks like coffee grounds (a sign of blood that has been partially digested).

TASTY Tidbits

As mentioned in Module 4.2b, taking antibiotics can destroy healthful bacteria that normally reside in your colon. This situation can cause an imbalance in the colon's bacterial populations, resulting in diarrhea. You may be able to reduce the risk of diarrhea by consuming foods or dietary supplements that contain probiotics.[9]

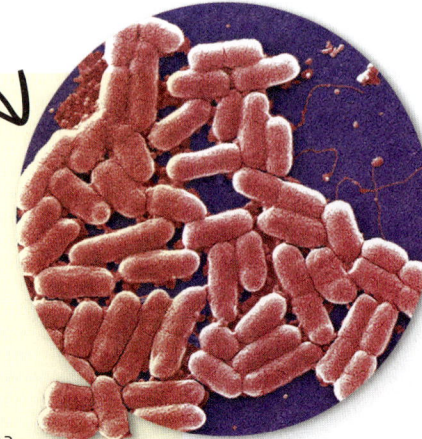
Janice Haney Carr/CDC

E. coli bacteria normally live in your colon.

4.3d Acid Reflux

If the lower esophageal sphincter doesn't function properly and opens when it should be closed, the stomach's contents can flow back into (reflux) the esophagus. This condition, gastroesophageal reflux (GER), irritates the lining of the esophagus, causing symptoms that are often referred to as "acid indigestion" or heartburn. **Heartburn** is a gnawing pain or burning sensation generally felt in the upper chest, under the breastbone. Despite the name, heartburn isn't a heart problem—it's the result of acid reflux.

Many factors can contribute to acid reflux or worsen the condition:

- being pregnant;
- having excess body fat, especially in the middle of the body;
- drinking alcohol;
- smoking cigarettes;
- lying down soon after eating a large meal; and
- consuming certain foods.

Commonly consumed foods and beverages that can contribute to acid reflux are

- fatty or greasy foods,
- tomatoes and tomato-based sauces,
- peppermint,
- coffee,
- alcohol, and
- chocolate.[11]

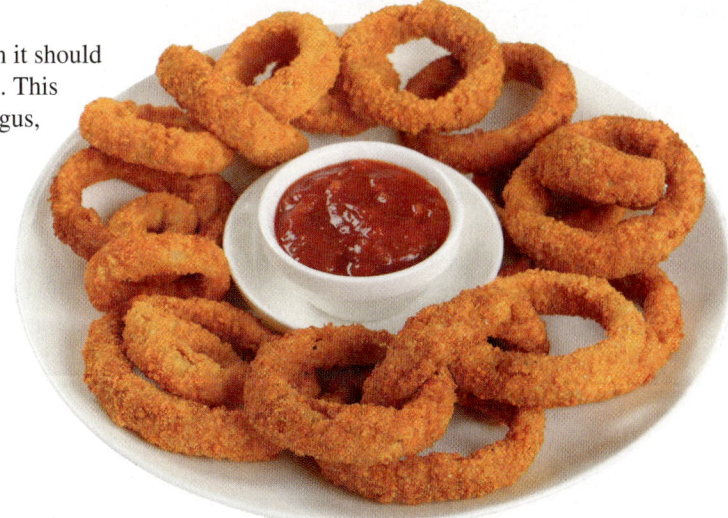

This combination is an invitation to acid reflux.

heartburn gnawing pain or burning sensation generally felt in upper chest

gastroesophageal reflux disease (GERD) chronic condition characterized by frequent heartburn

Gastroesophageal Reflux Disease

Many people think heartburn is a minor health problem that can be ignored. Frequent acid reflux, however, can be a symptom of a chronic condition—**gastroesophageal reflux disease (GERD).** Symptoms of GERD include

- acid reflux that occurs more than twice a week,
- nausea and vomiting,
- wheezing,
- chronic dry cough, and
- hoarse voice.[11]

Onion rings: from my point of view/Shutterstock;
Peppermint: Pixtal/AGE Fotostock;
Pasta with tomato sauce: Jonelle Weaver/Getty Images;
Chocolate: WR Publishing/Alamy

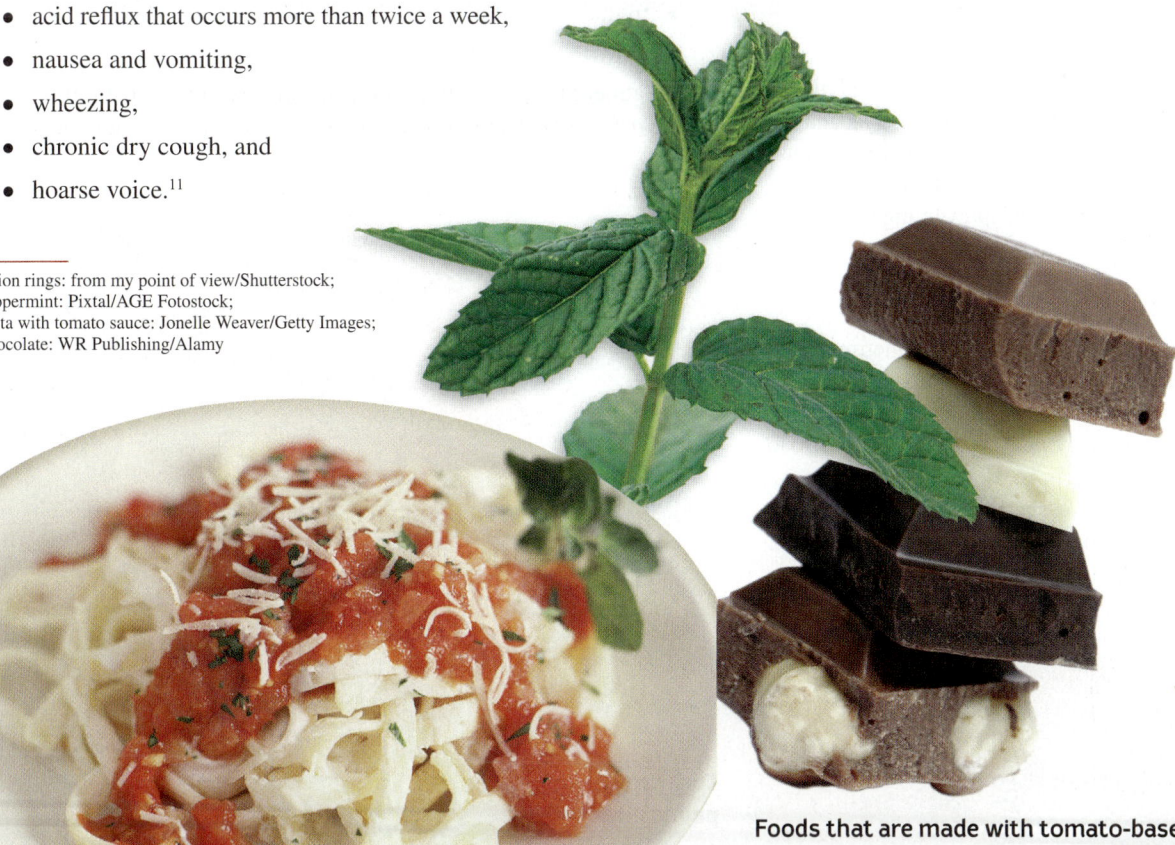

Foods that are made with tomato-based sauces, peppermint, or chocolate can contribute to acid reflux.

TASTY Tidbits

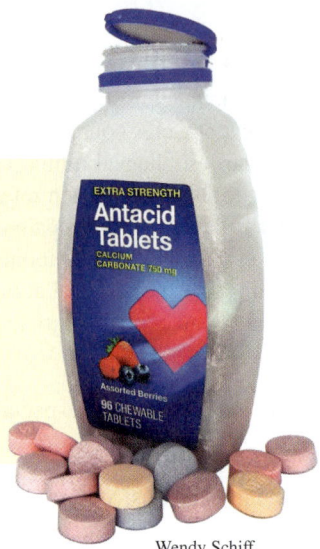

If you have mild heartburn, you can take an antacid to relieve the discomfort. Popular antacids usually include magnesium, calcium, and aluminum in forms that neutralize stomach acid. Antacids, however, can have side effects. Products that contain magnesium can cause diarrhea; aluminum- or calcium-containing antacids may cause constipation. In addition to neutralizing stomach acid, antacids that contain calcium can be a source of calcium, a mineral nutrient. Even though you can buy many kinds of antacids without prescriptions, it's a good idea to check with your physician before using them.

Wendy Schiff

To reduce your risk of heartburn and manage GERD:

- Take over-the-counter antacids to neutralize excess stomach acid and relieve heartburn after eating.
- Lose the excess weight, if you have too much belly fat.
- Do not lie down within 2 to 3 hours after eating.
- Do not overeat at mealtimes.
- Stop smoking cigarettes and avoid exposure to cigarette smoke.
- Elevate the head of your bed 6 to 8 inches higher than the foot of the bed.
- Do not wear tight belts, undergarments that flatten the abdomen, or clothes with tight waistbands.
- Avoid foods that often cause acid reflux.[11]

If you suffer from frequent heartburn and have other GERD symptoms, let your physician know about it. GERD can damage the lining of the esophagus and contribute to the development of sores called *ulcers*.

People who suffer from GERD have a higher risk of esophageal cancer than people who do not have a history of this condition. You can manage GERD by making lifestyle changes and taking medications that inhibit stomach acid production, thus preventing heartburn.

4.3e Peptic Ulcers

A **peptic ulcer** is a sore that occurs in the lining of the upper digestive tract, especially in the duodenum, stomach, and sometimes the esophagus. If the layer of mucus that protects the stomach and small intestine breaks down, HCl and protein-digesting enzymes can reach the stomach and intestinal walls, destroying the tissue. Such destruction can cause one or more ulcers to form in the damaged tissues. If an ulcer injures the wall of a blood vessel, the sore can cause serious, even life-threatening, bleeding. Therefore, it's important to recognize peptic ulcer signs and symptoms and obtain professional medical treatment.

peptic ulcer a sore that occurs in the lining of the upper GI tract

The typical sign of peptic ulcers is "dull" or burning pain that is felt in the stomach area. Pain typically begins when the stomach is empty, and the discomfort eases for a while after food is eaten or antacids are taken.[12] Uncommon but more serious signs are

- vomiting fresh blood or vomit that looks like "coffee grounds," and
- black tarry stools (sign of digested blood).

Factors that increase the risk of peptic ulcers include

- *H. pylori* infection (a bacterial infection),
- tumors of the pancreas or duodenum that cause excessive stomach acid production,
- cigarette smoking,
- heavy consumption of alcohol, and
- frequent use of nonsteroidal anti-inflammatory drugs (NSAIDs) such as aspirin, ibuprofen, and naproxen.

Treatment for peptic ulcers may include antibiotics that kill *H. pylori* and medications that control stomach acid production.

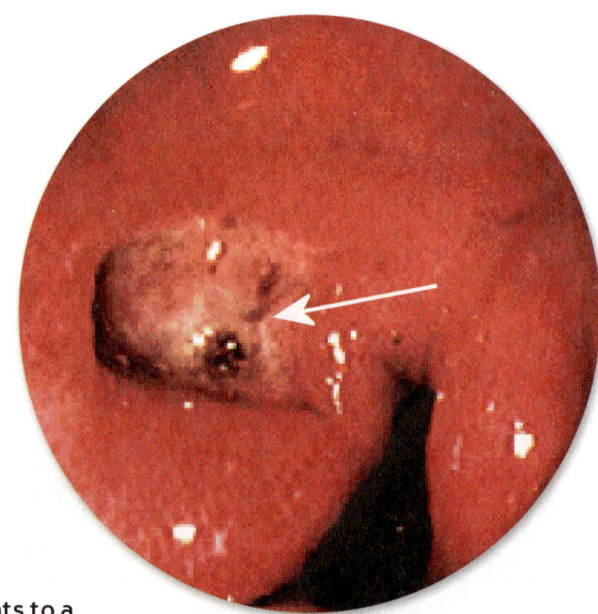

The arrow points to a peptic ulcer.

Image courtesy of Robert D. Fusco, MD, Three Rivers Endoscopy Center, Moon Township, PA www.gihealth.com

4.3f Gallstones

If you experience severe pain in the upper-right area of your midsection within an hour or two after eating a fatty meal, you may have gallstones.

Recall that the gallbladder stores bile, which is needed to digest fats properly. Gallstones form in the gallbladder (**Fig. 4.10**). The stones usually consist of cholesterol and can be small and grainy, like particles of sand, or as large as a coin or golf ball.[13] If a person has gallstones, they cause pain when the gallbladder contracts to release bile into the small intestine.

Sometimes a gallstone blocks the small passageway that carries bile to the duodenum. When this occurs, bile can back up into the liver or pancreas, injuring these organs. Surgery to remove the diseased gallbladder is necessary to relieve the pain and prevent damage to the liver or pancreas. After surgery, bile drips from the liver directly into the small intestine.

Having excess body fat increases the risk of gallstones. To reduce your risk of gallstones, keep your weight at a healthy level.

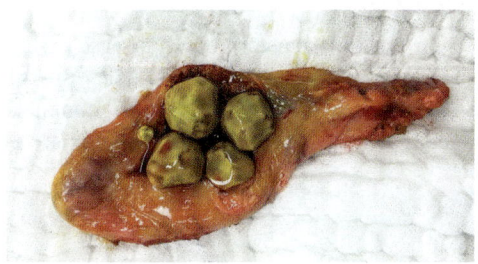

Figure 4.10 Gallbladder and gallstones. This diseased gallbladder has been cut to expose the gallstones that formed inside of it. Most gallstones contain cholesterol.

■ *Where do gallstones form?*

Q Answer This

Which of the following organs is not essential for good health: the liver, gallbladder, pancreas, or small intestine? You can find the answer on the last page of this unit.

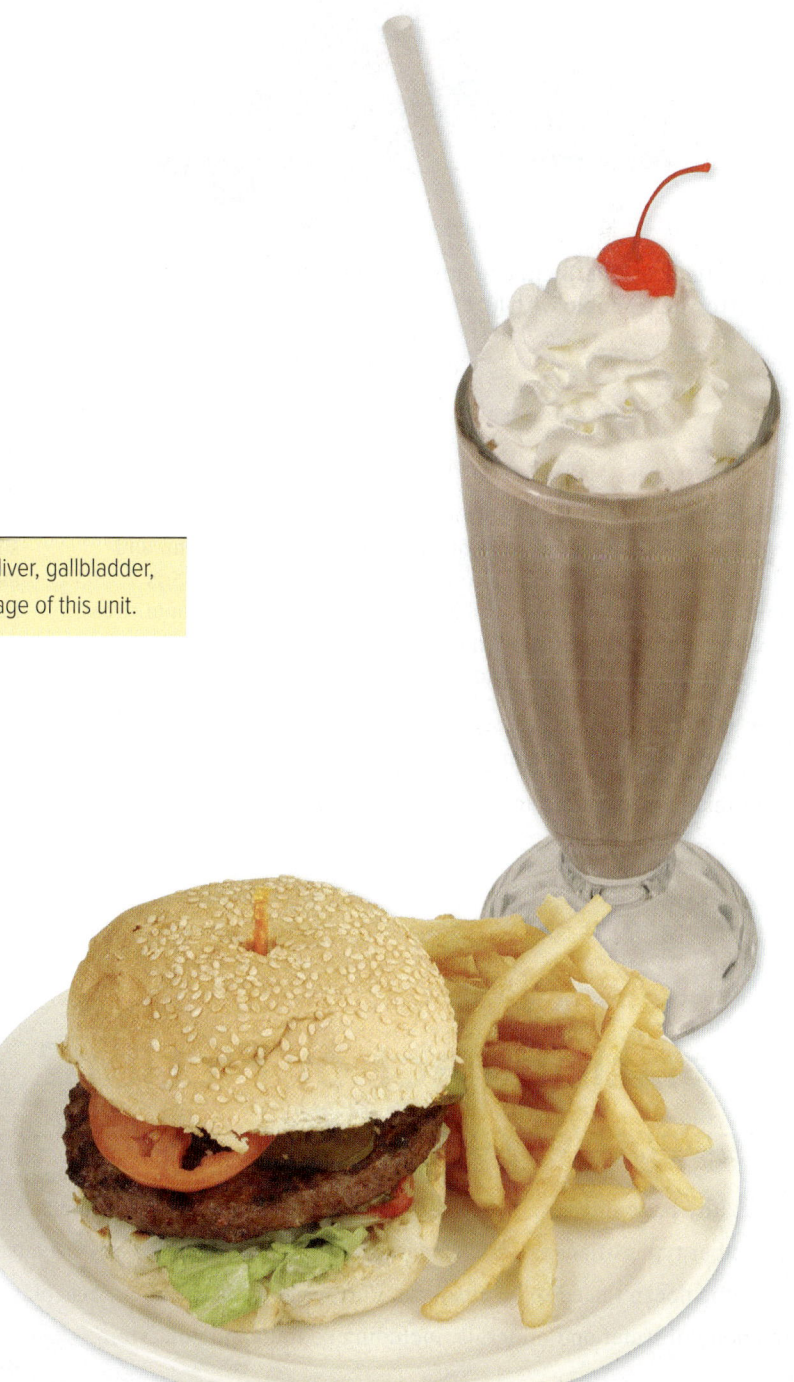

Eating a fatty meal might cause a gallbladder "attack" if you have gallstones.

Gallbladder and gallstones: Pthawatc/Shutterstock Milkshake: Ingram Publishing; Hamburger and French fries: Ingram Publishing/SuperStock

irritable bowel syndrome (IBS) chronic condition characterized by frequent bouts of intestinal cramps with diarrhea or constipation

ulcerative colitis (UC) form of inflammatory bowel disease

- learning stress management strategies;
- obtaining psychological counseling and taking antidepressants; and
- using certain probiotics.[14]

Although irritable bowel syndrome can be uncomfortable and upsetting, the condition doesn't appear to permanently harm the large intestine or increase the risk of colorectal cancer.[15]

4.3h Ulcerative Colitis

Ulcerative colitis (**UC**) is a chronic inflammatory bowel disease (IBD) that causes ulcers in the inner lining of the large intestine. As a result of the inflammation, the colon's lining erodes away, leading to abdominal cramping, rectal bleeding, and diarrhea. Other signs and symptoms include

- anemia,
- fatigue,
- fever,
- nausea, and
- appetite loss and weight loss.

Medical experts don't know what causes UC. People with the disease may have immune systems that react abnormally to bacteria in their digestive tract. UC tends to "run in families," so genetic factors are suspected to play a role in its development.[16] Although emotional stress doesn't cause UC, people with the disease report that stressful situations seem to worsen their symptoms. Furthermore, food allergies aren't the cause of UC. However, some people with the disease learn to avoid certain foods and beverages because consuming them seems to trigger bouts of the illness. Dietary recommendations generally include eating smaller meals more often, drinking more liquids but avoiding carbonated drinks, and avoiding high-fiber foods, especially when symptoms occur.

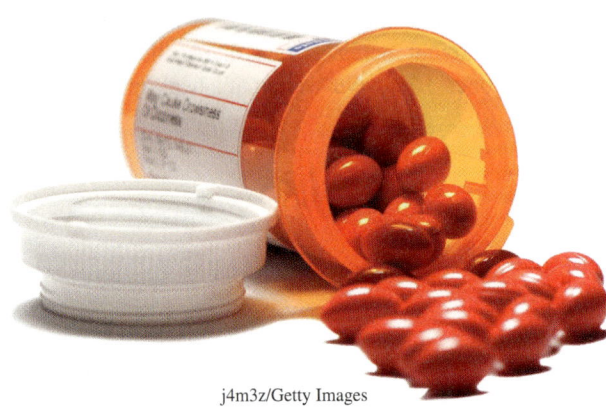

j4m3z/Getty Images

Taking medications, including antidepressants, can often help people with IBS.

4.3g Irritable Bowel Syndrome (IBS)

Many adult Americans suffer from **irritable bowel syndrome (IBS)**. People with IBS experience frequent bouts of abdominal pain and bloating with diarrhea and/or constipation. The cause of IBS is unknown, but certain foods and beverages as well as emotional stress, anxiety, and depression may trigger the disorder.

Treatment for IBS is individualized and may include

- eliminating foods that seem to trigger IBS symptoms (see Unit 5, section 5.3f, "What Are FODMAPs?");
- taking medications to relieve constipation, diarrhea, and abdominal pain;

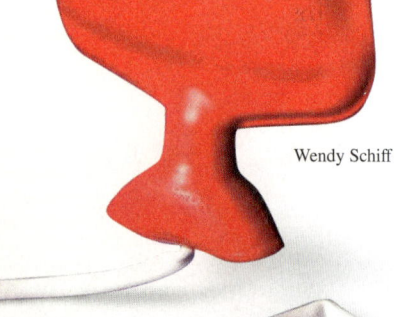

Wendy Schiff

Nutrition Fact or Fiction?

Regular colon cleansing is necessary for good health.

A healthy large intestine doesn't store toxins or large amounts of feces. Using "high colonics" and other types of enemas to "cleanse" your colon isn't necessary because the large intestine doesn't need to be cleansed. Furthermore, frequent enemas may deplete the body of water and minerals, including sodium and potassium.

Currently, scientists are studying probiotics to see if they can be helpful in treating UC.

There's no cure for UC. Treatment generally includes medications to reduce inflammation. People with UC generally must take the medication for the rest of their lives, unless their large intestine is so severely diseased that surgical removal of the organ is necessary.

Patients with UC have an increased risk of colon cancer, especially when their entire colon is affected and they've had the disease for 8 or more years.[16] Patients can reduce their risk of colon cancer by managing the inflammation with medication and having regular screening (testing) to detect colon cancer. Because of the risk of colon cancer, UC is a more serious medical condition than irritable bowel syndrome (IBS; see section 4.3g).

4.3i Colorectal Cancer

Normally, cells grow and divide to form new cells as the body needs them. When cells grow old, they die. Sometimes, new cells divide and grow more rapidly than normal cells. Furthermore, these cells don't function normally, and they invade nearby tissues, often forming a mass of tissue called a *tumor*. Such abnormal cells are cancer cells.

Cancerous (*malignant*) cells spread (*metastasize*) to other parts of the body, may grow back after being removed surgically, and can be life-threatening. Cancer that starts in either the colon or the rectum is often called **colorectal cancer (Fig. 4.11).**

In the United States, colorectal cancer is the third-leading cause of cancer deaths among adults.[17] Lung cancer is the leading cause of cancer deaths among Americans. Unit 8 provides more information about cancer and the role of diet in cancer development.

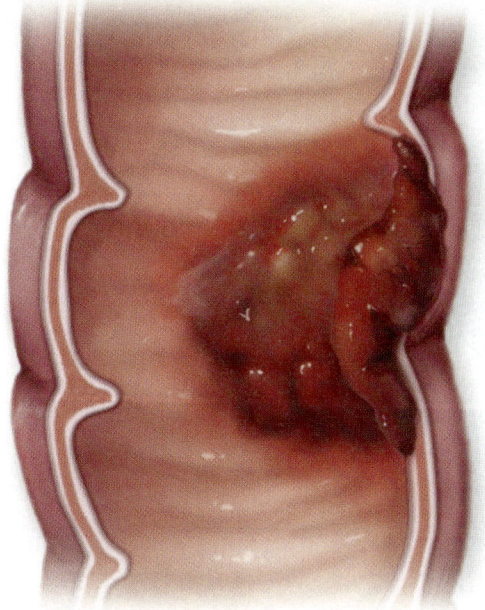

Figure 4.11 This illustration shows a large cancerous tumor in the colon.

■ *What steps can you take to reduce your risk of colorectal cancer?*

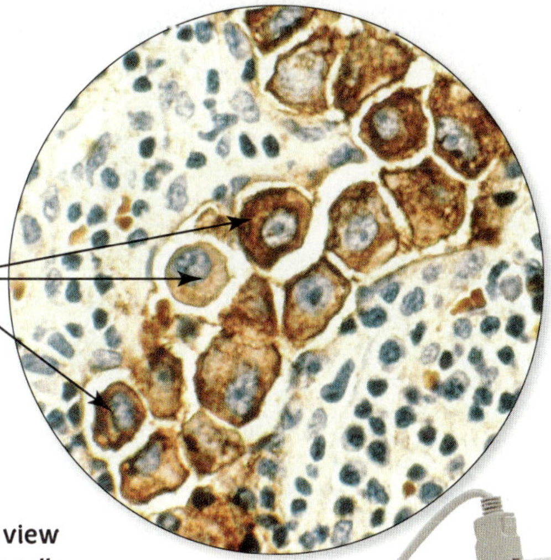

What Are the Signs and Symptoms of Colorectal Cancer?

Signs and symptoms of colorectal cancer include

- having diarrhea or constipation that persists,
- feeling that your bowel doesn't empty completely after bowel movements,
- finding blood (either bright red or very dark) in your stools,
- noticing that your stools are narrower than usual,
- losing weight without trying,
- feeling very tired all the time, and
- having abdominal cramps or pain.

Cancer cells

Microscopic view of cancerous cells

Dr. Lance Liotta Laboratory/National Cancer Institute

colorectal cancer cancer that starts in either the colon or the rectum

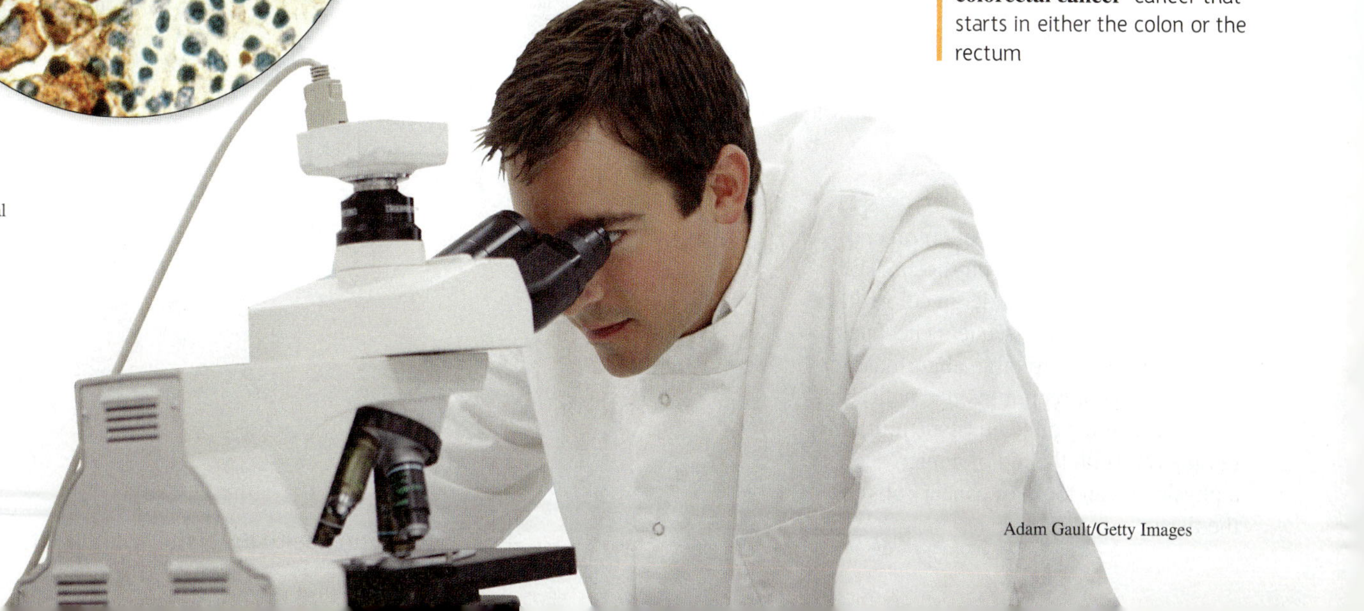

Adam Gault/Getty Images

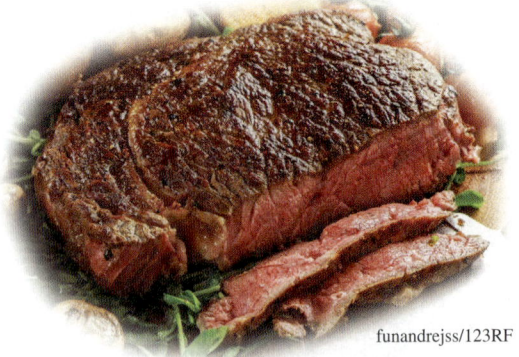

Eating lots of red meat may increase your risk of colorectal cancer.

Treatment Options

Treatment for colorectal cancer usually involves surgery, chemotherapy, biological therapy, or radiation therapy. Surgery removes the diseased areas of the large intestine. Chemotherapy uses drugs to kill cancer cells. Biological therapy involves using antibodies, which are special proteins that detect and bind to colorectal cancer cells. This treatment interferes with the cancer cells' ability to grow and spread. Radiation therapy uses high-energy rays to kill cancer cells. Although surgery is the most common treatment for colorectal cancer, people often undergo a combination of treatments.

Figure 4.12 shows the digestive system organs that are affected by the health problems discussed in this module. Some other disorders that affect the digestive system, such as food allergies and celiac disease, are discussed in Unit 7.

Who Is at Risk?

The following characteristics increase a person's risk of developing colorectal cancer:

- being over 50 years of age;
- having colorectal *polyps* (paw´-lips). Polyps are small clumps of tissue that grow on the inner wall of the colon or rectum. Most polyps are not cancerous, but some can become cancer;
- having a family history of colorectal cancer. If your close relatives have had colorectal cancer, your risk of the disease is high;
- having a personal history of cancer. If you've already had colorectal cancer, you're at risk of developing colorectal cancer again;
- having ulcerative colitis or Crohn's disease, another type of inflammatory bowel disease (IBD);
- eating a lot of red meat and processed meat, which includes ham, "deli" meat, and sausage;[17]
- having too much body fat and/or being physically inactive;
- smoking cigarettes; and
- drinking alcohol.

If you have a high risk of colorectal cancer, check with your physician. The doctor may have you undergo colorectal screenings and more frequent checkups. If tests show a polyp or an abnormal area in your colon or rectum, you may need to have some of the affected tissue removed (a *biopsy*). With the aid of a microscope, a physician can look for cancer cells in the tissue.

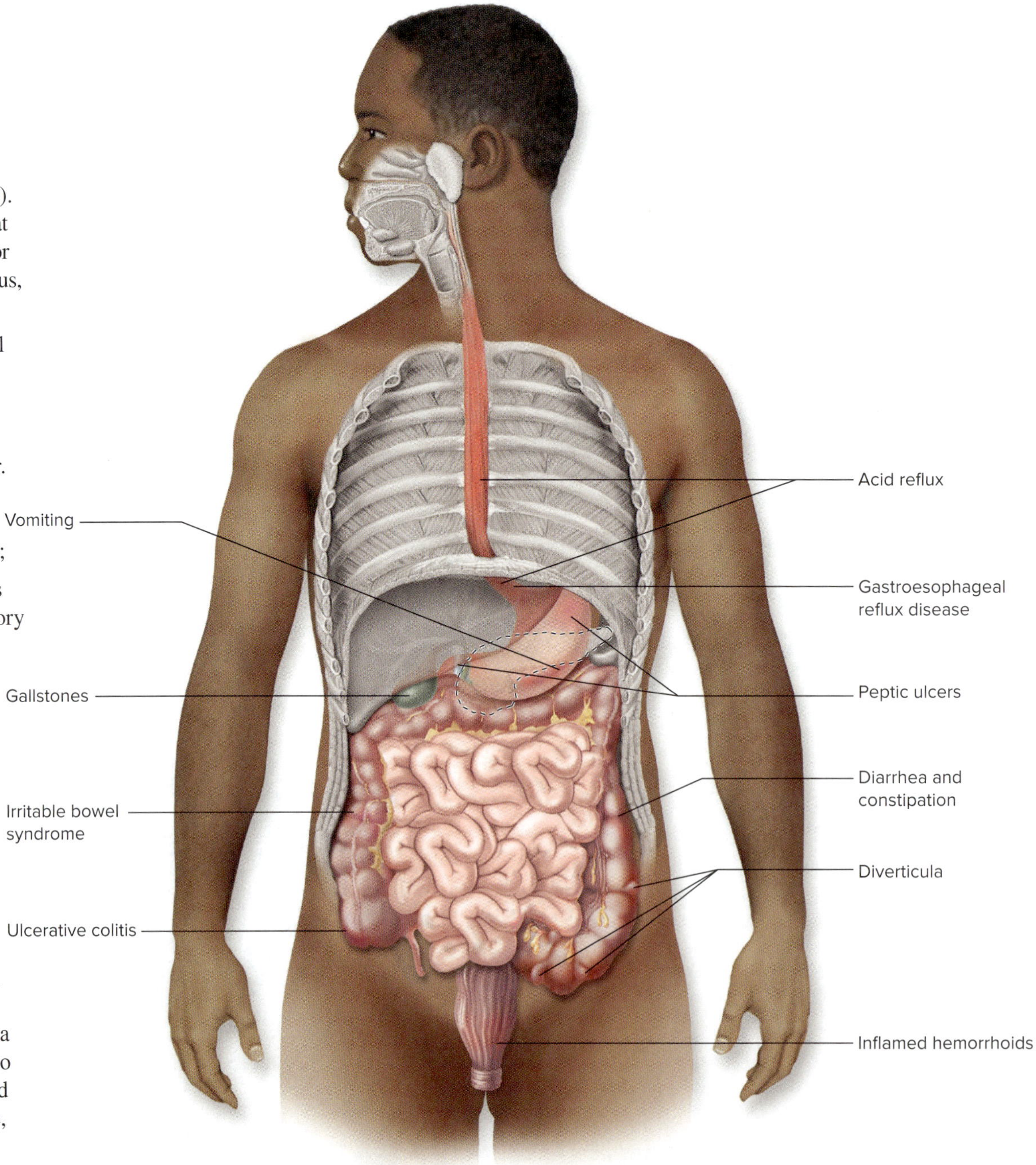

Figure 4.12 Sites of common health problems that affect the GI tract.

Module 4.4
Metabolism Basics

4.4 - Learning Outcomes
After reading Module 4.4, you should be able to
1. Define all of the **key terms** in this module.
2. Identify anabolic and catabolic processes.
3. Identify factors that influence the amount of ATP production.

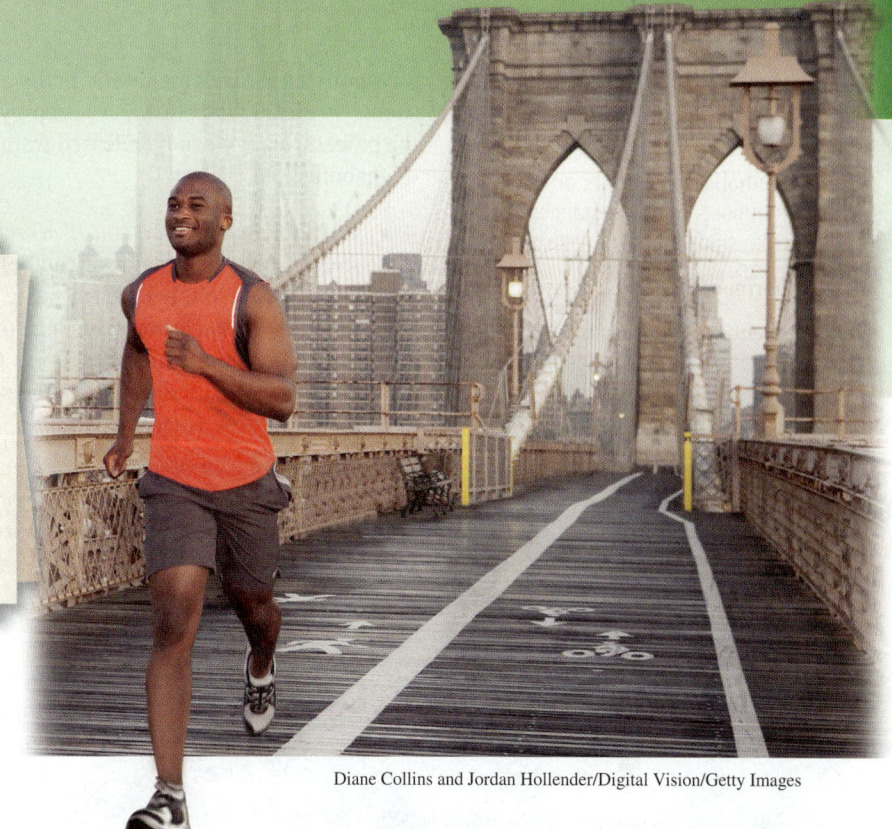

Diane Collins and Jordan Hollender/Digital Vision/Getty Images

4.4a A Remarkable Machine

In essence, your body is very much like a car engine—both are complex systems that need to generate energy, remove wastes, store excess energy until needed, and maintain a proper running temperature. Your body, the "human machine," is even more amazing than a car because it can repair, maintain, and even build itself. Furthermore, the human machine can run on a variety of "biological" fuels derived from the foods and beverages it consumes: glucose (a carbohydrate), fat, and protein. Although you don't have a section of your body that is a fuel reservoir (like a gas tank), you can store large amounts of energy in your liver, muscles, and body fat. When you use your muscles for a long period of time without consuming food, you may feel as though you've "run out of gas." You can, of course, replenish your fuel supply by resting and consuming food. Like a car, your body's performance can be improved dramatically when it has access to an adequate and high-quality fuel supply.

energy capacity to perform work

Energy Metabolism

Energy is the capacity to perform work. There are several forms of energy, including chemical, mechanical, electrical, heat, solar, and nuclear. Human cells use chemical energy to perform work. Although energy can neither be created nor destroyed, it can undergo transformations. Chemical energy, for example, can change into heat energy, which explains why a car's engine heats up as it burns gasoline and your muscles warm up during exercise.

The cells in your body release, transfer, and use energy constantly. Energy enables you to move, breathe, and perform other familiar activities. Your cells obtain energy by breaking down certain nutrients to release the chemical energy that's stored in them. It's important to remember that only carbohydrates, lipids, proteins, and alcohol can be *metabolized* ("burned") for energy; cells cannot release energy from vitamins, minerals, or water.

Metabolism is the sum of all chemical reactions that occur in living cells, including the reactions that release energy from macronutrients, make proteins, and eliminate waste products. Energy

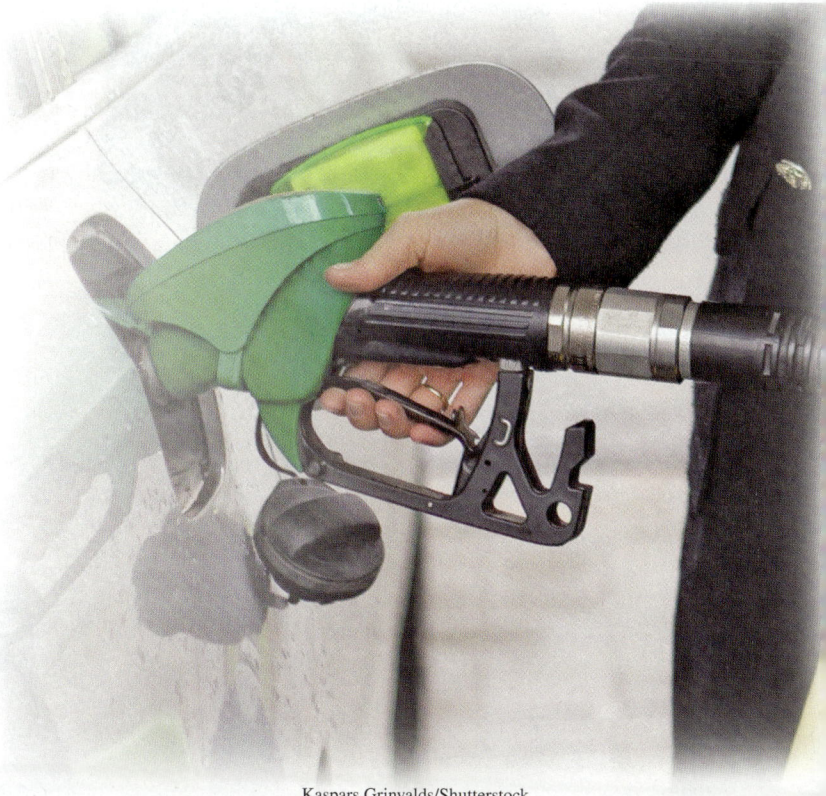

Kaspars Grinvalds/Shutterstock

catabolism metabolic processes that break down larger substances into smaller ones

anabolism metabolic processes that build larger substances from smaller ones

hormones chemical messengers

adenosine triphosphate (ATP) "energy currency" of cells

aerobic metabolism metabolic pathways that require oxygen

anaerobic metabolism metabolic pathway that functions without oxygen

metabolism involves metabolic pathways that enable your body to obtain and use energy from macronutrients. A metabolic pathway is a step-by-step process that converts compounds to new compounds. During the process, energy can be released from or gained by the compounds. Metabolic reactions may be catabolic or anabolic.

- **Catabolism** (*kuh-tab'-oh-lizm*) refers to metabolic processes that break down larger substances into smaller ones. Examples of catabolic reactions include the breakdown of a fatty acid to release energy. As a result, cells form waste products, carbon dioxide, and water. When you exhale, your lungs remove excess carbon dioxide. Your body can use the water that was formed during catabolic reactions in other chemical reactions. Otherwise, the excess water is removed when you exhale, sweat, or urinate. Heat comprises some of the energy that's released—"heat of metabolism" helps the body maintain its normal temperature.

- **Anabolism** (*an-ab'-oh-lizm*) refers to metabolic processes that build larger substances from smaller ones. Such processes generally store energy for future use. Anabolic reactions include those involved in making proteins, bones, and hormones. **Hormones** are chemicals that your body uses to transmit messages.

What Is ATP?

Much of the energy released by catabolic reactions is captured in a chemical form in the energy molecule **adenosine triphosphate** (*ah-den'-oh-seen try-fos'-fate*) **(ATP).** ATP is often referred to as "energy currency" because it functions like money. Just as you save money until it's needed to make a purchase, your cells save energy in ATP until it's needed to power cellular work. Your cells "earn" ATP in energy-releasing catabolic reactions and "spend" ATP in energy-requiring anabolic reactions.

Aerobic and Anaerobic Energy Metabolism

Cells require oxygen to produce the maximum number of ATP molecules from the catabolism of macronutrients. When adequate oxygen is present in a cell, the cell can make lots of ATP **(aerobic metabolism).** When the ATP supply is inadequate, cells can still obtain the molecule using a metabolic pathway that doesn't require oxygen **(anaerobic metabolism).** Compared to aerobic metabolism, however, much less ATP is made under low-oxygen conditions. When you exercise vigorously for an extended period, your lungs and circulatory system cannot deliver enough oxygen to your muscle cells to maintain adequate ATP production. As a result, you can't sustain the vigorous physical activity. You "run out of gas" and must slow down your pace. In Unit 10, Module 10.5 provides more information about energy metabolism, including how exercise can influence the proportions of macronutrients used for energy.

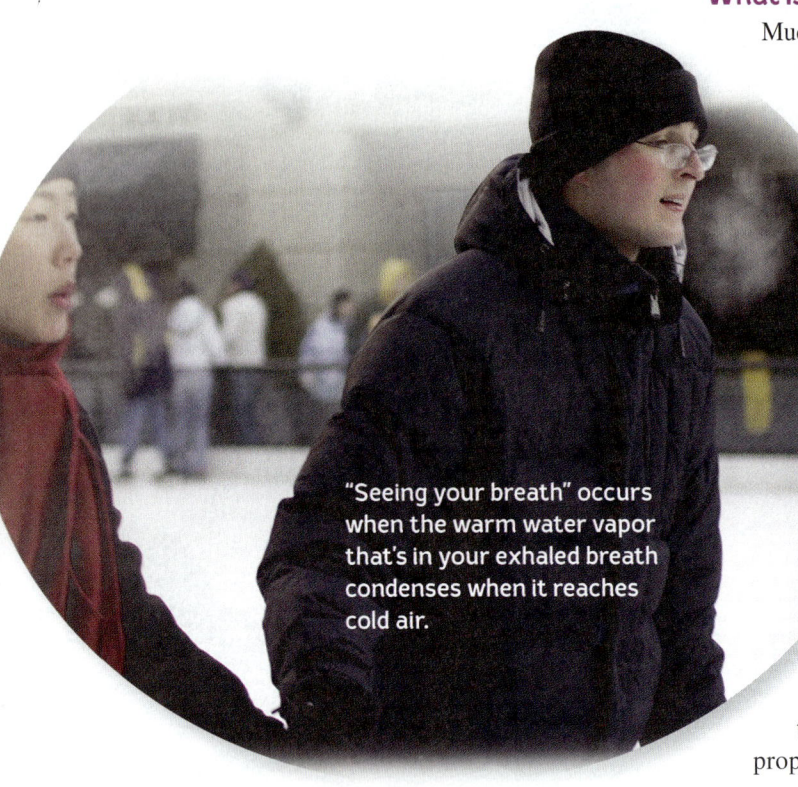

"Seeing your breath" occurs when the warm water vapor that's in your exhaled breath condenses when it reaches cold air.

Christopher Kerrigan/McGraw-Hill Education

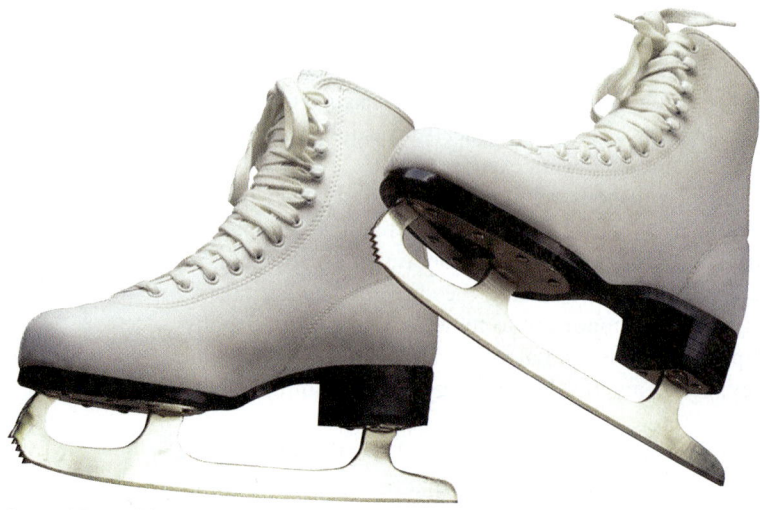

Comstock Images/Alamy

Biological Fuels

Your cells rely heavily on fat and glucose for energy. Under normal conditions, your cells don't metabolize much protein for energy. Cells in the central nervous system (CNS) depend primarily on glucose, rather than fats or proteins, to meet their energy needs. If glucose is unavailable, however, most cells (including those of the CNS) are resourceful in that they can burn more than one fuel, especially fat, for energy. **Figure 4.13** provides a basic summary of some metabolic pathways that dietary protein, carbohydrate, and fat follow during energy metabolism. For more detailed information about major metabolic pathways that cells use to obtain ATP, see **Appendix C.**

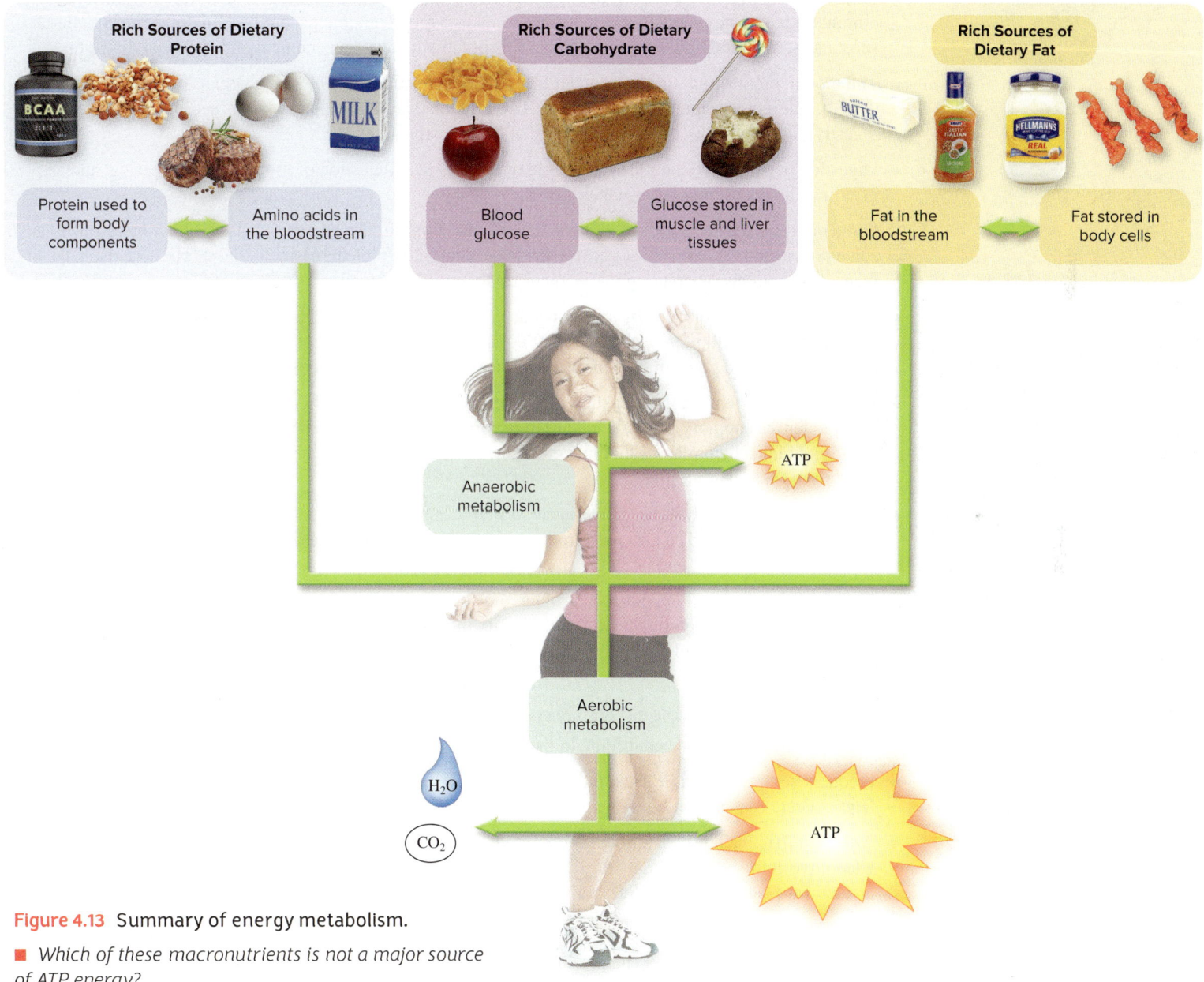

Figure 4.13 Summary of energy metabolism.

■ *Which of these macronutrients is not a major source of ATP energy?*

BCAA container: Alex Mit/Shutterstock; Mixed nuts: Sandra van der Steen/Alamy Stock Photo; Beef steaks: MaraZe/Shutterstock; Three white eggs: dancestrokes/123RF; Milk carton: Hurst Photo/Shutterstock; Pile of uncooked shell pasta: Jennifer Barrow/Alamy Stock Photo; Whole apple: Getty Images; Loaf of bread: Everyday Images/Alamy; Swirl lollipop: jirkaejc/123RF; Baked potato: Christopher Kerrigan/McGraw-Hill Education; A stick of butter: McGraw-Hill Education; Bottle of Italian dressing: Steve Cukrov/Shutterstock; Jar of Hellmann's mayonnaise: chrisdorney/Shutterstock; Bacon strips: Ingram Publishing/Alamy

In a Nutshell

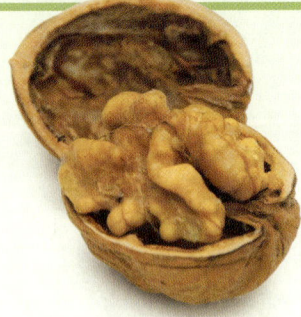

Module 4.1 From Cells to Systems
- Cells are the basic living units of the body. Masses of cells that have similar characteristics and functions form tissues. An organ is a collection of tissues that function in a related way. An organ system is a collection of organs that work together for a similar purpose.

Module 4.2 Digestive System
- Your digestive system processes food into nutrients, absorbs the nutrients into the bloodstream, and eliminates the waste products. During digestion, large food components are broken down into smaller substances, including individual nutrients. This process involves mechanical and chemical digestion.
- The mouth, esophagus, stomach, and small and large intestines are the major organs of the digestive system. The teeth, tongue, salivary glands, liver, gallbladder, and pancreas are accessory organs of the digestive system that assist the functioning of the digestive tract.
- Digestion begins in the mouth. Teeth begin the mechanical digestion of food by biting, tearing, and grinding chunks of food into smaller pieces.
- Some mechanical and chemical digestion occurs in the stomach. The enzymes in gastric juice break down some protein and fat; hydrochloric acid in the juice helps make proteins easier to digest. The acid also kills many dangerous disease-causing microorganisms that may be in food.
- Most nutrient digestion and absorption occur in the small intestine. The lining of the small intestine is covered by villi. Villi secrete enzymes that complete digestion. Proteins break down into amino acids, fats into fatty acids and glycerol, and most dietary carbohydrates into glucose.
- Absorptive cells remove the breakdown products of digestion from chyme. Nutrients that dissolve in water enter the capillary network and are transported to the liver by a large vein. Water-insoluble nutrients are formed into chylomicrons that move into lacteals. The lymphatic system transports chylomicrons away from the small intestine.
- The liver processes and stores many nutrients and makes cholesterol and bile. The gallbladder stores bile until it is needed. The pancreas produces and secretes most of the enzymes that break down carbohydrates, protein, and fat in the small intestine.
- Little additional absorption other than water and some minerals takes place in the large intestine. Feces consist primarily of bacteria that normally live in the large intestine. Feces also contain undigested fiber from plant foods; a small amount of fat, protein, and water; and mucus and cells shed from the walls of the intestinal tract.

Module 4.3 Common Digestive System Disorders
- Chronic constipation may contribute to the development of inflamed hemorrhoids and diverticula.
- Frequent acid reflux can be a symptom of GERD. People with GERD are at risk of esophageal cancer. Peptic ulcers can cause life-threatening bleeding.
- Although irritable bowel syndrome is common, the condition doesn't cause cancer of the large intestine. Ulcerative colitis is an inflammatory disease of the large intestine. In the United States, colorectal cancer is the third-leading cancer killer of adults.

Module 4.4 Metabolism Basics
- Metabolism is the sum of all chemical reactions that occur in living cells. Your cells obtain energy by breaking down macronutrients to release the chemical energy that's stored in them. Metabolic reactions can be catabolic or anabolic.
- Much of the energy released by catabolic reactions is captured in ATP. Cells use "ATP-energy" to power chemical reactions. Your cells "earn" ATP in energy-releasing catabolic reactions, and "spend" ATP in energy-requiring anabolic reactions. Glucose and fat are major sources of ATP-energy for your cells.

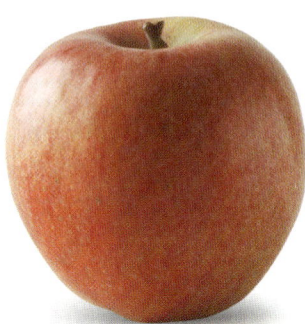

I. Rozenbaum/PhotoAlto

Design elements: Spiral notebook paper background, Stacked paper with clip background, Marginal note clip, and Culture & Cuisine globe icon: ©McGraw-Hill Education; In a Nutshell walnut; ©McGraw-Hill Education/Mark A. Dierker, photographer; Test Yourself red pepper: Iconotec/Glow Images

Consider This...

1. When you were 5 years old, why did you refuse to eat liver and onions?
2. Your sister hasn't been feeling well lately. This morning, she vomited what appears to be coffee grounds, but she doesn't drink coffee. Based on this information, your sister should see a physician because she might have which common digestive tract disorder?
3. Taylor had a serious condition that required removal of the upper third of his small intestine. Based on this information, is Taylor at risk for developing multiple nutrient deficiencies? Explain why or why not.
4. Your mother complains of having persistent heartburn, but she doesn't think her discomfort is serious enough to be investigated by her physician. Do you agree or disagree with her attitude about heartburn? Explain your position.
5. Twenty-year-old Barry is worried about his risk of colorectal cancer because one of his grandfathers died of the disease. What steps can he take to reduce his risk of the disease?
6. Mary is an 80-year-old woman who has a weak epiglottis. Based on this information, what would you expect to be her main sign of this condition?

Test Yourself

Select the best answer.

1. A _____ is a group of similar cells that perform similar functions.
   a. ribosome
   b. tissue
   c. cytoplasm
   d. system

2. Which of the following organs isn't an accessory organ of the digestive system?
   a. Stomach
   b. Pancreas
   c. Liver
   d. Gallbladder

3. Hydrochloric acid production occurs in the
   a. mouth.
   b. stomach.
   c. small intestine.
   d. liver.

4. Chemicals that help break down or make substances are called
   a. enzymes.
   b. cells.
   c. capillaries.
   d. hormones.

5. Tiny, fingerlike projections of the small intestine that absorb nutrients are called
   a. capillaries.
   b. villi.
   c. duodenum.
   d. chyme.

6. A lacteal is a
   a. special structure in the small intestine that digests milk proteins.
   b. form of carbohydrate in milk.
   c. muscular structure that regulates the movement of chyme in the large intestine.
   d. lymph vessel in a villus.

7. Glands in the mouth secrete
   a. saliva.
   b. hydrochloric acid.
   c. bile.
   d. hormones.

8. Peristalsis
   a. is a common intestinal infection.
   b. interferes with lipid absorption in the small intestine.
   c. stimulates cancer formation in the colon.
   d. helps move food/chyme through the digestive tract.

9. Your cells use ____ as a source of direct energy.
   a. ATP
   b. bile
   c. amino acids
   d. GERD

10. Which of the following practices increases the risk of peptic ulcers?
    a. Chewing gum
    b. Smoking cigarettes
    c. Drinking milk
    d. Eating probiotics

11. Catabolism includes which of the following situations?
    a. Production of red blood cells
    b. "Growth spurt" experienced by a 13-year-old
    c. Weight loss that occurs in a patient with cancer
    d. Increase in muscle tissue after 2 weeks of weight lifting

12. Which of the following recommendations may reduce your risk of colorectal cancer?
    a. Increasing sodium intake to 3500 mg/day
    b. Drinking at least 8 fl oz of beer or wine daily
    c. Eating less red meat and processed meat
    d. Reducing physical activity to 3 times per week

Answers: 1.b 2.a 3.b 4.a 5.b 6.d 7.a 8.d 9.a 10.b 11.c 12.c

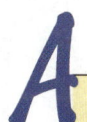

Answer This (Module 4.3f)

Gallbladder

References → See Appendix D.

Darren Greenwood/Design Pics

Unit 5
Carbohydrates
FUEL AND FIBER

What's on the Menu?

Module 5.1
Sugars, Sweeteners, Starches, and Fiber

Module 5.2
What Happens to the Carbohydrates You Eat?

Module 5.3
Carbohydrates and Health

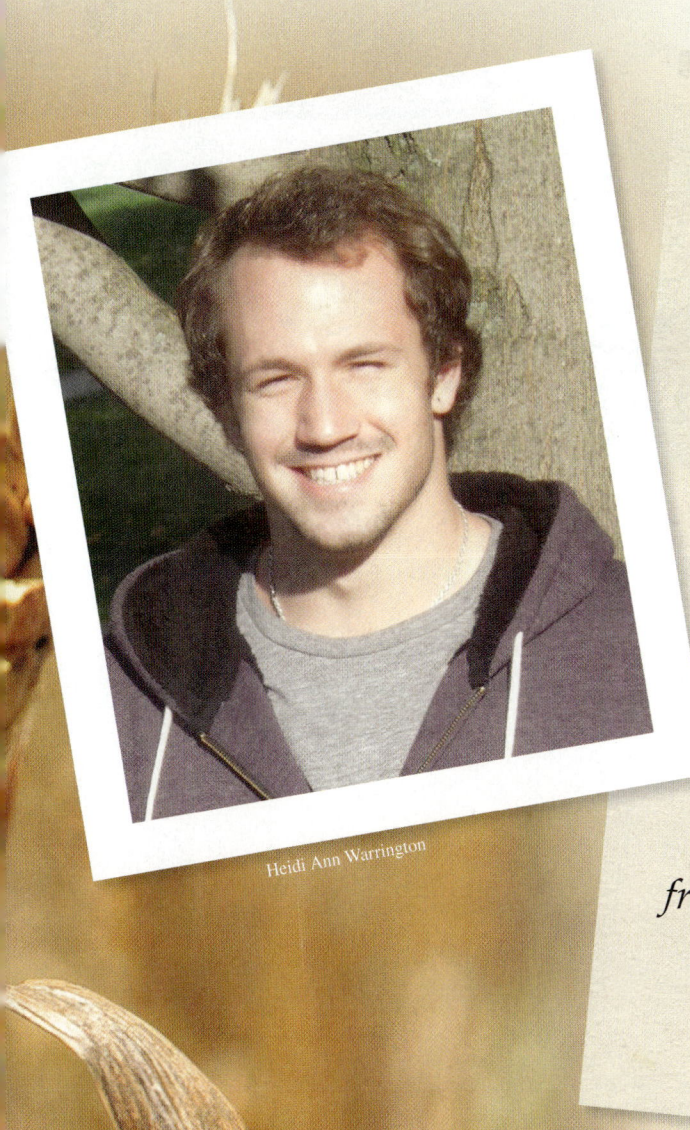
Heidi Ann Warrington

"I'd like to think my diet is pretty healthy. I like fruit, especially strawberries and bananas, and I love sandwiches made with whole-grain bread, turkey, and chicken. I try to avoid soft drinks because they have a lot of high-fructose corn syrup. From what I understand, high-fructose corn syrup is one of the leading causes of obesity. I avoid foods that contain the syrup, and I use honey to sweeten foods instead of sugar. I love honey! I think it's a healthier substitute for sugar, and I like the taste. I try not to eat sweets, but I'm not some kind of health guru. . . . I love cake! My favorite food is chocolate cake with white frosting and colored sprinkles."

Neill Warrington

If you're like **Neill Warrington,** a recent graduate of the University of Maryland, you enjoy eating cake and frosting, but you're concerned about your intake of other sugary baked goods and "sweets," especially "regular" soft drinks that are sweetened with manufactured high-fructose corn syrup. In 2017, each American consumed an estimated 73 pounds of added caloric sweeteners.[1] Such sweeteners include natural products such as honey and pure maple syrup as well as more refined sweeteners such as high-fructose corn syrup, table sugar, and powdered sugar, which is used to make cake frosting. Added caloric sweeteners are sources of "empty calories" that offer little nutritional value other than carbohydrates to your diet. Eating too much food that contains such sweeteners may reduce your desire to eat more nutrient-dense foods.

Are all carbohydrates unhealthy? How many "carbs" does the body need? Is honey a more nutritious sweetener than sugar? Does eating too much high-fructose corn syrup cause excess weight gain or any other health problems? What is lactose intolerance? What is dietary fiber? In Unit 5, you'll learn about carbohydrates, including which carbohydrate-rich foods are better sources of nutrients and healthier than others.

Module 5.1

Sugars, Sweeteners, Starches, and Fiber

5.1 - Learning Outcomes

After reading Module 5.1, you should be able to

1. Define all of the **key terms** in this module.
2. Identify the major carbohydrates in your diet as well as their primary food sources and functions in your body.
3. Recognize chemical and common names of nutritive sweeteners and identify common alternative sweeteners.

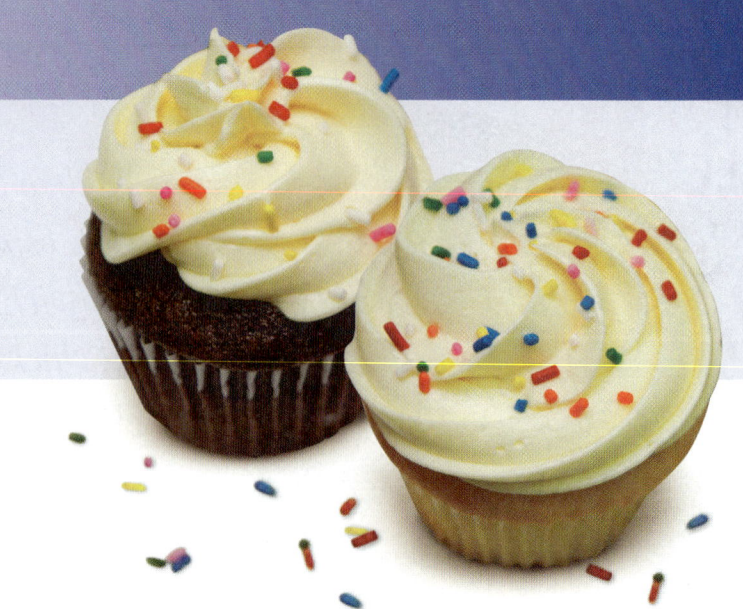

Why do people, even newborn infants, prefer foods that taste sweet? The pleasant and sometimes irresistible taste of sugar is a clue that the food contains **carbohydrates,** a major source of energy for cells. Without a steady supply of energy, cells cannot function and they die.

Sugars, starches, and most kinds of fiber are carbohydrates. Plants make carbohydrates by using the sun's energy to combine the carbon, oxygen, and hydrogen atoms from carbon dioxide (*carbo-*) and water (*-hydrate*). Thus, plants are rich sources of carbohydrates. A carbohydrate is an organic nutrient because it contains carbon.

Your cells can metabolize ("burn") the basic chemical units of most carbohydrates. This vital process releases energy that powers various forms of cellular work, including muscle contraction, enzyme production, and bone growth. Although you need some carbohydrates for energy, consuming too much carbohydrates, as well as the other macronutrients, can lead to extra body fat. This section of Unit 5 introduces the major types of carbohydrates and their primary food sources.

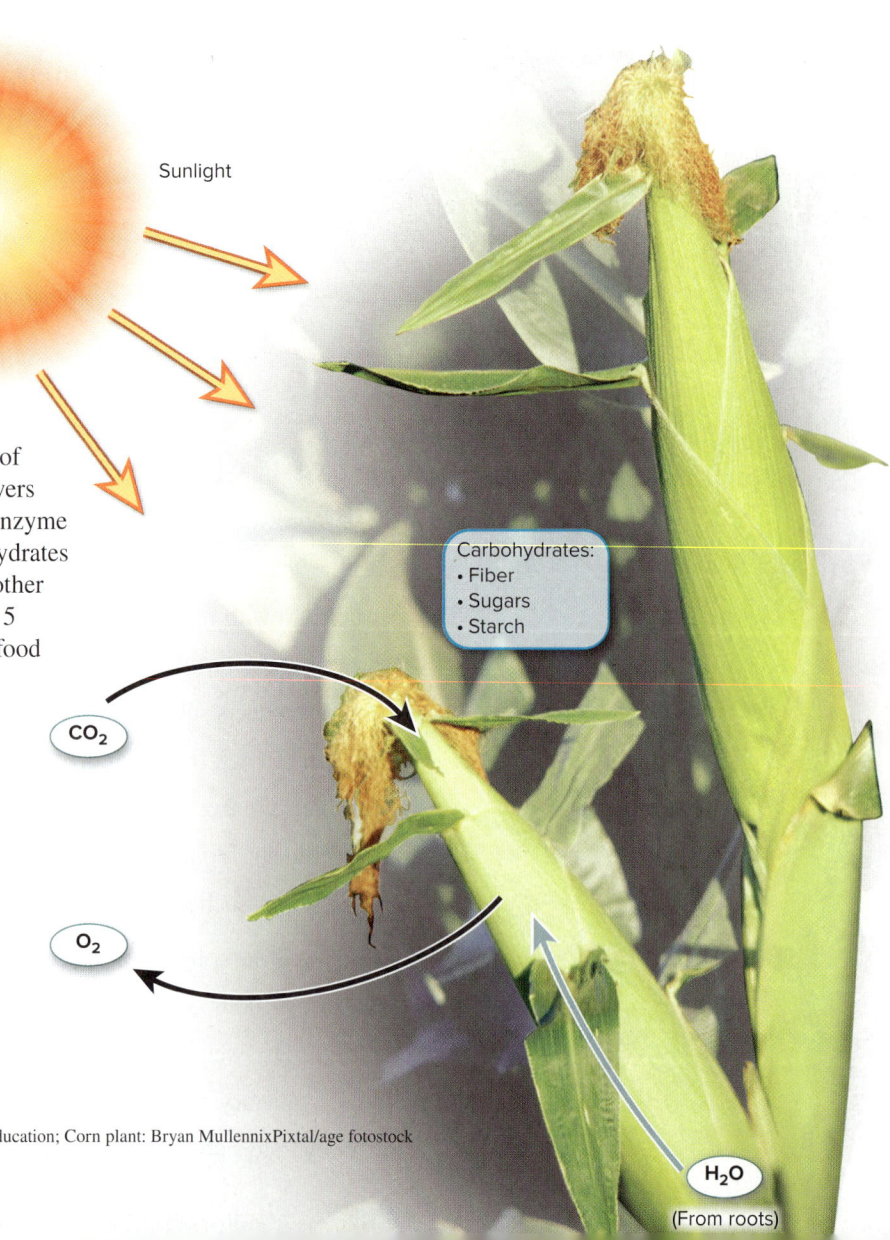

carbohydrates class of nutrients that is a major source of energy for the body

Cupcakes: McGraw-Hill Education; Corn plant: Bryan MullennixPixtal/age fotostock

5.1a Simple Carbohydrates: Sugars

You probably think of *sugar* as the sweet, white, granulated crystals that you sprinkle on cereal or into iced tea. However, this sweetener, which is commonly called "table sugar," is only one type of sugar. Sugars are a group of carbohydrates—simple carbohydrates.

You can often identify simple carbohydrates by their chemical names. If you read the ingredients on a food label and you see a substance that has "ose" at the end of its name, it's probably a carbohydrate. For example, the chemical name for table sugar is sucrose.

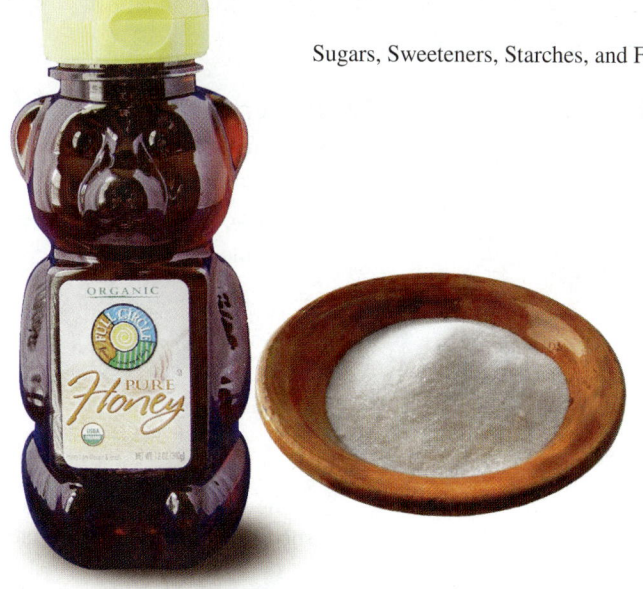

Monosaccharides

The simplest type of sugar, the **monosaccharide**, a "single sugar," is the basic chemical unit of carbohydrates. The three most important dietary monosaccharides are

- **Glucose,** which is commonly called "blood sugar," is a primary fuel for muscle and other cells. Red blood cells and nervous system cells, including your brain, must use glucose for energy under normal conditions. Thus, a healthy body maintains its blood glucose levels carefully. Fruits and vegetables, especially grapes, berries, corn, and carrots, are good food sources of glucose.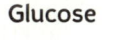

- **Galactose** isn't commonly found as a single sugar in foods. The monosaccharide, however, is a component of lactose, the form of carbohydrate in milk.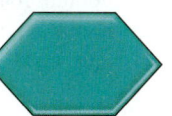

- **Fructose** ("fruit sugar" or levulose) is found naturally in fruit, honey, and a few vegetables, particularly cabbage, green beans, and asparagus. Your body has little use for fructose but can convert the simple sugar into glucose. Note that the chemical structure of fructose is different than that of glucose and galactose. This difference explains why fructose tastes sweeter than other natural sugars.

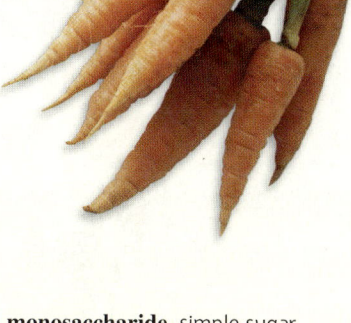

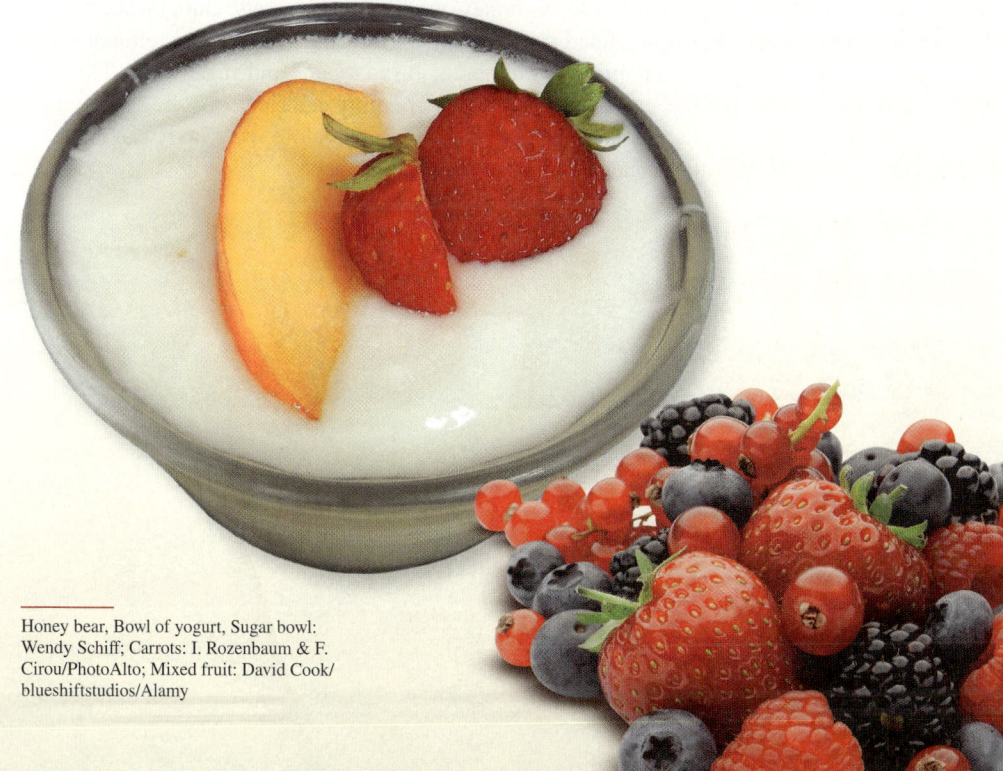

Honey bear, Bowl of yogurt, Sugar bowl: Wendy Schiff; Carrots: I. Rozenbaum & F. Cirou/PhotoAlto; Mixed fruit: David Cook/blueshiftstudios/Alamy

monosaccharide simple sugar that's the basic molecule of carbohydrates

glucose monosaccharide that is a primary fuel for muscles and other cells; "blood sugar"

galactose monosaccharide that is a component of lactose

fructose monosaccharide in fruits, honey, and certain vegetables; "levulose" or "fruit sugar"

disaccharide simple sugar comprised of two monosaccharides

lactose disaccharide comprised of a glucose and a galactose molecule; "milk sugar"

maltose disaccharide comprised of two glucose molecules; "malt sugar"

sucrose disaccharide comprised of a glucose and a fructose molecule; "table sugar"

Disaccharides

A **disaccharide** is a simple sugar comprised of two monosaccharides. Disaccharides include maltose, lactose, and sucrose.

- **Lactose,** which can be referred to as "milk sugar," is comprised of a galactose molecule and a glucose molecule.

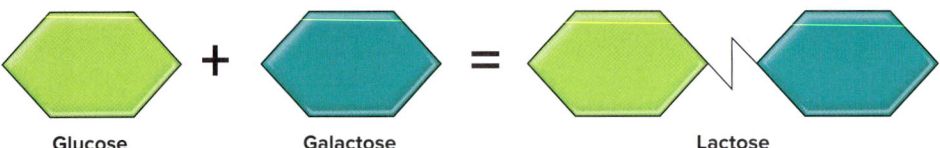

Glucose + Galactose = Lactose

Although most animal foods aren't sources of carbohydrate, milk and some products made from milk, such as ice cream, contain lactose.

- **Maltose** ("malt sugar") has two glucose molecules (chemical units) bonded together. Few foods contain maltose naturally, but the monosaccharide can be made from the breakdown of certain, more complex, carbohydrates. Food manufacturers use high-maltose syrup as a flavoring ingredient in sweets. High-maltose syrup is also used to brew beer.

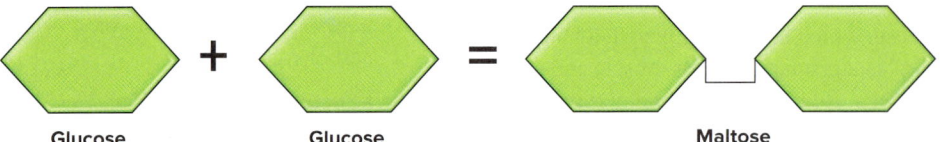

Glucose + Glucose = Maltose

- **Sucrose** ("table sugar"), a familiar sweetener, consists of one molecule of glucose and one of fructose.

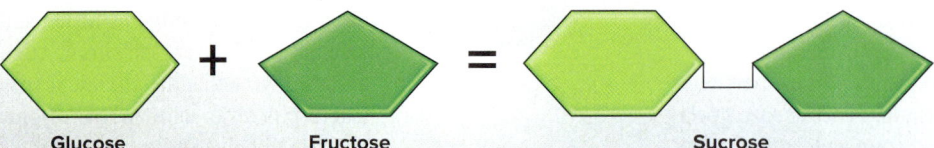

Glucose + Fructose = Sucrose

Although sucrose occurs naturally in foods such as honey, maple syrup, carrots, and pineapples, much of the sucrose in the American diet is refined from sugar cane and sugar beets. The refining process strips away the small amounts of vitamins and minerals in sugar cane and sugar beets. This explains why refined sugars such as table sugar are rich sources of empty calories.

The GI tract digests sucrose into glucose and fructose molecules. Therefore, your body can't distinguish whether the glucose or fructose came from table sugar or honey.

Sugar cane field in Hawai'i
Source: Richard Bain, NREL/DOE/U.S. Department of Agriculture

Nutrition Fact or Fiction?
Sugar makes children hyperactive.

If you've ever attended a child's birthday party, you can understand why people often blame sugary foods for causing "hyper" behavior. The results of scientific studies, however, don't indicate that sugar is a cause of *attention-deficit/hyperactivity disorder*, also known as *ADHD*.[2] There are a few different types of ADHD, but affected children generally have difficulty paying attention, following instructions, sitting quietly, and controlling their impulses. The cause of ADHD is uncertain, but genetic factors play an important role. Other risk factors include premature birth (being born too soon), low birth weight, and brain injury. Furthermore, pregnant women who smoke or drink alcohol increase their risk of having children with ADHD.

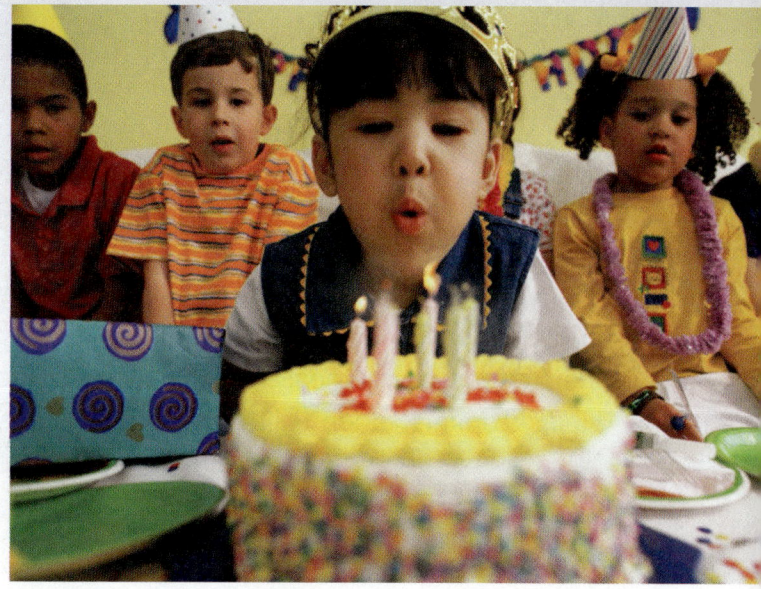

When children attend parties, their excitement and lower self-control are more likely caused by the situation than by their sugar intake. It's also possible that caffeine is responsible for children's "hyper" behavior. Caffeine is a stimulant drug. Sources of caffeine in children's diets include "energy drinks"; certain sugar-sweetened soft drinks, such as colas; and chocolate. Limiting children's intake of foods and beverages that contain caffeine may help boys and girls become more calm.

Natural sugars, such as the lactose in milk, fructose in orange juice, and glucose in grapes, make up a small percentage of all sugars in our diet. Most of the sugars that Americans eat are added to foods to sweeten them. Such refined sugars (**added sugars**) include sucrose and high-fructose corn syrup (HFCS), which Neill mentioned in the unit opener.

added sugars sugars added to foods during processing or preparation

Table 5.1 provides a comparison of the energy and selected nutrient contents of various sweeteners, including table sugar and honey. A tablespoon of white table sugar is almost 100% sucrose; a tablespoon of honey has glucose, fructose, water, and a small amount of sucrose. A tablespoon of honey contains more protein and micronutrients than a tablespoon of white sugar, but the amounts are insignificant. For example, you would have to eat about a cup of honey to obtain 1 g protein, 1.6 mg vitamin C, and 1.4 mg iron. That amount of honey supplies over 1000 kcal! Although honey contains beneficial phytochemicals, the amounts are too small to make the sweetener a valuable source of these substances. All of the sweeteners listed in Table 5.1 are sources of empty calories.

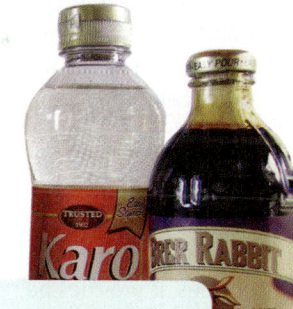

TABLE 5.1 NUTRITIONAL COMPARISON OF SELECTED SWEETENERS

Sugar/Syrup 1 Tablespoon	Water %	Kcal	Protein g	Carb g	Vit. C mg	Calcium mg	Niacin mg	Potassium mg	Iron mg	Zinc mg
Honey	17	64	0.06	17.3	0.1	1	0.025	11	0.09	0.05
White granulated sugar	0	49	0	12.6	0	0	0	0	0.01	0
Maple syrup (100% maple)	32	52	0.01	13.4	0	20	0.016	42	0.02	0.29
High-fructose corn syrup (HFCS)	24	53	0	14.4	0	0	0	0	0.01	0
Brown sugar	1	52	0.02	13.5	0	11	0.015	18	0.10	0
Molasses	22	58	0	15.0	0	41	0.186	293	0.94	0.06

Source: Data from U.S. Department of Agriculture, Agricultural Research Service: *USDA National Nutrient Database for Standard Reference Legacy Release, April 2018.* https://ndb.nal.usda.gov/ndb/search/list?home=true Accessed: November 2018

Children at party: Ryan McVay/Getty Images; Corn syrup, Molasses, Maple syrup: Wendy Schiff

What IS That?

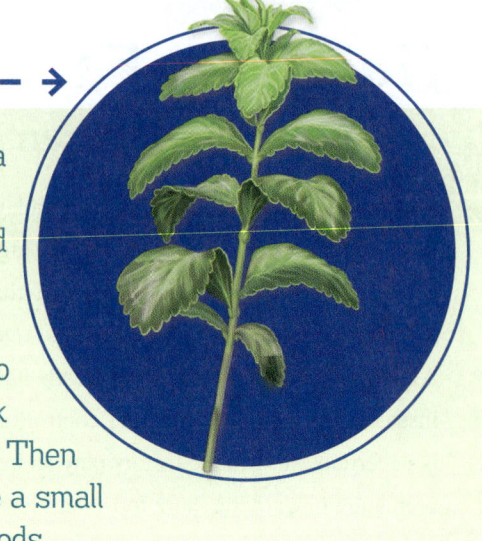

When dried, the leaves of the South American shrub *Stevia rebaudiana* Bertoni are very sweet. *Rebiana* is the common name for the highly purified form of the chemical (rebaudioside A) in stevia leaves that's responsible for their intense sweetness. The Food and Drug Administration (FDA) considers rebiana safe for use as an all-purpose sweetener.

You may be able to buy stevia plants at nurseries. By placing the plants in a sunny location and watering them when necessary, you can encourage the plants to grow in your garden or home. To enjoy this natural sweetener, pick the leaves and allow them to dry. Then crush some dried leaves and use a small amount to sweeten drinks and foods.

TASTY Tidbits

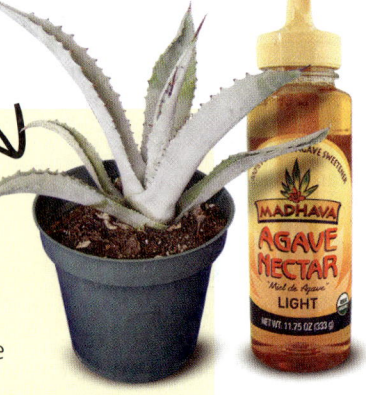

Wendy Schiff

Young blue agave

Agave nectar is a nutritive sweetener made from the blue agave, a plant that is native to southwestern United States and Mexico. The nectar is produced from mature agaves and refined into a mild-flavored syrup that can be used like honey to sweeten foods and beverages. Nutritionally, agave nectar is similar to honey, and as a source of empty calories, it provides no remarkable health benefits.[3] Because the body can convert excess carbohydrates, including fructose, to fat, you should use small amounts of the sweetener.

5.1b Nutritive Sweeteners

Sugars and syrups are nutritive sweeteners because they contribute energy to foods. Each gram of a mono- or disaccharide supplies 4 kcal. If one of the nutritive sweeteners listed in **Figure 5.1** is the first or second ingredient listed on a product's label, the food probably contains a high amount of sugar.

Fructose tastes much sweeter than glucose and is easily made from corn. Therefore, food manufacturers often add large amounts of HFCS when they make sugar-sweetened "regular" soft drinks, candies, and baked goods. **Table 5.2** indicates the amounts of added sugars, expressed as teaspoons of table sugar, that are in typical servings of commonly consumed foods and beverages.

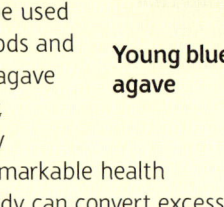

*The % DV (DV) tells you how much a nutrient in a serving of food contributes to a daily diet. 2000 calories a day is used for general nutrition advice.

INGREDIENTS: Raw sugar, brown sugar, table sugar, turbinado sugar, confectioner's or powdered sugar, coconut sugar, date sugar, corn syrup, high-fructose corn syrup (HFCS), cultured corn syrup, high-maltose corn syrup, agave nectar, maple syrup, molasses, honey, fruit juice concentrate, fruit juice sweetener, glucose, dextrose, polydextrose, fructose (levulose), invert sugar, lactose, maltose, maltodextrin, sorbitol, mannitol, xylitol, erythritol

Figure 5.1 Sugars and other nutritive sweeteners. You can determine the sources of added sugars and sugar alcohols in a product by reading the ingredients list on the label.

Q Answer This

According to Table 5.1, which nutritive sweetener provides the most potassium per tablespoon? You can find the answer on the last page of this unit.

TABLE 5.2

How Much Added Sugar Is in That Food?

Food	Serving Size	Kcal	Approximate Teaspoons Added Sugars
Doughnut, cake with frosting	1 small (55 g)	260	4
Chocolate chip cookies, commercial brand	1 snack package (39 g)	200	4
Sugar-frosted cornflakes	1 cup	150	3½
Chocolate-flavored soy milk	1 cup	150	3½
Ice cream, vanilla	2/3 cup	200	4
Chocolate candy bar with almonds	1.45 oz	210	5
Apple pie, double crust	⅛ 9″ diameter pie	600	6
Yogurt, vanilla low-fat	6 oz	150	4
Cola, canned	12 fl oz	150	10
Chocolate milkshake	16 fl oz	616	15
Tea, bottled	12 fl oz	120	13

Doughnut: Jules Frazier/Getty Images; Apple pie, Teaspoon of sugar: Wendy Schiff; Milkshake: Ingram Publishing

5.1c Alternative Sweeteners (Sugar Substitutes)

alternative sweeteners substances that are added to sweeten foods while providing few or no kilocalories

high-intensity ("artificial") sweeteners group of manufactured alternative sweeteners that are intensely sweet-tasting compared to sugar

Alternative sweeteners are substances added to food that sweeten the item while providing fewer calories per serving than sucrose or no calories. Alternative sweeteners that provide calories include sugar alcohols: *sorbitol, xylitol, erythritol,* and *mannitol.* Unlike sugars, sugar alcohols don't promote dental decay. Thus, these compounds are used to replace sucrose in products such as sugar-free chewing gums, breath mints, and "diabetic" candies. However, most "sugar-free" or "diabetic" foods supply some calories. Sugar alcohols aren't fully absorbed by the intestinal tract, and as a result, they supply an average of 2 kcal/g. Except for erythritol, sugar alcohols can cause diarrhea when consumed in large amounts.

High-Intensity Sweeteners

High-intensity ("artificial") sweeteners are a group of manufactured alternative sweeteners that include

- saccharin,
- aspartame,
- acesulfame-K,
- sucralose,
- neotame,
- monk fruit extract,
- steviol glycosides (high-purity substances from stevia leaves), and
- advantame.

High-intensity sweeteners live up to their name in that they taste very sweet when compared to the taste of the same amount of sugar **(Table 5.3).** Thus, a very small amount of a high-intensity sweetener is needed to sweeten a food. These sweeteners supply little or no energy per serving as a result.[4]

High-intensity sweeteners may help people control their energy intake and manage their body weight. Furthermore, researchers haven't been able to find clear evidence that using reasonable amounts of high-intensity sweeteners has any negative effects on the people who consume them.[5,6]

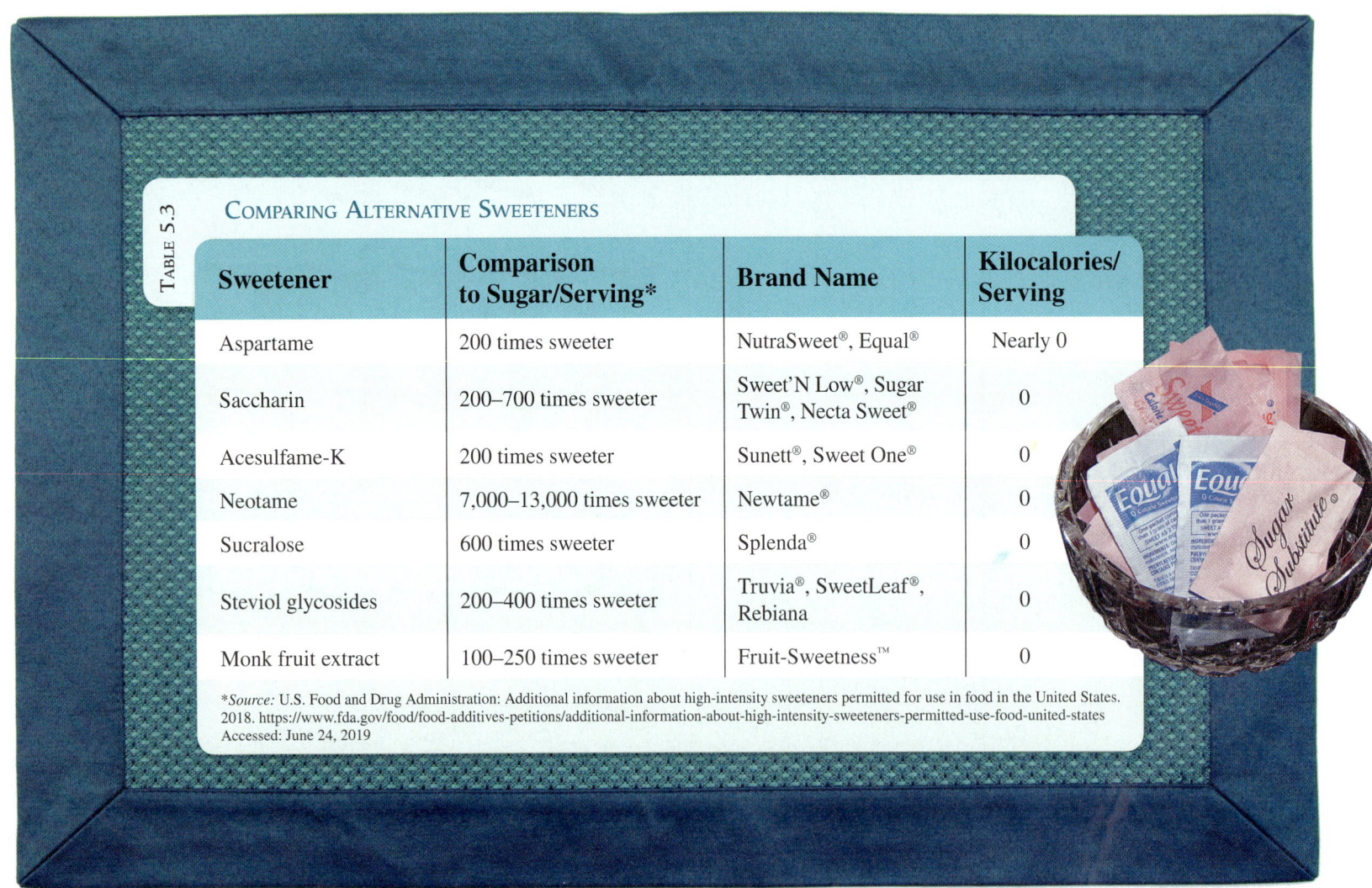

TABLE 5.3 COMPARING ALTERNATIVE SWEETENERS

Sweetener	Comparison to Sugar/Serving*	Brand Name	Kilocalories/Serving
Aspartame	200 times sweeter	NutraSweet®, Equal®	Nearly 0
Saccharin	200–700 times sweeter	Sweet'N Low®, Sugar Twin®, Necta Sweet®	0
Acesulfame-K	200 times sweeter	Sunett®, Sweet One®	0
Neotame	7,000–13,000 times sweeter	Newtame®	0
Sucralose	600 times sweeter	Splenda®	0
Steviol glycosides	200–400 times sweeter	Truvia®, SweetLeaf®, Rebiana	0
Monk fruit extract	100–250 times sweeter	Fruit-Sweetness™	0

*Source: U.S. Food and Drug Administration: Additional information about high-intensity sweeteners permitted for use in food in the United States. 2018. https://www.fda.gov/food/food-additives-petitions/additional-information-about-high-intensity-sweeteners-permitted-use-food-united-states Accessed: June 24, 2019

Placemat: Mark Dierker/McGraw-Hill Education; Bowl of sweeteners in packets: Wendy Schiff

TASTY Tidbits

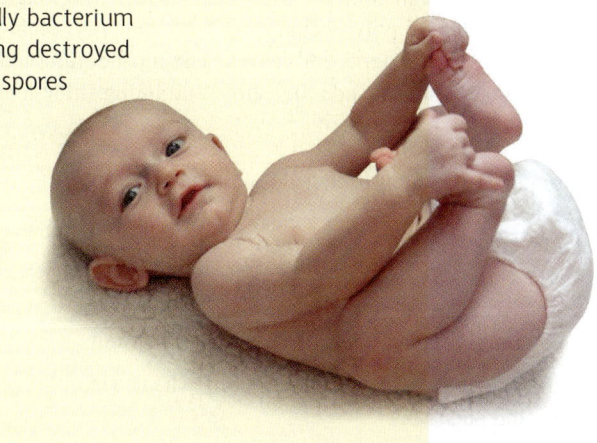

Honey can contain spores of the deadly bacterium *Clostridium botulinum* that resist being destroyed by food preservation methods. These spores can become active within an infant's intestinal tract and produce a poison that's extremely toxic to nerves. Therefore, honey shouldn't be fed to children younger than 12 months of age or used to sweeten infant foods because it may cause botulism poisoning.[7] Older children and adults can eat honey safely because the mature stomach produces enough acid to destroy the bacterial spores.

Are Artificial Sweeteners Safe? According to the U.S. Food and Drug Administration, all high-intensity sweeteners that have been approved by the agency are safe.[4] *Cyclamates* are a particular group of sweeteners that the FDA doesn't permit in foods. A group of international health and safety organizations, including the FDA, have established *Acceptable Daily Intakes* (*ADIs*) for certain high-intensity sweeteners **(Table 5.4)**. An ADI is the amount of an artificial sweetener that you can consume safely on a daily basis, throughout your life.[5]

What About Aspartame? Aspartame consists of two amino acids (the building blocks of proteins): phenylalanine and aspartic acid. Some people must avoid aspartame and certain protein-rich foods because they have *phenylketonuria* (*PKU*) (*fen´-il-kee´-toe-nur´-e-ah*). PKU is a rare, inherited disorder that results in the body's inability to use phenylalanine properly. To diagnose PKU, physicians generally rely on a simple blood test that's conducted on infants within 48 hours after their birth. If an infant with PKU isn't treated with a special diet, phenylalanine accumulates in the child's bloodstream and causes severe brain damage. The FDA requires the following warning statement on the label of any food that contains aspartame:

PHENYLKETONURICS: CONTAINS PHENYLALANINE.[8]

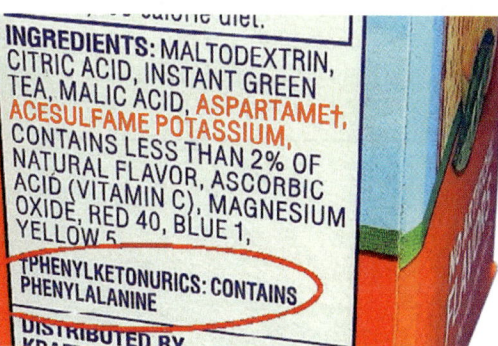

TABLE 5.4 ACCEPTABLE DAILY INTAKES FOR SOME HIGH-INTENSITY SWEETENERS

Food/Beverage	Sweetener	Amount
Diet cola	Aspartame	18 to 19 12-oz cans
Packets	Saccharin	9 to 12 packets
Lemon-lime soft drink	Acesulfame-K	30 to 32 12-oz cans
Diet cola	Sucralose	6 12-oz cans

Source: Mattes RD, Popkin BM: Non-nutritive sweetener consumption in humans: Effects on appetite and food intake and their putative mechanisms. *American Journal of Clinical Nutrition* 89(1):1, 2009.

Baby: Stacy Schmitt; Warning label: Wendy Schiff; Placemat: McGraw-Hill Education/Mark A. Dierker, photographer

polysaccharides compounds comprised of several monosaccharides bonded together

starch storage form of glucose in plants

glycogen storage form of glucose in humans and other animals

dietary fiber (fiber) indigestible plant material; most types are polysaccharides

soluble fiber forms of dietary fiber that dissolve or swell in water

insoluble fiber forms of dietary fiber that generally don't dissolve in water

5.1d Polysaccharides

Plant and animal cells can combine monosaccharides into long chains called **polysaccharides** (complex carbohydrates). Cells use polysaccharides to store energy; plant cells also use polysaccharides to make structural components such as stems and leaves. The most common dietary polysaccharides consist of hundreds of glucose molecules and include digestible and indigestible forms.

Starch and Glycogen

Plants store glucose as polysaccharides called **starch**. Your intestinal tract can digest starch into individual glucose molecules that can be absorbed. Each gram of starch supplies 4 kcal.

Seeds, roots, and fleshy underground stems called *tubers* often contain starch. Thus, starchy foods include

- bread and cereal products made from wheat, rice, barley, and oats;
- vegetables such as corn, squash, beans, and peas;
- *tubers* such as potatoes, yams, taro, cassava, and jicama.

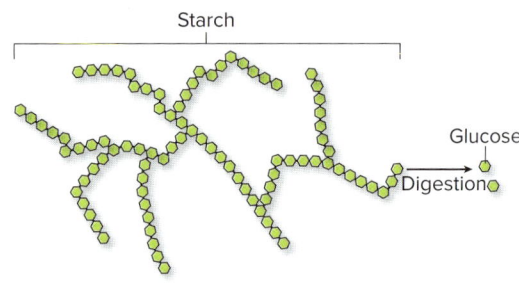

Starch digestion results in glucose molecules.

Animals store glucose as the polysaccharide **glycogen** ("animal starch"). The human body stores limited amounts of glycogen. Muscles and the liver are the major sites for glycogen formation and storage. Although muscles contain glycogen, most animal foods aren't sources of carbohydrate because muscle glycogen breaks down soon after an animal dies.

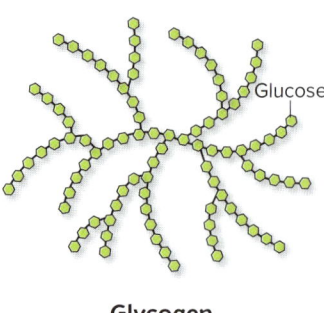

Glycogen

Culture & Cuisine

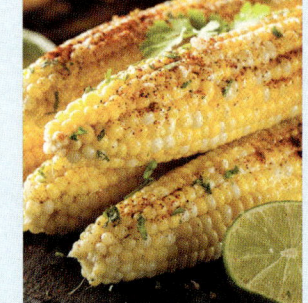

Brent Hofacker/Alamy Stock Photo
Mexican street corn

Throughout the world, populations rely on three starchy foods—rice, corn, and wheat—to supply the majority of their food energy intake. Other starchy foods, especially millet, sorghum, cassava, taro, potatoes, and yams, are often consumed along with the three starchy *staple* foods. A staple food forms the foundation of a population's diet and provides a large share of their calorie and nutrient needs. Rice, for example, is a staple food for almost 50% of the world's population.

5.1e Fiber

In addition to starches, plants make **dietary fiber (fiber)**; most forms of fiber are polysaccharides. *Cellulose*, for example, is made up of repeating glucose units. However, the links that connect the glucose units are in a form that people can't digest (see **Essential Concept 5.1**). Hemicellulose, pectin, gums, and mucilages are also polysaccharides that humans cannot digest. Lignin is the only type of fiber that's not carbohydrate.

When the undigested fiber is in the large intestine, it serves as an energy source for the bacteria that normally live there. Any fiber that the bacteria don't use is eliminated in feces. Keep in mind that only plant foods provide fiber; animal flesh contains *muscle* fibers, which are digestible proteins.

Essential Concept

5.1 Why You Can't Digest Fiber

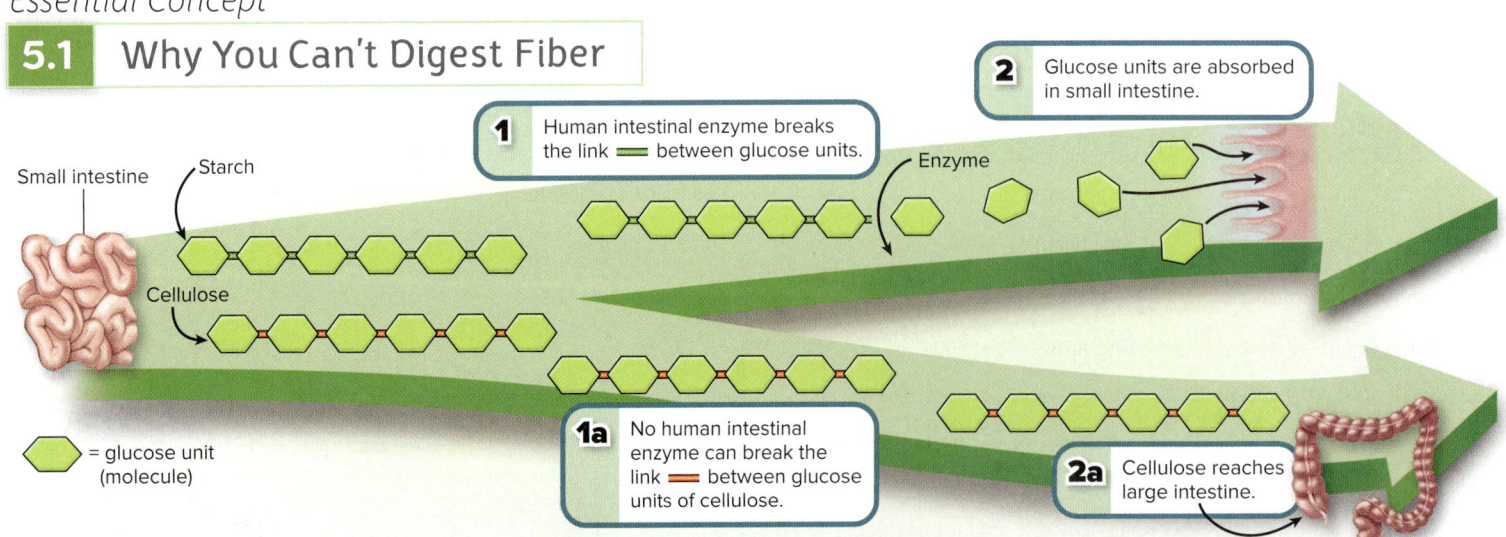

There are two types of fiber—**soluble fiber** and **insoluble fiber**:

- Soluble fiber dissolves or swells in water.
- Insoluble fiber generally doesn't dissolve in water.

Although fiber isn't digested by humans, soluble and insoluble fiber provide important health benefits. Soluble fiber binds cholesterol and slows glucose absorption. As a result, soluble fiber can help reduce blood cholesterol and glucose levels. Insoluble fiber increases fecal "bulk," which contributes to good health by easing bowel movements. **Table 5.5** provides information about the effects of fiber in the body as well as major food sources of soluble and insoluble fiber. It's important to note that plant foods usually contain both forms. **Table 5.6** lists some foods and their total dietary fiber contents.

Table 5.5 Classifying Fiber

Type	Physiological Effects	Food Sources
Insoluble	Increases fecal bulk and speeds fecal passage through large intestine	All plants Wheat, rye, brown rice, vegetables
	Increases fecal bulk; may ease bowel movements	Whole grains, wheat bran
Soluble	Delays stomach emptying; slows glucose absorption; can lower blood cholesterol	Apples, bananas, citrus fruits, carrots, oats, barley, psyllium seeds, beans, and thickeners added to foods

Table 5.6 Dietary Fiber Content of Common Foods

Food	Fiber (g)	Food	Fiber (g)
Split peas, cooked (1 cup)	16.3	Green peas, frozen, cooked (½ cup)	3.6
Chickpeas, canned, drained (1 cup)	16.2	Almonds, 23 whole kernels (1 oz)	3.5
Black beans, cooked (1 cup)	15.0	Prunes, dried uncooked (5 prunes)	3.4
Oat bran, raw (1 cup)	14.5	Orange, raw (1 orange)	3.4
Kidney beans, canned (1 cup)	11.0	Carrots, raw, grated (1 cup)	3.1
Baked beans, plain, canned (1 cup)	10.4	Barley, cooked (½ cup)	3.0
Raspberries, raw (1 cup)	8.0	Broccoli, chopped, cooked (½ cup)	2.6
Blackberries (1 cup)	7.6	Strawberries, 10 medium	2.4
Kellogg's Raisin Bran® cereal (1 cup)	7.0	Whole-grain bread, toasted (1 slice)	1.9
Apple, raw, with skin (3″ diameter)	4.4	Romaine lettuce, shredded (1 cup)	1.0
Baked potato, Russet, with skin (approx. 6.5 oz)	4.0	Iceberg lettuce, shredded (1 cup)	0.9
Beans, green snap, cooked (1 cup)	4.0	White bread (1 slice)	0.8
Banana, sliced (1 cup)	3.9		

Source: Data from U.S. Department of Agriculture, Agricultural Research Service: *USDA National Nutrient Database for Standard Reference Legacy Release, April 2018.* https://ndb.nal.usda.gov/ndb/search/list?home=true Accessed: November 2018

Fruit, nut and vegetable display: Source: Photo by Keith Weller, USDA-ARS; Pea pod: Danny Smythe/Shutterstock; Almonds: Jula Store/Shutterstock; Romaine lettuce: Danny Smythe/Alamy Stock Photo

5.1f How Much Carbohydrate Should You Eat?

According to the DRIs, nutritionally adequate diets should provide 45 to 65% of total energy from carbohydrates (see Unit 3).[9] The average diet of adult Americans supplies about 47% of total calories from carbohydrates (**Fig. 5.2**).[10] This amount includes calories from complex carbohydrates as well as sugars.

Added Sugars

In 2017, Americans, on average, consumed about 22 teaspoons of added sugars per person per day, which is 17.6% of the energy in a diet that supplies 2000 kcal/day.[1] Diets that contain a lot of added sugars, especially sugar-sweetened soft drinks, may increase the risk of heart disease.[11] According to the U.S. Dietary Guidelines, people should limit their added sugars intake to less than 10% of total calories. If you follow a 2000 kcal/day diet, you should limit your added sugars intake to 12 teaspoons per day.[12]

A major source of added sugars in Americans' diets is sugar-sweetened beverages, which include regular soft drinks, fruit "ades," sweetened coffees and teas, and energy drinks. A 12-ounce serving of an orange-flavored, sugar-sweetened soft drink that isn't made with orange juice contains about 45 g of added sugars, primarily HFCS.[13] This amount of HFCS equals about 11.5 teaspoons of table sugar. A 12-ounce serving of 100% orange juice supplies about 31 g of natural sugars, which equals almost 8 teaspoons of table sugar. Both beverages contain sugars, so should you drink the sugar-sweetened, orange-flavored soft drink instead of the orange juice? Unlike typical sugary soft drinks, 100% fruit juices, such as orange, grapefruit, and cranberry juice, contribute less sugar and more water-soluble vitamins and antioxidant phytochemicals to your diet. According to MyPlate, adults should consume 1½ to 2 cups of fruit or fruit equivalents each day, some of which can be 100% fruit juice.

TASTY Tidbits

Canned fruit is often packed in a sugary syrup. Consider buying canned fruit that's packed in water or its own juice. If you have canned fruit that's in syrup, rinse the fruit in plain water before serving it. Also choose frozen fruit that has no sugar added.

Wendy Schiff

The following tips can help you reduce your intake of sugar-sweetened drinks:

- Replace soft drinks with a naturally calorie-free thirst-quencher—plain water. Make plain water more interesting to drink by adding to it a slice of lemon or lime, or a few fresh or frozen berries.
- Add 1 part club soda to 1 part orange or other 100% fruit juice to make a refreshing carbonated drink.
- Avoid fruit "drinks," "punches," "blends," "cocktails," or "ades" because they often contain high amounts of added sugars and little or no fruit juice. Check the ingredients list to see which fruit juices are in the product.
- Limit your intake of pre-sweetened flavored coffees and teas. Make your own coffee and tea, so you can control the amount of table sugar added. An even better idea: Learn to drink tea and coffee without sugar!

Appendix F has tips for reducing the amount of sugar in your favorite recipes.

Percentage of Total Calories from Macronutrients per Person (adults, one day)

- Protein
- Carbohydrates
  - Complex carbohydrates
  - Sugars, including added sugars
- Fat

Protein: 16.2%
Complex carbohydrates: 25.8%
Sugars, including added sugars: 20.8%
Fat: 37.2%

Figure 5.2 Macronutrient intakes. This graph shows adult Americans' average intake of macronutrients as percentages of approximate total calories from macronutrients (2036 kcal) on one day in 2015–2016.

Source: U.S. Department of Agriculture, Agricultural Research Service: *What we eat in America, NHANES 2015–2016.* July 2018. www.ars.usda.gov/northeast-area/beltsville-md-bhnrc/beltsville-human-nutrition-research-center/food-surveys-research-group/docs/wweia-data-tables/ Accessed June 21, 2019

Module 5.2

What Happens to the Carbohydrates You Eat?

5.2 - Learning Outcomes

After reading Module 5.2, you should be able to

1. Define all of the **key terms** in this module.
2. Describe how the body digests and absorbs carbohydrates and uses glucose for energy.
3. Explain how the body regulates its blood glucose level.

John A. Rizzo/Getty Images

Essential Concept

5.2 Carbohydrate Digestion, Absorption, and Elimination

If you eat cooked oatmeal made with milk and sweetened with a little brown sugar for breakfast, what happens to the carbohydrates in these foods? The carbohydrates in oats are primarily starch and fiber; mixing milk and brown sugar with the cereal adds lactose and sucrose. **Essential Concept 5.2** indicates the main steps of digesting carbohydrates, including the kinds that are in this meal.

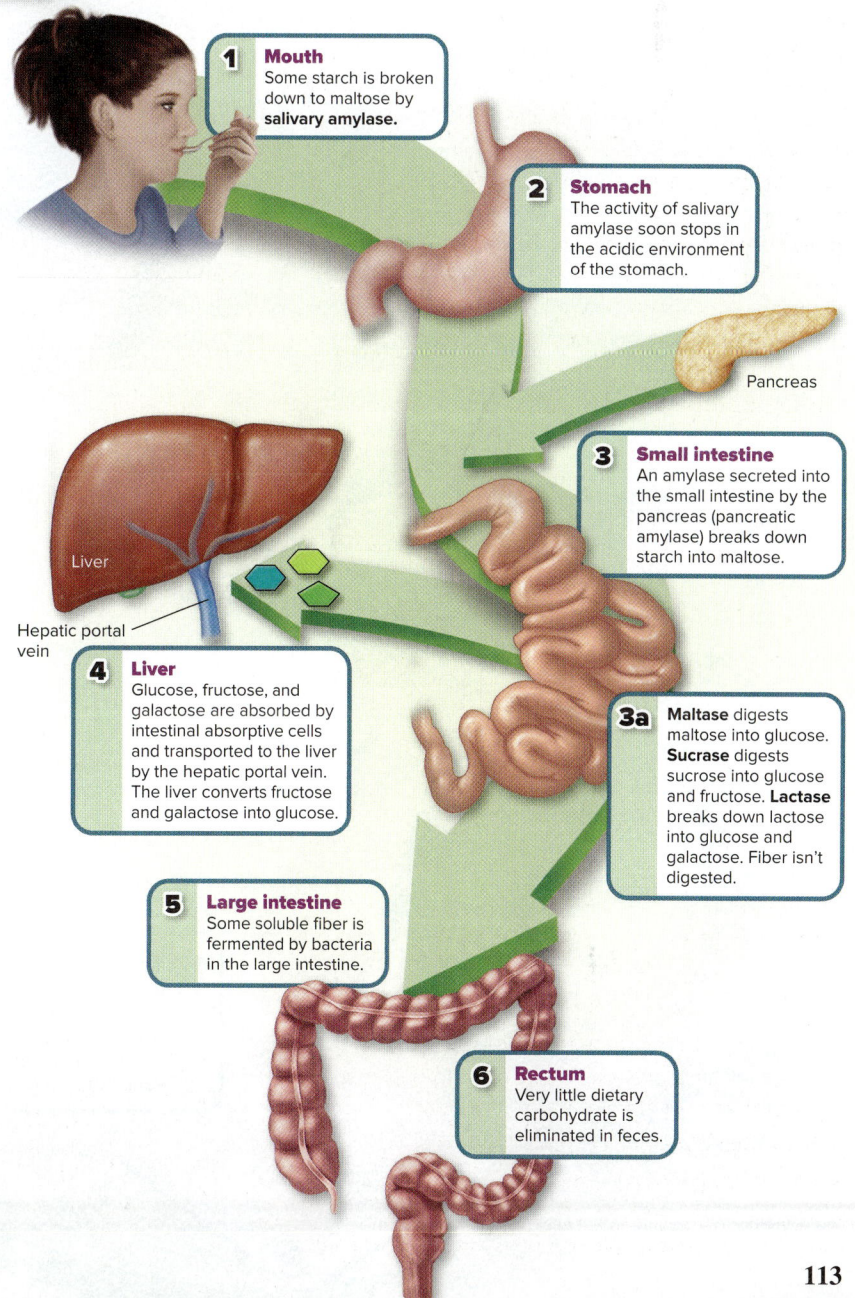

1 Mouth Some starch is broken down to maltose by **salivary amylase**.

2 Stomach The activity of salivary amylase soon stops in the acidic environment of the stomach.

3 Small intestine An amylase secreted into the small intestine by the pancreas (pancreatic amylase) breaks down starch into maltose.

4 Liver Glucose, fructose, and galactose are absorbed by intestinal absorptive cells and transported to the liver by the hepatic portal vein. The liver converts fructose and galactose into glucose.

3a **Maltase** digests maltose into glucose. **Sucrase** digests sucrose into glucose and fructose. **Lactase** breaks down lactose into glucose and galactose. Fiber isn't digested.

5 Large intestine Some soluble fiber is fermented by bacteria in the large intestine.

6 Rectum Very little dietary carbohydrate is eliminated in feces.

salivary amylase enzyme secreted by the salivary glands that begins starch digestion in the mouth

maltase enzyme that breaks down maltose into two glucose molecules

sucrase enzyme that breaks down sucrose into a glucose and a fructose molecule

lactase enzyme that breaks down lactose into glucose and galactose

Unit 5 Carbohydrates: Fuel and Fiber

5.2a Maintaining Normal Blood Glucose Levels

Glucose is a major fuel for your cells. Therefore, hormones carefully maintain your blood glucose level. Your pancreas contains various types of cells, including beta and alpha cells. Beta cells produce **insulin,** and alpha cells make **glucagon.** Insulin helps lower the blood glucose level by signaling cells to allow glucose to enter them. Glucagon signals certain cells to release glucose into the bloodstream. This action raises the level of glucose in the bloodstream. Thus, these two hormones play key roles in regulating blood glucose levels.

If you're healthy, insulin and glucagon help maintain your fasting (before breakfast) blood glucose level between 70 and 100 milligrams per deciliter of blood (mg/dl).[14] **Essential Concept 5.3** illustrates how insulin and glucagon help regulate your body's blood glucose level.

insulin hormone that helps lower blood glucose levels

glucagon hormone that helps raise blood glucose levels

Essential Concept

5.3 How Your Body Regulates Your Blood Glucose

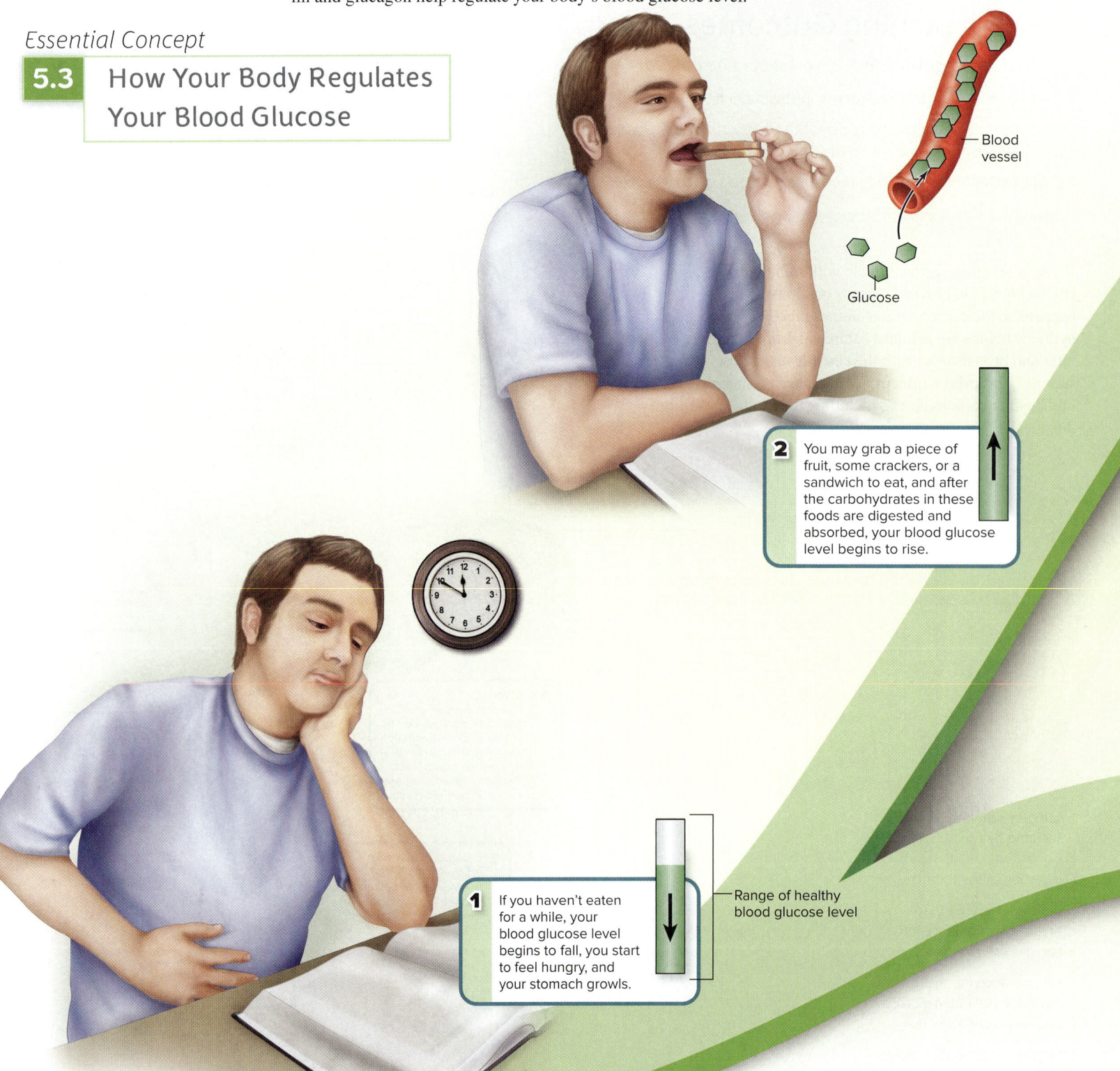

Blood vessel

Glucose

2 You may grab a piece of fruit, some crackers, or a sandwich to eat, and after the carbohydrates in these foods are digested and absorbed, your blood glucose level begins to rise.

1 If you haven't eaten for a while, your blood glucose level begins to fall, you start to feel hungry, and your stomach growls.

Range of healthy blood glucose level

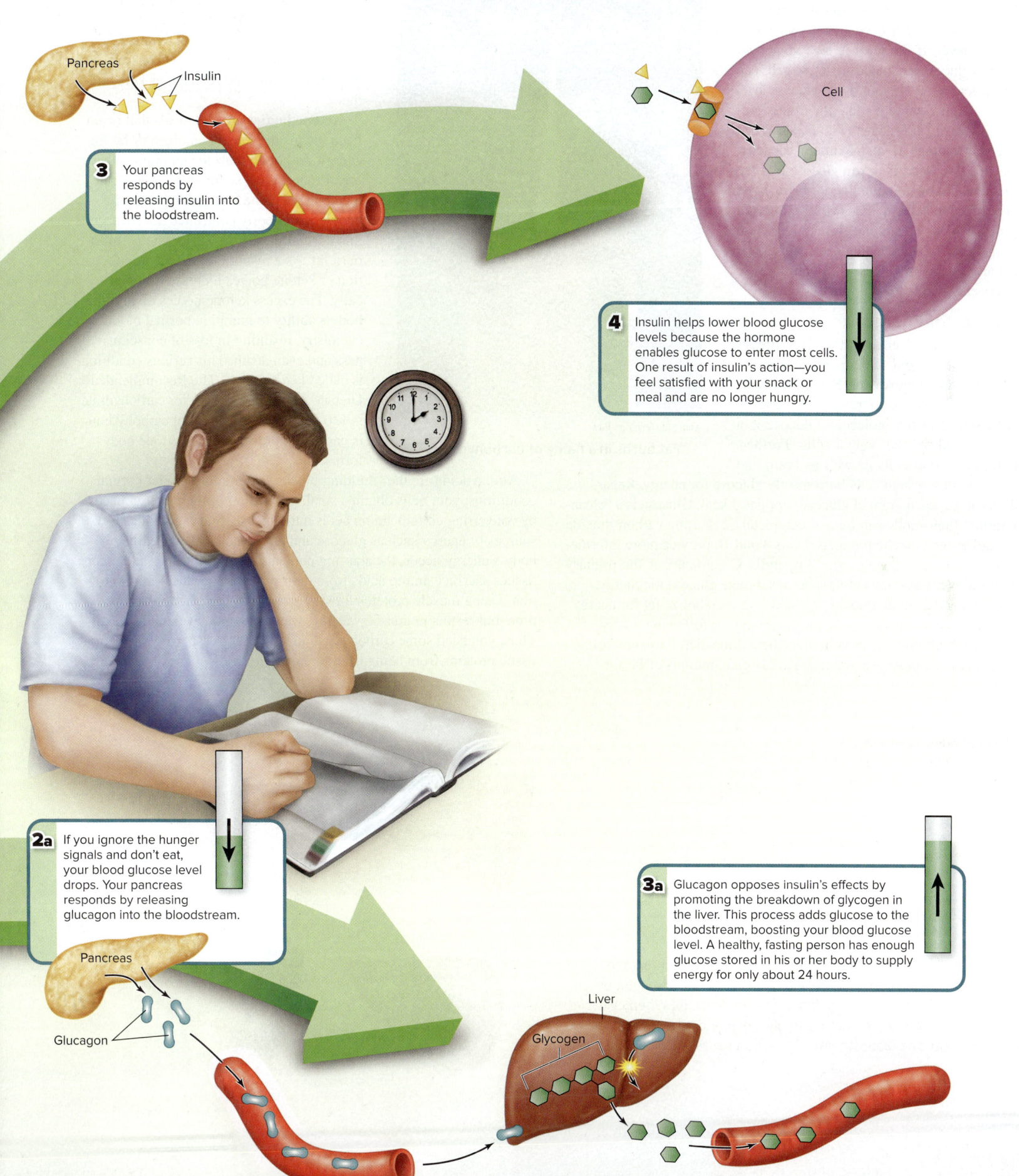

5.2b The Fate of Glucose

What happens to glucose after it's absorbed and in your liver? It depends on your blood glucose level. If the level is low, your liver releases glucose into bloodstream, so cells can burn it for energy. If your blood glucose level is normal and you're resting, the excess glucose is stored as glycogen (**Fig. 5.3a**). When glycogen storage is at maximum capacity, your liver converts the extra glucose into fat. The fat can remain in the liver or be released into the bloodstream. Fat cells remove fat from the bloodstream and store it for future energy needs. Thus, eating too many foods that are sources of glucose may contribute to excess energy intakes and weight gain.

Glucose for Energy

When cells need energy, the liver breaks down glycogen and releases glucose molecules into the bloodstream (**Fig. 5.3b**). Cells metabolize glucose to release the energy that's stored in the molecule. Glucose is a primary fuel for the body's cells. Furthermore, red blood cells as well as brain and other nervous system cells burn mostly glucose for energy. Regardless of its source, each gram of glucose supplies 4 kcal. Glucose is a "clean-burning" fuel—cells can burn it completely, releasing carbon dioxide gas and water as waste products. Units 4 and 10 provide more information about energy metabolism. **Appendix C** summarizes the primary chemical pathways that cells use to metabolize glucose for energy.

Cells need a small amount of glucose to metabolize fat for energy properly. When a person is fasting, starving, or following a very low-carbohydrate/high-protein diet (the Atkins diet, for example), his or her cells must use greater-than-normal amounts of fat for energy. When this situation occurs, there isn't enough glucose available for cells to metabolize the fat efficiently. As a result, excessive amounts of *ketone bodies* ("ketones") form. Thus, very low-carbohydrate diets may be referred as ketogenic diets.

Ketone bodies are chemicals that result from the incomplete metabolism of fat for energy. Although muscle and brain cells prefer to use glucose for energy, they can metabolize ketone bodies for energy. In people with poorly controlled diabetes, cells that normally use glucose for energy must burn fat. As a result, the body's production of ketone bodies increases dramatically. The excess ketone bodies disrupt the body's ability to maintain normal blood chemistry, resulting in loss of consciousness and even death. This serious condition is called ketoacidosis. The Recommended Dietary Allowance (RDA) for carbohydrate is 130 g/day.[9] This amount of carbohydrate is enough to prevent excess ketone body formation.

Amino acids are the "building blocks" of proteins. Under normal conditions, your cells obtain a small proportion of their energy needs by converting certain amino acids into glucose. Starvation diets lack sources of energy such as glucose and amino acids. To meet the body's energy needs, the starving person's skeletal muscles and other tissues sacrifice amino acids from their proteins for glucose production. Using muscle proteins for energy extends the person's survival time, but results in muscle wasting, weakness, and, eventually, death. Thus, you need some carbohydrate in your diet to "spare" your body's tissue proteins from being used for energy.

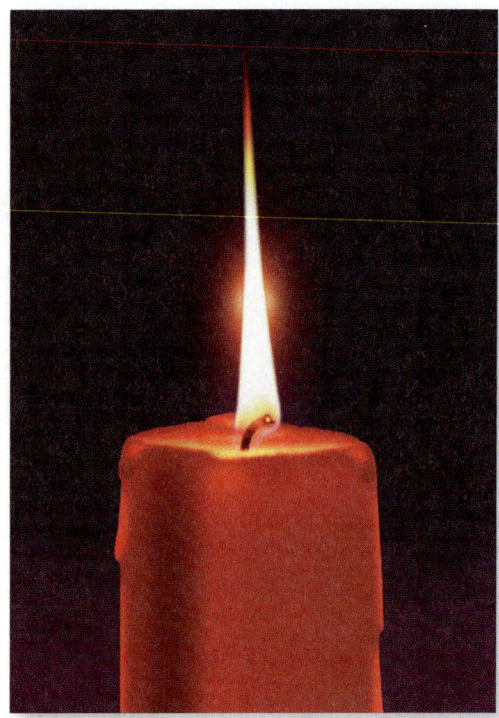

Alan Marsh/Design Pics

"Fat burns in a flame of carbohydrate."

ketone bodies chemicals that result from the incomplete breakdown of fat for energy

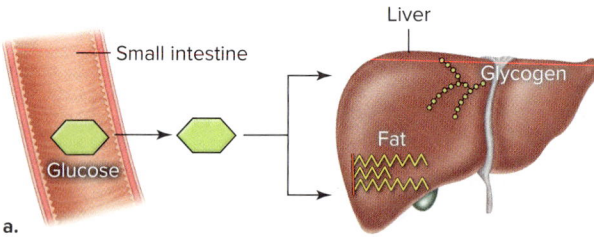

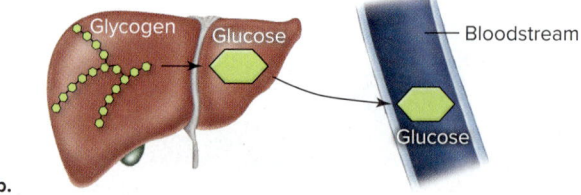

Figure 5.3 Fate of glucose. (a) After a meal, glucose enters the liver of a well-fed and resting person and is stored as glycogen or fat. This action helps lower the blood glucose level. (b) When cells need glucose, the liver breaks down glycogen and releases glucose molecules into the bloodstream. This action raises the blood glucose level.

Module 5.3

Carbohydrates and Health

5.3 - Learning Outcomes

After reading Module 5.3, you should be able to

1. Define all of the **key terms** in this module.
2. Discuss the effects of excess carbohydrate consumption on health.
3. Discuss differences between type 1 and type 2 diabetes and list common signs and symptoms of each disorder.
4. Identify risk factors for type 2 diabetes and measures that may prevent this disease.
5. Explain how carbohydrates can contribute to dental decay.
6. Explain the health benefits of soluble and insoluble fiber.
7. Explain why lactose intolerance occurs, and discuss dietary measures that will reduce signs and symptoms of the disorder.

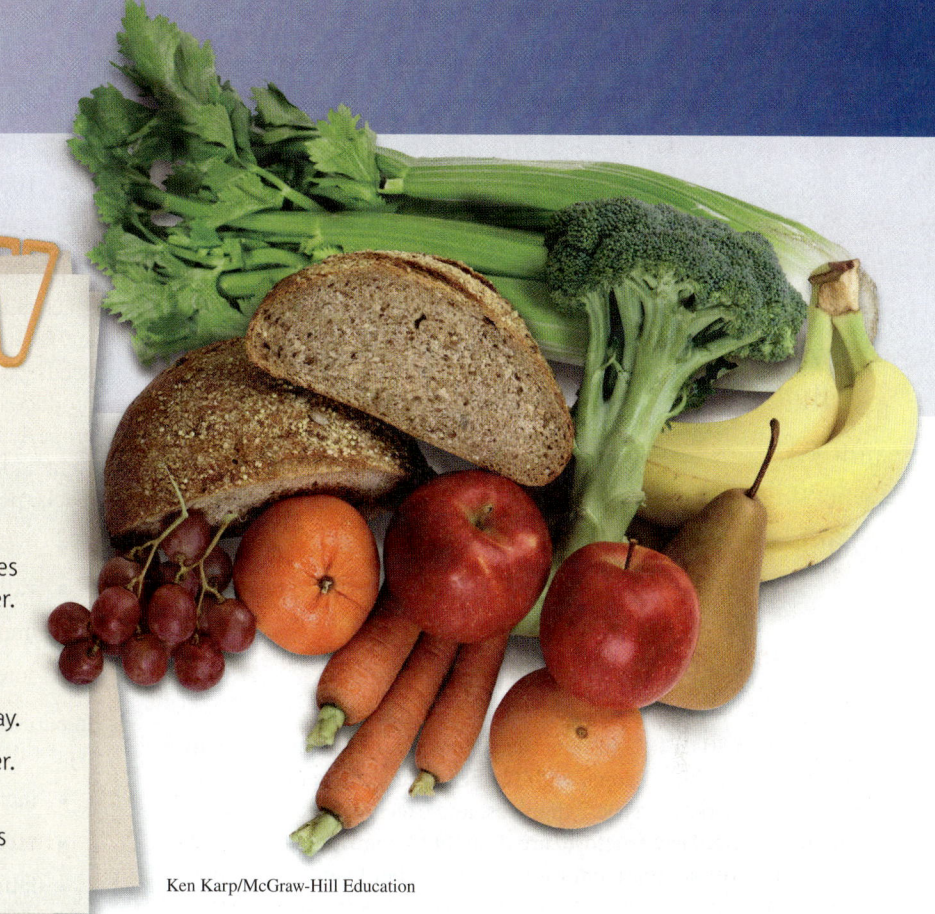

Ken Karp/McGraw-Hill Education

5.3a Are Carbohydrates Fattening?

Americans are fatter now than they were 20 years ago. Do carbohydrates cause obesity? When a well-fed person consumes excess digestible carbohydrates (starches and sugars), his or her body converts some of the glucose into fat, but much of the excess is "burned" as a biological fuel. As a result, dietary fat is spared from being used as a fuel, and it's stored in fat cells. Thus, eating too much digestible carbohydrate contributes to unwanted weight gain.

Foods that contain large amounts of refined carbohydrates, especially added sugars, may not satisfy hunger as well as those that contain more protein, fat, and/or fiber. As a result, you may want to eat sooner after having a meal or snack that contains a lot of added sugars and refined starches than if you ate a high-protein, high-fat, or high-fiber meal or snack.

Excess calorie intake from all energy sources (sugars, starches, fat, protein, and alcohol) contributes to excess body fat. Recall that each gram of fat supplies more than twice the calories as a gram of carbohydrate. People, however, often blame carbohydrates for their unwanted weight gain. Why? Starches and sugars are often combined with "hidden fats" such as butter, oil, or shortening in processed foods. By adding sugar to the food, the sweet taste masks the bland taste of fat. Furthermore, adding a little salt to the fat and carbohydrate mixture often enhances the food's taste. How easy is it for you to limit your intakes of eating energy-dense foods that combine "carbs" with fat and some salt, such as snack chips, candy bars, cakes, cookies, and pies?

Sugar-sweetened drinks, including teas, coffees, and energy drinks, are major sources of added sugars in the diets of Americans.[15] Some nutrition experts think Americans' intake of added sugars is largely responsible for the population's high rate of obesity. People who drink sugar-sweetened beverages don't reduce their consumption of solid foods enough to avoid gaining weight.[16] Scientists, however, haven't found a clear link between drinking regular soft drinks and weight gain.[17] On the other hand, there's a lot of evidence that consuming high amounts of fructose can harm the liver.[18]

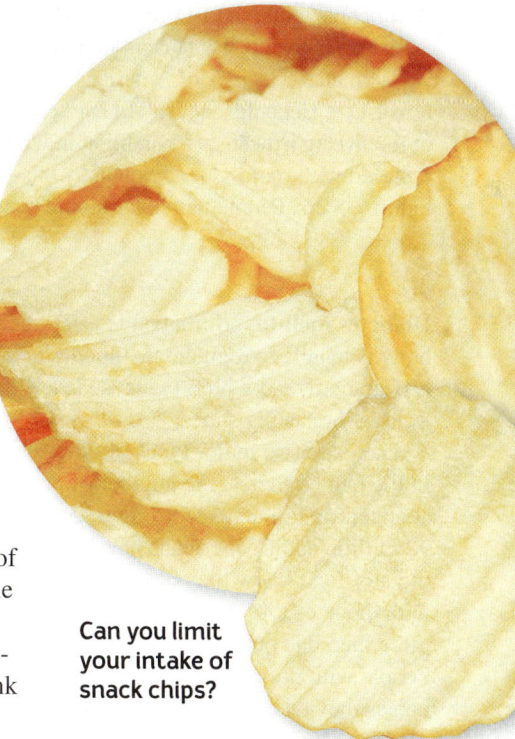

Can you limit your intake of snack chips?

Darren Greenwood/DesignPics

117

Should you be like Neill Warrington, who was quoted in the opener of this unit, and use honey to sweeten foods? Is honey a more nutritious sweetener than table sugar? Would you recommend that Neill use agave syrup as a sweetener instead of honey? Explain why you would or wouldn't make this recommendation.

5.3b What Is Non-alcoholic Fatty Liver Disease?

An estimated 30 to 40% of Americans have **non-alcoholic fatty liver disease (NAFLD)**.[19] People with NAFLD accumulate too much fat in their liver. Obesity, type 2 diabetes, and excess intake of carbohydrates, particularly fructose, are thought to contribute to NAFLD. There's no specific treatment for the disease, but losing excess body fat and following a healthy diet pattern may allow the liver to stop accumulating fat and become healthy again.

If people with NAFLD continue to have fat build up in their liver, the fat damages liver cells, causing inflammation of the organ (*hepatitis*). An estimated 3 to 12% of Americans have hepatitis that resulted from NAFLD.[19] Hepatitis can lead to liver cancer or *cirrhosis (sear-hoe´-sis)* of the liver. Cirrhosis is a condition in which liver cells have died and are replaced with scar tissue. Eventually the scar tissue hardens, and liver failure occurs. People with liver failure need a liver transplant to survive.

5.3c What Is Diabetes?

Diabetes mellitus (diabetes) is a serious chronic disease in which the body is unable to regulate its blood glucose level properly. The disease is characterized by blood glucose levels that remain abnormally high, even in the fasting state.

There are two major types of diabetes mellitus—type 1 and type 2. In the United States, the number of people with diabetes is increasing at an alarming rate. According to government estimates, more than 30 million adult Americans have diabetes, but about 25% of these individuals don't know they have the condition.[20] The majority of adults with diabetes (90%) have type 2.[20] According to government estimates, more than one out of three adult Americans have pre-diabetes.[21] People with pre-diabetes are very likely to develop type 2 diabetes, unless they take steps to lower their risk.

non-alcoholic fatty liver disease (NAFLD) accumulation of fat in the liver that's not caused by alcohol consumption

diabetes mellitus (diabetes) group of serious chronic diseases characterized by abnormal glucose, fat, and protein metabolism

Fasting blood glucose levels that are
- 70 to 99 mg/dl are normal;
- 100 to 125 mg/dl indicate pre-diabetes;
- 126 mg/dl or more indicate diabetes.

People with untreated diabetes have high blood glucose levels because their bodies don't produce any insulin or don't produce enough to meet their needs. In other cases, the people with the disease produce insulin, but their cells don't respond properly to the hormone (insulin resistance).

In addition to high fasting blood glucose levels, people with diabetes usually experience

- excessive thirst and frequent urination,
- vaginal yeast infections (adult women),
- impotence (male), and
- sores that don't heal.

Device that's used for testing blood glucose level

In addition to these health problems, people with poorly controlled type 1 diabetes tend to have

- increased appetite with weight loss,
- breath that smells "fruity,"
- fatigue and confusion.

Over time, untreated or poorly controlled diabetes damages nerves, organs, and blood vessels. For adult Americans, diabetes is a major cause of heart disease, kidney failure, blindness, and lower limb amputations. The disease is the seventh-leading cause of death in the United States (see Figure 1.2).

Type 1 Diabetes

Type 1 diabetes is an *autoimmune* disease. Such diseases occur when certain immune system cells don't recognize the body's own insulin-producing cells of the pancreas (beta cells). As a result, the immune system cells attack and destroy the pancreatic cells. It isn't clear why the immune cells malfunction, but genetic susceptibility and environmental factors, particularly exposure to certain viral infections, are associated with the development of type 1 diabetes.[22]

At the present time, most people with type 1 diabetes obtain insulin by injections or other means, such as an inhaler or a device that's commonly called an "insulin pump." The device, which is usually worn on a waistband or belt, has a container for insulin. The insulin pump is programmed to deliver the hormone through a small tube that's inserted under the patient's skin. Scientists are developing a similar device (an "artificial pancreas") that would continuously monitor the patient's blood glucose level and deliver insulin in amounts that are needed to maintain a specific range of blood glucose level.

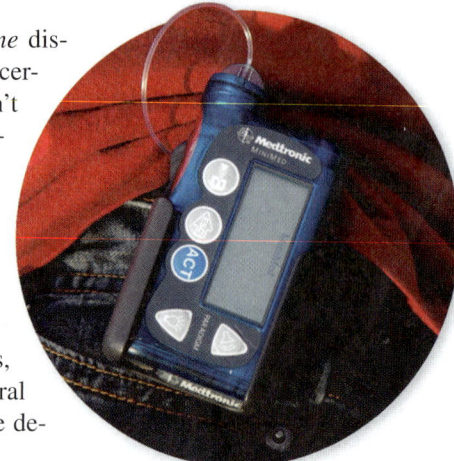

An insulin pump in use

Type 2 Diabetes

The most common form of diabetes is type 2 diabetes. Beta cells of people with type 2 diabetes usually produce insulin, but the body's cells are *insulin-resistant*, which means they don't respond properly to the hormone. As a result, the blood glucose level rises to abnormal levels, and the signs of diabetes occur.

People at high risk for type 2 diabetes are

- physically inactive,
- overweight or obese,
- genetically related to a close family member with type 2 diabetes, or
- Americans with Hispanic, Native American, certain Asian, African, or Pacific Islander ancestry.[23]

Some people with type 2 diabetes can control their disease by exercising regularly and losing weight. Other persons with the condition rely on a special diet as well as medications that reduce cells' insulin resistance or stimulate the pancreas to secrete insulin. The American Diabetes Association (www.diabetes.org) has more in-depth information about both types of diabetes. The association also has an online questionnaire ("Type 2 Diabetes Risk Test") that you can take to determine your risk of type 2 diabetes.

Diabetes During Pregnancy

A woman who has poorly controlled diabetes can experience serious health problems, such as high blood pressure, during pregnancy. Her developing offspring (*embryo* or *fetus*) can also be harmed by its mother's lack of good blood glucose control. The first 8 weeks of pregnancy are a critical period in a human embryo's development because its organs are forming. If a pregnant woman with diabetes has poor control of her blood glucose level, her embryo/fetus can develop birth defects, grow too fat, and have abnormal blood glucose levels as a result.[24]

Women may develop diabetes during pregnancy (*gestational diabetes*). This type of diabetes usually begins around the middle of pregnancy and ends with the birth of the baby. However, women who've had gestational diabetes often experience the condition again with future pregnancies. They also have a higher risk of developing type 2 diabetes later in life, when compared to women who had healthy pregnancies.

A pregnant woman with poorly controlled diabetes or gestational diabetes is more likely to have miscarriages (death of an embryo/fetus before the 20th week of pregnancy), stillbirth (delivery of a dead baby), and premature delivery (fetus born before the 37th week of pregnancy) than a pregnant woman with diabetes who manages her blood glucose properly. Thus, pregnant women who have diabetes should monitor their blood glucose levels carefully to increase their chances of having trouble-free pregnancies and healthy newborns.

Monitoring Diabetes

To avoid or delay serious health complications, people who have diabetes need to achieve and maintain normal or near-normal blood glucose levels. This can be accomplished by carefully planning and spacing out meals and snacks as well as following treatment that is individualized to meet the patient's needs.

Many people with diabetes rely on daily blood testing to monitor their blood glucose levels (**Fig. 5.4**). Such blood tests provide a "snapshot" of a single blood glucose value at a moment in time. Physicians should also measure their patients' hemoglobin A1c ("A1c").

Hemoglobin is the compound in red blood cells that carries oxygen. Normally, some of the glucose that's in the bloodstream attaches to hemoglobin. The higher the level of glucose in the bloodstream, the higher the level of hemoglobin that has glucose attached to it. The A1c test shows how well the body has controlled its blood glucose level over the past 90 days. **Table 5.7** indicates how diabetes is classified according to A1c values.[25]

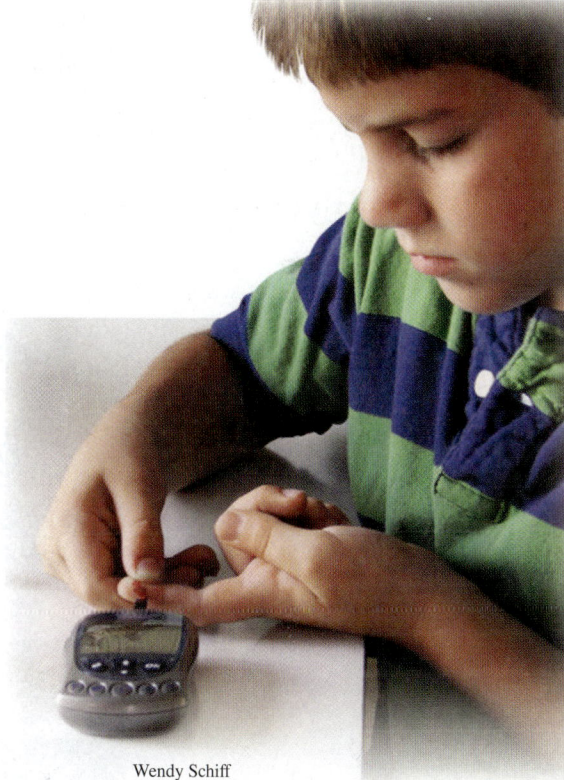

Wendy Schiff

Figure 5.4 Carson Smith has type 1 diabetes. He tests his blood glucose level at least four times a day.

■ *Why do many people with diabetes monitor their blood glucose levels?*

Table 5.7 CLASSIFYING DIABETES ACCORDING TO A1c VALUES

Diagnosis*	A1c Level
No diabetes	Below 5.7%
Pre-diabetes	5.7 to 6.4%
Diabetes	6.5% or above

*Any test for diagnosing diabetes requires a second test to confirm the diagnosis, unless the patient has signs and symptoms of diabetes.

glycemic index (GI) measure of the body's blood glucose response after eating a food that supplies 50 g of digestible carbohydrates as compared to a standard amount of glucose or white bread

Can Diabetes Be Prevented?

There is no way to prevent type 1 diabetes. However, you may reduce your risk of type 2 diabetes by

- losing excess weight (if necessary),
- exercising regularly, and
- following a diet that contains less processed meats, refined grains, and added sugars; and more fish; fiber-rich whole grains; beans; dairy products, especially yogurt; fruits; and vegetables.[26]

What's the Glycemic Index? The body digests carbohydrate-rich foods at different rates, and its blood glucose response to each food varies. This response can be rated by the glycemic index. The **glycemic index (GI)** is a value that reflects the body's blood glucose response after eating a food that supplies 50 g of digestible carbohydrates as compared to a standard amount of glucose or white bread. Foods with high GIs have values of 70 or more.[27] Foods with low GIs have values of 55 or less. A carbohydrate-rich food such as cornflakes (GI = 81) contains large amounts of refined carbohydrates, so the cereal is digested rapidly. As a result, glucose enters the bloodstream quickly, raising blood glucose and insulin levels rapidly. Carbohydrate-rich foods that have high fiber content, such as raw carrots (GI of 39), are digested slowly. By slowing down the rate of carbohydrate digestion,

Essential Concept

5.4 Glycemic Index and Glycemic Load: Average Values of Selected Foods

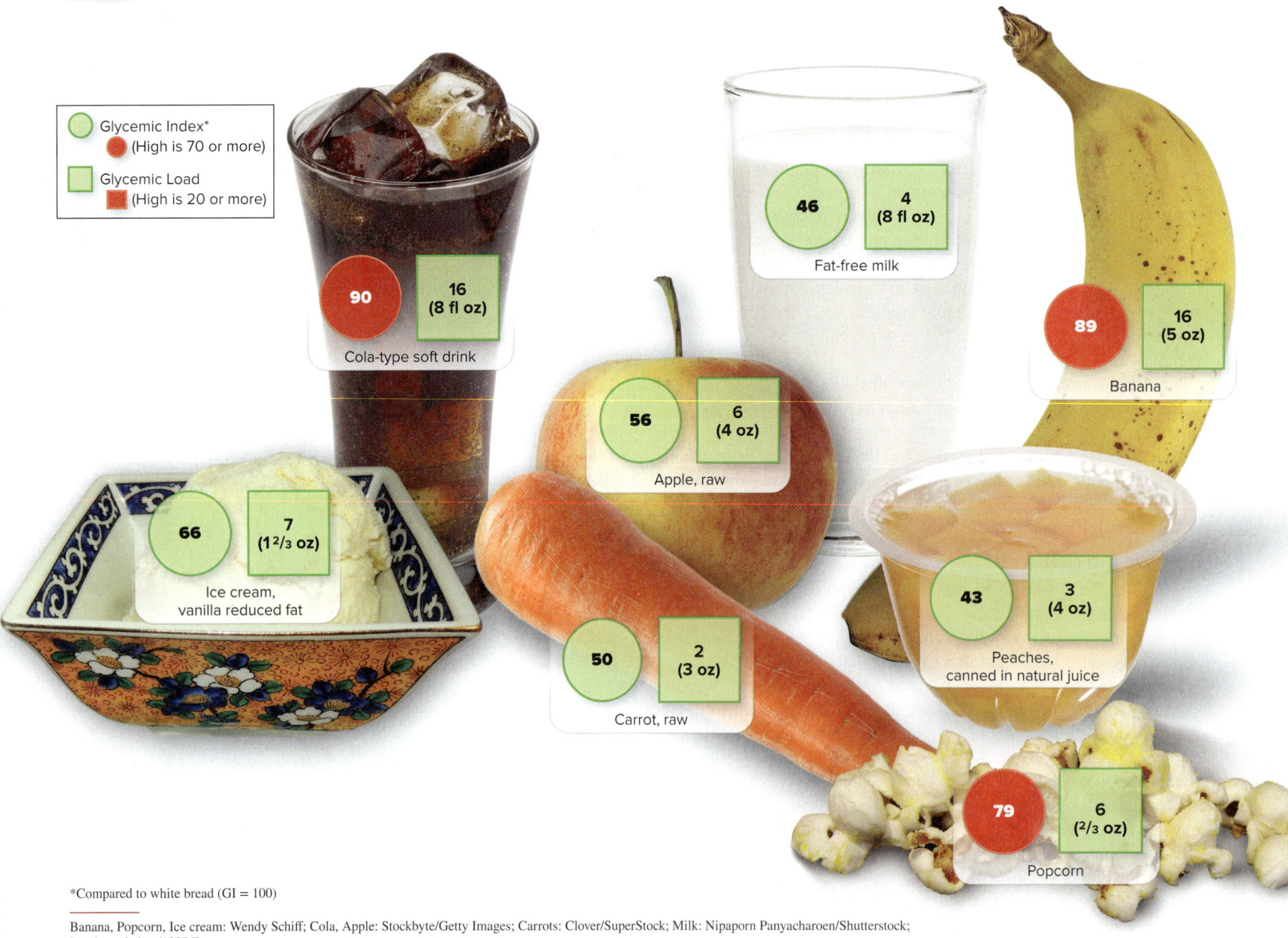

*Compared to white bread (GI = 100)

Banana, Popcorn, Ice cream: Wendy Schiff; Cola, Apple: Stockbyte/Getty Images; Carrots: Clover/SuperStock; Milk: Nipaporn Panyacharoen/Shutterstock; Peaches: shakzu/123RF

low-GI foods don't cause a dramatic increase in blood glucose and insulin levels. As a result, a person's blood glucose level is more likely to remain in the healthy range.

A related value, the **glycemic load (GL),** is determined by multiplying a food's glycemic index by the amount of carbohydrate that's in a typical serving of the food. **Essential Concept 5.4** lists average GIs and GLs of several commonly eaten foods. High-GL foods have values of more than 20; low-GL foods have values of less than 10.[27, 28]

GI and GL values can vary greatly, depending on where the food was grown, its degree of ripeness, or the extent of its processing. Furthermore, GI and GL values reflect a *single* food's effect on blood glucose levels. The increase in blood glucose levels is often less dramatic when the food is eaten as part of a meal that contains a mixture of macronutrients. Nevertheless, you may be able to reduce your risk of type 2 diabetes by following a low GI/GL diet.

5.3d What Is Hypoglycemia?

If you're healthy and haven't eaten for a while, your blood glucose level falls, and you become hungry. Eating a meal or snack raises your blood glucose. (See Essential Concept 5.3 in Module 5.2a.) **Hypoglycemia** occurs when the blood glucose level is less than 70 mg/dl.[29] In response to rapidly declining blood glucose levels, the body secretes the hormone epinephrine, which is also called *adrenaline*. Like glucagon, epinephrine increases the supply of glucose and fatty acids in the bloodstream, but the hormone can also make a person feel irritable, restless, shaky, and sweaty. If the blood glucose level drops too low, brain cells cannot obtain enough glucose for energy. Treatment involves giving the affected person a rapidly absorbed source of sugar, particularly fruit juice, glucose tablets, or honey. If untreated, the person with hypoglycemia becomes confused, and he or she may lose consciousness and die.

glycemic load (GL) value determined by multiplying the glycemic index of a carbohydrate-containing food by the amount of carbohydrate in a typical serving of the food

hypoglycemia condition that occurs when the blood glucose level is abnormally low

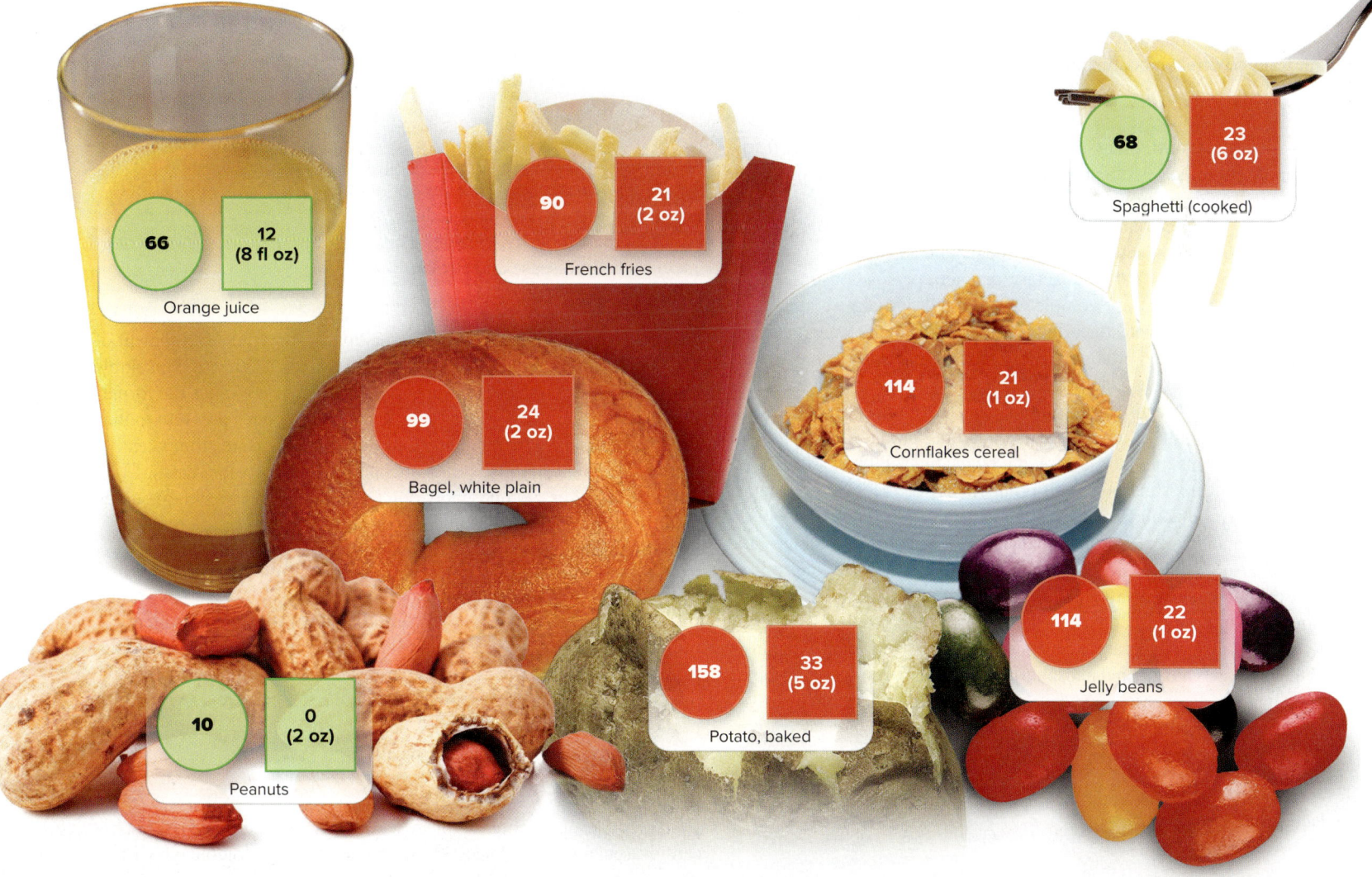

Source: Data from Atkinson FS and others: International tables of glycemic index and glycemic load values: 2008. *Diabetes Care* 31(12):2281, 2008.

Peanuts: multik/123RF; Orange juice, French fries, Spaghetti: Ingram Publishing/SuperStock; Bagel: Wendy Schiff; Cornflakes: CS-Stock/Alamy; Baked potato: Christopher Kerrigan/McGraw-Hill Education; Jelly beans: Burke/Triolo Productions/Getty Images

Hypoglycemia is a serious condition for people with diabetes, but it rarely affects healthy persons. Some people develop *reactive hypoglycemia* after they eat a lot of highly refined carbohydrates because the pancreas responds by releasing too much insulin. People with reactive hypoglycemia may feel better if they avoid eating large amounts of sugary foods and instead eat smaller, more frequent meals that contain a mixture of macronutrients.

5.3e Carbohydrates and Tooth Decay

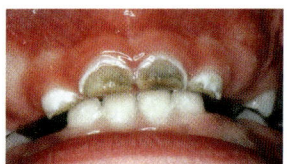

Child with nursing bottle syndrome
Ted Croll/Science Source

Carbohydrates, especially simple sugars that stick to your teeth, contribute to tooth decay. Bacteria that live on your teeth and gums use the carbohydrate in foods for their energy needs. The bacteria produce acid that damages tooth enamel and results in decay. Good dental hygiene habits, including brushing teeth after meals and eating sweet snacks, helps remove the harmful bacteria from teeth.

Infants and young children who drink bedtime bottles of milk, juice, or other beverages that contain sugars are likely to have "nursing bottle syndrome." When a sleepy child sucks slowly on the bottle, the carbohydrate-rich solution stays in contact with teeth, increasing the likelihood of dental decay. To reduce the risk of nursing bottle syndrome, offer a young child a bottle that contains a small amount of plain water to drink at bedtime.

5.3f Carbohydrate Intolerance

Throughout the world, many people are unable to digest lactose, fructose, and/or other kinds of carbohydrates completely. This condition is called *carbohydrate intolerance*. One form of this condition, **lactose intolerance,** is quite common among adults. Lactose-intolerant people don't produce enough lactase, the enzyme that breaks down lactose into glucose and galactose. When a lactase-deficient person consumes lactose, the disaccharide isn't completely digested and absorbed by the time it enters the large intestine. Bacteria that reside in the large intestine break down lactose and produce irritating gases and acids as metabolic by-products. As a result, a lactose-intolerant person usually experiences intestinal cramps, bloating, gas, and diarrhea within a couple of hours after consuming milk or other lactose-containing products.

Normally, infants produce lactase, but by the time children are 2 years old, their small intestine begins to produce less of the enzyme. Many older children and adults, particularly those with African, Asian, Native American, and Eastern European ancestry, are lactose intolerant and experience some degree of abdominal discomfort after drinking milk. Lactose intolerance isn't the same as milk allergy. Milk allergy is an immune system response to proteins in cow's milk.

Milk and milk products are excellent sources of protein, many vitamins, and the minerals calcium and phosphorus. Some lactose-intolerant people can eat hard (aged) cheeses and yogurt without experiencing any digestive tract problems.[30] Why? Milk loses most of its lactose content when it's processed to make aged cheeses, such as cheddar and Swiss, and yogurt.

lactose intolerance inability to digest lactose properly

FODMAPs carbohydrates and sugar alcohols that the GI tract doesn't digest and fully absorb

If you suspect you cannot digest lactose, try consuming a smaller-than-usual size serving of milk and note if you have intestinal discomfort within a few hours. If you cannot tolerate even small amounts of fresh fluid milk, you can substitute soy milk for cow's milk because soy milk doesn't contain lactose. Another choice is to drink milk or other lactose-containing dairy foods that have been pretreated with lactase. Most supermarkets sell fresh lactase-treated milk in the dairy food section.

What Are FODMAPs?

Can you recall having a bellyache and/or diarrhea after eating too much candy on Halloween? FODMAPs in candy may have been the source of your discomfort. **FODMAPs** are carbohydrates and sugar alcohols that your GI tract may not fully digest or absorb, especially when you eat too much of them. These substances attract water while passing through the intestines, and the bacteria that reside in the intestines can ferment FODMAPs for their energy needs. Side effects of the bacteria's activity often include abdominal cramps, intestinal bloating and gas, and diarrhea.

FODMAPs include fructose, lactose, and sugar alcohols such as xylitol and sorbitol. Wheat products, various kinds of fruit, high-lactose dairy foods, and onions are often excluded in low-FODMAP diets because they are rich sources of FODMAPs. Although a low-FODMAP diet can be difficult to follow for a long period, people with irritable bowel syndrome (IBS)[31] and, possibly, ulcerative colitis[32] may benefit from such diets. See Unit 4, sections 4.3g and 4.3h, for information about IBS and ulcerative colitis.

5.3g Fiber and Health

Fiber isn't an essential nutrient because you can live without it. You can live *better,* however, by adding fiber-rich foods to your diet. Eating high-fiber foods may reduce your risk of certain intestinal tract disorders, obesity, diabetes, and cardiovascular disease, which includes heart disease and stroke.

Fiber and the Digestive Tract

A high-fiber diet can help prevent constipation and the development of diverticula and inflamed hemorrhoids (see Unit 4). When the insoluble fiber in undigested food is in the large intestine, it promotes the formation of a large, soft fecal mass. This fecal mass applies pressure to the inner muscular walls of the large intestine. The pressure stimulates the muscles to push the residue quickly through the colon, easing elimination. Thus, you probably don't need to rely on over-the-counter laxatives to treat constipation. Try consuming more fiber-rich foods along with adequate amounts of water—it's the natural way to become "regular."

Fiber and Colorectal Cancer Eating a diet that contains plenty of dietary fiber may reduce your risk of colorectal cancer.[33] According to some studies, the fiber in cereal grains and fruit is more protective than the fiber in vegetables. As is often the case, more research is needed to determine which forms of fiber protect against colorectal cancer and how much should be eaten.

Fiber and Heart Health

High blood levels of cholesterol are associated with increased risks of cardiovascular disease. Diets rich in fiber, particularly soluble types of fiber, can reduce the risk of cardiovascular disease by reducing blood cholesterol levels.[33] In Unit 4, we mentioned that the intestinal tract breaks bile down and absorbs its components, which eventually enter the

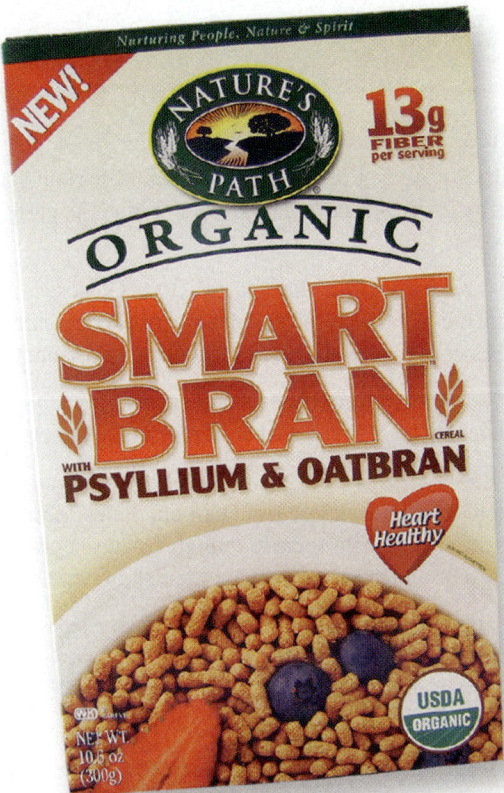
Wendy Schiff

liver. The liver recycles bile components to make new bile. When you eat sources of soluble fiber, however, the fiber binds to the bile components and prevents them from being absorbed. Thus, the bile components are eliminated in bowel movements. As a result, blood cholesterol levels drop as the liver removes cholesterol from the blood to make new bile. Unit 6 provides more information about soluble fiber intake and the risk of heart disease.

Fiber and Weight Control

Populations that consume high amounts of dietary fiber tend to have healthier body weights than populations with low fiber intakes.[33] Furthermore, people who want to lose excess weight may experience some greater weight loss by increasing their intake of dietary fiber. The reasons for this healthful effect are unclear, so more research is needed to understand the relationship between dietary fiber intake and body weight.

Increasing Your Fiber Intake

The Adequate Intakes (AIs) for fiber are 38 and 25 g/day for young men and women, which is much higher than what the typical American eats.[10] According to the Dietary Guidelines, fiber is a nutrient of "public health concern" because Americans generally don't eat enough of it.[12] The following tips can help you increase your fiber intake:

- Read the ingredient label to find out if a bread or cereal product is whole grain; *whole grain* or *bran* should be the first ingredient.
- When comparing bread or cereal products, don't rely on the product's name or appearance. Check the ingredients. Terms such as "100% wheat," "multigrain," or "stone-ground wheat" are misleading because the product may contain little or no whole grain.
- Brown rice has more fiber and flavor than white rice. Instant-cooking brown rice takes less time to cook than regular brown rice.
- Substitute whole-wheat pasta for regular pasta or use half whole-wheat and half regular pasta in pasta dishes.
- Snack on pieces of fresh, frozen, or dried fruit.
- Instead of removing them, eat the edible peels, pulp, and seeds of fruits and vegetables. Eat vegetables as snacks.
- Include more nuts, beans, and seeds in your diet.
- Spread peanut or soy butter on whole-grain crackers for a fiber-filled snack.
- Sprinkle unsalted nuts or hulled sunflower seeds on pancakes, waffles, or salads.
- Add frozen, dried, or fresh fruit such as berries, raisins, or bananas instead of sugar or honey to sweeten cereal or plain yogurt.
- Add a small amount of uncooked oatmeal and wheat germ to raw ground meats when making hamburgers or meatloaf.
- Add bran, wheat germ, and uncooked oatmeal to pancake or waffle batter.
- Choose packaged foods that contain at least 2.5 g of fiber per serving. You can determine the food's fiber content by reading the Nutrition Facts panel on the product label.

Eating excessive amounts of fiber may interfere with the intestinal absorption of certain minerals. You can estimate your daily carbohydrate intake, which includes fiber, by completing the What's in Your Diet?! feature at the end of this unit or in Connect®.

Bacteria that live in the colon produce gases when they metabolize fiber, so high-fiber diets can increase intestinal gas. To reduce the likelihood of experiencing *flatulence* (uncomfortable and embarrassing intestinal gas), you can add products such as Beano® to dishes that contain beans before eating them. Beano® contains natural enzymes that break down undigested complex carbohydrates before they can be metabolized by intestinal bacteria. Practices that result in swallowing air, such as eating quickly, drinking carbonated beverages (especially with a straw), and chewing gum, also contribute to intestinal gas.

In a Nutshell

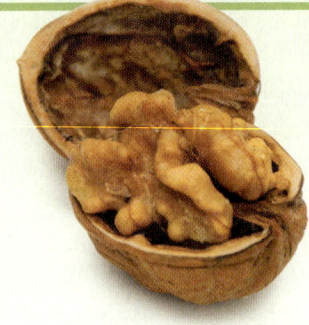

Module 5.1 Sugars, Sweeteners, Starches, and Fiber

- Sugars, starches, and most kinds of fiber are carbohydrates. Carbohydrates are an important source of energy for the body. Plants make carbohydrates by using the sun's energy to combine the carbon, oxygen, and hydrogen atoms from carbon dioxide and water.

- The three most important dietary monosaccharides are glucose, fructose, and galactose. Glucose is a primary fuel for muscles and other cells; nervous system and red blood cells rely on glucose for energy under normal conditions. Fruits and vegetables, especially grapes, berries, corn, and carrots, are good food sources of glucose.

- Lactose and sucrose are major dietary disaccharides. Most animal foods aren't sources of carbohydrate, but milk and some products made from milk contain lactose. Much of the sucrose in the American diet is refined from sugar cane and sugar beets.

- Nutritionally adequate diets should provide 45 to 65% of total energy from carbohydrates. A major source of added sugars in Americans' diets is beverages sweetened with sucrose or high-fructose corn syrup. High intakes of added sugars, especially sugar-sweetened beverages, may increase the risk of heart disease.

- Alternative sweeteners sweeten food while providing fewer calories per serving than sucrose. Alternative nutritive sweeteners include sugar alcohols: sorbitol, xylitol, and mannitol. High-intensity sweeteners may help people control their energy intake and manage their body weight. People with PKU must avoid consuming the high-intensity sweetener aspartame.

- Starch, glycogen, and most forms of dietary fiber are polysaccharides. Your intestinal tract can digest starch into individual glucose molecules that can be absorbed. Muscles and the liver are the major sites for glycogen formation and storage. Fiber isn't digested by humans, but soluble and insoluble fiber provide important health benefits. Soluble fiber can help reduce blood cholesterol levels, insoluble fiber may ease bowel movements, and fiber promotes a healthy balance of gut bacteria.

Module 5.2 What Happens to the Carbohydrates You Eat?

- Glucose is the primary end product of carbohydrate digestion and an important cellular fuel. Insulin and glucagon maintain normal blood glucose levels. Cells need a small amount of glucose to metabolize fat for energy properly. When glucose is unavailable, ketone bodies result from the incomplete metabolism of fat.

Module 5.3 Carbohydrates and Health

- Excess calorie intakes from carbohydrates, as well as fat, protein, and alcohol, contribute to excess body fat. The body converts some excess dietary glucose into fat, but much of it is burned as a biological fuel. As a result, dietary fat is spared from being used as a fuel, and it's stored in fat cells. Thus, eating too many carbohydrates indirectly contributes to unwanted weight gain.

- Foods that contain large amounts of refined carbohydrates may contribute to unwanted weight gain because they are often combined with hidden fats in processed foods.

- Diabetes is characterized by high blood glucose levels. Type 1 and type 2 are the two major types of diabetes. Most people with diabetes have type 2. Poorly controlled diabetes can result in cardiovascular disease, kidney failure, blindness, and lower limb amputations. Signs and symptoms of diabetes include excessive thirst and urination, sores that don't heal, vaginal yeast infections (women), and impotence (men). Signs of poorly controlled type 1 diabetes include breath that smells "fruity" and increased appetite accompanied by weight loss. People who are physically inactive, are overweight, and have a close relative with type 2 diabetes are at risk of developing this form of the disease.

- The glycemic index (GI) and glycemic load (GL) are ways of classifying certain foods by their effect on blood glucose levels. By following a low GI/GL diet, you may be able to reduce your risk of type 2 diabetes.

- Consumption of simple sugars that stick to the teeth as well as poor dental hygiene practices contribute to tooth decay. Many people are unable to digest lactose, fructose, and/or other kinds of carbohydrates completely. A low-FODMAPs diet may benefit such persons.

- Eating fiber-rich foods may reduce your risk of obesity, type 2 diabetes, cardiovascular disease, and certain intestinal tract disorders. Eating more foods that contain insoluble fiber may lower your risk of constipation and swollen hemorrhoids. Eating foods that contain soluble fiber may improve your cardiovascular health by reducing cholesterol absorption in the small intestine.

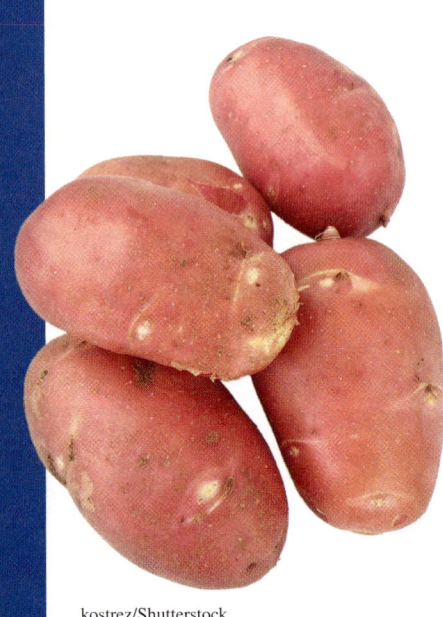

kostrez/Shutterstock

What's in Your Diet?!

1. Refer to the 3-day food log from the "What's in Your Diet?" feature in Unit 3. List the total number of kilocalories you consumed for each day of recordkeeping. Add the figures to obtain a total, divide the total by 3, then round the figure to the nearest whole number to obtain your average daily energy intake for the 3-day period.

   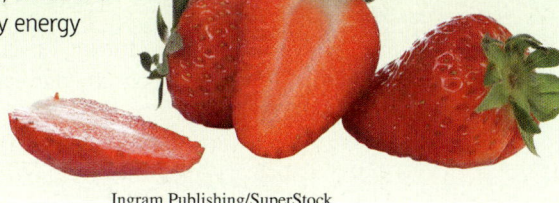
   Ingram Publishing/SuperStock

   ### Sample Calculation:

Day 1	2500 kcal
Day 2	3200 kcal
Day 3	2750 kcal
Total kcal	8450 kcal ÷ 3 days = 2817 kcal/day

   (average kilocalorie intake, rounded to the nearest whole number)

   ### Your Calculation:

Day 1	_____ kcal
Day 2	_____ kcal
Day 3	_____ kcal
Total kcal	_____ ÷ 3 days = _____ kcal/day

   (average kilocalorie intake, rounded to the nearest whole number)

2. Add the number of grams of carbohydrate eaten each day of the period. Divide the total by 3 and round to the nearest whole number to calculate the average number of grams of carbohydrate consumed daily.

   ### Your Calculation:

Day 1	_____ g
Day 2	_____ g
Day 3	_____ g
Total g	_____ ÷ 3 days = _____ g of carbohydrate/day

   (average, rounded to the nearest whole number)

3. Each gram of carbohydrate provides about 4 kcal; therefore, you must multiply the average number of grams of carbohydrate obtained in step 2 by 4 to obtain the number of kcal from carbohydrates.

   ### Your Calculation:

   _____ g/day × 4 kcal/g = _____ kcal from carbohydrates

4. To calculate the average daily percentage of kilocalories that carbohydrates contributed to your diet, divide the average kilocalories from carbohydrate obtained in step 3 by the average total daily kilocalorie intake obtained in step 1; round figure to the nearest one-hundredth. Multiply the value by 100, drop the decimal point, and add the percent symbol.

   ### Sample Calculation:

   1692 kcal ÷ 2817 kcal = 0.60

   0.60 × 100 = 60%

   ### Your Calculation:

   _____ kcal ÷ _____ kcal = _____

   _____ × 100 = _____ %

5. On average, did you consume *at least* the RDA of 130 g of carbohydrate? Yes _____ No _____

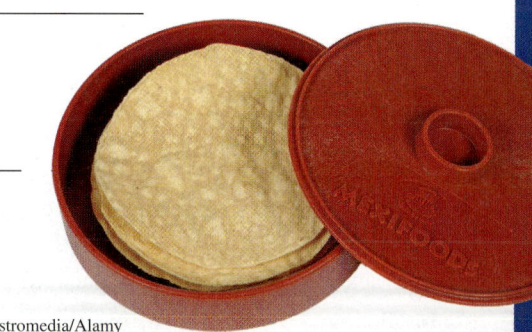
Gastromedia/Alamy

6. Did your average carbohydrate intake meet the recommended 45 to 65% of total energy? Yes ____ No ____

   a. If your average carbohydrate intake was less than 130 g or below 45% of total calories, list five nutrient-dense, carbohydrate-rich foods you could eat that would boost your intake of carbohydrates.

   Foods: _____

7. Review the log of your 3-day food intake. Calculate your average daily intake of fiber by adding the grams of fiber consumed over the 3-day period and dividing the total by three.

   Your Calculation: _____

   Day 1 ____ g
   Day 2 ____ g
   Day 3 ____ g
   Total = ____ g
   Total g ____ ÷ 3 days = ____ g of fiber daily

   a. What was your average daily fiber intake? ____ g

   b. Did your average daily fiber intake meet the Adequate Intakes of 38 and 25 g/day for young men and women, respectively? Yes ____ No ____

   c. If your response is yes, list foods that contributed to your fiber intake.

   d. If you did not meet the recommended level of fiber intake, list at least five foods that you would eat to increase your fiber intake to the recommended level.

8. Review the log of your 3-day food intake. Calculate your average daily intake of sugars by adding the grams of sugars consumed over the 3-day period and dividing the total number by three.

   a. What was your average daily intake of sugars? ____ g

   b. Calculate the average number of kcal that you consumed from sugars. ____ kcal

Consider This...

1. One of your friends thinks honey is more nutritious and safer to eat than table sugar. He wants you to avoid table sugar and use only honey as a sweetener. What would you tell this person about the nutritive value and safety of honey compared to sugar?

2. Prepare a pamphlet that describes the health benefits of dietary fiber. In addition to English, you may prepare the pamphlet in Spanish, Vietnamese, or another modern language.

3. How did you feel about drinking sugar-sweetened soft drinks before reading Unit 5? Has your opinion changed? If so, explain how.

4. If you were 25 pounds overweight, explain why you would or wouldn't follow a weight-loss diet that supplied less than 15% of calories from carbohydrate.

5. Consider the fiber content of your diet. Do you consume enough fiber each day? If your fiber intake is adequate, what foods do you eat regularly that contribute fiber to your diet? If your dietary fiber intake is low, list foods you would consume to increase your intake.

Test Yourself

Select the best answer.

1. Which of the following substances is a disaccharide?
   a. Fructose
   b. Glucose
   c. Galactose
   d. Lactose

2. Which of the following substances is a primary fuel for muscles and other cells?
   a. Glucose
   b. Glycerol
   c. Fructose
   d. Mannitol

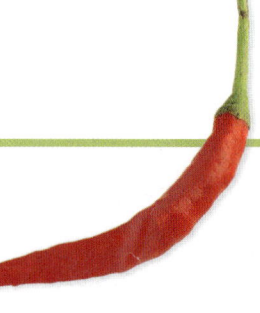

3. Which of the following substances is a polysaccharide?
   a. Glucagon
   b. Starch
   c. Lactose
   d. Aspartame

4. Dietary fiber
   a. is a source of energy for bacteria in the large intestine.
   b. is fully digested by enzymes produced by the human intestinal tract.
   c. promotes tooth decay.
   d. is only in animal sources of food.

5. Dietary fiber is
   a. in beef and pork.
   b. the primary carbohydrate in dairy foods.
   c. needed for good bowel health.
   d. an essential nutrient.

6. Which of the following substances is the hormone that enables glucose to enter cells?
   a. Glucagon
   b. Adrenaline
   c. Glycerol
   d. Insulin

7. Which of the following substances is an enzyme that breaks down lactose?
   a. Galactose
   b. Hydrochloric acid
   c. Lactase
   d. Lactic acid

8. Type 1 diabetes is
   a. a disease that primarily affects elderly people.
   b. characterized by severe hypoglycemia.
   c. often associated with excess body weight.
   d. an autoimmune disease.

9. Which of the following signs is generally associated with type 2 diabetes?
   a. Swollen hemorrhoids
   b. Elevated blood glucose
   c. Low glycemic index
   d. Dental decay

10. A major source of added sugars in the typical American diet is
    a. sweetened yogurt.
    b. whole fruit.
    c. sugar-sweetened soft drinks.
    d. pickled vegetables.

11. Recently, 5-year-old Lane tires easily, is unusually thirsty, and makes frequent trips to the bathroom to relieve his urinary bladder. According to his mother, Lane's breath smells like over-ripe bananas. Based on this information, Lane's parents should have him tested for
    a. diverticular disease.
    b. type 1 diabetes.
    c. GERD.
    d. peptic ulcers.

12. Wynona avoids drinking more than a few ounces of milk at a time because she develops bloating, intestinal cramps, and diarrhea after consuming the beverage. Based on this information, Wynona probably has
    a. diverticular disease.
    b. maltase toxicity.
    c. glucose resistance.
    d. lactose intolerance.

Answers: 1. d 2. a 3. b 4. a 5. c 6. d 7. c 8. d 9. b 10. c 11. b 12. d

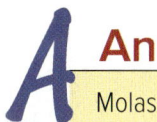

Answer This (Module 5.1b)

Molasses

References → See Appendix D.

Wendy Schiff

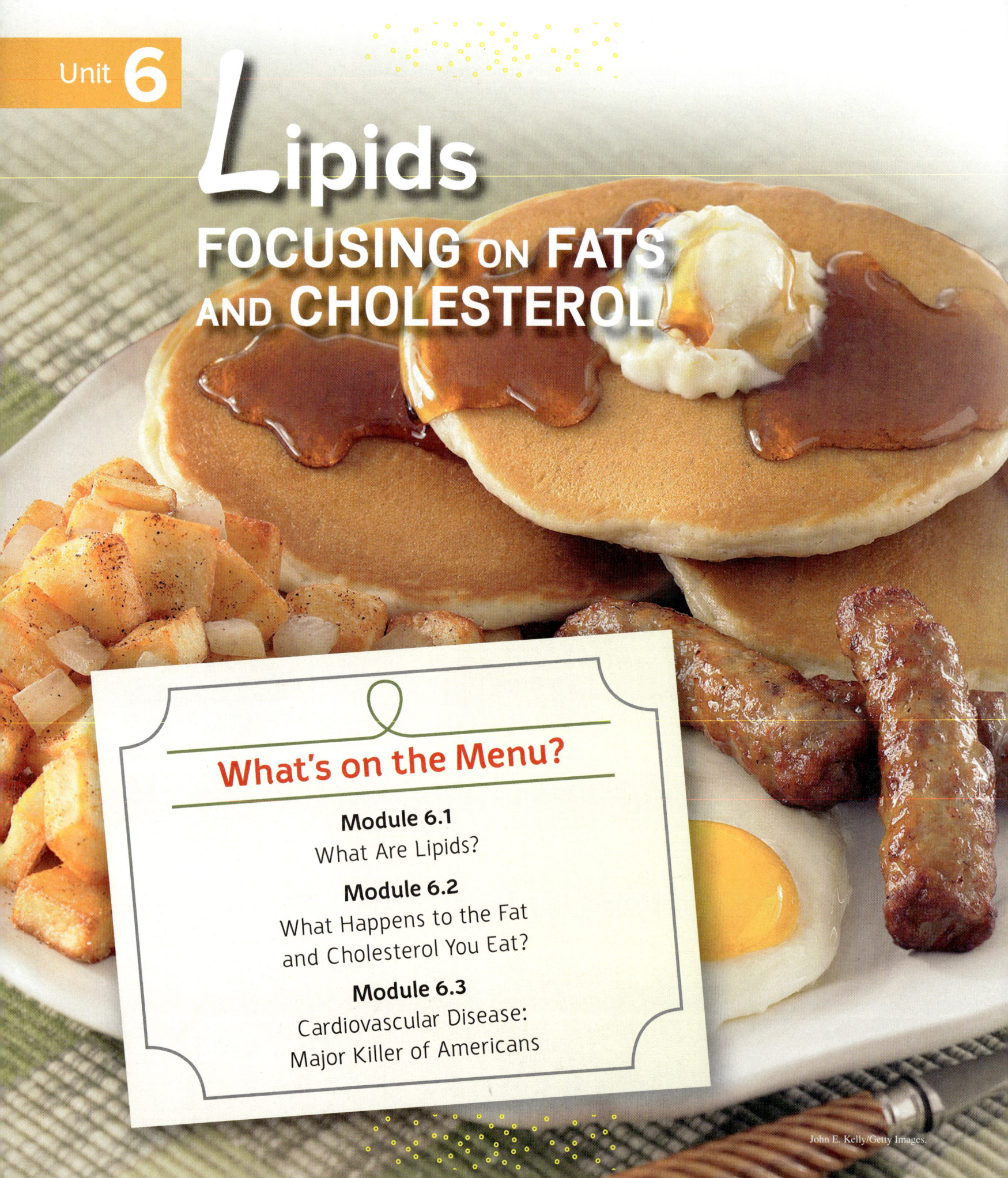

Unit 6

Lipids
FOCUSING ON FATS AND CHOLESTEROL

What's on the Menu?

Module 6.1
What Are Lipids?

Module 6.2
What Happens to the Fat and Cholesterol You Eat?

Module 6.3
Cardiovascular Disease: Major Killer of Americans

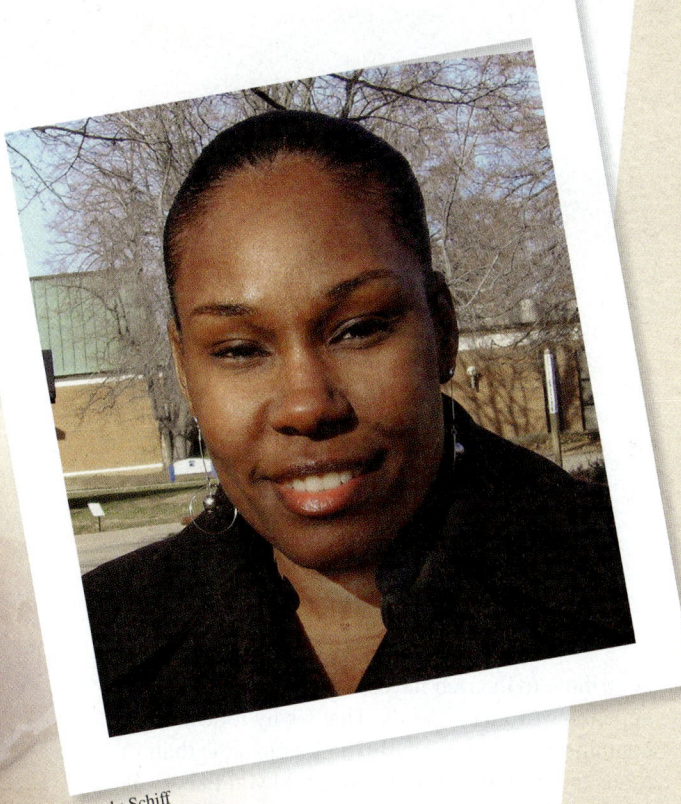
Wendy Schiff

"I eat all the wrong foods. I like butter on everything! For breakfast, my mom usually makes sausage, fried eggs, and pancakes. For lunch, I try to eat salads, but sometimes, I just grab some potato chips or "hot fries." We eat dinner late—around 10 at night—when my mother brings fast food home. I eat cereal daily; I'm trying to get more fiber in my system. I like the high-fiber, high-antioxidant cereals.

My mother takes medication to control her high cholesterol and blood pressure.... I'm healthy, but I don't like my pudgy belly. I would like to lose 20, maybe 30 pounds. I just don't have the motivation to eat better and exercise more."

Nancy Scott

Nancy Scott majored in nursing at Florissant Valley Community College. As the mother of two school-aged children, Nancy is extremely busy with her job and family. It's difficult for her to plan nutritious meals for herself and her children. Should she be more concerned about her diet, especially her fat intake? Should Nancy be concerned about her family history of high cholesterol and blood pressure levels?

What do you think when you hear the word *fat* or *cholesterol?* Does "bad" or "overweight" or "heart disease" enter your mind? If your answer is yes, are you concerned about the amounts and types of fat in your diet? Why?

You may be surprised to learn that having some fat ("healthy fats") in your diet is essential to good health. However, consuming high amounts of certain fats ("unhealthy fats") may increase your risk of serious health conditions, especially heart disease.[1] By reading Unit 6, you'll learn about fats and other lipids in your food and body as well as their major food sources. Additionally, you'll learn how these nutrients may influence your health.

Module 6.1
What Are Lipids?

6.1 - Learning Outcomes

After reading Module 6.1, you should be able to

1. Define all of the **key terms** in this module.
2. Identify the major lipids in your diet as well as their primary food sources and functions in your body.
3. Explain the difference between a saturated and an unsaturated fatty acid.
4. Identify foods that are rich sources of saturated fat, monounsaturated fat, or polyunsaturated fat.
5. Identify the two essential fatty acids and foods that are rich sources of these nutrients.
6. Identify sources of trans fats, and explain why partially hydrogenated oils have been banned from foods.

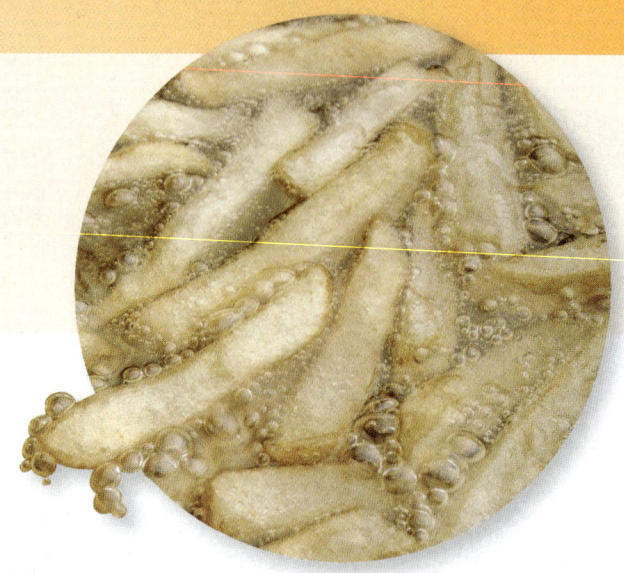

Ed Bock Photography Studio/Ingram Publishing

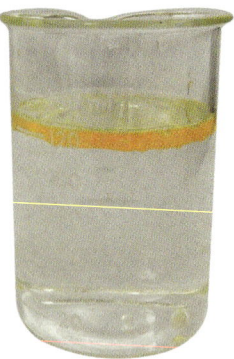

Wendy Schiff

Lipids generally don't dissolve in water or watery solutions such as vinegar.

Fats, oils, and cholesterol are **lipids,** a class of organic nutrients that generally don't dissolve in water (*water insoluble*). Despite all the "bad press," fat and cholesterol are very important nutrients. Fat is a major source of energy for the body; recall from Unit 1 that each gram of fat supplies 9 kcal. Fats and other lipids play many other important roles in your body, including

- maintaining cell membranes,
- producing certain hormones,
- insulating against cold temperatures,
- regulating blood pressure and inflammation, and
- cushioning against bumps, blows, and falls.

Dietary fat helps your body absorb fat-soluble vitamins and phytochemicals. Dietary lipids also contribute to the rich flavor, smooth texture, and appetizing aroma of foods. That's why foods that contain some fat often taste more enjoyable than foods that lack the nutrient. What do you like to add to a baked potato—butter, margarine, sour cream, or some other fatty food?

6.1a Fatty Acids and Triglycerides

Most lipids have fatty acids in their chemical makeup. Each **fatty acid (FA)** has a chain of carbon atoms bonded to each other and to hydrogen atoms (**Fig. 6.1**). At one end of the chain, the first carbon has three hydrogen atoms attached to it. This part of the chain is called the *omega end*. At the other end of the fatty acid chain, the last carbon has two oxygen atoms and one hydrogen atom in a special arrangement that's called an "acid group."

A **triglyceride** is composed of three fatty acid molecules attached to a glycerol (*glis'-er-ol*) "backbone" molecule (**Fig. 6.2**).

Triglycerides comprise about 95% of lipids in your body and food. Triglycerides are often referred to as *fats* and *oils*. In this textbook, triglycerides, fats, and oils may be referred to simply as "fats."

lipids class of organic nutrients that generally don't dissolve in water (water insoluble)

fatty acid (FA) chain of carbon atoms bonded to each other and to hydrogen atoms with an acid group on one end

triglyceride lipid that has three fatty acids attached to a three-carbon compound called glycerol; fats and oils

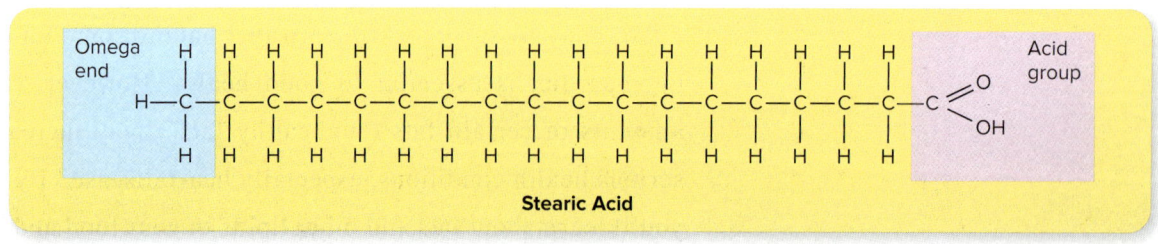

Stearic Acid

Figure 6.1 Fatty acid. This particular fatty acid is stearic acid. Chemists often use straight lines to show bonds between carbon, hydrogen, and oxygen atoms.

What Are Saturated Fat and Unsaturated Fat?

Fatty acids can be saturated or unsaturated. Furthermore, unsaturated fatty acids can be either monounsaturated or polyunsaturated. In foods, the three different types of fatty acids usually occur in different proportions.

The fatty acid shown in Figure 6.1 (stearic acid) has single bonds holding each carbon in the carbon chain together. Note that each of these carbons has two hydrogen atoms attached to it. This is a **saturated fatty acid (saturated FA)** because each carbon within the chain is completely filled (*saturated*) with hydrogen atoms. Animal fats tend to contain more saturated FAs, such as stearic acid, than plant oils. Important exceptions are the highly saturated "tropical" plant oils—cocoa butter and coconut, palm, and palm kernel oils.

A **monounsaturated fatty acid (monounsaturated FA)** has two neighboring carbons within the carbon chain that each lacks a hydrogen atom. When this occurs, a double bond holds those particular carbons together (**Fig. 6.3**). Oleic acid is a monounsaturated FA. Avocados and olive, peanut, and canola oils are rich sources of monounsaturated FAs.

A **polyunsaturated fatty acid (polyunsaturated FA)** has more than one double bond in the carbon chain (**Fig. 6.4**). Safflower (high-linoleic), grapeseed, sunflower seed (high-linoleic), and soybean oils are rich sources of polyunsaturated FAs. **Essential Concept 6.1** compares certain sources of saturated and unsaturated FAs. **Table 6.1** compares the percentages of saturated FAs, monounsaturated FAs, and polyunsaturated FAs in commonly eaten fats.

Liquid or Solid Fat? Saturated fatty acid molecules can pack together tightly because they are straighter than unsaturated fatty acids. This structural difference allows animal fats that are rich sources of saturated FAs, such as beef fat and butter fat, to be fairly solid at usual room temperatures. On the other hand, the double bonds of unsaturated fatty acids cause the molecules to have "bends" or kinks in their chemical structures. Such bends prevent the molecules from being arranged tightly together and forming solids. That's why a fat that contains a high proportion of unsaturated fatty acids, such as sunflower seed oil or corn oil, tends to be liquid when it's stored at room temperature.

Essential Fatty Acids The body cannot make two polyunsaturated FAs. These **essential fatty acids** are **linoleic** (*lin'-o-lay'-ik*) **acid** and **alpha-linolenic** (*al-fah lin-o-len'-ik*) **acid**. Linoleic acid is an **omega-6 fatty acid** (see Figure 6.4). Alpha-linolenic acid is an **omega-3 fatty acid** (Fig. 6.5). The "6" and "3" in the names identify the position of the first double bond that appears in the fatty acids' carbon chains, when you start counting carbons at the omega end of the molecules.

Corn oil, seeds, and nuts are naturally rich sources of linoleic acid. Seafood is generally a rich source of alpha-linolenic acid (see Table 6.4).

Cells use alpha-linolenic acid to produce two other omega-3 fatty acids: **eicosapentaenoic** (*eye'-ko-seh-pen'-tah-ee-no'-ik*) **acid (EPA)** and **docosahexaenoic** (*doe'-ko-seh-hex'-uh-ee-no'-ik*) **acid (DHA)**. Cells can

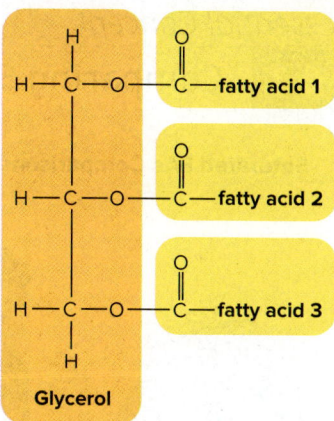

Figure 6.2 Basic parts of a triglyceride.

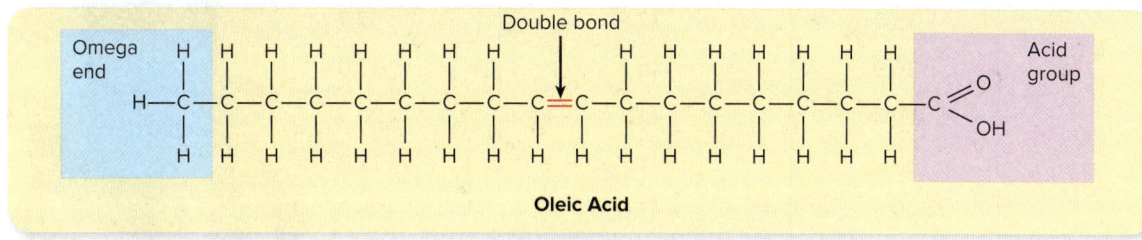

Figure 6.3 Monounsaturated fatty acid. This particular fatty acid is oleic acid.

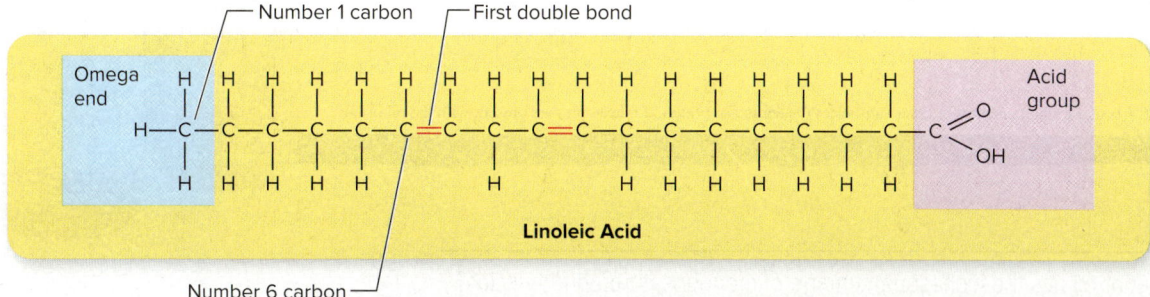

Figure 6.4 Polyunsaturated fatty acid. This particular fatty acid is linoleic acid, an omega-6 fatty acid.

■ *What is the basic structural difference between a polyunsaturated FA and a monounsaturated FA?*

---

saturated fatty acid (saturated FA) fatty acid that has only single bonds holding each carbon in the carbon chain together

monounsaturated fatty acid (monounsaturated FA) fatty acid that has one double bond within the carbon chain

polyunsaturated fatty acid (polyunsaturated FA) fatty acid that has two or more double bonds within the carbon chain

essential fatty acids lipids that must be supplied by the diet

linoleic acid an essential omega-6 fatty acid

alpha-linolenic acid an essential omega-3 fatty acid

omega-3 fatty acid type of polyunsaturated fatty acid that has its first double bond at the number 3 carbon

omega-6 fatty acid type of polyunsaturated fatty acid that has its first double bond at the number 6 carbon

eicosapentaenoic acid (EPA) omega-3 fatty acid derived from alpha-linolenic acid

docosahexaenoic acid (DHA) omega-3 fatty acid derived from alpha-linolenic acid

Essential Concept

6.1 Comparing Sources of Saturated and Unsaturated FAs

Saturated FAs Comparisons

Beef fat has more **saturated FAs** than corn oil.

Polyunsaturated FAs Comparisons

Corn oil has some **saturated FAs**, but it's a richer source of **polyunsaturated FAs** than beef fat.

Monounsaturated FAs Comparisons

Olive oil has a lot more **monounsaturated FAs** than beef fat or corn oil.

Table 6.1 — Comparing Fatty Acid Contents of Fats and Oils*

Fat/Oil	% Saturated	% Monounsaturated	% Polyunsaturated
Safflower oil (high linoleic)	6.2	14.4	74.6
Canola oil	7.4	63.3	28.1
Walnut oil	9.1	22.8	63.3
Grapeseed oil	9.6	16.1	69.9
Sunflower oil (high linoleic)	10.3	19.5	65.7
Corn oil	12.9	27.6	54.7
Olive oil	13.8	73.0	10.5
Soybean oil	15.7	22.8	57.7
Peanut oil	16.9	46.2	32.0
Chicken fat	29.8	44.7	20.9
Lard (pork fat)	39.2	45.1	11.2
Palm oil	49.3	37.0	9.3
Beef fat	49.8	41.8	4.0
Butter	50.4	23.4	3.0
Cocoa butter	59.7	32.9	3.0
Coconut oil	82.5	6.3	1.7

*Values don't total 100% because small amounts of other substances (water and/or protein, for example) are present with the oil or fat.

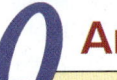 **Answer This**

Based on Table 6.1, which fat or oil has the highest percentage of monounsaturated fatty acids? You can find the answer on the last page of this unit.

Raw meat, Corn oil, Olive oil: Wendy Schiff; Blue placemat: McGraw-Hill Education/Mark A. Dierker, photographer; Cooking oils: Elite Images/McGraw-Hill Education convert linoleic acid to another omega-6 fatty acid, **arachidonic** (air-ik'-ah-don'-ik) **acid (AA)**. **Figure 6.6** shows relationships among the essential fatty acids.

Essential fatty acids are necessary in small amounts for good health. The body uses EPA, DHA, and AA to make several hormone-like substances. These

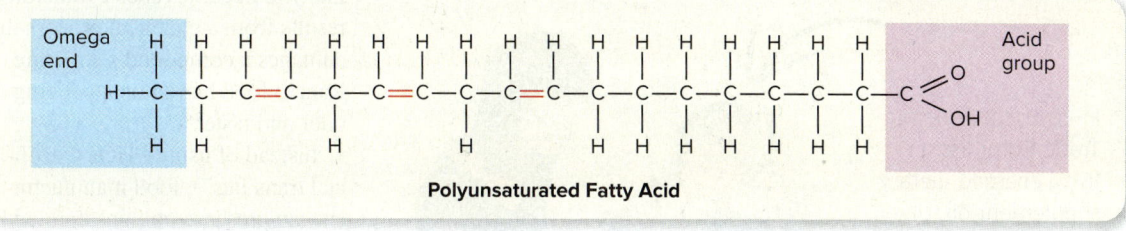

Figure 6.5 Alpha-linolenic acid (an omega-3 fatty acid).

compounds have a variety of important effects, such as regulating blood pressure and the immune system's inflammatory response. Infants require DHA and EPA for nervous system development, and babies don't grow properly when their diets lack essential fatty acids. Other signs of essential fatty acid deficiency include scaly skin, hair loss, and poor wound healing. In the United States, essential fatty acid deficiency is uncommon because most Americans eat plenty of fat, especially linoleic acid.

What Are Trans Fats? **Trans fatty acids** ("trans fats") are unsaturated fatty acids that have an unusual type of chemical structure **(Fig. 6.7)**. Some carbons with double bonds have hydrogens on the opposite instead of the same side. This structure enables the carbon chain to be relatively straight, compared to other types of unsaturated fatty acids.

Prior to 2018, processed foods contributed the largest share of trans fat in the American diet. *Partially hydrogenated oils (PHOs)* were the major kind of trans fat in processed foods. **Partial hydrogenation** is a food manufacturing process that converts many of an oil's naturally occurring unsaturated fatty acids into trans fatty acids and saturated fatty acids.

For several years, medical experts had been growing increasingly concerned about the negative effects of trans fat on health, especially PHOs. In 2015, the FDA banned the use of PHOs in foods.[2] This ban went into effect for most foods in 2018.

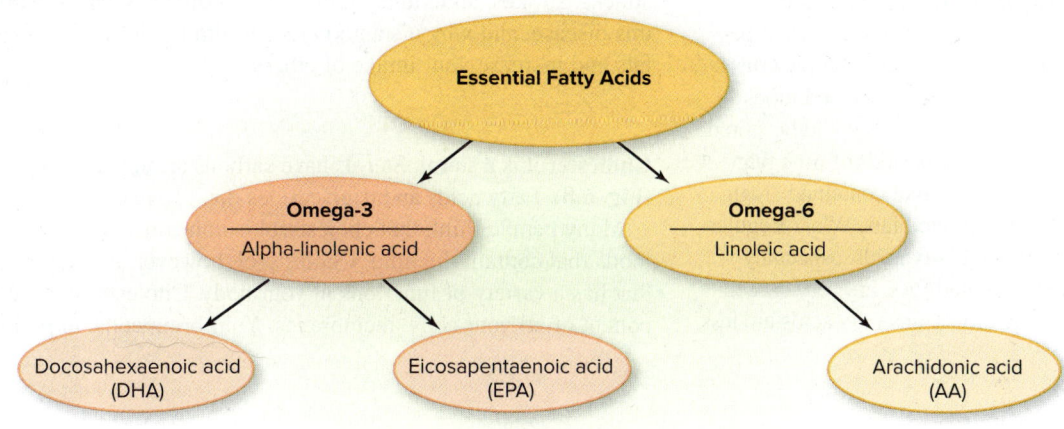

Figure 6.6 Relationships among essential fatty acids.

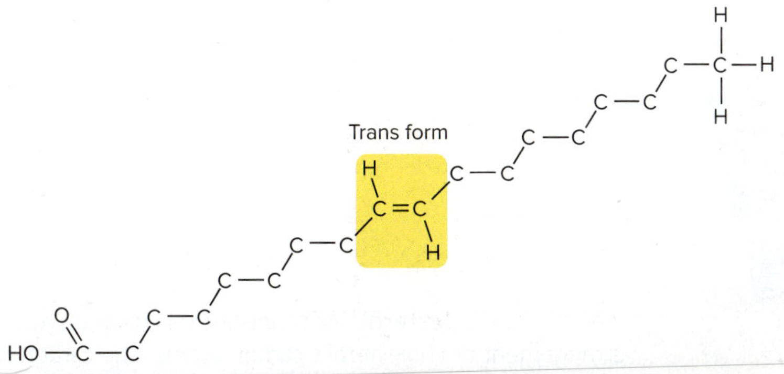

Figure 6.7 **Trans fatty acid.** For simplicity, this diagram doesn't show all of the hydrogens within the carbon chain.

arachidonic acid (AA) omega-6 fatty acid derived from linoleic acid

trans fatty acids unsaturated fatty acids that have an unusual structure

partial hydrogenation food manufacturing process that adds hydrogen atoms to liquid vegetable oil, forming trans fats and saturated fats

TASTY Tidbits

In 2010, the Federal Trade Commission (FTC) charged dietary supplement distributor NBTY, Inc. and two related companies, NatureSmart LLC and Rexall Sundown, Inc., with making false claims about the amount of DHA in their Disney- and Marvel Heroes–licensed children's multivitamin supplements. The companies also claimed that a daily serving of the multivitamin promoted healthy brain and eye development in children. According to the FTC, such claims were not supported by scientific evidence. The companies were required to refund $2.1 million to consumers who purchased the vitamins.[3]

Why were PHOs used by food manufacturers? Because the shape of a trans fatty acid is like that of a saturated fat, a partially hydrogenated vegetable oil is more solid at room temperature. This feature enabled food manufacturers to make shortening and sticks of margarine. Shortening was used to fry foods and make pastries, especially flaky biscuits and pie crusts. Furthermore, processed foods made with PHOs could be stored for longer periods of time than could foods that contained "regular" unsaturated fats. Why? Regular unsaturated fatty acids, especially polyunsaturated FAs, are very susceptible to rancidity. Trans fatty acids are less likely to become rancid. Rancidity results from a chemical process that damages a compound's structure. Rancid food has an unappetizing odor and taste.

Instead of using PHOs ("artificial trans fats"), food manufacturers can preserve polyunsaturated FAs in foods by adding antioxidants, such as butylated hydroxyanisole (BHA) and butylated hydroxytoluene (BHT), to them. Additionally, highly saturated tropical oils, particularly coconut oil and palm oil, are often used to replace PHOs in processed foods.

Although PHOs have been banned, trans fat is not likely to disappear completely from your diet. Some foods (particularly, beef and whole-fat dairy foods) naturally contain small amounts of this type of fat.

The U.S. Food and Drug Administration (FDA) requires food manufacturers to show their products' trans fat content in the Nutrition Facts panel. According to the Dietary Guidelines, Americans should keep their trans fat intake as low as possible while eating a healthy diet.[1]

Why is it important to understand the differences among saturated, unsaturated, and trans fats, and identify foods that contain high amounts of these fats? Populations that consume diets rich in saturated fat and trans fat have higher risk of cardiovascular disease than populations whose diets contain more unsaturated fat.[1] **Cardiovascular disease (CVD)** is a group of diseases that affect the heart and blood vessels. Cardiovascular disease can result in heart attacks, strokes, and kidney failure. In Module 6.3, you'll learn about this disease, and why it's a good idea to limit your intake of certain fats and increase your intake of others.

cardiovascular disease (CVD) group of diseases that affect the heart and blood vessels

cholesterol sterol in animal foods that's made by your body

6.1b Cholesterol

Cholesterol is a sterol. Sterols have carbons arranged in rings (Fig. 6.8). Fatty acids and triglycerides don't have carbon rings.

Many people think that cholesterol is unhealthy, so they avoid foods that contain the lipid. Cholesterol, however, is a key nutrient that has a variety of functions in your body. Cholesterol is a component of all your cells' membranes. Your brain cells, in particular,

TASTY Tidbits

Before the ban on PHOs, fast-food outlets relied on shortening that contained PHOs for deep-fat frying items such as French fries and breaded chicken. Because PHOs can no longer be used in processed or commercially prepared foods, the food industry is now relying on other oils, including high oleic oils, which are rich sources of monounsaturated FA.

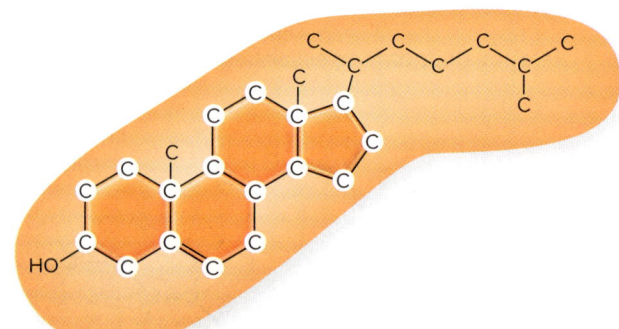

Figure 6.8 Cholesterol. For simplicity, this diagram just shows the arrangement of cholesterol's carbon atoms. The carbon rings are highlighted.

■ *Why do your cells need cholesterol?*

Woman and girl: - I: zorani/Getty Images; Pie: Wendy Schiff; French fries: Mixa/Alamy

contain high amounts of cholesterol. Although cholesterol isn't metabolized for energy, cells use the lipid to produce a variety of substances, including vitamin D, and steroid hormones such as estrogen and testosterone. Your liver uses cholesterol to make bile salts, which help the small intestine digest lipids.

Although triglycerides are widespread in foods, dietary sources of cholesterol are only in animal foods. Egg yolk, liver, meat, poultry, whole milk, shrimp, cheese, and ice cream are rich sources of cholesterol **(Table 6.2)**. Even if you don't eat animal foods, your body produces all the cholesterol you need, primarily in the liver. If your body makes too much cholesterol, the excess can increase your risk of CVD.

6.1c What Are Phospholipids?

A **phospholipid** is chemically similar to a triglyceride, except that one of the fatty acids is replaced by chemical groups that contain phosphorus and, often, nitrogen. Phospholipids are needed for normal functioning of nerve cells, including those in the brain. Phospholipids are also major structural components of cell membranes. Cell membranes are comprised of a double layer that is mostly phospholipids **(Fig. 6.9)**. The phosphate "head" of a phospholipid is water soluble. The two fatty acid "tails" of a phospholipid are not water soluble. Thus, phospholipids are soluble in both water and fat. In a cell membrane, the phosphate heads of phospholipids face the watery environments that are inside and outside the cell. The fatty acid tails of phospholipids avoid such watery environments, so they face each other within the membrane (see Figure 6.9). The two fatty acids that comprise a phospholipid may be saturated and/or unsaturated. Compared to saturated fatty acids, unsaturated fatty acids help make the membrane more flexible.

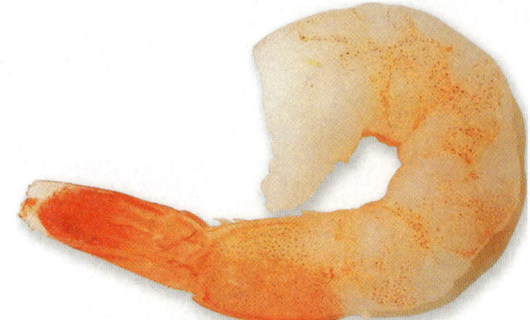

Shrimp is a rich source of cholesterol.

phospholipid type of lipid needed to make cell membranes and for proper functioning of nerve cells

TABLE 6.2 APPROXIMATE CHOLESTEROL CONTENT OF SOME FOODS/SERVING

Food	Serving Size	Cholesterol (mg)
Liver, beef, braised	3 oz	337
Egg, hard cooked	1 large	186
Egg yolk, hard cooked	1	184
Shrimp, cooked	3 oz	161
Sardines, Atlantic, canned in oil, drained	3 oz	121
Turkey, cooked, dark meat, no skin	3 oz	109
Turkey patty, ground, lean, broiled	3 oz	89
Beef patty, ground, 85% lean, broiled	3 oz	75
Chicken breast, meat only, cooked	3 oz	73
Salmon, Atlantic, cooked	3 oz	54
Ham, smoked, extra lean	3 oz	42
Hot dog	1	28
Chocolate milkshake, thick	8 fl oz	25
Whole milk	8 fl oz	24
Egg noodles, cooked	½ cup	23
Ice cream, vanilla, light, soft-serve	½ cup	11

Source of data: U.S. Department of Agriculture, Agricultural Research Service: *USDA National Nutrient Database for Standard Reference Legacy Release, April 2018.* https://ndb.nal.usda.gov/ndb/search/list?home=true Accessed: September 2018

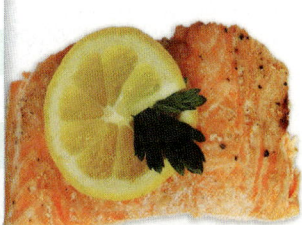

Shrimp, Salmon: Wendy Schiff; Ice cream cone: Ingram Publishing

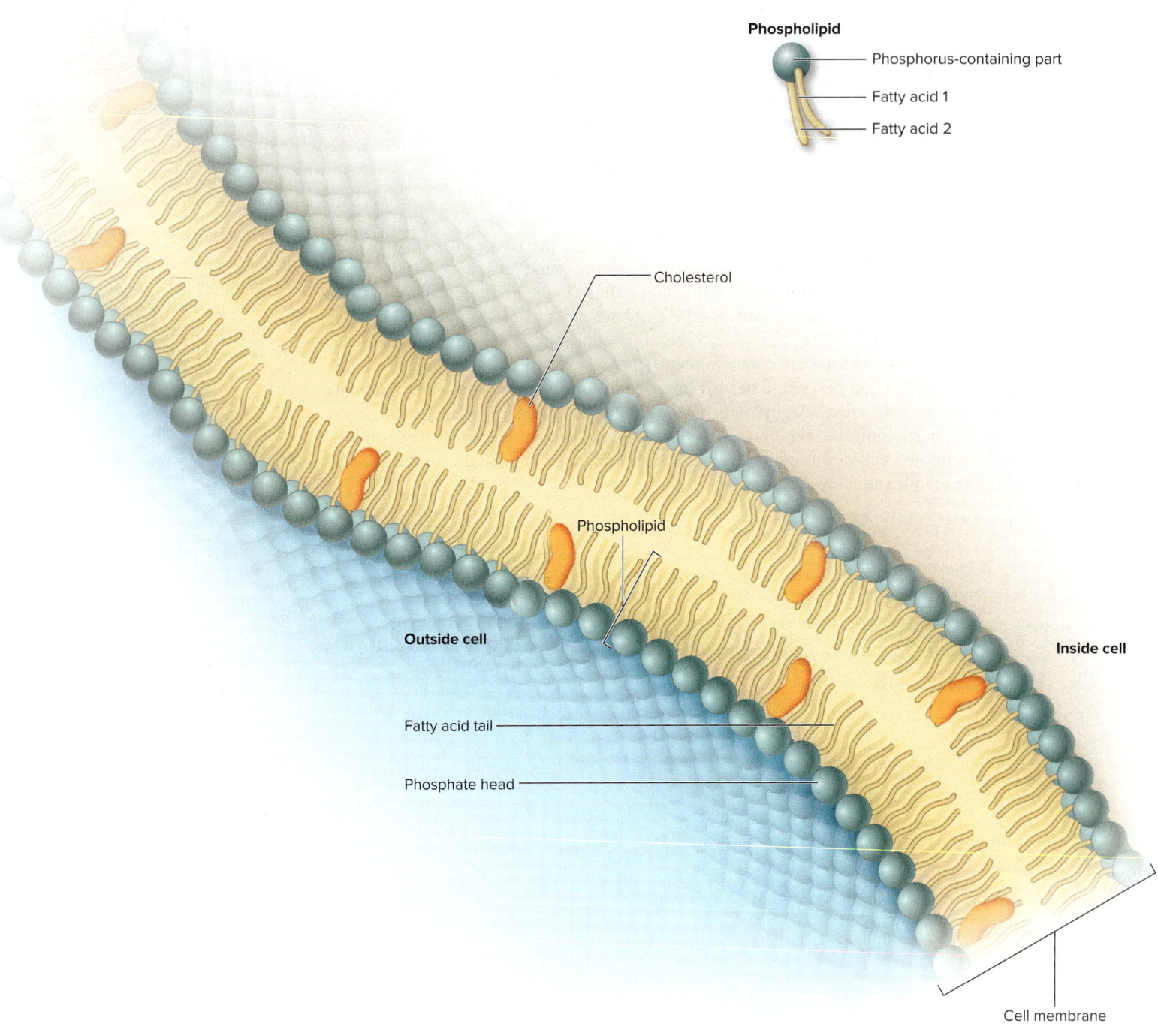

Figure 6.9 Phospholipids in a cell membrane.

■ *What is a major structural component of cell membranes?*

lecithin major phospholipid in food

choline vitamin-like nutrient

Phospholipids are found naturally in plant and animal foods. **Lecithin** (*less'-uh-thin*) is the primary phospholipid in food; egg yolks, liver, wheat germ, peanut butter, and soybeans are rich sources of lecithin. Lecithin contains **choline** (*co'-leen*). Nerves use choline to produce acetylcholine (*ah-see'-till-co'-leen*), a chemical that transmits messages between nerve cells.

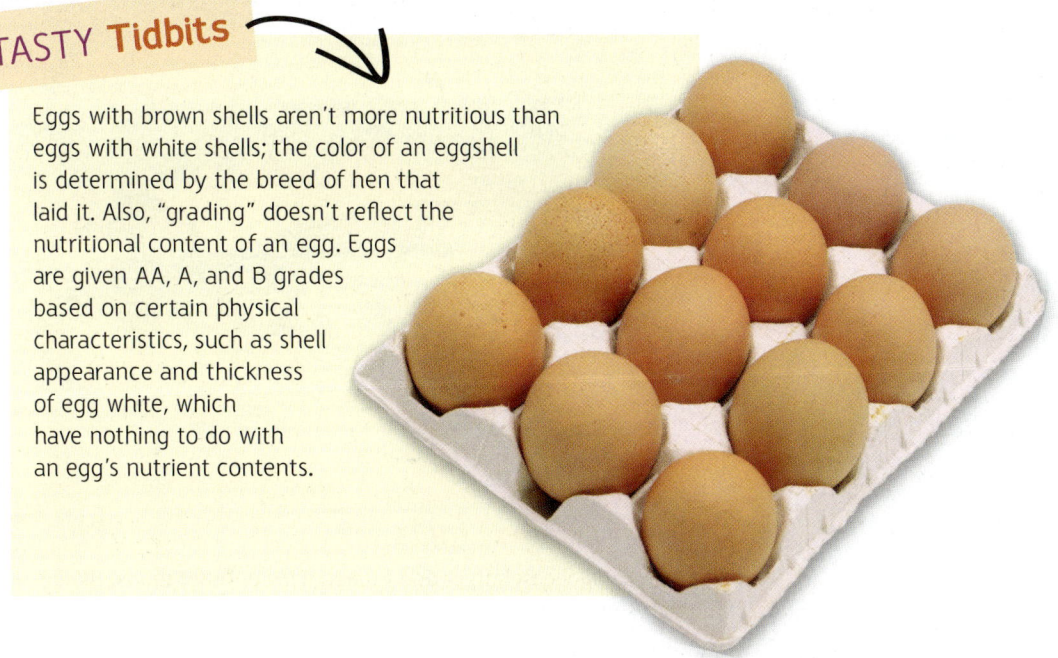

TASTY Tidbits

Eggs with brown shells aren't more nutritious than eggs with white shells; the color of an eggshell is determined by the breed of hen that laid it. Also, "grading" doesn't reflect the nutritional content of an egg. Eggs are given AA, A, and B grades based on certain physical characteristics, such as shell appearance and thickness of egg white, which have nothing to do with an egg's nutrient contents.

A healthy adult's body makes phospholipids, so deficiencies among adults are uncommon. Nutrition experts, however, classify choline as a vitamin-like nutrient because deficiency symptoms can occur under certain conditions, including pregnancy.[4] Unit 8 provides more information about choline.

In foods, phospholipids can serve as an **emulsifier**, a substance that keeps fat-soluble and water-soluble compounds together. Manufacturers may add emulsifiers to foods to keep oily and watery ingredients from separating during storage. Egg yolk naturally contains phospholipids. Eggs are often used to emulsify oil and vinegar when making mayonnaise and mixing oil and milk in cake or pancake batters.

emulsifier substance that helps fat-soluble and water-soluble compounds mix with each other

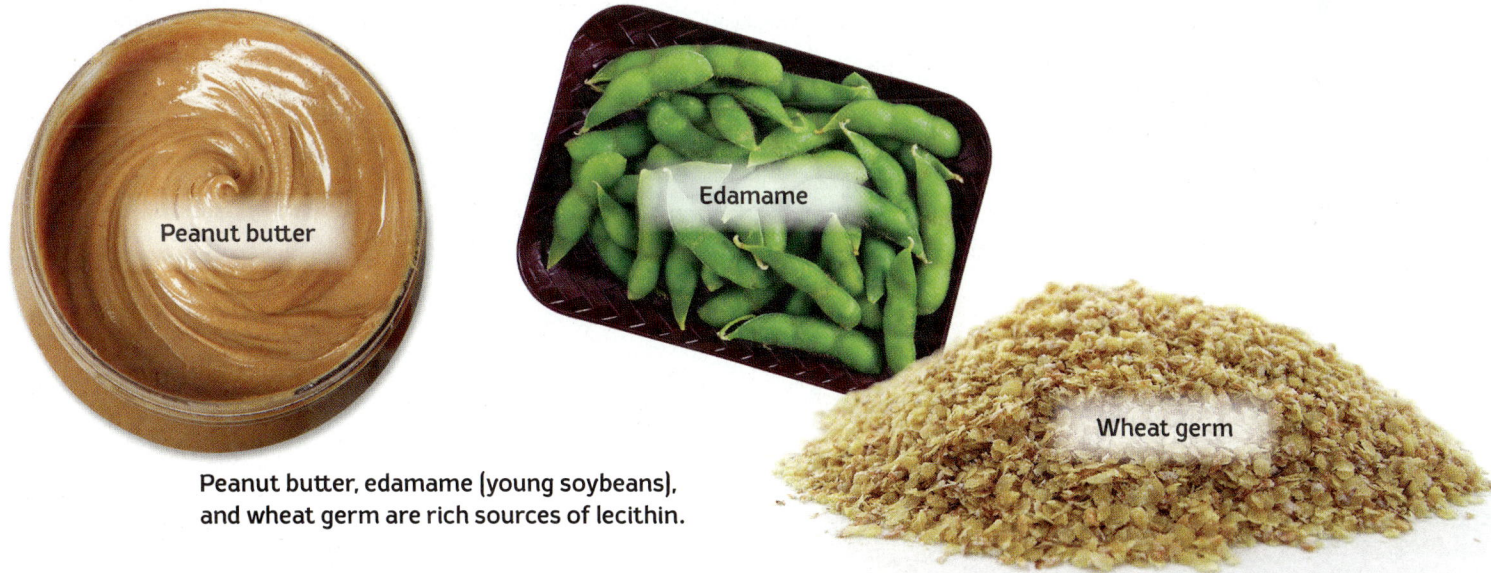

Peanut butter, edamame (young soybeans), and wheat germ are rich sources of lecithin.

Eggs: Pixtal/AGE Fotostock; Peanut butter: D. Hurst/Alamy Images; Edamame: C Squared Studios/Getty Images; Wheat germ: Wendy Schiff

Module 6.2

What Happens to the Fat and Cholesterol You Eat?

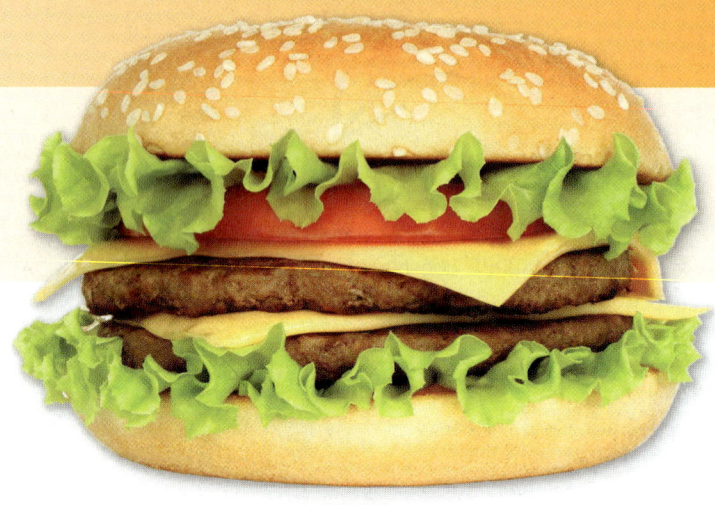
rvlsoft/123RF

6.2 - Learning Outcomes

After reading Module 6.2, you should be able to

1. Define all of the **key terms** in this module.
2. Describe what happens to the fat and cholesterol in food as they undergo digestion and absorption in your intestinal tract.
3. Describe the function of a chylomicron.

6.2a Digesting Lipids

When you eat a cheeseburger and French fries or other foods, the fat in the items undergoes a little digestion in the stomach. However, the small intestine is the primary site of lipid digestion. The pancreas releases enzymes (**lipases**) into the small intestine that digest fats and phospholipids. Because fats don't dissolve well in watery chyme, fat digestion involves the need for an emulsifier (see **Essential Concept 6.2**).

Essential Concept

6.2 Digesting Fat

1. In response to the presence of the fatty chyme in the duodenum, the gallbladder releases bile into the chyme. Bile contains **bile salts**, which emulsify the lipids—that is, keep lipids suspended as small particles in chyme.

Legend:
- Glycerol
- Free fatty acids
- Monoglycerides
- Triglycerides
- Bile salts

2. The presence of chyme in the small intestine also stimulates the pancreas to secrete **pancreatic lipase.** Pancreatic lipase gains greater access to the fat molecules because of the action of bile salts. As a result, the lipase digests the molecules more easily. Without the presence of bile salts, lipids in chyme would clump together in large fatty globules, making lipid digestion less efficient.

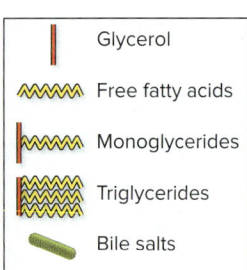

Bile salts in bile

Large fat droplet → Emulsified lipids

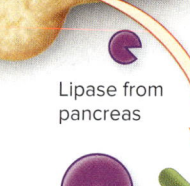
Lipase from pancreas

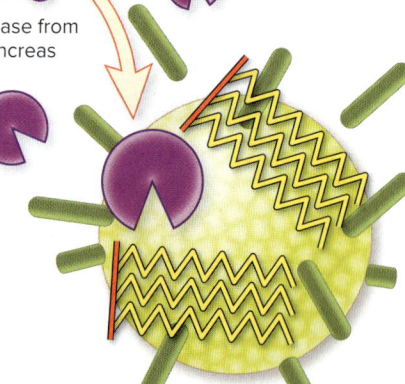

lipases enzymes that break down lipids

bile salts component of bile

pancreatic lipase digestive enzyme that removes two fatty acids from each triglyceride molecule

138

What Happens to the Fat and Cholesterol You Eat?

monoglyceride single fatty acid attached to a glycerol backbone

micelle lipid-rich particle that is surrounded by bile salts; transports lipids to absorptive cells

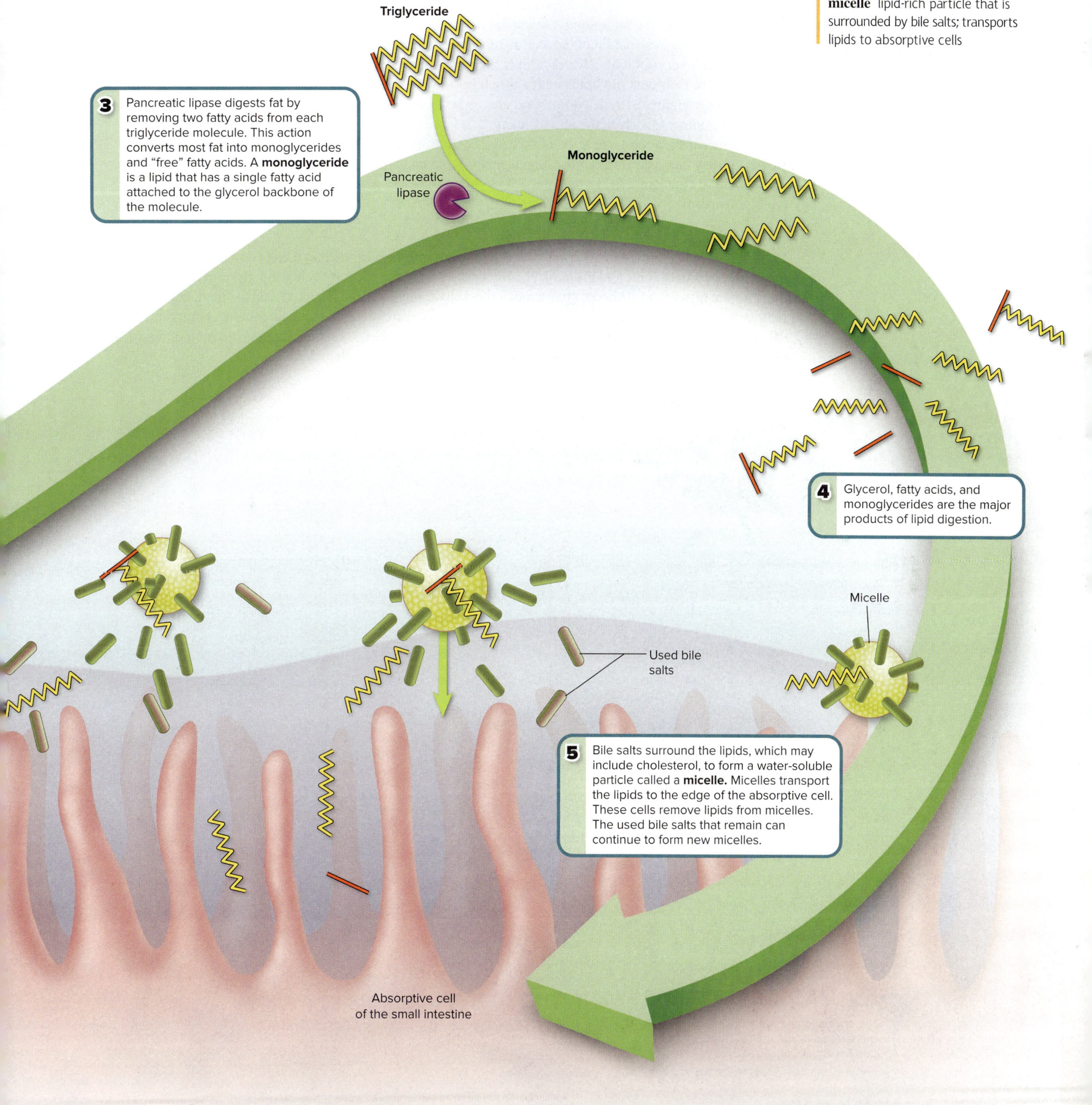

Triglyceride

3 Pancreatic lipase digests fat by removing two fatty acids from each triglyceride molecule. This action converts most fat into monoglycerides and "free" fatty acids. A **monoglyceride** is a lipid that has a single fatty acid attached to the glycerol backbone of the molecule.

Pancreatic lipase

Monoglyceride

4 Glycerol, fatty acids, and monoglycerides are the major products of lipid digestion.

Micelle

Used bile salts

5 Bile salts surround the lipids, which may include cholesterol, to form a water-soluble particle called a **micelle.** Micelles transport the lipids to the edge of the absorptive cell. These cells remove lipids from micelles. The used bile salts that remain can continue to form new micelles.

Absorptive cell of the small intestine

lipoprotein structure that transports lipids through the bloodstream and lymph

very-low-density lipoprotein (VLDL) lipoprotein that transports a high proportion of lipids in the bloodstream

6.2b Absorbing and Transporting Fat and Cholesterol

In the small intestine, absorptive cells remove monoglycerides, fatty acids, glycerol, and cholesterol from micelles. (Cholesterol doesn't undergo digestion.) Under normal conditions, the small intestine digests and absorbs nearly all of the fat in food, but only about 50% of the dietary cholesterol is absorbed. In the absorptive cells, the fatty acids and monoglyceride molecules are reassembled into triglycerides **(Fig. 6.10)**.

Lipids aren't very soluble in watery fluids such as lymph (fluid that's in the lymphatic system) and blood. The absorptive cells coat the lipids with a thin layer of protein, phospholipids, and cholesterol to form chylomicrons (see Figure 6.10). Chylomicrons are a type of **lipoprotein.** A lipoprotein transports lipids through watery environments such as the bloodstream.

Chylomicrons are too large to be absorbed directly into the bloodstream from absorptive cells. However, they can pass through the larger openings of lacteals, lymphatic system vessels in each villus (see Essential Concept 4.5). Lymph carries chylomicrons to a major vein in the chest, where they enter the bloodstream.

What Happens to Chylomicrons?

Cells in the walls of tiny blood vessels called capillaries release a lipase that breaks down the chylomicron's load of fat into fatty acids and glycerol. Nearby cells can pick up the fatty acids and glycerol and metabolize them for energy. Ten to 12 hours after a meal, most chylomicrons have been reduced to small, cholesterol-rich particles. The liver clears these particles from the bloodstream and uses their contents to produce various substances, including **very-low-density lipoprotein (VLDL).** VLDL carries a high proportion of lipids in the bloodstream. Module 6.3 provides more details about lipoproteins such as VLDL.

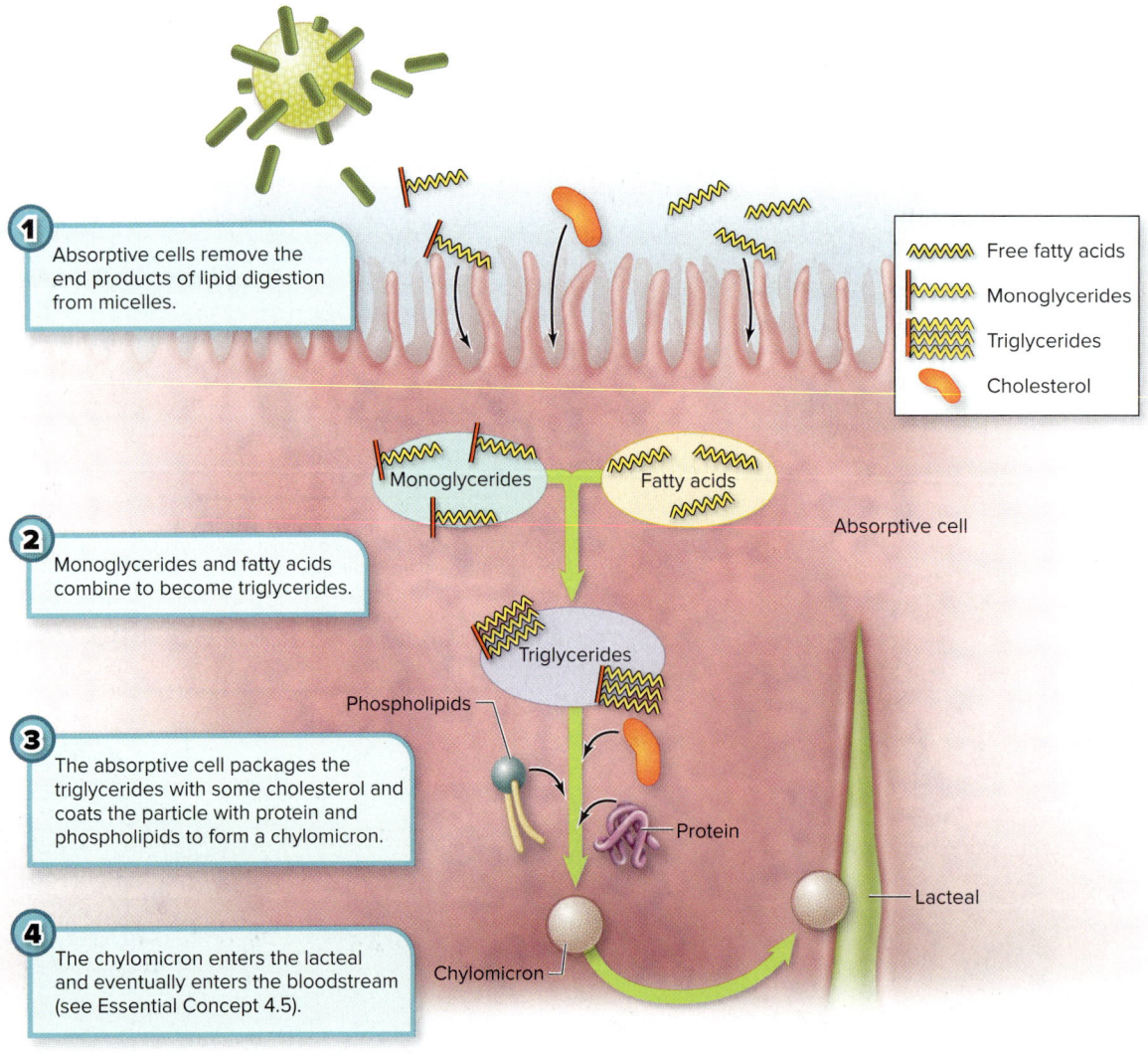

Figure 6.10 Chylomicron formation.

6.2c What Happens to the Used Bile Salts?

After the absorptive cells remove lipids from micelles, the used bile salts remain within the small intestine. **Essential Concept 6.3** explains what happens to the used bile salts.

Essential Concept 6.3 Fate of Bile Salts

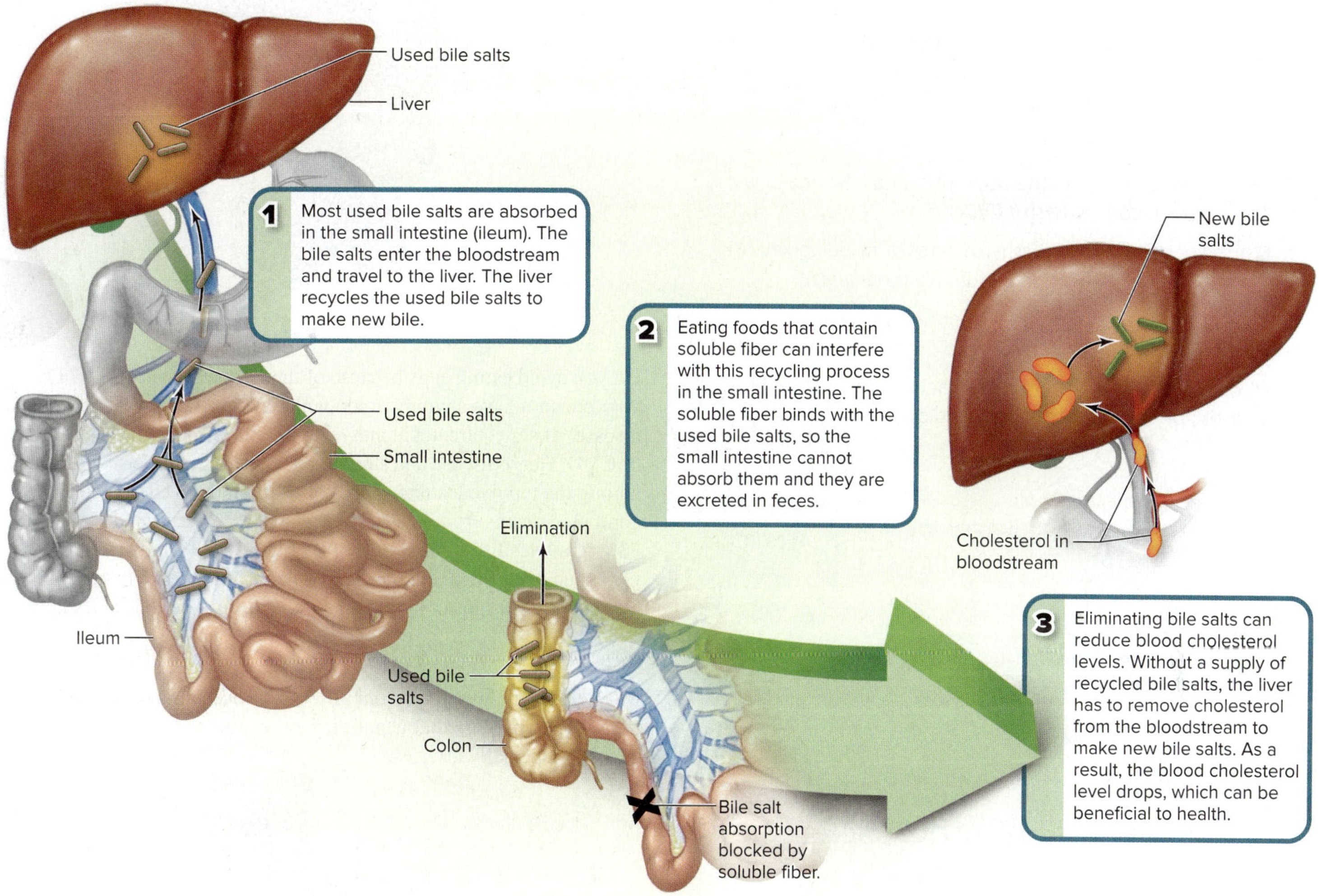

1. Most used bile salts are absorbed in the small intestine (ileum). The bile salts enter the bloodstream and travel to the liver. The liver recycles the used bile salts to make new bile.

2. Eating foods that contain soluble fiber can interfere with this recycling process in the small intestine. The soluble fiber binds with the used bile salts, so the small intestine cannot absorb them and they are excreted in feces.

3. Eliminating bile salts can reduce blood cholesterol levels. Without a supply of recycled bile salts, the liver has to remove cholesterol from the bloodstream to make new bile salts. As a result, the blood cholesterol level drops, which can be beneficial to health.

adipose cells fat cells

6.2d What Happens to Excess Fat That You Eat?

Most cells can metabolize ("burn") fatty acids to release the energy that's stored in the molecules. Sometimes your body doesn't need the energy from the fat you have just eaten. When this happens, **adipose** (*ad'-eh-pose*) **cells** remove fatty acids and glycerol from the bloodstream and reassemble them into fat for storage.

Adipose cells are commonly called "fat cells" because they are designed to store large amounts of fat (**Fig. 6.11**). When your body needs energy, adipose cells break down some stored triglycerides into fatty acid and glycerol molecules and release these substances into your bloodstream. Muscle and other cells then remove the fatty acids from circulation and metabolize them. The liver clears the glycerol molecules from the bloodstream and converts them into glucose molecules that cells can also use for energy.

Eating too much fat contributes to unwanted weight gain, but consuming too much energy from carbohydrates or protein also increases body fat. Why? The body can convert excess glucose and certain amino acids into fatty acids that are used to make fat. Additionally, the nonnutrient alcohol stimulates fat production, so fat can be stored in the liver as a result of drinking alcohol. For more information about alcohol, see Unit 9.

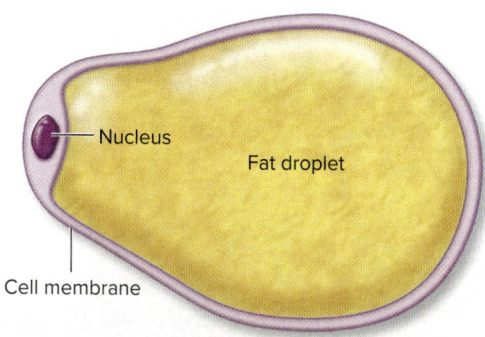

Figure 6.11 Fat cell.

■ *What is the primary lipid that's stored in fat cells?*

Module 6.3

Cardiovascular Disease: Major Killer of Americans

6.3 - Learning Outcomes

After reading Module 6.3, you should be able to

1. Define all of the **key terms** in this module.
2. Explain the process of atherosclerosis, and describe how the condition contributes to CVD.
3. List major risk factors for atherosclerosis, including key risk factors, and indicate which factors are modifiable.
4. Explain the roles that various lipoproteins play in the development of CVD.
5. Discuss dietary and other lifestyle actions that can reduce your risk of atherosclerosis and cardiovascular disease.

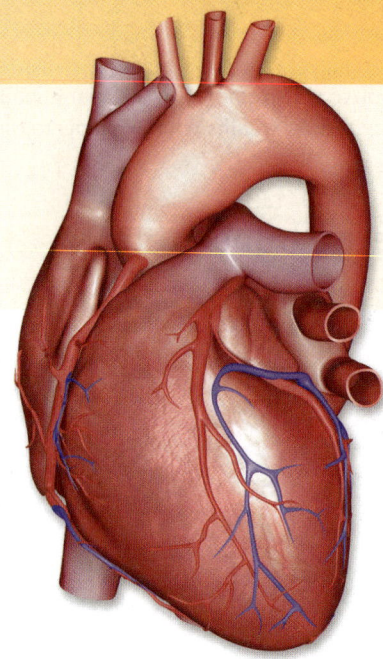

MedicalRF.com

Do you avoid eating eggs because of their cholesterol content? Does your concern have anything to do with having a family history of heart disease? If so, you're not alone—one in three Americans has some form of CVD. Heart disease and stroke, the most common forms of CVD, are among the top five leading causes of death in the United States. In 2017, combined deaths from heart disease and stroke accounted for nearly 30% of all deaths in this country (see Figure 1.2).[5] In many instances, CVD begins during adolescence and young adulthood, but people usually don't have signs or symptoms of the disease until decades later.

6.3a The Road to Cardiovascular Disease (CVD)

Most cases of CVD result from **atherosclerosis** (*ath'-er-oh-skler-oh'-sis*), a long-term process that negatively affects the functioning of blood vessels, especially arteries.

atherosclerosis long-term disease process in which plaque builds up inside arterial walls, causing hardening of the arteries

Essential Concept

6.4 The Process of Atherosclerosis

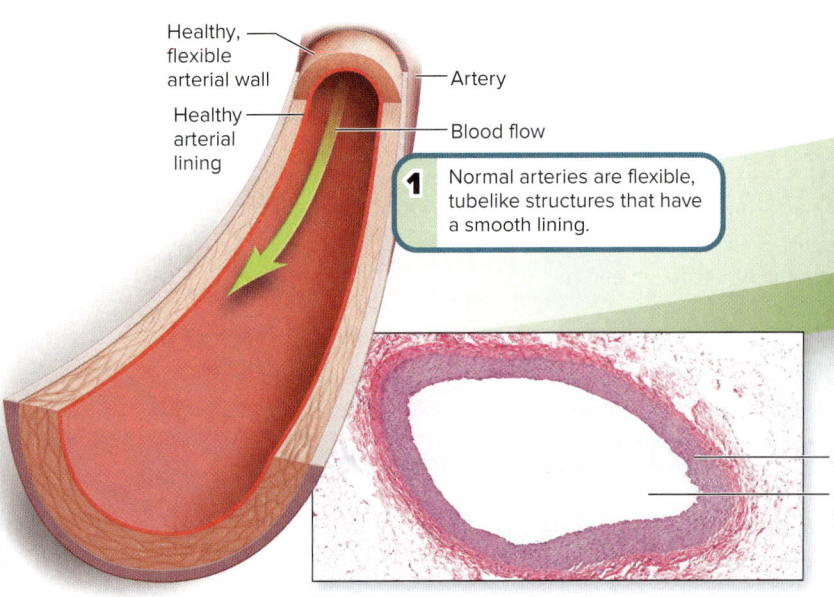

1. Normal arteries are flexible, tubelike structures that have a smooth lining.

2. Atherosclerosis can begin when something in the bloodstream, such as excess cholesterol or glucose, compounds from cigarette smoke, or certain bacteria, irritates the lining of an artery. The body's immune system responds to the irritation by producing inflammation within the artery.

vetpathologist/Shutterstock

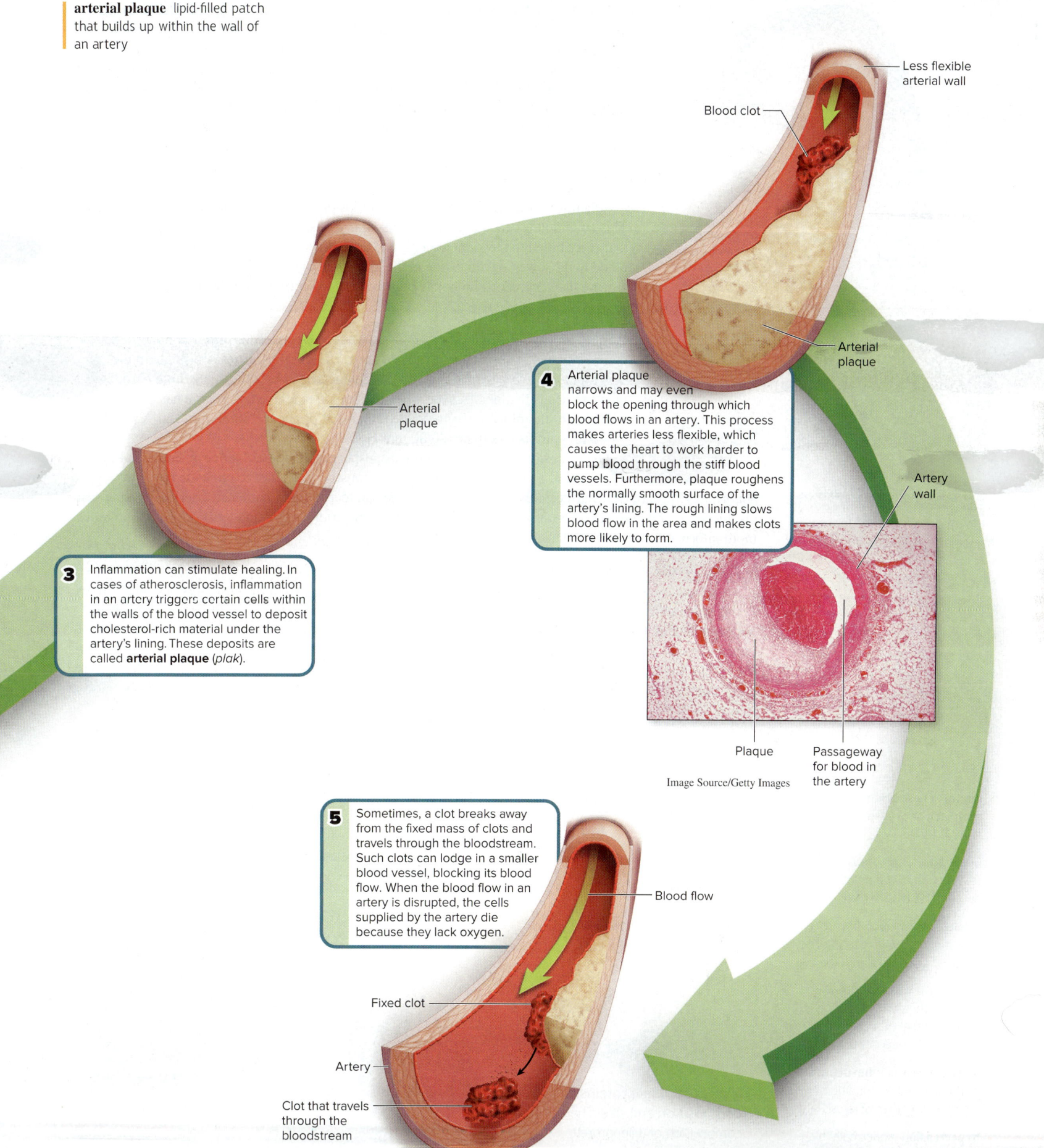

144 Unit 6   Lipids: Focusing on Fats and Cholesterol

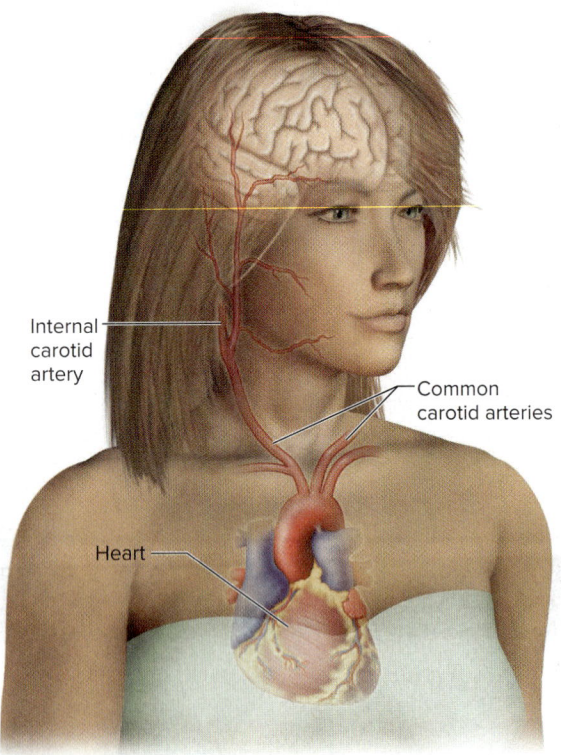

Figure 6.12 Carotid arteries.

■ *Why are clots that form in the carotid arteries dangerous?*

If a clot or a bunch of clots form in one of the arteries that supplies the heart, they can partially close off the artery. When this happens, the affected section of the heart muscle is unable to receive enough oxygen and nutrients to function properly. As a result, the person with the partially blocked artery typically experiences bouts of chest pain called **angina.** If the plaque or clot completely blocks blood flow to a section of the heart muscle, the tissue dies and a **heart attack** occurs.

A **stroke** ("brain attack") can happen when a clot blocks an artery in the brain, and brain cells that are nourished by the blood vessel die. Plaque can form in the common carotid arteries in the neck (**Fig. 6.12**). Clots that form in those arteries can travel to the brain, causing a stroke.

Atherosclerosis can also develop in arteries that don't carry blood to the heart or brain. This condition is called **peripheral vascular disease (PVD).** PVD often affects arteries that carry blood to the kidneys, legs, and arms. When a clot blocks an artery that carries blood to the lower leg, the tissue in the limb dies, causing gangrene to occur. Surgery to remove the gangrenous limb may be necessary to prevent a life-threatening infection.

What's "Hardening of the Arteries"?

Plaques reduce the flexibility of arteries, causing **arteriosclerosis,** a condition that's commonly called "hardening of the arteries." Inflexible arteries contribute to the development of **hypertension,** which is characterized by abnormally high blood pressure levels that persist even when the person is relaxed. A person has hypertension when his or her blood pressure value remains at or above 130/80 mm Hg. A healthy blood pressure is less than 120/80 mm Hg.[6]

Hypertension often damages organs, especially the heart, kidneys, brain, and eyes. The heart of a person with hypertension must work harder to circulate blood through abnormally stiff arteries. Furthermore, high blood pressure can tear or burst hardened arteries, causing serious bleeding problems and even sudden death, depending on the artery's size and location. Unit 9 provides more information about hypertension.

Lipoproteins and Atherosclerosis

Lipoproteins transport cholesterol and triglycerides in the bloodstream, so these structures play major roles in the development of atherosclerosis. In addition to chylomicrons, the body makes three major types of lipoprotein (**Fig. 6.13**). Each type carries different proportions of protein, cholesterol, triglycerides, and phospholipids. The protein content of a lipoprotein contributes to its density. A chylomicron, for example, is the largest and least dense of these lipoproteins. Compared to the other types of lipoproteins, chylomicrons carry much more fat and very little protein. HDL is the smallest and densest of these lipoproteins because it transports more protein and less lipids than the other lipoproteins.

angina chest pain that results from lack of oxygen to heart muscle tissue

heart attack loss of blood flow to a section of the heart muscle, causing the tissue to die

stroke loss of blood flow to a region of the brain, causing the death of brain cells in that area

peripheral vascular disease (PVD) atherosclerosis affecting a blood vessel that doesn't carry blood to the heart or brain

arteriosclerosis ("hardening of the arteries") condition that results from atherosclerosis

hypertension abnormally high blood pressure levels that persist

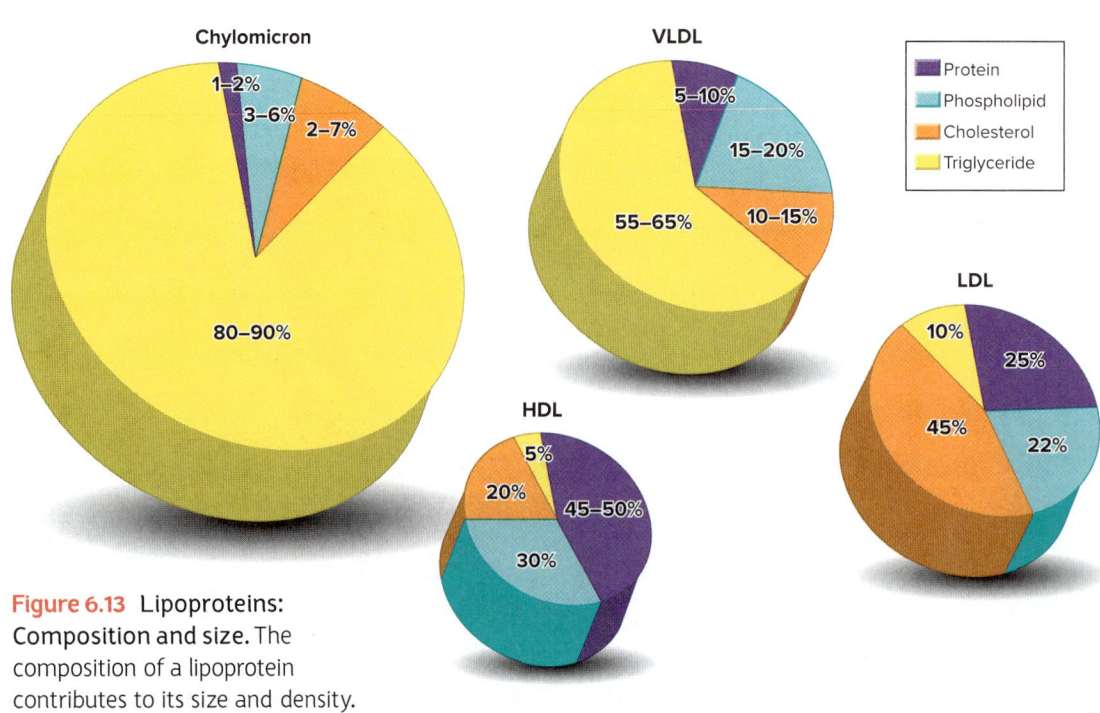

Figure 6.13 Lipoproteins: Composition and size. The composition of a lipoprotein contributes to its size and density.

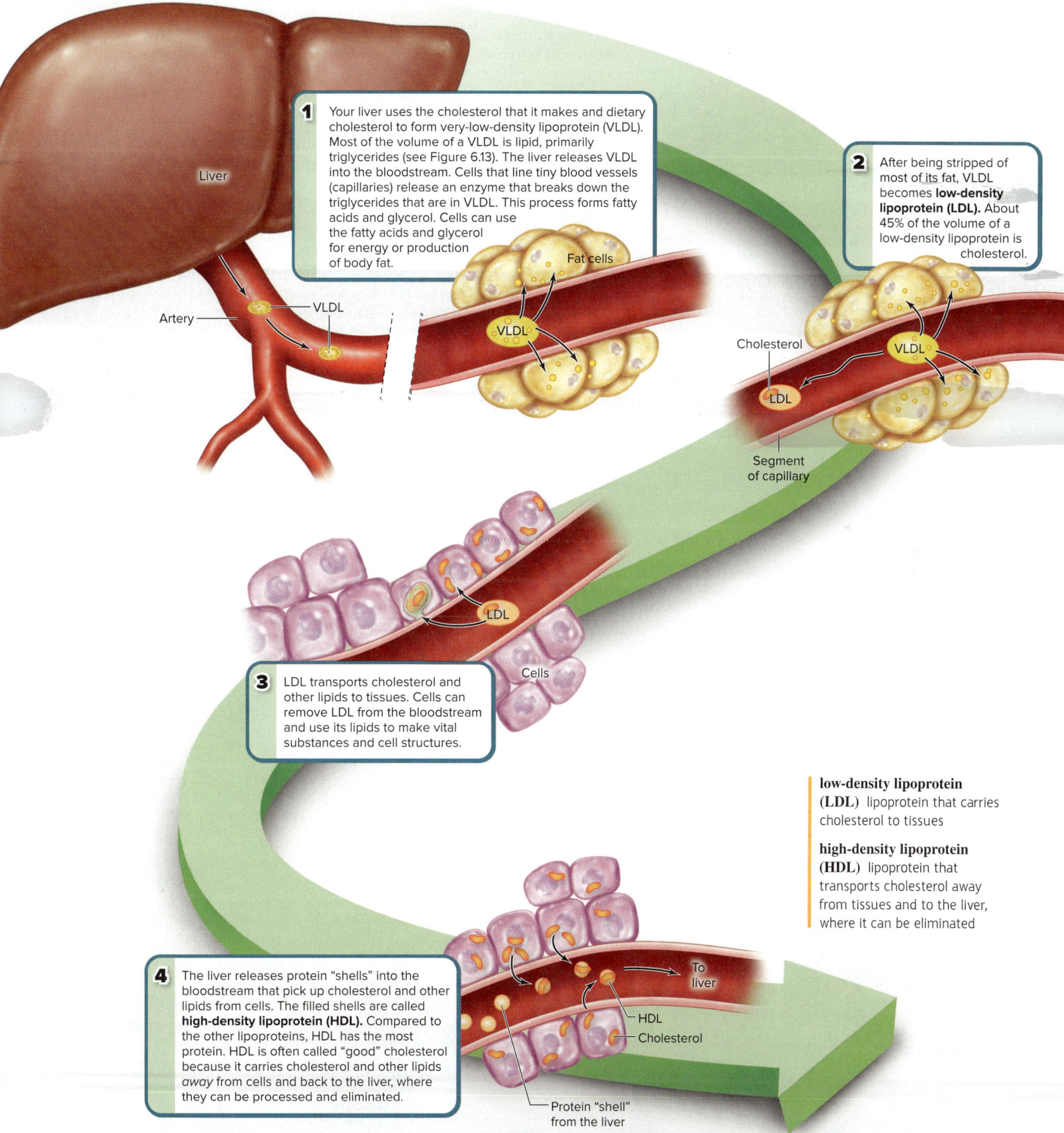

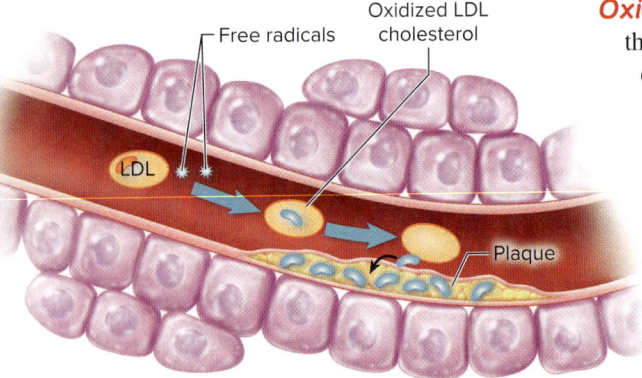

Figure 6.14 Oxidized LDL cholesterol. Cells that line the artery remove LDL from the bloodstream. If the cholesterol in the LDL has been oxidized by free radicals, the oxidized cholesterol enters arterial cells that form plaque.

■ Why is oxidized LDL cholesterol harmful?

Oxidized LDL Cholesterol LDL cholesterol is often referred to as "bad" cholesterol because the lipoprotein carries the lipid to cells in the arterial walls that make plaques. However, there are different types of LDL, and not all forms of the lipoprotein are unhealthy. Chemically unstable substances ("free radicals") can damage LDL. The damage results in *oxidized LDL cholesterol*, which is taken up by the plaque-forming arterial cells **(Fig. 6.14)**. The body's immune system responds to the buildup of plaque, and the affected artery becomes inflamed as a result. Cigarette smoking increases the production of oxidized LDL cholesterol.[7]

High Triglycerides Excessive intake of alcohol and refined carbohydrates,[5] especially added sugars, stimulates VLDL production in the liver. VLDL carries a larger amount of triglycerides than cholesterol (see Figure 6.13). As blood triglyceride levels increase, the amount of cholesterol that's carried by HDL (HDL cholesterol) tends to decrease. Low HDL cholesterol is a risk factor for atherosclerosis. Therefore, high triglyceride levels contribute to the development of CVD.

6.3b Risk Factors for Atherosclerosis

Although atherosclerosis can begin during adolescence and young adulthood, the disease usually doesn't produce signs or symptoms of CVD until decades later. Medical experts haven't been able to determine a cause of atherosclerosis. However, they have identified risk factors and some health conditions that may increase your risk of the disease. The more risk factors you have, the greater your chances of developing CVD. The three key risk factors for heart disease are hypertension, unhealthy blood cholesterol levels, and smoking.[8]

The following points are other known risk factors for atherosclerosis:

- *Poor diet*
  Diets that supply high amounts of:
  Saturated fat and trans fat;
  Added sugars, especially in sugar-sweetened beverages;
  Processed meat;
  Alcohol; and
  Sodium ("salt").
  Diets that don't supply enough:
  Nuts and seeds,
  Fruits and vegetables,
  Omega-3 fat,
  Whole grains.[9, 10]

- *Insulin resistance*
  If your cells don't respond to insulin normally, your blood glucose level increases as a result.

- *Diabetes*
  Diabetes often results from insulin resistance.

- *Excess body fat*
  Too much body fat can contribute to insulin resistance, type 2 diabetes, high triglyceride levels, and hypertension.

- *Lack of physical activity*
  Physical inactivity contributes to excess body fat, hypertension, high LDL cholesterol levels, insulin resistance, and type 2 diabetes.

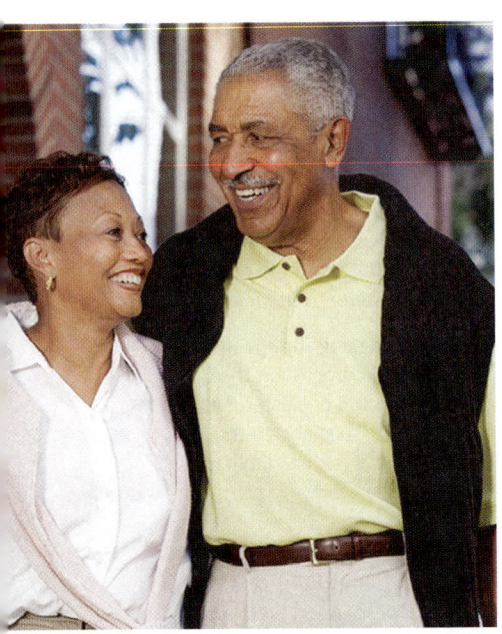

Age is a major risk factor for CVD.

David Buffington/Blend Images

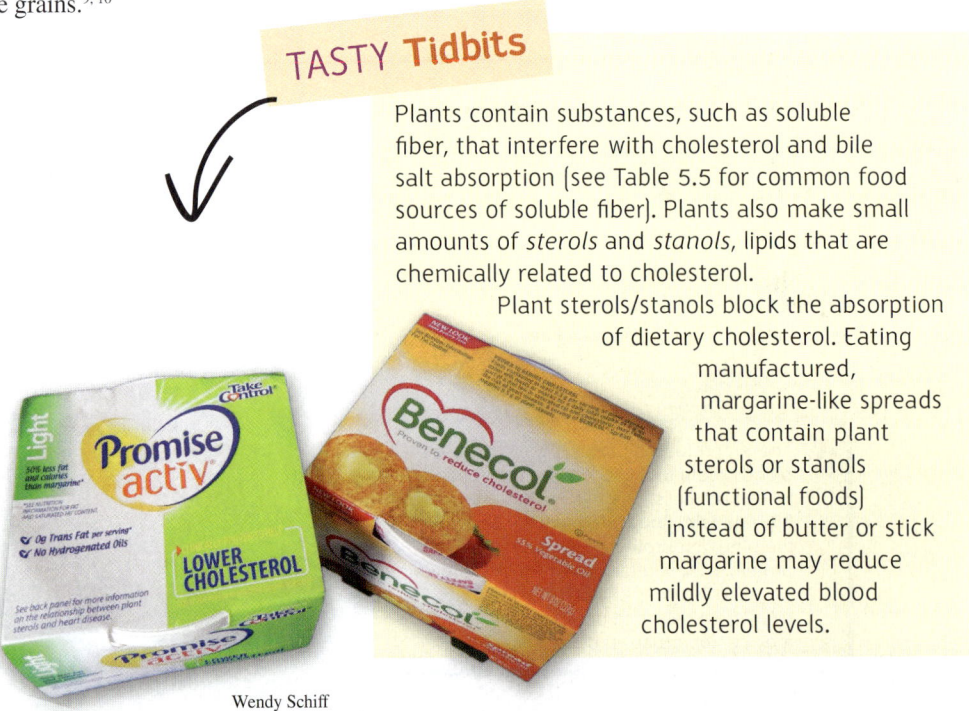

TASTY Tidbits

Plants contain substances, such as soluble fiber, that interfere with cholesterol and bile salt absorption (see Table 5.5 for common food sources of soluble fiber). Plants also make small amounts of *sterols* and *stanols*, lipids that are chemically related to cholesterol.

Plant sterols/stanols block the absorption of dietary cholesterol. Eating manufactured, margarine-like spreads that contain plant sterols or stanols (functional foods) instead of butter or stick margarine may reduce mildly elevated blood cholesterol levels.

Wendy Schiff

- *Increasing age*

  Risk increases after age 45 for men and after age 55 for women.

- *Family history of CVD*

  Risk increases if your father or a brother developed heart disease by age 55 or your mother or a sister developed the disease by age 65.

You may have inherited factors that increase your risk of atherosclerosis. Nevertheless, modifying the key risk factors, such as lowering high blood cholesterol levels, may reduce the possible negative effects of genetics on your cardiovascular health. The following conditions may also be risk factors for atherosclerosis:

- *C-reactive protein*

  High blood levels of C-reactive protein are an indication that inflammation is occurring in your body. Recall that inflammation within arteries is an early step in the process of atherosclerosis.

- *Triglycerides*

  Excessive alcohol and refined carbohydrate intakes stimulate VLDL production in the liver. VLDL carries a larger amount of triglycerides than cholesterol (see Figure 6.13). As mentioned earlier in this module, high triglyceride levels are a risk factor for CVD.

- *Sleep apnea*

  While asleep, a person with sleep apnea stops breathing intermittently or doesn't breathe deeply. As a result, this person doesn't feel refreshed after sleeping. Untreated sleep apnea may contribute to hypertension, heart attack, and stroke.

- *Emotional stress*

  Emotional stress, particularly anger, may also play a role in the development of atherosclerosis.

- *Alcohol*

  Drinking too much alcohol can damage your heart and worsen some of the other risk factors for atherosclerosis. You can learn more about alcohol in Unit 9.

6.3c Reducing Your Risk of Atherosclerosis and CVD

You may not be able to prevent having a heart attack or stroke someday, but there's plenty of scientific evidence that suggests you can forestall CVD and live a longer, more satisfying life by reducing or eliminating modifiable risk factors for atherosclerosis. Modifiable risk factors are personal characteristics and behaviors you can change.

You can lower your chances of developing atherosclerosis, usually by changing your lifestyle:

- Be more physically active. Regular physical activity can increase your HDL cholesterol level, lower your LDL cholesterol level, and help you lose excess body fat.

- Quit smoking and avoid exposure to tobacco smoke.

- Limit salt intake and manage your blood pressure.

- Achieve and maintain a healthy weight for height.

- Eat more fiber-rich foods.

Nancy, the young woman featured in the unit opener, should be concerned about her risk of CVD because she may have inherited CVD risk factors from her mother. Based on what you've learned by reading this unit, what lifestyle changes could Nancy make to reduce her risk of CVD?

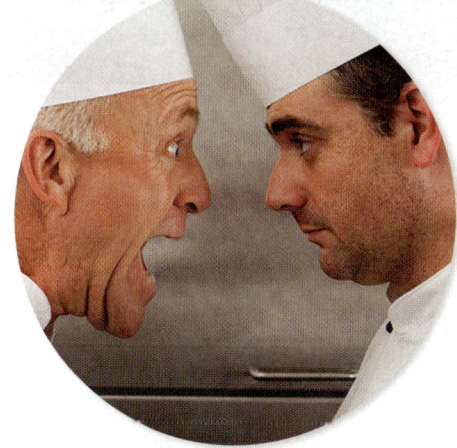

Emotional stress may be a risk factor for CVD.

Juice Images/Juice Images/Getty Images

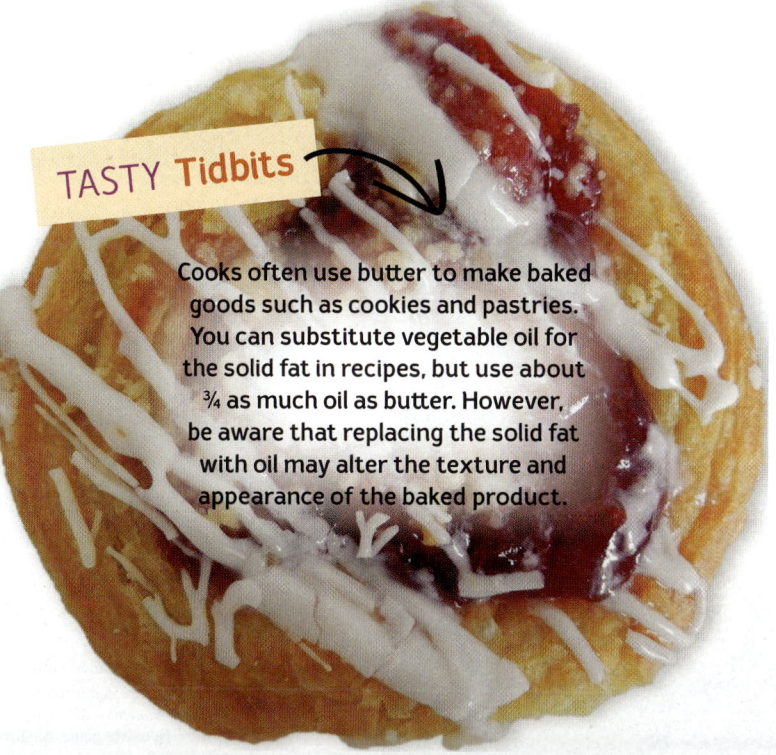

TASTY Tidbits

Cooks often use butter to make baked goods such as cookies and pastries. You can substitute vegetable oil for the solid fat in recipes, but use about ¾ as much oil as butter. However, be aware that replacing the solid fat with oil may alter the texture and appearance of the baked product.

Wendy Schiff

- Learn to relax and manage your emotional stress.
- Reduce added-sugar and alcohol intake.
- Replace saturated FAs with monounsaturated FAs and polyunsaturated FAs, especially the essential fatty acids.

Focus on Types of Dietary Fats

In the past, medical experts recommended reducing total fat intake as a way of lowering the risk of CVD. Today, the focus is on eating reasonable amounts of fat, while limiting intake of saturated FAs. Recall from Unit 3 that the AMDR for total fat is 20 to 35% of total calories.

Although oils, fatty spreads, and salad dressings are obvious sources of dietary fat, much of the fat you eat isn't visible. Saturated fat contributes much of the calories in fatty meats, luncheon meats, sausages, hot dogs, and "full-fat" dairy products such as hard cheeses and whole milk. Tropical fats, which include palm oil, cocoa "butter," and, especially, coconut oil, are highly saturated, too. (See Table 6.1.) Populations that consume diets rich in saturated FAs (SFAs) generally have higher rates of heart disease than populations that eat less saturated fat.[9]

You can reduce your risk of CVD by replacing foods that are rich sources of saturated FAs with foods that contain more polyunsaturated and monounsaturated FAs.[9] Replacing fat with carbohydrate, especially refined carbohydrates (added sugars, for example), doesn't help reduce your risk of CVD.[9] **Essential Concept 6.6** illustrates the general effects of saturated, trans, and unsaturated FAs on blood LDL and HDL levels.

A healthy eating pattern (see Unit 3) and the traditional Mediterranean Diet are heart-healthy diets because they limit saturated FA intakes and emphasize seafood, unsaturated fats, whole grains, nuts, beans, fruits, and vegetables (see Figure 3.6).[9]

6.3d Assessing Your Risk of Atherosclerosis

To determine your risk of atherosclerosis, it's a good idea to have regular medical checkups. Your physician should measure your blood pressure and listen to blood flow in your carotid arteries to assess whether those particular arteries are becoming blocked. The physician may request a blood test to assess your total blood cholesterol level as well as HDL cholesterol, LDL cholesterol, and triglyceride levels. Ask your physician for a copy of the laboratory results; keep them in your personal "medical file" for future reference.

Table 6.3 presents classifications for blood lipid levels for healthy persons. The desirable range for total cholesterol is less than 200 mg/dl. Do you know what your blood cholesterol level is? Even if it's below 200 mg/dl, you may still have a high risk of

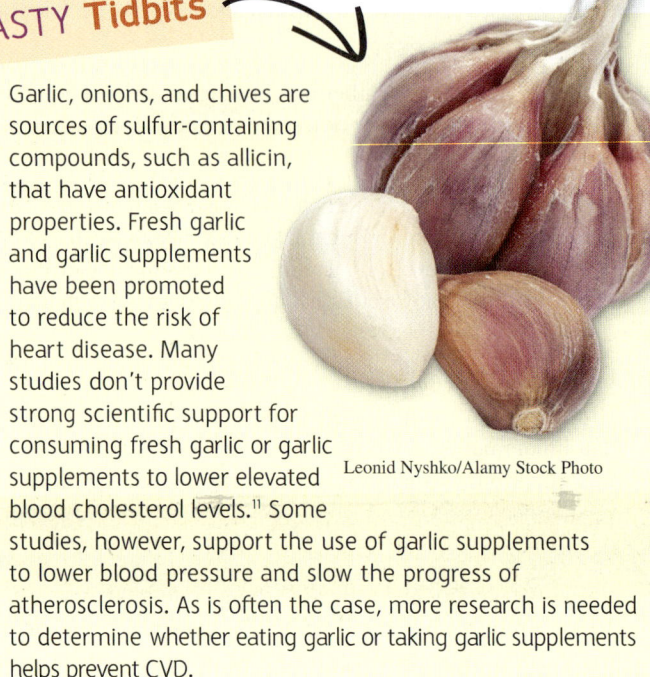

TASTY Tidbits

Garlic, onions, and chives are sources of sulfur-containing compounds, such as allicin, that have antioxidant properties. Fresh garlic and garlic supplements have been promoted to reduce the risk of heart disease. Many studies don't provide strong scientific support for consuming fresh garlic or garlic supplements to lower elevated blood cholesterol levels.[11] Some studies, however, support the use of garlic supplements to lower blood pressure and slow the progress of atherosclerosis. As is often the case, more research is needed to determine whether eating garlic or taking garlic supplements helps prevent CVD.

Leonid Nyshko/Alamy Stock Photo

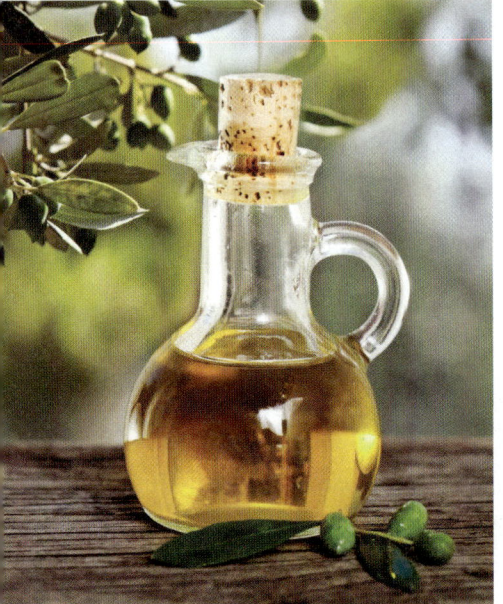

Olives and olive oil are associated with the Mediterranean Diet.

Dasha Petrenko/Shutterstock

Table 6.3 Classification of Blood Lipid Levels for Healthy Persons

Total Cholesterol (mg/dl)	Classification
125 to 200	Desirable
LDL cholesterol (mg/dl)	**Classification**
< 100	Optimal for health
HDL cholesterol (mg/dl)	**Classification**
< 40 (Men) < 50 (Women)	Increases risk of heart disease
≥ 50	Protects against heart disease*
Triglycerides (mg/dl)	**Classification**
< 150	Acceptable
≥ 200	Unhealthy

*People with certain medical conditions and very high HDL levels may have *increased* risk of CVD.[12]

Sources of data: National Institutes of Health, National Heart, Lung, and Blood Institute: *High blood cholesterol, also known as hypercholesterolemia: Screening and prevention.* ND; www.nhlbi.nih.gov/health-topics/high-blood-cholesterol; U.S. National Library of Medicine, MedlinePlus: *Triglycerides.* Updated June 25, 2019. https://medlineplus.gov/triglycerides.html Accessed: June 26, 2019

Essential Concept

6.6 General Effects of Dietary Fatty Acids on LDL and HDL

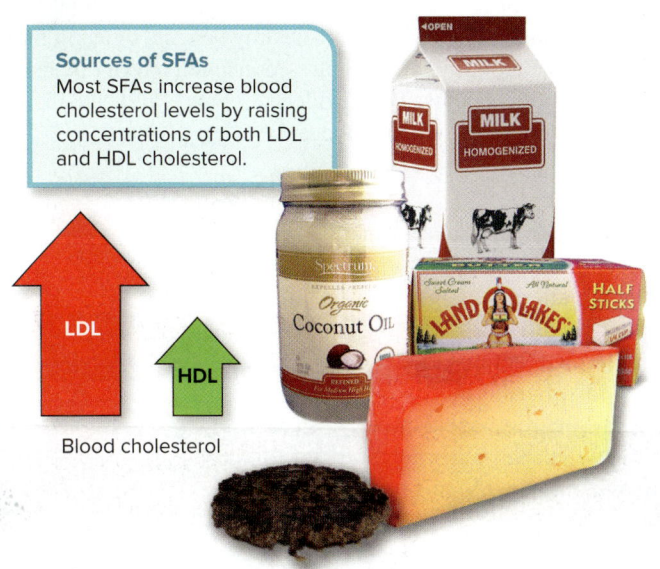

Sources of SFAs
Most SFAs increase blood cholesterol levels by raising concentrations of both LDL and HDL cholesterol.

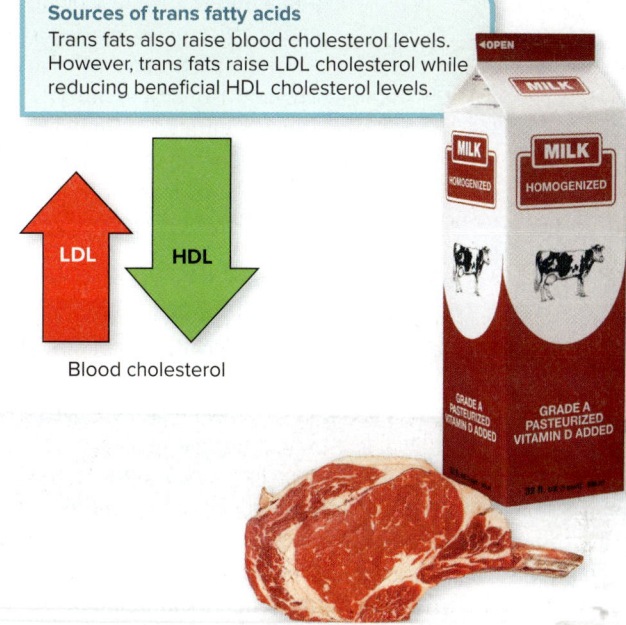

Sources of trans fatty acids
Trans fats also raise blood cholesterol levels. However, trans fats raise LDL cholesterol while reducing beneficial HDL cholesterol levels.

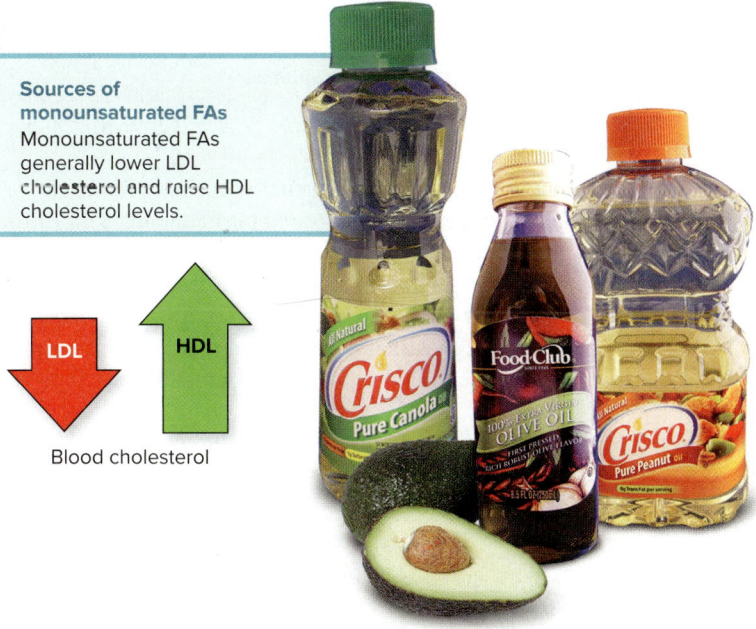

Sources of monounsaturated FAs
Monounsaturated FAs generally lower LDL cholesterol and raise HDL cholesterol levels.

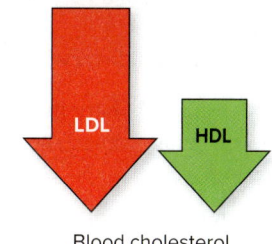
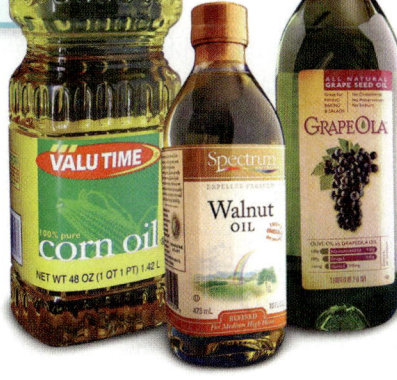

Sources of polyunsaturated FAs
Diets containing more polyunsaturated FAs than saturated FAs reduce LDL cholesterol more than monounsaturated FAs.[9] Replacing saturated FAs with polyunsaturated FAs may also slightly reduce beneficial HDL cholesterol.[9] Nevertheless, polyunsaturated FAs tend to be good for you because they don't promote inflammation and atherosclerosis.

atherosclerosis. Why? Although knowing the concentration of cholesterol carried by all lipoproteins is important, the amounts of certain lipoproteins in your blood, particularly LDL and HDL, are more critical risk factors. For healthy persons, it's generally better to have higher levels of HDL cholesterol than to have higher levels of LDL cholesterol. For reasons that are unclear, having very high HDL levels is linked to increased risk of early death.[12] To calculate your risk of having a future heart attack, use the risk assessment tool (*Check. Change. Control. Calculator™*) at the American Heart Association's website (https://ccccalculator.ccctracker.com/).

6.3e Recommendations for Fat and Cholesterol Intakes

On average, fat contributes a little more than 37% of adult Americans' daily energy intake from macronutrients (see Figure 5.2). The Acceptable Macronutrient Distribution Range (AMDR) for fat is 20 to 35% of total calories.

The *Dietary Guidelines for Americans* recommends that less than 10% of your energy intake should be from saturated FAs. In 2015–2016, American adults consumed an average of about 11.8% of their

Quart of milk: PhotoSpin, Inc/Alamy; Coconut oil, Butter, Cheese, Hamburger patty, Canola oil, Olive oil, Peanut oil, Corn oil, Walnut oil, grapeseed oil: Wendy Schiff; Avocados: Ken Cavanagh/McGraw-Hill Education; Prime rib steak: aoldman/Getty Images

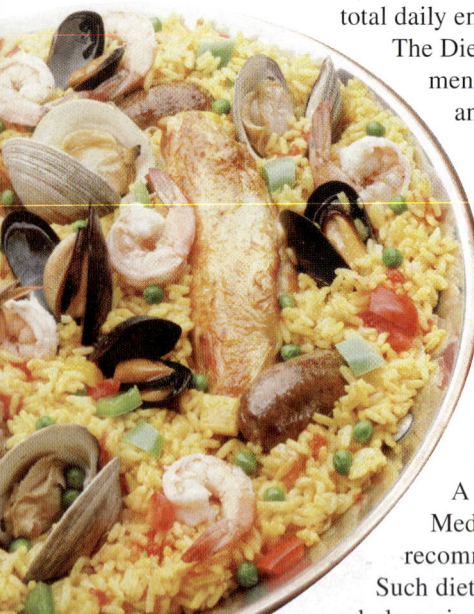

total daily energy intake from saturated fat.[13] The Dietary Guidelines also recommends that you keep your cholesterol and trans fat intakes as low as possible while following a healthy eating pattern. To estimate your average percentage of total energy from fat as well as your saturated fat intake per day, complete the "What's in Your Diet?!" activity at the end of this unit.

How to Increase Your Essential Fat Intake

A heart-healthy diet, including the Mediterranean Diet (see Figure 3.6), recommends eating less red meats. Such diets emphasize fruits, vegetables, whole grains, low-fat dairy products, and foods that are rich sources of the essential omega-3 and omega-6 fatty acids. According to the Dietary Guidelines, you can meet the recommended amounts of essential fatty acids by consuming the equivalent of about 5 teaspoons of vegetable oil daily (2000 kcal diet).[14] Fats and oils are energy dense (9 kcal/g). Therefore, it is important to *replace* foods that are high in unhealthy saturated fats with foods that are high in unsaturated fats, instead of simply adding oil-rich foods to your diet.

Your body can make only small amounts of DHA and EPA. Therefore, it's a good idea to include sources of DHA and EPA, such as many kinds of fish and seafood, in your diet. Shark, swordfish, king mackerel, and tilefish contain high levels of methylmercury, which is toxic, especially for growing bodies. Therefore, pregnant women, breastfeeding women, and young children should avoid those kinds of fish. Food sources of omega-3 fats, including DHA and EPA, are listed in **Table 6.4**.

To increase your intake of essential fatty acids from dietary sources,

- Eat approximately 8 ounces of seafood, especially fatty fish, a week (see Table 6.4). Pregnant or breastfeeding women should limit their seafood intake to 12 ounces per week.[1]
- Add water-packed canned tuna or salmon to salads, or mix the fish with a little vegetable oil to make a spread for toast or crackers.
- Sprinkle chopped walnuts on salads, yogurt, or cereal, or simply eat the nuts as a snack. However, control your portion sizes because nuts are an energy-dense food.

What About Fish Oil? What if you don't like to eat fish? Should you take fish oil supplements? The heart-healthy benefits of using fish oil supplements that are available without prescription haven't been supported by scientific studies.[15] The evidence seems to indicate that eating fish is the best way to obtain omega-3s.

If you decide to take fish oil supplements, it's a good idea to check with your physician first. People who are allergic to fish and/or shellfish may have allergic reactions to the supplements. Furthermore, taking high doses of omega-3 FAs may cause serious side effects, including reducing the blood's ability to clot.

6.3f Heart-Healthy Food Selection and Preparation Tips

You can change your food selection and preparation practices to reduce the amount of saturated fat, salt, and calories in your diet.

- If you eat meat, choose lean cuts such as
  - Round and top round, loin, and top sirloin steaks, as well as chuck and arm roasts.
- When buying ground beef, consider choosing "lean" and "extra lean" products. Lean ground beef contains 8% or less fat. Ground beef that is called "extra lean" has no more than 4% fat. To keep the ground beef from tasting "dry," add a small amount of olive or canola oil to the raw meat before shaping it into a meatloaf or hamburger patties. This practice replaces some saturated fat with unsaturated fats.

TABLE 6.4 FOOD SOURCES OF OMEGA-3 FATS

Fish/Shellfish (DHA and EPA)	Oils	Nuts and Seeds	Other
Herring, salmon, sablefish, anchovies, tuna, bluefish, sardines, catfish, striped bass, mackerel, trout, halibut, pollock, flounder, shrimp, mussels, crab	Flaxseed, walnut, canola, soybean, chia seed	Walnuts, flaxseeds, chia	Algae

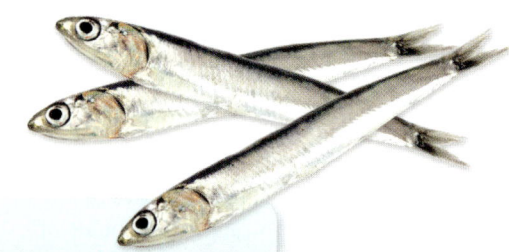

Seafood dish: Kevin Sanchez/Cole Group/Getty Images; Fish oil, Can of tuna: Wendy Schiff; Sardines: Antonio Gravante/Alamy Stock Photo

TASTY Tidbits

About 80% of stick margarine is fat—the same percentage of fat as in butter. A pat of stick margarine (approximately a teaspoon) also supplies about the same amount of energy as a pat of butter—35 kcal. Compared to a teaspoon of tub margarine, a teaspoon of butter provides less unsaturated fat and more saturated fat and cholesterol. But occasionally having some butter is unlikely to clog your arteries.

- The fat in meat contributes to its "juiciness" and tenderness, so when cooking lean cuts of meat:
  - Use moist heat cooking methods, such as pot roasting, which is adding some water to the meat and covering the pot with a lid or tightly covering the baking dish with foil. Moist heat cooking methods help tenderize meats without adding fat.
- Reduce the oven temperature from 350°F to less than 325°F. The meat will take longer to cook, but it's less likely to toughen and dry out.
- After cooking, trim away much of the visible fat from the meat.
- Don't use pan drippings to make sauces or gravies.
- Stir-fry pieces of raw vegetables, lean meat, fish, shellfish, and poultry in small amounts of hot vegetable oil. This method cooks the foods quickly and preserves micronutrients.
- Brown ground beef in a pan, then drain the beef fat before you add other ingredients to the meat. If more fat is needed, add a little vegetable oil to the pan. This practice replaces some saturated fat with unsaturated fats.
- Avoid dipping raw foods in batter or breading and deep-fat frying them. Such coatings absorb the oil, adding extra calories to your diet.
  - If you deep-fat fry foods, place the items on paper towels after cooking them to soak up as much excess fat as possible.
  - Peel greasy breading from fried fish and poultry before eating them.
- Don't add salt while you're preparing food or before you eat it.
- Switch from drinking whole or 2% milk to 1% or fat-free milk. Whole milk is 3.25% fat by volume. Fat-free milk ("skim milk") contains less than 0.5% fat. Switch from using regular cream cheese to reduced-fat cream cheese.

Culture & Cuisine

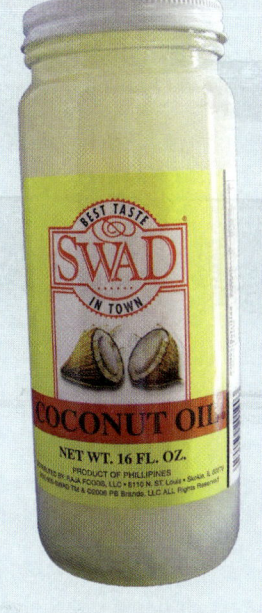

For thousands of years, people have prepared foods using fats and oils derived from locally available plants and animals. In India, *ghee* is made by gently heating butter and then straining it to remove milk solids (primarily protein and lactose) from the oily butter. In Japan and other Asian countries, sesame seed oil is popular in sauces, in dips, and for frying foods. People from the Mediterranean region harvest olives for eating as well as pressing to extract the fruit's flavorful oil for preparing and cooking foods. Coconut oil is often used in tropical countries, where coconut palms grow. Another tropical oil, palm oil, is made from the fruit of the African oil palm. Both coconut and palm oils are highly saturated (see Table 6.1), so unlike other plant oils, they're semisolid at typical room temperatures. In the United States, both coconut oil and palm oil are often used in processed foods as substitutes for partially hydrogenated oils, which have been banned from foods.

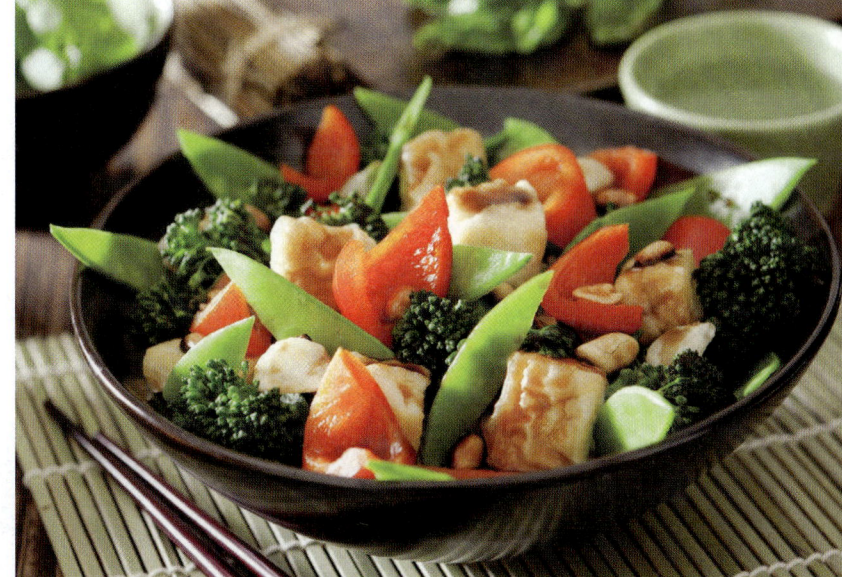

Stir-fried vegetables

Corn: Purestock/SuperStock; Coconut oil: Wendy Schiff; Tofu and vegetable stir fry: nicolebranan/Getty Images

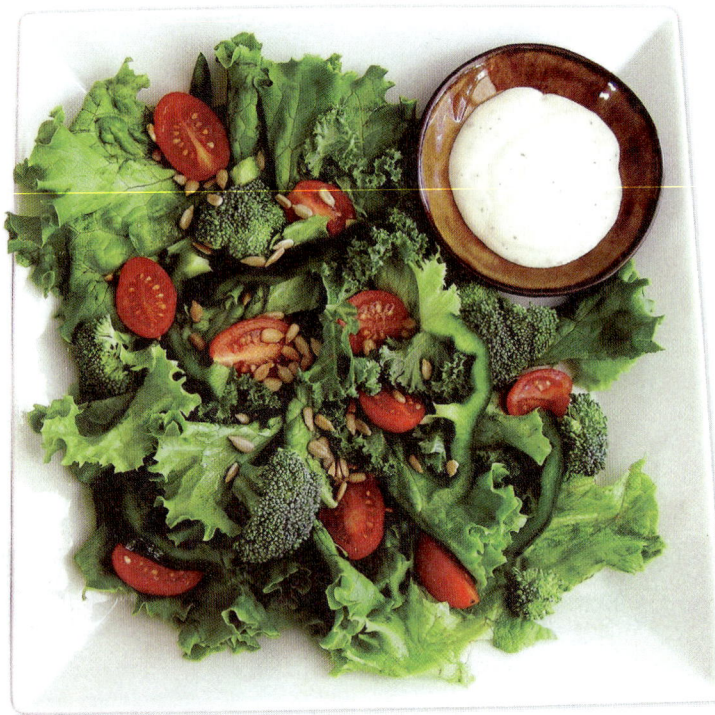

Salad dressing "on the side"

- Use less salad dressing on salads. When in restaurants, order salad dressings "on the side" so you can control the amount that's added. Make your own salad dressing by combining vegetable oil and vinegar with some herbs and spices, such as oregano, basil, and black pepper.

- To lower the fat content of their products, manufacturers of "lite" spreads may have water as the first ingredient. Therefore, replacing the margarine, butter, oil, or shortening in a recipe with a reduced-fat spread could alter the product's taste, texture, and appearance. It's a good idea to read the reduced-fat spread's label to determine whether the product is suitable to use in recipes.

- When ordering food at a restaurant, request that no salt be added during its preparation.

- Purchase brands of microwave popcorn that have little added fat and no salt. Buy plain popcorn, and use a small amount of hot oil in a covered saucepan to pop the kernels or use a hot-air machine.

- Replace half or all of the solid fat or oil in recipes for baked goods with unsweetened applesauce. If a recipe, for example, calls for 1 cup butter, you can replace half of the butter with ½ cup of applesauce. Substituting oil for all of the solid fat in a recipe for a baked product is often not recommended. Instead, try replacing up to ¾ of the solid fat with oil.

- Substitute plain, fat-free yogurt in recipes that call for sour cream. Place a spoonful of the yogurt, instead of butter or sour cream, on a baked potato.

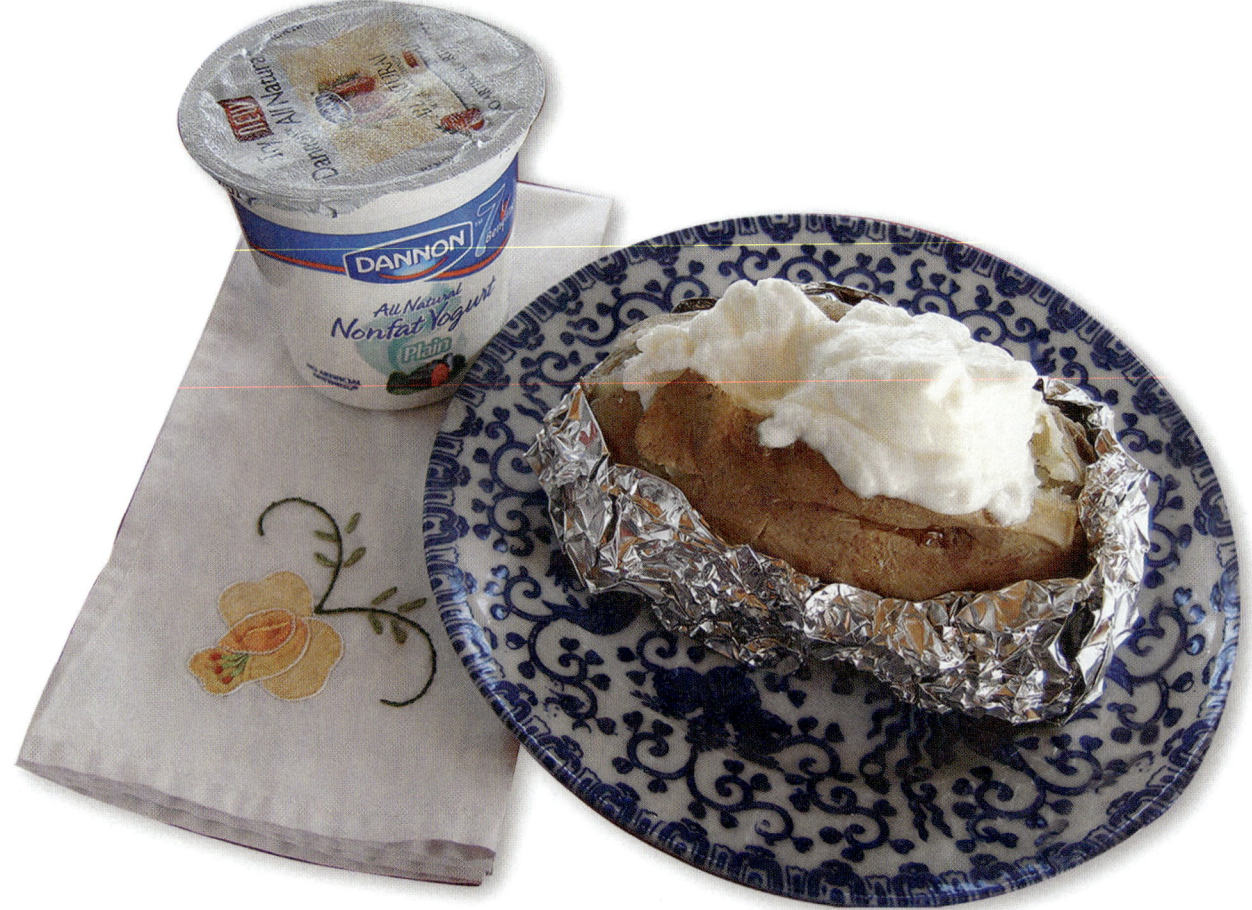

Plain yogurt is a low-fat substitute for sour cream.

What *IS* That?

If you need to reduce your cholesterol intake, you can use commercially available egg substitutes to replace whole eggs in recipes. Such products are made from eggs, but they include only the egg whites, which are free of cholesterol and fat. One-fourth cup of an egg substitute replaces one whole egg. If you don't have an egg substitute on hand, you can use two egg whites for each whole egg in a recipe.

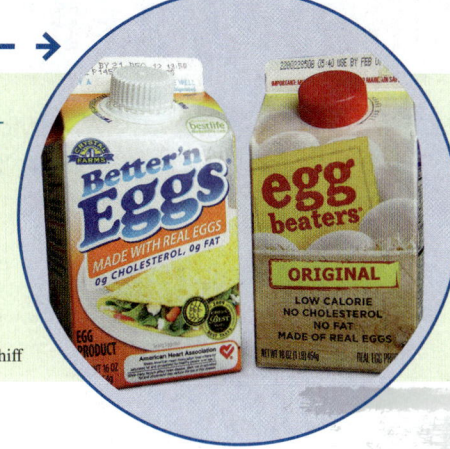
Wendy Schiff

- Use peanut, soy nut, or other nut butters instead of cheese or luncheon meat in sandwiches. Some nut butters contain added salt and sugar, so read the Nutrition Facts panel and ingredients list before selecting these products.

Appendix F has more tips for reducing the amount of unhealthy solid fats in your favorite recipes.

What If Lifestyle Changes Don't Work?

Some people are unable to lower their risk of CVD by making dietary changes, exercising regularly, and losing excess body fat. If you've made these lifestyle changes and your blood lipids are still too high, it's important to discuss additional treatment options with your physician. Millions of Americans take a class of prescription drugs called statins to reduce their high blood lipid levels. Statins interfere with the liver's metabolism of cholesterol, effectively reducing LDL cholesterol and triglyceride levels as a result. The results of research, however, don't clearly indicate that statins lower the risk of CVD. Statins are relatively safe when taken as directed.

Zetia® (ezetimebe) is a drug that works differently from a statin. Zetia® inhibits intestinal absorption of cholesterol and, as a result, lowers LDL cholesterol levels.

Nutrition Fact or Fiction?

Eggs are loaded with cholesterol, so you should avoid eating them.

Having too much cholesterol in your blood may increase your risk of heart disease and stroke. Egg yolks are a rich source of cholesterol, but yolks contain more of the "healthy" unsaturated fats than the "unhealthy" saturated fats. Furthermore, whole eggs are nutrient dense and relatively low in cost. If you're healthy, you probably can eat one egg a day without worrying.[16] Why? For most healthy people, the saturated fat content of a food has more of an effect on their blood cholesterol levels than does the food's cholesterol content.[17] Nevertheless, results of a recent major study indicated that eating eggs increases the risk of CVD.[18] It's important to note that researchers often find conflicting results when studying the relationship between egg consumption and risk of CVD. Therefore, it's wise for healthy people to practice "moderation" when eating all foods, including eggs.

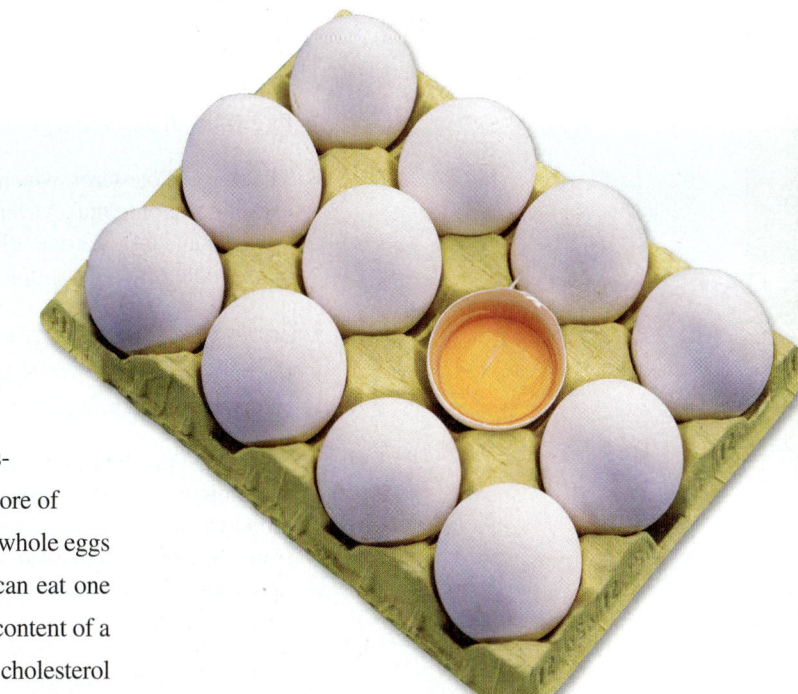
Pixtal/AGE fotostock

In a Nutshell

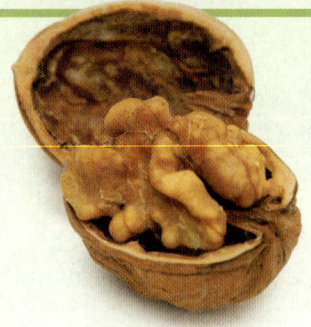

Module 6.1: What Are Lipids?

- The body needs lipids for many functions, including energy, maintaining cell membranes, producing bile and certain hormones, insulating against cold temperatures, regulating blood pressure and inflammation, and cushioning against bumps, blows, and falls. Major lipids are triglycerides, sterols, and phospholipids.

- The fat in food enhances absorption of fat-soluble vitamins and phytochemicals. Dietary lipids also contribute to the appealing flavor, texture, and aroma of foods. Consuming some lipids is essential for health, but high amounts of certain lipids may increase your risk of serious health conditions, particularly heart disease, stroke, and obesity.

- Triglycerides comprise most of the lipid content of your food and body. A triglyceride molecule has three fatty acids in its chemical structure. Fatty acids can be saturated or unsaturated. Unsaturated fatty acids can be either monounsaturated or polyunsaturated.

- The body cannot make the omega-6 fatty acid linoleic acid and the omega-3 fatty acid alpha-linolenic acid; these essential fatty acids must be supplied by the diet. The richest sources of essential fats include canola, soybean, and corn oils and products made with these oils, such as salad dressings. You can also meet your essential fatty acid needs by eating nuts, seeds, whole grains, and, especially, fatty fish.

- Triglycerides usually contain mixtures of unsaturated and saturated fatty acids, but one type of fatty acid tends to predominate. In general, animal fats contain more saturated fatty acids than plant oils. Important exceptions are palm oil, cocoa butter, and the highly saturated coconut oil.

- The partial hydrogenation of unsaturated fats is a commercial process that converts unsaturated fatty acids into saturated fats and trans fats. The trans fats in partially hydrogenated oils (PHOs) are "bad" fats because they're associated with an increased risk of heart disease and stroke. PHOs have been banned from being used in foods. However, meat and dairy products naturally contain some trans fat.

- Phospholipids are the major structural component of cell membranes and are needed for proper functioning of nerve cells, including those in the brain. Lecithin is the major phospholipid in food. Egg yolks, liver, wheat germ, peanut butter, and soybeans are rich sources of lecithin compound.

- The sterol cholesterol, which is found only in animal foods, is a component of every cell membrane. Cells use cholesterol to make a variety of substances, including vitamin D, bile, and steroid hormones such as estrogen and testosterone. Plants make sterols and stanols that may be beneficial to health because they block cholesterol absorption in the GI tract.

Module 6.2: What Happens to the Fat and Cholesterol You Eat?

- Fat undergoes digestion primarily in the upper part of the small intestine. Cholesterol isn't broken down and is absorbed through the intestinal wall.

- Before leaving the small intestine, triglycerides, cholesterol, and other lipids are formed into chylomicrons. Chylomicrons enter the lymphatic system of the small intestine and eventually reach the bloodstream. The liver removed lipids from chylomicrons to make various lipoproteins—substances that transport lipids in the bloodstream.

- The small intestine absorbs bile components for the liver to recycle to make new bile.

- Triglycerides are major sources of cellular energy. If energy isn't needed, fat cells store the energy in triglycerides. When cells need energy, fat cells break down some stored triglycerides and release glycerol and fatty acids into the bloodstream.

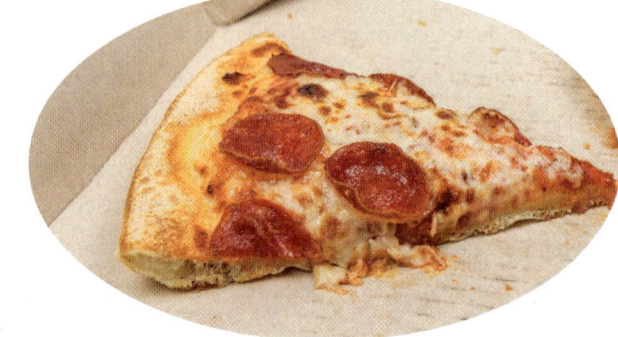

Elizabeth Cummings/123RF

Module 6.3: Cardiovascular Disease: Major Killer of Americans

- CVD affects the heart and blood vessels. In the United States, heart disease is the leading cause of death; stroke is the fifth-leading cause of death. Atherosclerosis is a long-term process that can result in arteriosclerosis and CVD.

- Numerous risk factors are associated with atherosclerosis; some risk factors are inherited and difficult to modify, but many are related to lifestyle practices that can be altered. The three key risk factors are hypertension, unhealthy blood cholesterol levels, and smoking.

- Lipoproteins transport much of the lipid content of the blood. Having high blood levels of HDL cholesterol is healthier than having high LDL cholesterol levels. Elevated LDL cholesterol contributes to atherosclerosis, whereas having a healthy HDL cholesterol level generally reduces the risk of this condition.

- Exercising and replacing saturated fats with unsaturated fats may reduce your LDL cholesterol levels and increase HDL cholesterol levels. On the other hand, physical inactivity and eating high amounts of saturated fat can raise LDL cholesterol, increasing your risk of atherosclerosis. Many healthy people, however, do not experience an increase in their blood cholesterol levels when they eat cholesterol in foods.

- Fat contributes more than 37% of the average American's daily energy intake. The AMDR for fat is 20 to 35% of total calories.

- If you make recommended dietary modifications, lose excess weight, and exercise regularly, and your blood lipid levels still remain high, you should discuss additional treatment options with your physician. Millions of Americans take prescription statin medications to reduce their elevated blood lipid levels.

What's in Your Diet?!

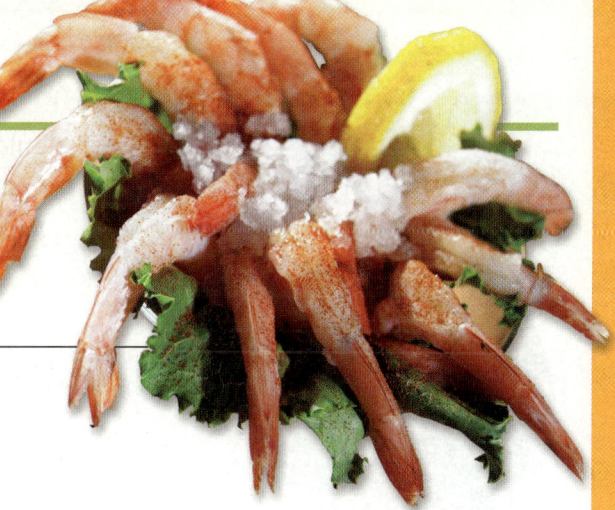

Purestock/SuperStock

1. Refer to the 3-day food log from the "What's in Your Diet?!" feature in Unit 3. List the total number of kilocalories you consumed for each day of recordkeeping. Add the figures to obtain a total, divide the total by 3, then round the figure to the nearest whole number to obtain your average daily energy intake for the 3-day period.

   ### Sample Calculation:

Day 1	2000 kcal
Day 2	1700 kcal
Day 3	2350 kcal
Total kcal	6050 ÷ 3 days = 2017 kcal/day

   (average kilocalorie intake, rounded to the nearest whole number)

   ### Your Calculation:

Day 1	_____ kcal
Day 2	_____ kcal
Day 3	_____ kcal
Total kcal	_____ ÷ 3 days = _____ kcal/day

   (average kilocalorie intake, rounded to the nearest whole number)

2. Add the number of grams of fat eaten each day of the period. Divide the total by 3 and round to the nearest whole number to calculate the average number of grams of fat consumed daily.

   ### Sample Calculation:

Day 1	50 g
Day 2	57 g
Day 3	42 g
Total =	149 g
Total grams	149 ÷ 3 days = 50 g/day (average)

Your Calculation: _____

Day 1	_____ g
Day 2	_____ g
Day 3	_____ g
Total =	_____ g
Total grams	_____ ÷ 3 days = _____ g of fat/day

(average, rounded to the nearest whole number)

3. Each gram of fat provides about 9 kcal; therefore, you must multiply the average number of grams of fat that you ate daily (step 2) by 9 to obtain the average number of kilocalories from fat.

Sample Calculation: _____

50 g/day × 9 kcal/g = 450 kcal from fat

Your Calculation: _____

_____ g/day × 9 kcal/g = _____ kcal from fat

4. To calculate the average percentage of calories that fat contributed to your diet, divide the average number of calories from fat obtained in step 3 by the average total daily calorie intake obtained in step 1, and round to the nearest one-hundredth. Multiply the value by 100, drop the decimal point, and add the percent symbol.

Sample Calculation: _____

450 kcal ÷ 2017 kcal = 0.22

0.22 × 100 = 22%

Your Calculation: _____

_____ kcal ÷ _____ kcal = _____

_____ × 100 = _____ %

5. Did your average daily fat intake meet the AMDR of 20 to 35% of total energy?   Yes _____   No _____

6. If your average fat intake was more than 35% of your total energy intake, which foods contributed to your high intake of fats?

Foods: _____

7. Review the log of your 3-day food intake. Calculate your average daily intake of saturated fat by adding the grams of saturated fat consumed over the 3-day period and dividing the total by 3.

Your Calculation: _____

Day 1	_____ g
Day 2	_____ g
Day 3	_____ g
Total =	_____ g
Total g	_____ ÷ 3 days = _____ g of saturated fat daily

a. What was your average daily saturated fat intake? _____ g

b. Was your average daily saturated fat intake less than the Dietary Guidelines' recommended limit for a healthy adult (less than 10% of total calories)?

c. If your average saturated fat intake was more than the recommended percentage, list foods that contributed to your high saturated fat intake.

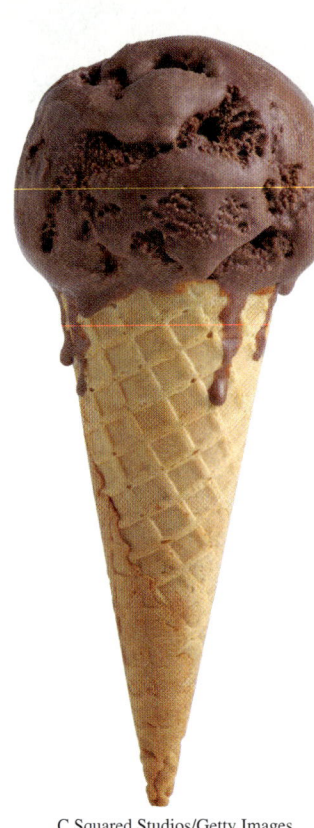
C Squared Studios/Getty Images

Using Nutrient Labels: Total Fat and Saturated Fat

1. Remove the labels from two different packaged foods that contain fat. Using information from each of the product's Nutrition Facts panel, answer the following questions.

   a. Name of product #1 _____

      Name of product #2 _____

   b. How many kcal are in one serving of each food?

      Product 1 _____ kcal

      Product 2 _____ kcal

   c. How many grams of fat and saturated fat are in a serving?

      Product 1

      _____ grams of fat

      _____ grams of saturated fat

      Product 2

      _____ grams of fat

      _____ grams of saturated fat

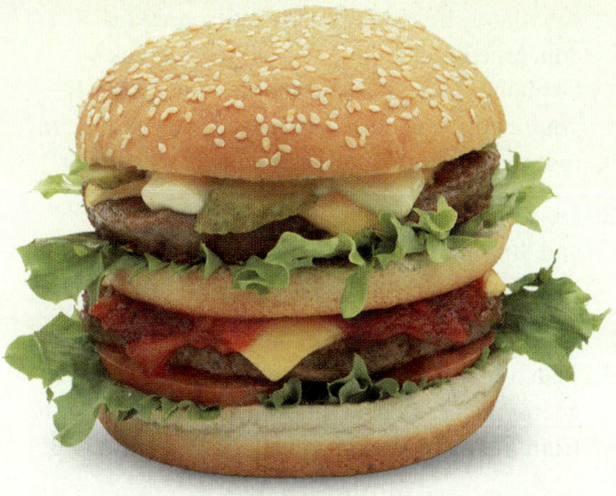

   d. Calculate the percentage of total kcal/serving that are from saturated fat. First, multiply the number of grams of saturated fat by 9 (number of kcal per gram of fat). Then, divide the number of kcal contributed by saturated fat by the total number of kcal per serving. (The Nutrition Facts panel uses the term "Calories" for kcal.) To obtain the percentage, move the decimal point two places to the right, remove the decimal point, and insert % symbol.

      Product 1

      _____ grams of saturated fat × 9 kcal = _____ kcal of saturated fat/serving

      _____ % total kcal/serving contributed by saturated fat

      Product 2

      _____ grams of saturated fat × 9 kcal = _____ kcal of saturated fat/serving

      _____ % total kcal/serving contributed by saturated fat

   e. Read the list of ingredients for each product. If the food contained saturated fat, identify ingredients that contributed this type of fat to the product.

      Saturated fat ingredients in Product 1 _____

      Saturated fat ingredients in Product 2 _____

Ingram Publishing

Consider This...

1. Visit the American Heart Association's "*Check. Change. Control. Calculator*™" at https://ccccalculator.ccctracker.com/. Take the risk calculator. Based on your results, are you concerned about your risk of heart attack? Explain why you are or are not concerned. If you're concerned, discuss steps you can take to reduce your risk of atherosclerosis.

2. Do you avoid fried foods and look for "lite" and "fat-reduced" foods when shopping for groceries? Explain why you do or do not take these actions.

3. Plan a main meal that supplies 20 to 35% of energy from fat. The meal should include foods from the major food groups, incorporate foods that are sources of healthy fats, and provide 700 to 900 kcal.

4. Suggest at least four ways you can reduce your intake of saturated fat and increase your intake of unsaturated fat.

5. Develop a lesson for high school–aged youth that describes atherosclerosis and the role that personal choices (lifestyles) play in the development of the disease.

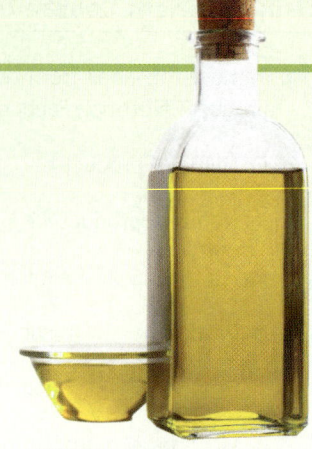

JUPITERIMAGES/ Brand X / Alamy

Test Yourself

Select the best answer.

1. Fats in foods
   a. contribute 7 kcal per gram.
   b. are digested and absorbed in the stomach.
   c. help the body absorb fat-soluble vitamins.
   d. need to be limited to less than 20% of total kcal to have a healthful diet.

2. Liquid fats generally have a high proportion of _____ fatty acids.
   a. unsaturated
   b. saturated
   c. trans
   d. partially hydrogenated

3. A monounsaturated fatty acid has
   a. one double bond within the carbon chain.
   b. two double bonds within the carbon chain.
   c. no double bonds within the carbon chain.
   d. three double bonds within the carbon chain.

4. Which of the following statements is true?
   a. Walnuts are a rich source of PHOs.
   b. Omega-3 fatty acids decrease the risk of cardiovascular disease.
   c. Trans fats are rich sources of omega-3 fatty acids.
   d. The human body converts dietary fiber into omega-3 fatty acids.

5. Fatty fish, including salmon and sardines,
   a. contain too much methylmercury to be eaten.
   b. should be eaten daily, according to the Dietary Guidelines (U.S. version).
   c. are not sources of cholesterol.
   d. are sources of omega-3 fatty acids.

6. Cholesterol is
   a. metabolized for energy.
   b. found only in animal foods.
   c. not made by the human body.
   d. harmful to health.

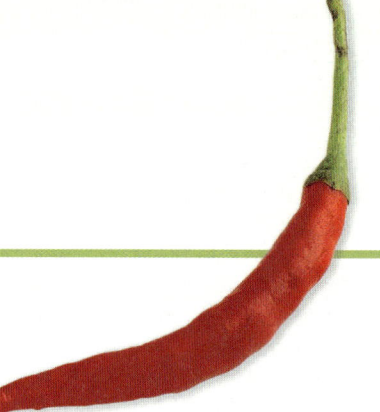

7. The primary site of fat digestion and absorption is the
   a. stomach.
   b. liver.
   c. small intestine.
   d. gallbladder.

8. Lipoproteins
   a. are made in the kidneys.
   b. transport fat and cholesterol in the bloodstream.
   c. contain oxidized glucose.
   d. are toxic to cells.

9. Key risk factors for atherosclerosis include
   a. educational background.
   b. occupation.
   c. income.
   d. hypertension.

10. Atherosclerosis contibutes to
    a. dental decay.
    b. type 2 diabetes.
    c. gallbladder disease.
    d. cardiovascular disease.

11. According to nutrition scientists, you may reduce your risk of CVD by replacing calories from added sugars and saturated fats with foods that are rich sources of
    a. polyunsaturated fats.
    b. trans fats.
    c. partially hydrogenated fats.
    d. phospholipids.

12. Eliot's HDL cholesterol level is 30 mg/dl and his LDL cholesterol level is 185 mg/dl. According to this information, Eliot has _____ of CVD.
    a. very low risk
    b. low risk
    c. high risk
    d. no risk

Answers: 1. c 2. a 3. a 4. b 5. d 6. b 7. c 8. b 9. d 10. d 11. a 12. c

Answer This (Module 6.1a)

Olive oil

References → See Appendix D.

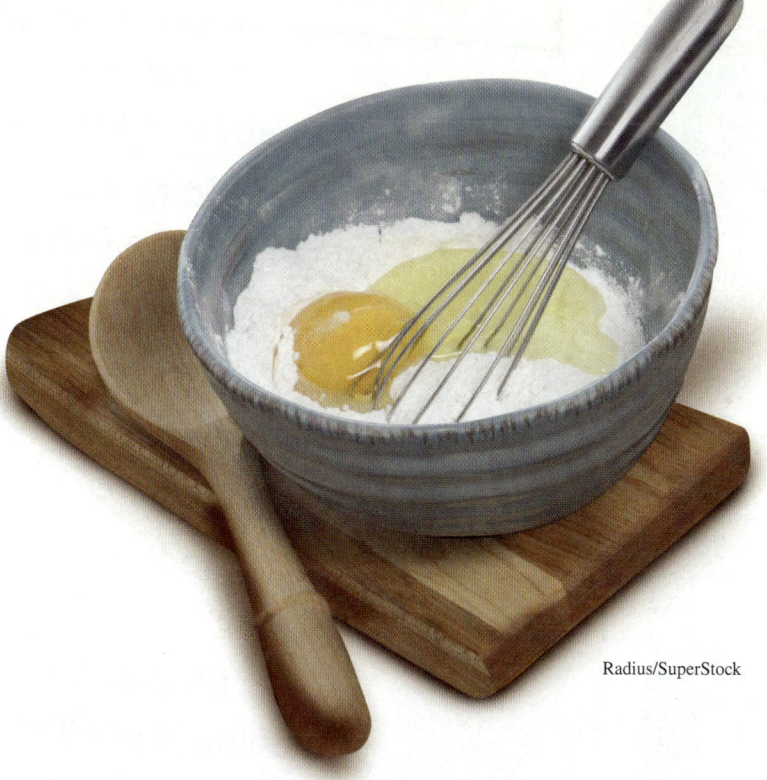

Radius/SuperStock

Design elements: Spiral notebook paper background, Stacked paper with clip background, Marginal note clip, and Culture & Cuisine globe icon: ©McGraw-Hill Education; In a Nutshell walnut: ©McGraw-Hill Education/Mark A. Dierker, photographer; Test Yourself red pepper: Iconotec/Glow Images

Unit 7

Proteins
LIFE'S BUILDING BLOCKS

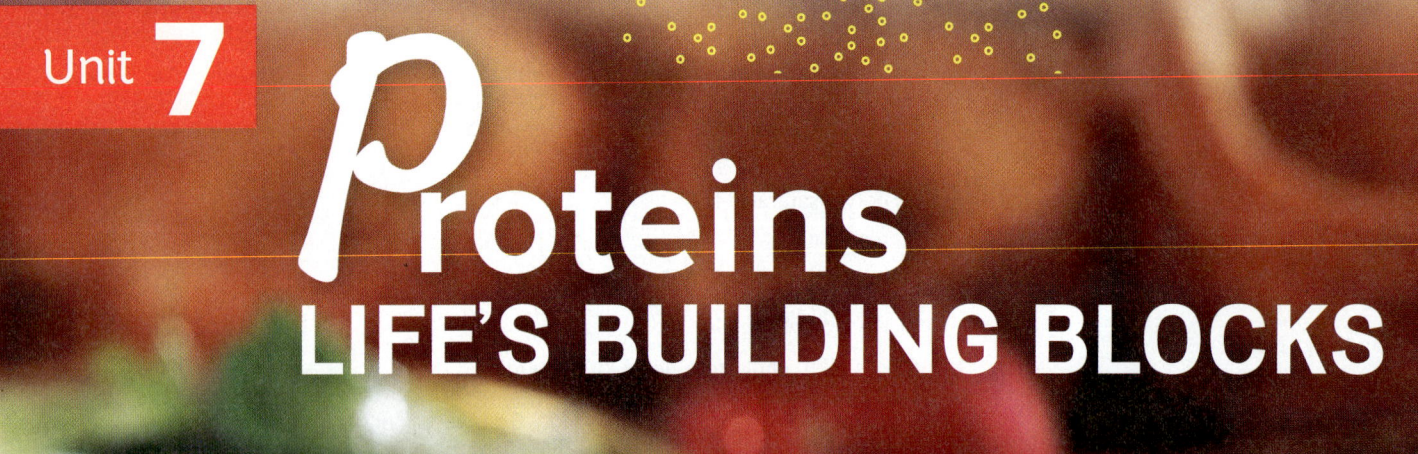

What's on the Menu?

Module 7.1
What Are Proteins?

Module 7.2
What Happens to the Protein You Eat?

Module 7.3
Proteins in Foods

Module 7.4
What's Vegetarianism?

Module 7.5
Proteins and Health

Module 7.6
Stretching Your Food Dollars

Ingram Publishing/SuperStock

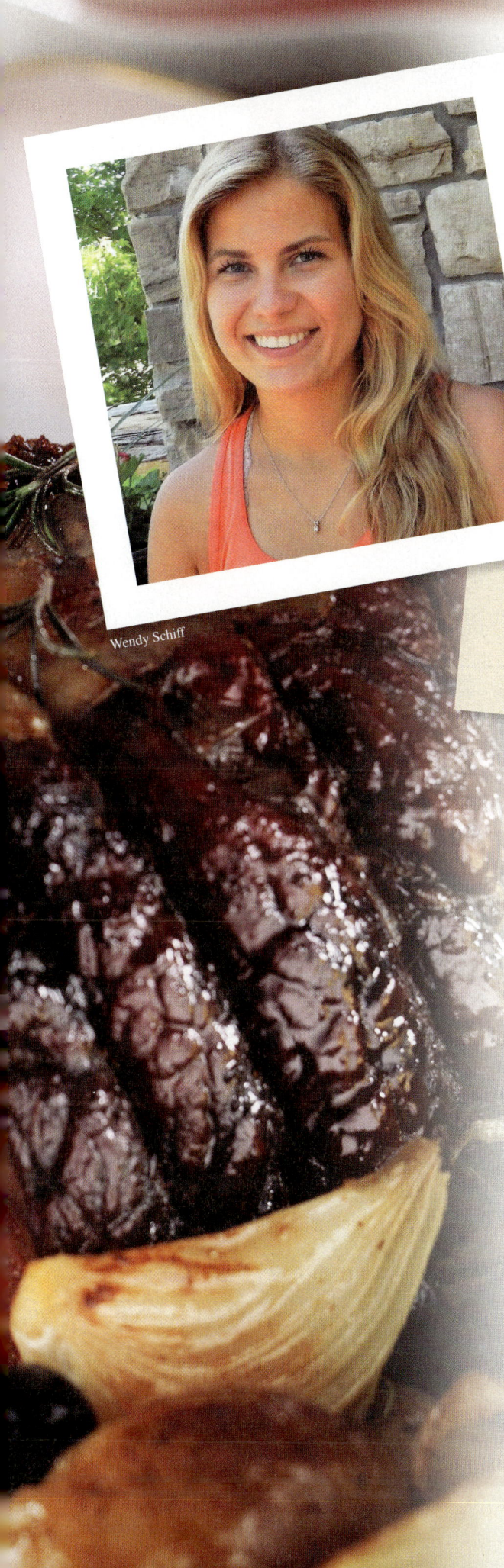

"I'm very physically active. When I was in high school, I ran cross-country, swam competitively, and played lacrosse. I also did strength and conditioning training. Now that I'm in college, I have to prioritize my time around my class schedule so I can work out and train for half-marathons. This year, I ran a half-marathon and came in second for my age group. . . . I find running is a great stress reliever. I eat more when I'm in training, and my performance suffers when I don't eat the right foods. . . . I have enough 'likes' in each food group; I think my diet is well rounded."

Olivia Coomes

Olivia Coomes is majoring in accounting at Auburn University. She is so physically active, she doesn't have to worry about her weight. She says, "I work out and eat healthy." Although she describes herself as a "picky eater," she has become more willing to try new foods since she left home to begin college.

Unlike many athletic persons, Olivia doesn't focus on eating protein-rich foods to ensure her optimal physical performance. Is it necessary for athletes to consume more protein than nonathletes consume? Does eating a high-protein diet help people build muscle tissue?

Many Americans think a meal isn't a meal unless it contains large portions of beef, pork, or poultry. Although it's true that these foods are rich sources of protein, other foods, including those from plants, are often overlooked as sources of protein. Protein is an important nutrient, but it isn't more valuable to your health than other nutrients. Nutrients work together in your body like members of a well-trained lacrosse team on the playing field. Making one player the star while neglecting to develop the other athletes' skills can have disastrous effects on the team's success. Similarly, overemphasizing one class of nutrients in your diet, such as protein, while ignoring other nutrients can lead to nutritional imbalances that result in serious health problems. By reading Unit 7, you'll learn about the roles of proteins in your body and their major food sources. You'll also learn how eating too much or not enough dietary protein can influence your health.

Module 7.1

What Are Proteins?

7.1- Learning Outcomes

After reading Module 7.1, you should be able to

1. Define all of the **key terms** in this module.
2. List the primary functions of proteins in the body.
3. Identify the basic structural unit of proteins.
4. Distinguish between essential and nonessential amino acids.

Proteins are organic nutrients that are chemically similar to lipids and carbohydrates because they contain carbon, hydrogen, and oxygen atoms. Proteins, however, contain nitrogen, the element cells need to make a wide array of important biological compounds. Plants, animals, bacteria, and even viruses contain hundreds of proteins.

7.1a What Roles Do Proteins Play in the Body?

All cells in your body contain proteins. The thousands of different proteins in your body have a wide variety of functions. Your body uses protein to

- *Make, maintain, and repair cells.*

  Cells have proteins in their membranes and other cellular structures. When cells divide, such as during periods of growth, they need protein to form cell membranes and other protein-containing components of the new cells.

- *Build structures.*

  Structural proteins such as *collagen* are in your cartilage, ligaments, and bone tissue. *Keratin* is another structural protein—it's in your hair, nails, and skin. Keratin is tough and water-resistant. Contractile proteins in your muscles enable you to move.

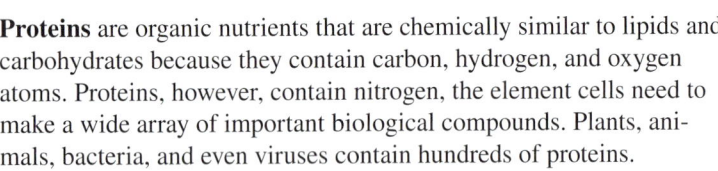
Your hair contains a protein called keratin.

- *Produce enzymes, lubricants, and clotting compounds.*
  - Nearly all enzymes are proteins. Enzymes speed up the rate of (*catalyze*) chemical reactions without becoming a part of the products.
  - Lubricants include *mucin,* which is in mucus and saliva.
  - *Fibrin* is a tough protein that forms when a blood clot is needed to stop bleeding.

- *Transport substances.*
  - Transport proteins include hemoglobin, which transports oxygen in red blood cells, and *retinol binding protein,* which carries vitamin A in the bloodstream.
  - Proteins in cell membranes control the movement of substances in and out of cells.

- *Make antibodies and certain hormones.*
  - **Antibodies** are structures in the bloodstream that help prevent and combat infections.
  - Many hormones (chemical messengers), including insulin and glucagon, are proteins.

- *Maintain proper fluid balance and acid-base balance.*
  - Proteins in blood, such as *albumin*, help maintain the proper distribution of fluids in blood and body tissues. The force of blood pressure moves watery fluid out of the bloodstream and into tissues. Blood proteins help counteract the effects of blood pressure by attracting the fluid, returning it to the bloodstream. In starvation, the level of protein in blood decreases and, as a result, some water leaks out of the bloodstream and enters spaces between cells. The resulting accumulation of fluid in tissues is called **edema** (*eh-dee'mah*) (**Fig. 7.1**).
  - Proteins also help maintain **acid-base balance,** the proper

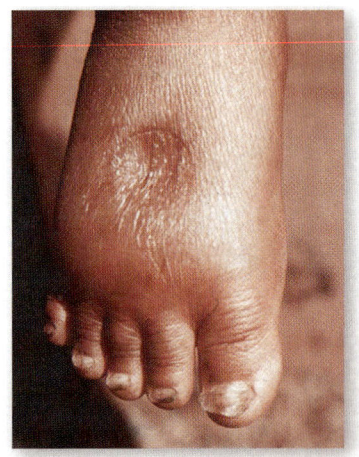

Figure 7.1 "Pitting" edema.

■ *How does a protein-deficient diet contribute to edema?*

Beans: Pixtal/AGE fotostock; Hair: Joe DeGrandis/McGraw-Hill Education; Foot: Centers for Disease Control and Prevention/Dr. Lyle Conrad

concentration of hydrogen ions (H⁺), in body fluids. To function properly, blood and tissue fluids need to be slightly basic (alkaline). If the H⁺ concentration of these fluids increases above normal levels, the tissues become too acidic. If the H⁺ concentration decreases too much, the blood and tissues become too basic. When a particular body fluid becomes too acidic or too basic, cells can have difficulty functioning and may die. A *buffer* helps maintain the proper H⁺ concentration of fluids. Proteins can act as buffers because they have acidic and basic components. If cells form an excess of H⁺, the basic portions of protein molecules bind to the excess H⁺, neutralizing the excess and reducing the concentration of H⁺ back to normal.

- *Provide energy.*

    Although cells can use the basic components of proteins for energy, normally they metabolize very little for energy. As a result, cells save protein for other important functions that carbohydrates and lipids are unable to perform.

proteins large, complex organic nutrients made up of amino acids

antibodies proteins that help prevent and fight infection

edema accumulation of fluid in tissues

acid-base balance maintaining the proper hydrogen concentration of body fluids

amino acids nitrogen-containing chemical units that comprise proteins

nonessential amino acids group of amino acids that the body can make

essential amino acids amino acids the body can't make or can't make enough to meet its needs

7.1b What Are Amino Acids?

The basic building blocks of proteins are **amino acids.** Each amino acid has four parts:

- a carbon atom that anchors a hydrogen atom,
- the amino (nitrogen-containing) group,
- the R-group that varies with each type of amino acid, and
- the acid group.

The chemical structure of the amino acid alanine indicates these three groups **(Fig. 7.2)**.

When the nitrogen-containing amino group is removed, the R-group, the acid group, and the anchoring carbon atom form the "carbon skeleton" of an amino acid (see Figure 7.2). The body can convert the carbon skeletons of certain amino acids to glucose and use the simple sugar for energy. Recall from Unit 1 that each gram of protein provides about 4 kcal.

Classifying Amino Acids

Your body contains proteins made from 20 different amino acids. Nutritionists often classify amino acids as either nonessential or essential according to the body's ability to make them. A healthy human body can make 11 of the 20 amino acids. These compounds are the **nonessential amino acids.** The remaining 9 amino acids are **essential amino acids** that must be supplied by foods because your body cannot make them or produce enough to meet its needs. **Table 7.1** classifies amino acids as either essential or nonessential.

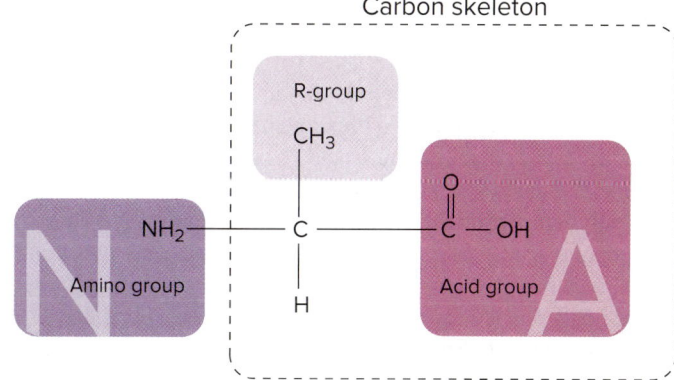

Figure 7.2 Components of an amino acid (alanine).

Table 7.1 Amino Acids

Essential		Nonessential	
Histidine	Phenylalanine	Alanine	Glutamine*
Isoleucine	Threonine	Arginine*	Glycine*
Leucine	Tryptophan	Asparagine	Proline*
Lysine	Valine	Aspartic acid	Serine
Methionine		Cysteine*	Tyrosine*
		Glutamic acid	

*Under certain conditions, this amino acid can become essential.

McGraw-Hill Education/Mark Dierker, photographer Pixtal/AGE Fotostock

Module 7.2

What Happens to the Protein You Eat?

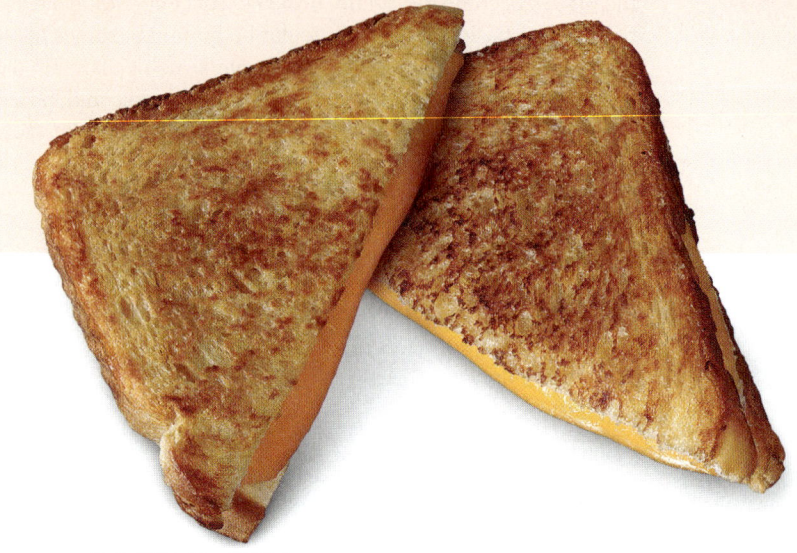

7.2 - Learning Outcomes

After reading Module 7.2, you should be able to

1. Define all of the **key terms** in this module.
2. Explain what happens to proteins as they undergo digestion and absorption in the human digestive tract.
3. Explain how cells make proteins.
4. Describe what happens to excess amino acids.
5. Calculate your Recommended Dietary Allowance (RDA) for protein based on your body weight.

Burke/Triolo/Brand X Pictures

7.2a Protein Digestion and Absorption

An amino acid can connect to another amino acid by a **peptide bond,** a chemical attraction between two amino acids. To illustrate how amino acids bind together, we'll use a protein "necklace" that contains amino acid "beads" **(Fig. 7.3).** In our example of the necklace, the string that connects two beads is a peptide bond.

A **polypeptide** forms when two or more amino acids join to form chains (see Figure 7.3). A dipeptide is a very simple polypeptide that has only two amino acids linked together. A tripeptide is a polypeptide that has only three amino acids bonded together. A protein is a polypeptide that may be comprised of hundreds of amino acids connected to each other by peptide bonds.

When you eat a toasted cheese sandwich for lunch, the large proteins in the bread and cheese must be digested before undergoing absorption. **Essential Concept 7.1** describes what happens to proteins during digestion and absorption.

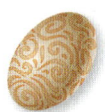

Amino acid

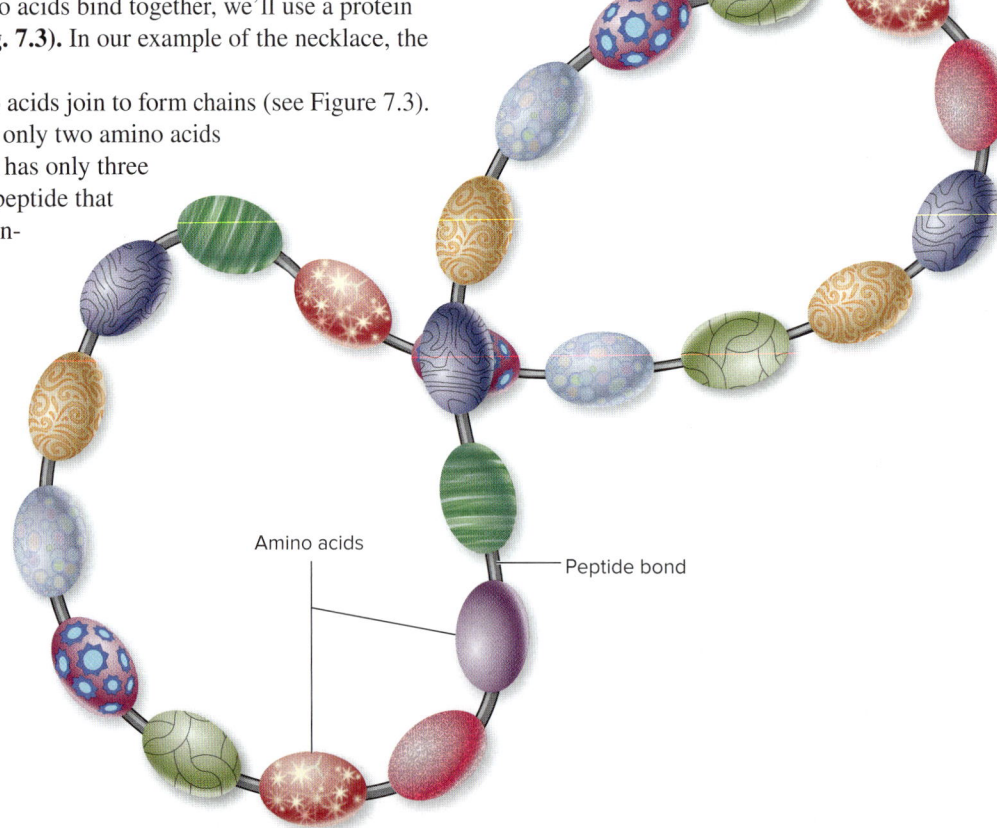

Amino acids

Peptide bond

peptide bond chemical attraction that connects two amino acids together

polypeptides chains of two or more amino acids

Figure 7.3 Amino acids make up proteins. Human cells use 20 different amino acids to make proteins. In this illustration, amino acids are represented by beads.

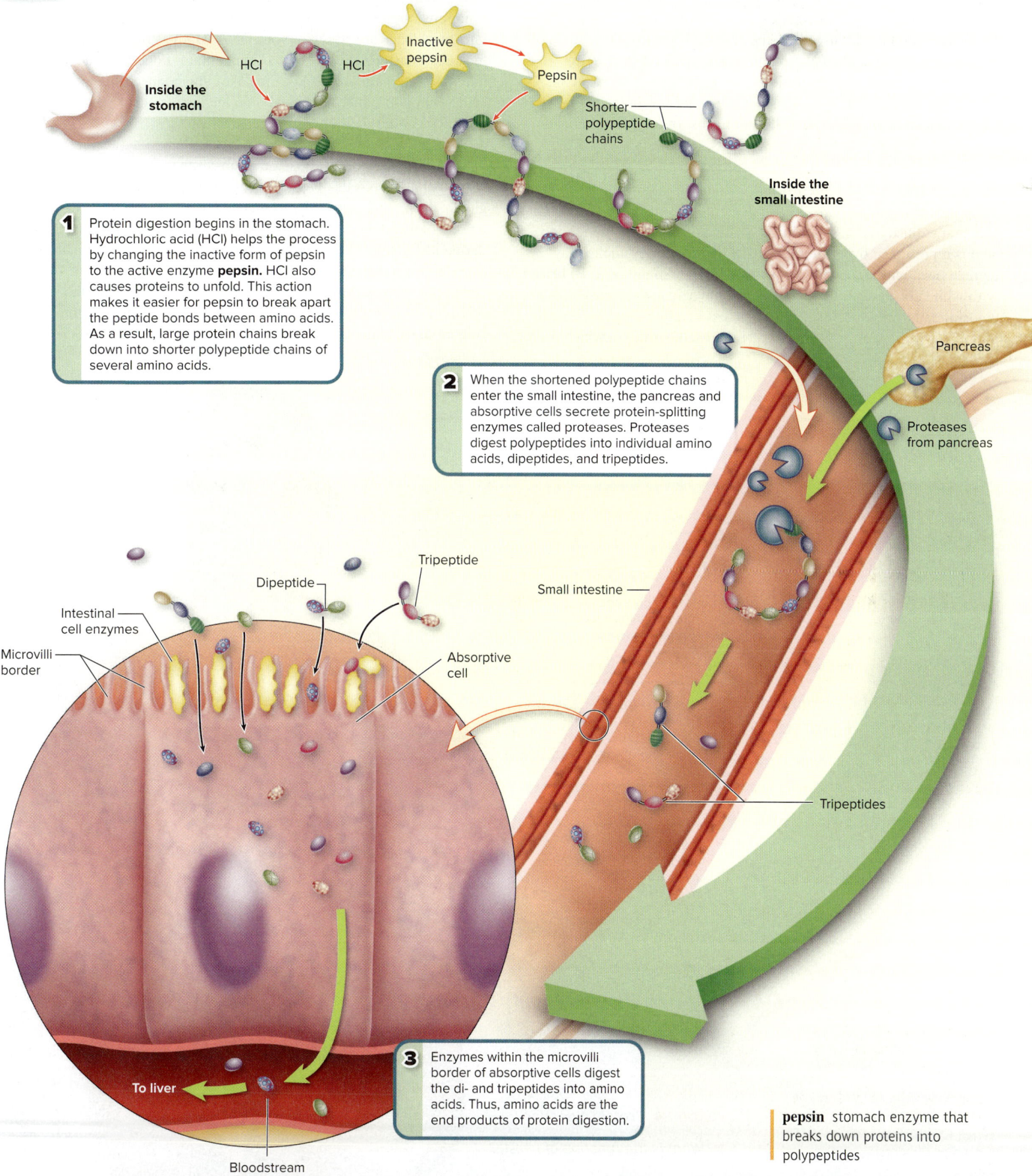

After being absorbed, the amino acids enter the large vein (hepatic portal vein) that takes absorbed water-soluble nutrients to the liver. The liver keeps some amino acids for its needs and releases the rest into the general circulation. By the time cells obtain amino acids from blood, they cannot distinguish the ones that were originally in the bread from those that were in the cheese. The cells, however, now have all the amino acids they need to make your body's proteins.

Protein digestion and absorption is very efficient—only a small amount of dietary protein escapes digestion and is eliminated in feces. **Figure 7.4** summarizes protein digestion, absorption, and elimination.

7.2b Using Amino Acids to Build Proteins

To understand how your body uses the 20 different amino acids to make thousands of proteins, let's consider the protein "beaded" necklace that's illustrated in Figure 7.3. Assume that each type of amino acid is represented by a different bead. Alanine, for example, may be a green bead with fine white stripes; methionine might be a red bead with white dots. Each of the other 18 amino acids would have its own colorful pattern. A specific protein, such as insulin or sucrase, can be identified by the kinds of "beads" it contains, the order in which the beads are strung, and the number of beads that are used. The wide variety of proteins in your body reflects the numerous ways your cells can connect amino acids to form proteins.

If you have a box of 1000 amino acid "beads," how do you form functional proteins from them? The instructions for making each protein "necklace" are stored in your DNA. **DNA** is often referred to as the cells' master molecule because it contains coded instructions for making proteins. If cells make mistakes and connect the wrong amino acids, they'll produce abnormal proteins that can cause birth defects, chronic health conditions, and even death.

Sickle cell disease is an inherited disorder that primarily affects people with African ancestry. The disease results from a single *mutation* (a change) in the DNA that provides instructions for making a part of hemoglobin, the protein that carries oxygen in your red blood cells (RBCs). As a result of the mutation, the wrong amino acid is added to hemoglobin during its formation. The disease gets its name from the abnormal crescent ("sickle") shape that the RBCs develop when they're in low-oxygen conditions. The sickle-shaped RBCs don't move through tiny blood vessels as easily as normal, round RBCs pass through them. The abnormal cells clump together and block blood flow in the blood vessels, causing tissue damage. In some cases, sickle cell disease is deadly.

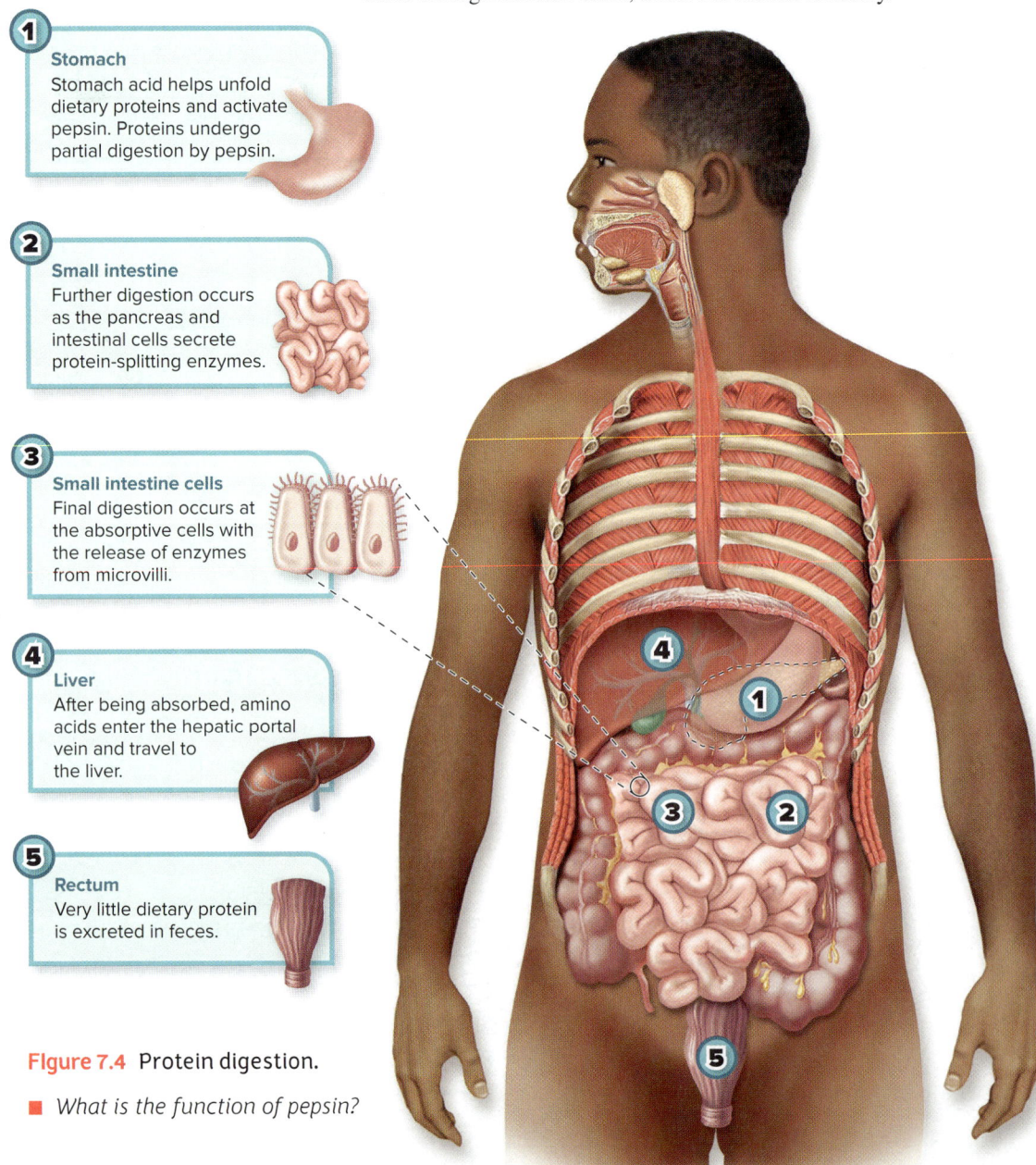

1 Stomach
Stomach acid helps unfold dietary proteins and activate pepsin. Proteins undergo partial digestion by pepsin.

2 Small intestine
Further digestion occurs as the pancreas and intestinal cells secrete protein-splitting enzymes.

3 Small intestine cells
Final digestion occurs at the absorptive cells with the release of enzymes from microvilli.

4 Liver
After being absorbed, amino acids enter the hepatic portal vein and travel to the liver.

5 Rectum
Very little dietary protein is excreted in feces.

Figure 7.4 Protein digestion.

■ *What is the function of pepsin?*

DNA master molecule that has the instructions for making proteins

7.2c The Fate of Excess Amino Acids

Your body doesn't store excess amino acids in muscle or other tissues. If you consume more protein than you need, what happens to the extra amino acids? **Essential Concept 7.2** illustrates how your body handles the unneeded amino acids. Module 7.5 provides more information about the effects of excess amino acid intakes on the body.

Essential Concept

7.2 What Can Happen to Unneeded Amino Acids?

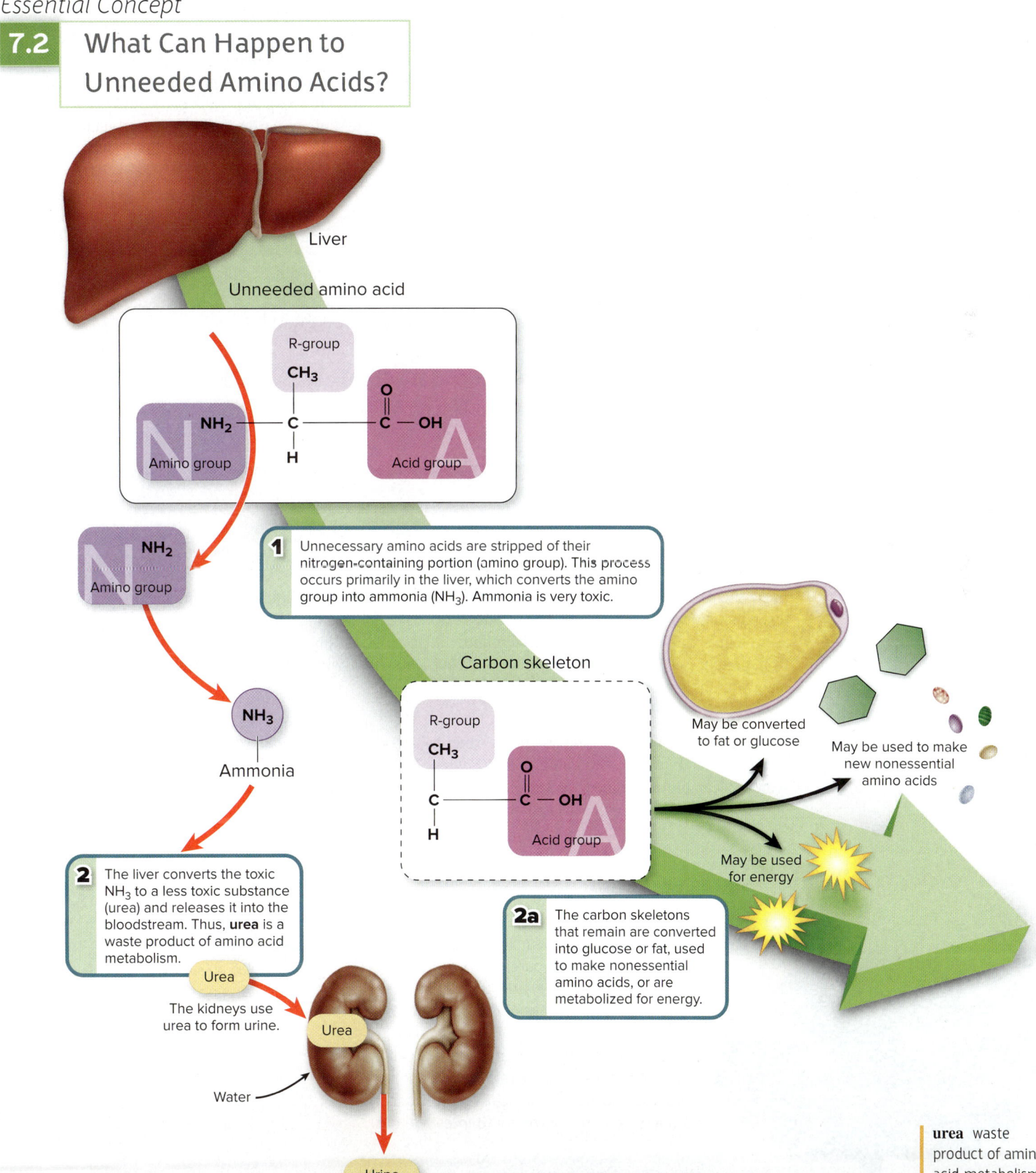

1. Unnecessary amino acids are stripped of their nitrogen-containing portion (amino group). This process occurs primarily in the liver, which converts the amino group into ammonia (NH_3). Ammonia is very toxic.

2. The liver converts the toxic NH_3 to a less toxic substance (urea) and releases it into the bloodstream. Thus, **urea** is a waste product of amino acid metabolism.

The kidneys use urea to form urine.

2a. The carbon skeletons that remain are converted into glucose or fat, used to make nonessential amino acids, or are metabolized for energy.

May be converted to fat or glucose

May be used to make new nonessential amino acids

May be used for energy

urea waste product of amino acid metabolism

Your body can recycle nitrogen from amino acids to make nonessential amino acids. Each day, however, you lose some protein and the nitrogen it contains from your body. Your urine contains most of the lost nitrogen. Daily nitrogen losses also occur as your nails and hair grow, and when you shed the outermost layer of your skin and cells from your intestinal tract. To be healthy, your body needs amino acids from foods to replace the lost nitrogen.

7.2d How Much Protein Do You Need?

A healthy adult's Recommended Dietary Allowance (RDA) for protein is 0.8 g/kg of body weight. To determine your RDA for protein, first divide your weight in pounds by 2.2 to obtain your weight in kilograms. If, for example, you weigh 145 pounds, you weigh about 66 kg (145 ÷ 2.2). Now, multiply 0.8 g protein times 66 kg body weight. Based on these calculations, you should consume about 53 g of protein daily (66 kg × 0.8 g/kg) to meet your RDA for the nutrient. The body's need for protein increases during pregnancy, when breastfeeding, and in periods of growth, extreme physical exertion, and recovery from serious illnesses, blood losses, and burns.

Your weight in pounds is _____ lbs.

Now, divide this weight by 2.2 to obtain your weight in kg.

My weight is _____ kg.

Multiply _____ (your weight in kg) by 0.8 g/kg to obtain _____ g.

This amount is your RDA for protein.

How Much Protein Do Americans Eat?

In 2015–2016, adult Americans consumed an average of 82.5 g protein/day.[1] This amount is about 15.7% of this population's total energy intake for a day. For healthy adults, diets that supply this percentage of calories as protein is within the Acceptable Macronutrient Distribution Range (AMDR), which is 10 to 35% of energy from protein (see Table 3.1). The "What's in Your Diet?!" activity at the end of this unit can help you estimate your daily protein intake.

MyPlate: Recommendations for Protein Intake Animal foods, including eggs and milk products, supply almost two-thirds of the protein in America's food supply.[2] Animal sources of protein are often rich sources of saturated fat. According to the *Dietary Guidelines for Americans,* you should choose fish and seafood, lean or low-fat meat, and poultry.[3] MyPlate recommends including more plant sources of protein in your diet, especially dried beans and peas, nuts, and seeds.

TASTY Tidbits

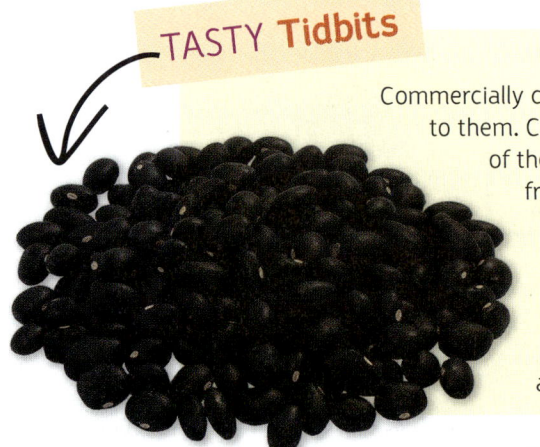

Commercially canned beans may have a lot of salt added to them. Consider rinsing the beans to remove much of the salt. Also, consider purchasing canned or frozen beans that have little or no added salt. Dried beans don't have added salt, but to shorten their cooking time, you can soak them in water several hours before cooking and then discard the water. The soaking process also makes the beans more digestible and less likely to contribute to intestinal gas.

 **Answer This**

Josh is a nonathlete who weighs 165 pounds. What is his RDA for protein? You can find the answer on the last page of this unit.

McGraw-Hill Education/Jacques Cornell

Module 7.3
Proteins in Foods

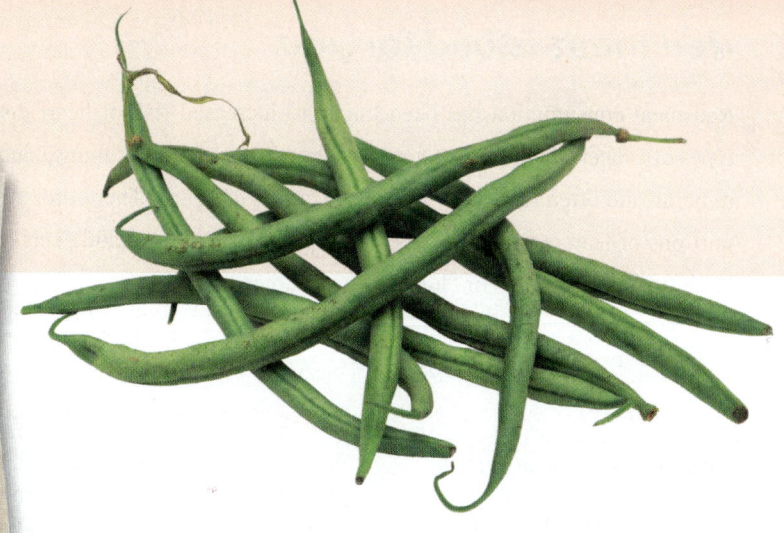

7.3 - Learning Outcomes

After reading Module 7.3, you should be able to

1. Define all of the **key terms** in this module.
2. Identify foods that are legumes.
3. Explain the difference between a high-quality protein and a low-quality protein, and identify foods that are rich sources of high-quality proteins.
4. Plan nutritious meals and snacks that reduce animal protein intake.
5. Develop strategies for increasing your intake of plant protein without sacrificing the overall protein quality of your diet.

legumes plants that produce pods with a single row of seeds

People often associate animal foods with protein, but dry beans and peas, nuts, seeds, grains, and certain vegetables are good sources of protein, too. In fact, nearly all foods contain protein, but no naturally occurring food is 100% protein. **Table 7.2** lists some commonly eaten foods and their approximate protein content per serving.

Not all plant foods are good sources of protein. Legumes (*lay'-gumes*), seeds, and tree nuts supply more protein per serving than do servings of fruit or the edible leaves, roots, flowers, and stems of vegetables. **Legumes** are plants that produce pods that have a single row of seeds, such as soybeans, peas, peanuts, lentils, and beans. Tree nuts include walnuts, cashews, pecans, and almonds.

TABLE 7.2 APPROXIMATE PROTEIN CONTENT OF SOME COMMONLY EATEN FOODS/PORTION

Food	Serving Size	Protein g/serving	Food	Serving Size	Protein g/serving
Pepperoni pizza, regular crust, 14" pie	2 slices (220 g)	27	Milk, fat-free	1 cup	8
Chicken, breast, cooked, meat only	3 oz	27	Peanut butter, smooth	2 Tbsp	7
Tofu, firm, made with calcium sulfate	½ cup	22	Baked beans, vegetarian	½ cup	6
Hamburger patty, 85% lean, broiled	3 oz	22	Egg, large, hard cooked	1	6
Tuna, canned, water-packed, drained	3 oz	20	American processed cheese	1 oz	5
Ham, lean, cooked	3 oz	16	Vanilla ice cream	1 cup	4
Almonds, whole	½ cup	15	Peas, green, cooked	½ cup	4
Bagel, plain	1 (3½" diam.)	11	White rice, cooked	½ cup	2
Cottage cheese, 2% low-fat	3 oz	9	Banana, medium	1	1

Source: U.S. Department of Agriculture, Agricultural Research Service: *USDA National Nutrient Database for Standard Reference Legacy Release, April 2018.* https://ndb.nal.usda.gov/ndb/search/list?home=true Accessed: September 2018.

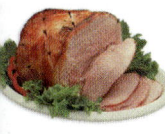

Green beans: Pixtal/AGE Fotostock; Ham: Ingram Publishing; Peas: C Squared Studios/Getty Images

Nutrition Fact or Fiction?
Red meat is bad for you.

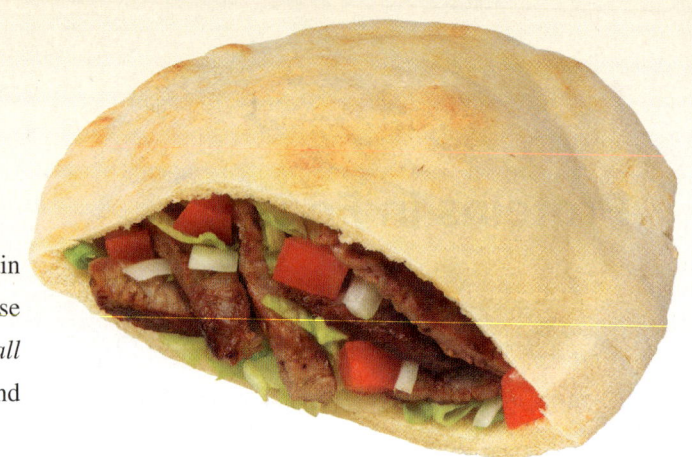

Red meat consumption has been linked to increased risk of heart disease and certain types of cancer. However, meat is also a good source of B vitamins, zinc, and iron. These minerals are often less easily absorbed from plant foods. Therefore, it's OK to eat *small* portions of lean red meats occasionally. Lean red meats include cuts of beef, pork, and lamb that have "round" or "loin" in their names.

7.3a Protein Quality

high-quality protein protein that contains all essential amino acids in amounts that support the deposition of protein in tissues and the growth of a young person

low-quality protein protein that lacks or has inadequate amounts of one or more of the essential amino acids

Foods differ not only in the amount of protein they contain but also in their protein quality. A **high-quality protein** contains all essential amino acids in amounts that support the health of your muscles and other tissues, as well as a young child's growth. High-quality proteins are well digested and absorbed by your body. Meat, fish, poultry, eggs, milk, and milk products contain high-quality proteins. A **low-quality protein** lacks or contains inadequate amounts of one or more of the essential amino acids. High-quality protein and low-quality protein may be referred to, respectively, as *complete* and *incomplete* protein.

The essential amino acids that are in relatively low amounts are referred to as *limiting amino acids*. A protein that has limiting amino acids may be unable to provide the amino acids that your cells need to support growth, repair, and maintenance of tissues.

Most plant foods aren't sources of high-quality proteins. Quinoa (*keen'-wa*) and soy protein are among the few exceptions. Quinoa is related to sugar beets and spinach, but the quality and amount of protein in quinoa seeds are superior to those of most other plant sources of protein.[4] Cooked quinoa is often used as a cereal (**Fig. 7.5**). After being processed, the quality of soy protein is comparable to that of most animal proteins. Processed soybeans are used to make a variety of nutritious foods, including soy milk (soy beverage), infant formula, and meat substitutes.

Understanding the concept of protein quality is important. Regardless of how much protein is eaten, a child will fail to grow properly if his or her diet lacks essential amino acids.

TASTY Tidbits

A 3-ounce serving of almonds, dry-roasted peanuts, or sunflower seed kernels supplies about 20 g of protein. Many seeds and nuts are rich sources of "healthy" fats (discussed in Unit 6). Because of their high fat content, seeds and nuts pack a lot of calories. Snack on just 3 ounces of almonds, dry-roasted peanuts, or sunflower seed kernels, and you'll add almost 500 kcal to your diet!

Sunflower seeds

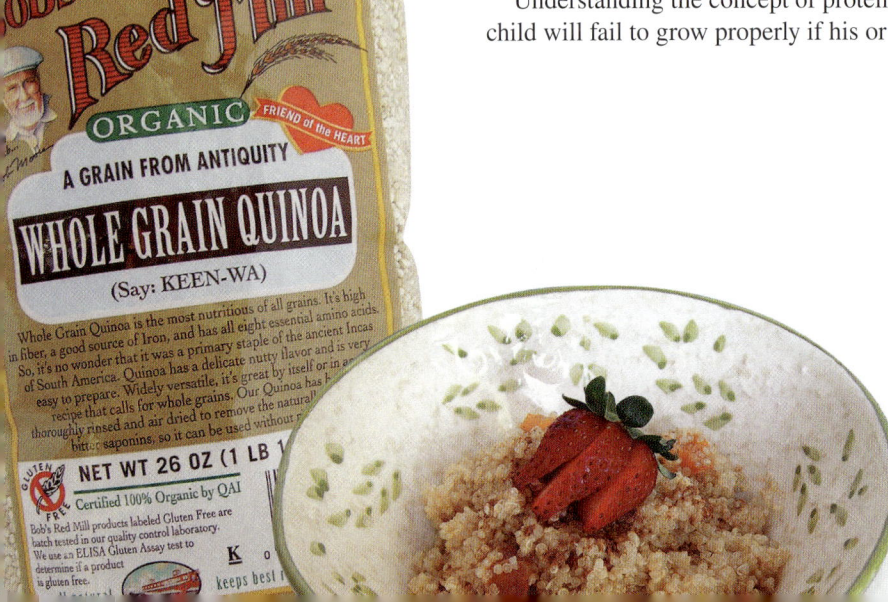

Figure 7.5 Quinoa.

■ *Why is quinoa a good source of high-quality protein?*

Pita sandwich: Ingram Publishing/Alamy; Sunflower seeds, Quinoa package, Cooked quinoa: Wendy Schiff

Combining Complementary Proteins

It's not necessary to consume all essential amino acids during the same meal for your body to use them to make proteins. However, nutrition experts recommend that you consume adequate amounts of the essential amino acids each day. Most plant foods are poor sources of one or more essential amino acids, particularly tryptophan, lysine, and methionine (see Table 7.1). If you eat only plant foods, you need to plan your meals and snacks carefully. **Complementary combinations** are mixtures of certain plant foods that provide all essential amino acids without adding animal proteins.

Figure 7.6 shows three categories of plant proteins (legumes, grains, and tree nuts and seeds) that make complementary combinations when legumes are mixed with one or more items from the other groups. Legumes, for example, are good sources of lysine, but they contain low amounts of tryptophan and methionine. Cereal grains, such as wheat, rice, and corn, are good sources of tryptophan and methionine, but they are low in lysine. A meal that combines legumes and grains is "complementary," because it provides satisfactory amounts of limiting essential amino acids.

Examples of complementary combinations include

- black or red beans and rice;
- vegetable lasagna with layers of pasta, bits of tofu (a food made from soybeans), thinly sliced zucchini, mushrooms, and bell peppers;
- grilled vegetable kabobs served over rice and black beans; or
- bean burritos.

Most fruits and many kinds of vegetables are poor sources of protein. Therefore, not every mixture of plant foods creates a complementary combination. For example, making a fruit salad by combining apples, grapes, and oranges will not provide a complementary mixture of essential amino acids. Furthermore, combining Boston, iceberg, and romaine varieties of lettuce with carrots and onions makes a tasty salad, but simply mixing leafy greens with other vegetables doesn't make a complementary combination. Why? Leafy vegetables have small amounts of protein that tend to contain low amounts of essential amino acids. However, adding sunflower seed kernels, kidney or black beans, cashews, cooked quinoa, and bread cubes to the vegetable salad boosts the amount of protein and provides a complete mix of amino acids.

Although fruits and many kinds of vegetables are poor protein sources, these foods add appealing colors and textures as well as vitamins, minerals, and phytochemicals to plant-based meals. Module 7.4 explains how you can obtain a nutritionally adequate diet by increasing your intake of protein-rich plant foods and reducing your intake of animal foods.

Legumes

Primary limiting amino acids:
Methionine
Tryptophan

Mature split peas and lentils
Peanuts and peanut butter
Soybeans, soy products, and other mature beans

Seeds and Tree Nuts

Primary limiting amino acid:
Lysine

Sesame seeds, sunflower seed kernels, pumpkin seeds
Cashews, pistachios, walnuts, pine nuts, almonds, pecans

Grains

Primary limiting amino acid:
Lysine

Wheat and products made from wheat flour
Rice, oats, millet, barley, bulgur
Corn and products made from corn

Figure 7.6 Complementary combinations. Combining legumes with grains and/or seeds and nuts can result in complementary combinations of essential amino acids.

■ *To improve the protein quality of mature split peas without using animal proteins, you could mix the split peas with what food?*

complementary combinations mixing certain plant foods to provide all essential amino acids without adding animal protein

Plate of plant foods, Pecans, Corn: Wendy Schiff; Peanuts: C Squared Studios/Getty Images

Module 7.4

What's Vegetarianism?

7.4 - Learning Outcomes

After reading Module 7.4, you should be able to

1. Define all of the **key terms** in this module.
2. Distinguish among the various types of vegetarianism.
3. Discuss the pros and cons of vegetarian diets.

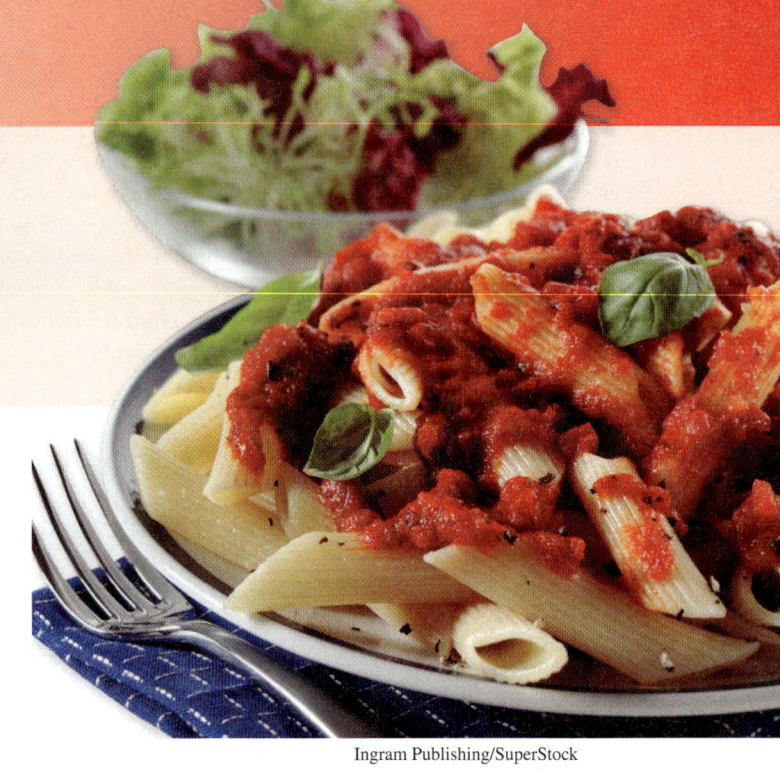

Penne pasta with tomato sauce

Ingram Publishing/SuperStock

7.4a Vegetarianism

In 2018, about 5% of American adults described themselves as vegetarians; about 3% of adults reported being vegans.[5] **Vegetarians** rely heavily on plant foods and may or may not include some animal foods in their diets. *Vegans* don't eat any animal products. There are different types of vegetarian diets, including some that combine plant foods with certain animal foods:

- A **semivegetarian** (or **flexitarian**) eats eggs, fish, and dairy foods but generally avoids meat.
- A **lactovegetarian** (*lacto* = milk) consumes milk and milk products, including yogurt, cheese, and ice cream, to obtain animal protein.
- An **ovovegetarian** (*ovo* = egg) eats eggs.
- A **lacto-ovovegetarian** consumes milk products and eggs.
- A **vegan,** or total vegetarian, eats only plant foods.

vegetarians people who eat plant-based diets

semivegetarian or flexitarian person who eats eggs, fish, and dairy foods but generally avoids meat

lactovegetarian vegetarian who consumes milk and milk products for animal protein

ovovegetarian vegetarian who eats eggs for animal protein

lacto-ovovegetarian vegetarian who consumes milk products and eggs for animal protein

vegans vegetarians who eat only plant foods

7.4b Is Vegetarianism a Healthy Lifestyle?

Vegetarian diets are often lower in fat and energy than "Western diets" that contain animal foods, particularly plenty of red meat. Compared to people who eat meat, vegetarians tend to have a lower risk of obesity, cardiovascular disease, type 2 diabetes, hypertension, and certain cancers.[6] It's difficult, however, to pinpoint diet as being solely responsible for vegetarians' health status. Why? Vegetarians often adopt other healthy lifestyle practices, such as exercising regularly, practicing relaxation activities such as meditation, and avoiding tobacco products and excess alcohol.

What IS That?

Tofu is made from pureed soybeans; the food is available in firm, extra-firm, and liquid forms. Plain tofu has little flavor, and when used in recipes, this protein-rich food tends to absorb flavors of the other ingredients.

Firm tofu has the consistency of thick gelatin. Add small pieces of firm tofu to soups, salads, and stir-fried vegetables.

You can use liquid tofu to make protein-rich smoothies and "creamy" soups.

A half cup of firm tofu that's made with calcium sulfate is high in calcium and iron and supplies about 180 calories, 22 g protein, 11 g fat (primarily unsaturated fat), 2 mg zinc, and 3 g fiber.

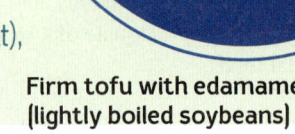

Firm tofu with edamame (lightly boiled soybeans)

D. Hurst/Alamy Stock Photo

Compared to the typical American diet, vegetarian diets generally provide more fiber, phytochemicals, vitamins K and C, and the minerals potassium and magnesium.[7] Furthermore, vegetarian diets often supply less saturated fat than do diets that include animal foods.

In general, plant foods add bulk to the diet without adding a lot of calories. Thus, vegetarians may feel "full" soon after eating a meal of plant foods, and they may not consume as much energy and nutrients as they need. Poorly planned plant-based diets may not contain nutritionally adequate amounts of

- omega-3 fatty acids,
- vitamins B-12 and D, and/or
- minerals iron and calcium.[7]

Vegans, even some vegan athletes, can obtain adequate amounts of nutrients, with proper dietary planning.[7] To ensure that their diets supply adequate amounts of the essential amino acids, vegans can focus on eating processed soybean products and meals that combine complementary plant proteins. Vegetarians who don't consume fish may need to obtain omega-3 fatty acids by eating certain algae or taking supplements that contain the algae (see Table 6.4). Vegans can obtain vitamin B-12, vitamin D, iron, calcium, and other micronutrients by consuming fortified foods such as soy and rice beverages. Vegans and other vegetarians can also take a multiple vitamin/mineral supplement to provide an additional source of micronutrients. **Table 7.3** summarizes the nutritional advantages and possible nutritional disadvantages of vegetarian, especially vegan, diets.

Children have higher protein and energy needs per pound of body weight than an adult. Because plant foods add bulk to the diet, vegan children are likely to eat far less food than adult vegans because they become full sooner during meals. Thus, very young vegans may be unable to eat enough plant foods to meet their protein and energy needs. Therefore, it's very important for parents or other caretakers to plan nutritionally adequate diets for vegetarian children and monitor the youngsters' growth rates.

Vegan women who breastfeed their infants may produce milk that's deficient in vitamin B-12, particularly if the mothers' diets lack the vitamin. Such babies have a high risk of developing severe growth and developmental delays associated with nerve damage, especially when breast milk is their only source of vitamin B-12.[8] Vegan mothers who breastfeed their infants may need to provide their babies with a dietary supplement that contains vitamin B-12.

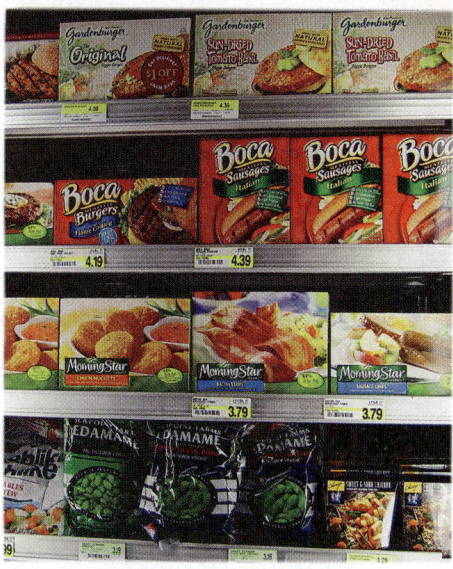

Commercially prepared vegetarian foods in the frozen food section of a supermarket.

Commercially prepared vegetarian foods that substitute for meat, fish, and poultry items are often available in the frozen food section of supermarkets. These vegetarian products (meat analogs) can look and taste like their nonvegetarian counterparts, but they generally don't contain cholesterol and may be lower in saturated fat. Such foods include soy-based sausage patties or links, soy hot dogs, "veggie" burgers, and soy "crumbles" that look like bits of cooked ground beef.

With careful planning, vegetarians can overcome the nutritional limitations of a plant-based diet and consume adequate diets. If you're interested in learning more specific details about vegetarian cookery and menu planning, contact a registered dietitian or university extension nutritionist in your area. The MyPlate website also offers "Tips for Vegetarians" at www.choosemyplate.gov/tips-vegetarians.

TABLE 7.3 VEGETARIAN DIETS: NUTRITIONAL ASPECTS

Advantages	Possible Disadvantages
High in:	**Low in:**
Vitamins C and K	Vitamins B-12 and D
Fiber	Iron and calcium
Magnesium and potassium	Omega-3 fatty acids
Phytochemicals	
Low in:	
Fat (saturated)	
Cholesterol (particularly, a vegan diet)	

Vegetarian pizza

Placemat: McGraw-Hill Education/Mark Dierker, photographer; Pizza: Lucky Business/Shutterstock; Vegetarian foods: Wendy Schiff

Module 7.5

Proteins and Health

7.5 - Learning Outcomes

After reading Module 7.5, you should be able to

1. Define all of the **key terms** in this module.
2. Calculate the AMDR for protein intake.
3. Identify people who have a high risk of protein deficiency.
4. Explain the cause of a food allergy, identify foods that are most likely to cause food allergies, and list three common signs or symptoms of a food allergy.
5. Explain what causes celiac disease, identify foods that a person with celiac disease must avoid, and list three common signs or symptoms of the disease.

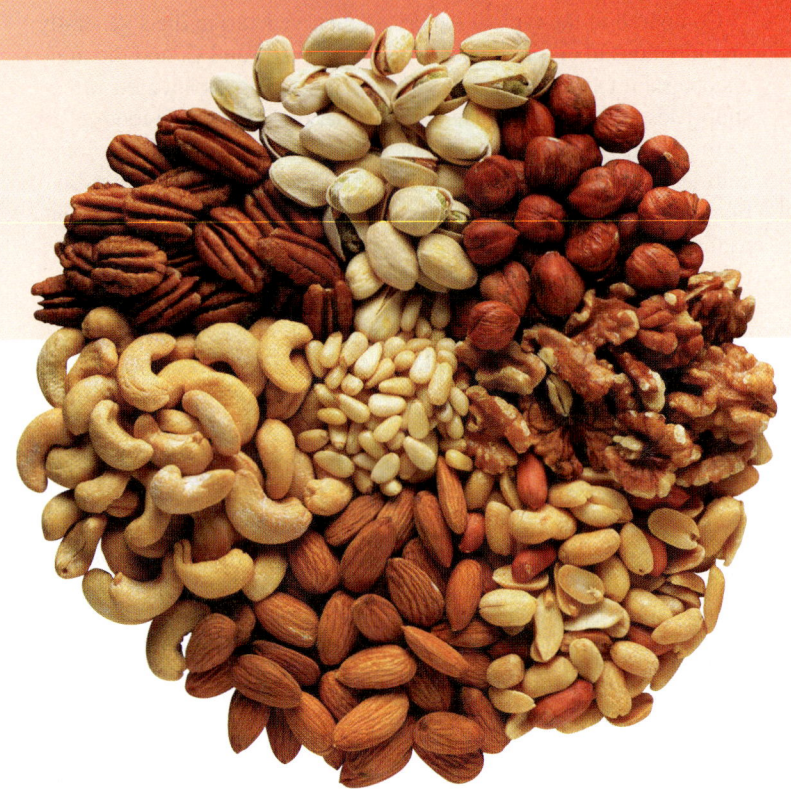

C Squared Studios/Photodisc/Getty Images

7.5a High Protein Intakes

If some protein is essential for proper growth and good health, can eating extra amounts of the nutrient make you extra healthy or physically fit? If your diet contains adequate amounts of protein, then eating more isn't necessary. As mentioned earlier in this unit, the RDA for protein is 0.8 g/kg/day. (This value applies to healthy adults, who aren't athletes.) As mentioned earlier in this unit, adult Americans consumed 82.5 g protein/day[1] in 2015–2016. This amount of protein is the RDA for a person who weighs 227 pounds!

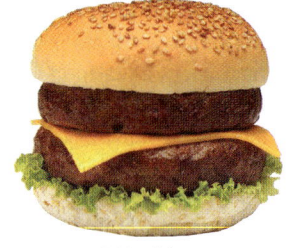

Ingram Publishing/Alamy

Recall that the Acceptable Macronutrient Distribution Range (AMDR) for protein is 10 to 35% of total daily calories. Thus, you're eating a high-protein diet if protein supplies more than 35% of your daily energy intake.[9] High-protein diets are generally not necessary for healthy individuals.

Recall from Essential Concept 7.2 that excess amino acids undergo removal of their nitrogen-containing groups. The reaction forms ammonia, a toxic compound. The liver uses the ammonia to make urea, a less toxic substance. The kidneys remove urea from the bloodstream and eliminate it in urine. People who have a history of kidney stones, have kidney disease, or are at risk of kidney disease should check with their physician before eating a high-protein diet.[9, 10]

Do Athletes Need More Protein?

About 70% of muscle tissue is water, and only about 22% is protein. An effective way to increase muscle mass safely is to combine a nutritionally adequate diet with a program of muscle-strengthening exercises. During resistance exercise, proteins in working muscles break down. The rebuilding of these proteins occurs during the recovery period that follows.[11] As a result, muscles grow larger and stronger.

During high-intensity as well as long-duration physical training, an athlete's diet should supply enough calories to maintain good health and support increased energy needs. If protein intake is high, but overall calorie intake, particularly from carbohydrate, is too low, the body uses the protein for energy.[11] Healthy people, including athletes, may adapt to protein intakes that are higher than the AMDR for the macronutrient and not experience health problems as a result.

Eating a snack that supplies some high-quality protein before, during, and immediately after exercise is recommended.[12] Nutritious choices include a bowl of cereal, chocolate milk, low-fat cottage cheese and a whole-wheat bagel, or a sandwich made with lean meat or poultry. Unit 10 provides more information about nutrition for physically active people, including protein needs for athletes.

What About Protein Supplements? Approximately 43% of the protein in an average person's body is in his or her skeletal muscle mass. Not surprisingly, athletes and other people interested in building their muscle mass often eat large portions of animal foods and consume amino acid and protein supplements to boost their protein intakes. However, consuming more protein than the body can use at one time doesn't stimulate increased muscle size and strength.

For thousands of years, people have obtained amino acids directly by eating plants and animals. The use of amino acid and protein supplements as sources of the nutrient is a relatively recent development, and more research is necessary to determine the long-term safety of using these products.

What About High-Protein Weight-Loss Diets?

Certain popular weight-loss diets, such as the Atkins, "Keto," and Paleo diets, promote high intakes of protein. People who follow high-protein diets to lose weight often report decreased feelings of hunger and increased sense of stomach fullness (*satiety*) after meals.[9] This response probably occurs because protein contributes to satiety to a greater extent than does fat or carbohydrate.[9] Unit 10 provides information about the safety and effectiveness of various popular weight-loss diets.

Olivia, the young woman featured in the unit opener, often trains for half-marathons. While preparing for competition, Olivia eats rich sources of carbohydrates, such as pasta and "a lot of bananas" to support her performance. After running, she chooses protein-rich foods, including peanut butter and chicken. "I tried protein shakes but didn't see any benefits, so I quit using them," she said.

TASTY Tidbits

Whey is the watery fluid that forms when milk curdles during cheese and yogurt production. The fluid is dried and used to make whey protein powder.

The use of dietary supplements that contain the milk protein whey to help build muscle mass in athletes is controversial. Results of some studies indicate that whey protein supplements can help increase muscle mass and strength.[13]

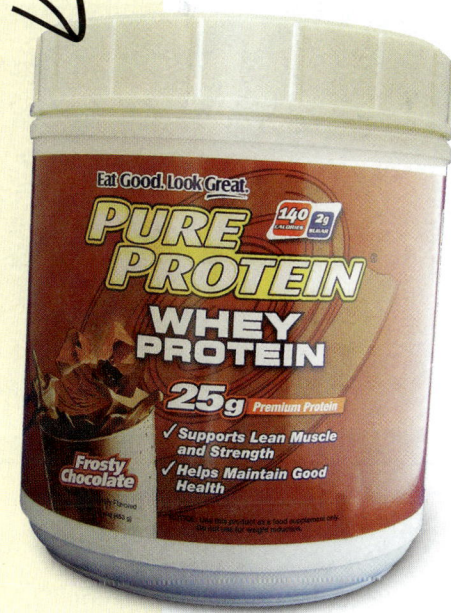
Wendy Schiff

7.5b Protein Deficiency

In the United States, protein deficiency is uncommon. However, certain populations, especially chronically ill, older adults, often have diets that are low in protein. Why? Many older adult Americans have limited incomes and must make difficult choices concerning their expenses. If you were older, on a low fixed income, and taking several prescription medications to control your chronic health problems, what would you think was more important? Would you decide to purchase nutritious foods or the costly medications?

In children, stunting (poor growth in height) and being underweight are signs of protein deficiency. In 2017, the World Health Organization (WHO) estimated that there were 151 million children, 5 years of age or younger, who were too short (stunted) because of poor nutrition.[14] Impoverished children in southern Asia and western Africa are most likely to be stunted and underweight. The effects of protein malnutrition are especially devastating for the very young. Children whose diets lack sufficient protein as well as energy don't grow well and are very weak, irritable, and vulnerable to dehydration and infections, such as measles, that can kill them. If these children survive, their growth may be permanently stunted. Furthermore, their intelligence may be lower than normal because protein deficiency during early childhood can cause permanent brain damage. Unit 11 provides more information about poor nutrition, including protein deficiency.

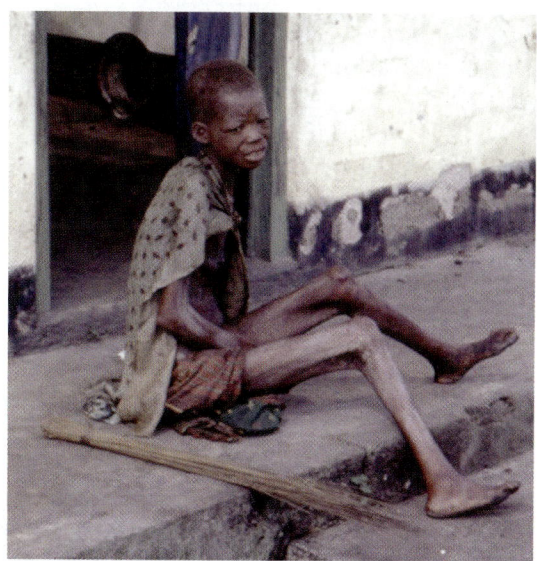
This photograph (late 1960s) shows a starving person being cared for at a relief camp located near the Nigerian-Biafran war zone in Africa.

Source: Centers for Disease Control and Prevention/Dr. Lyle Conrad

Culture & Cuisine

Globally, people eat over 1900 different kinds of insects, primarily beetles; caterpillars; wasps, ants, and bees; and grasshoppers, locusts, and crickets.[15] Populations in Africa, Asia, and South America are more likely to consume insects than people living in other parts of the world. In most instances, the edible insects are gathered, prepared, and consumed where they naturally live. Insect "farming," however, is becoming more common where people enjoy eating the little animals in meals or for snacks. When compared to raising conventional kinds of livestock for food (especially cattle and hogs), raising edible insects doesn't require as much land, water, and feed. Furthermore, farming the insects isn't as harmful to the environment as conventional methods of livestock production.[15]

In some regions of Africa, Cambodia, and the Philippines, many people eat desert locusts, especially when the insects are plentiful. Popular ways to cook the locusts include removing the wings and legs before frying with seasonings or placing the insects on skewers and roasting them over hot embers. Desert locusts are an excellent source of high-quality protein. In addition to being a relatively inexpensive source of protein, edible insects such as desert locusts supply diets with essential fatty acids, and several vitamins and minerals.[15] In parts of the world where meat, pork, and fish are too costly for impoverished people to purchase, collecting and using edible insects as protein substitutes offer a nutrient-dense dietary option.

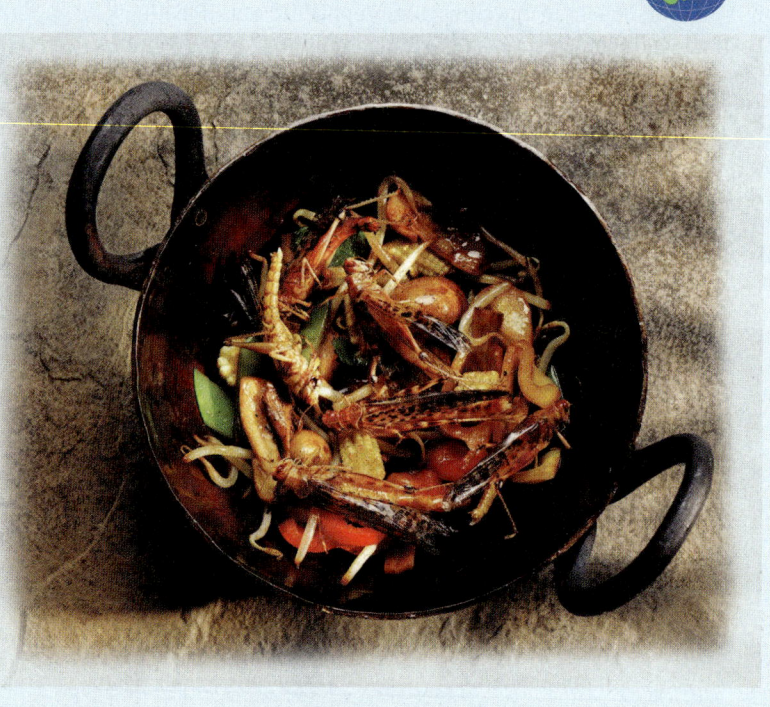

IT Stock Free/Alamy

7.5c What's a Food Allergy?

Have you ever experienced an allergic reaction after eating certain foods or drinks? A food allergy occurs when the body's immune system reacts to one or more harmless substances (allergens) in the food. In most instances, the allergen is a protein.

Allergic reactions generally occur within a few minutes to a couple of hours after eating the offending food. Some protein in the food doesn't undergo digestion, and it enters intestinal tissues without passing through absorptive cells. When this occurs, immune system cells in the small intestine recognize the food protein as a foreign substance. These cells try to protect the body by mounting a defensive response. As a result of the immune response, the person who is allergic to the food typically experiences one or more of the following signs and symptoms:

- Hives—red raised bumps that usually appear on the skin
- Swollen or itchy lips
- Skin flushing
- A scaly skin rash (eczema)
- Difficulty swallowing
- Wheezing and difficulty breathing
- Abdominal pain, vomiting, and diarrhea

In severe cases, sensitive people who are exposed to food allergens can develop anaphylactic (*an-a-pha-lak'-tic*) shock, a serious drop in blood pressure that affects the whole body. This kind of shock can be deadly, unless emergency treatment is provided.

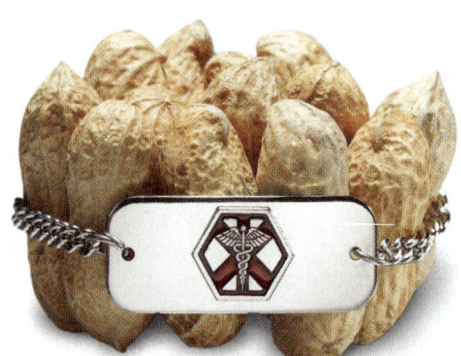

Corbis Super RF/Alamy

Although any food protein can cause an allergic reaction in a susceptible person, the most allergenic proteins are in cow's milk, eggs, peanuts and tree nuts, wheat, soy, fish, and shellfish.[16]

In the United States, approximately 4 to 8% of children[16] and 4% of adults[17] suffer from food allergies. Children tend to outgrow their food allergies by the time they're young adults. Allergies to peanuts and tree nuts, however, usually persist into adulthood.

Accurate diagnosis of a food allergy should be undertaken by a physician who specializes in the diagnosis and treatment of allergies. Skin testing is a reliable way to identify allergens. Although hair analysis, cytotoxic or electrodermal testing, and kinesiology are promoted by unconventional health care practitioners (people who aren't physicians) to diagnose allergies, these are unproven diagnostic methods.

Treatment of food allergies involves strict avoidance of the offending foods. Food manufacturers must identify any of the leading allergenic ingredients, such as soy, milk, and peanuts, on product labels (**Fig. 7.7**). Parents or caregivers of young children with food allergies should read food labels carefully to check for allergens listed among ingredients.

For decades, health care providers recommended that parents delay introducing foods that were likely to cause an allergic response to infants. Now, some medical researchers think food allergies can be *prevented* if such foods are given to infants when they can swallow them, which is about 4 to 6 months of age.[18] However, caregivers of infants who have a high risk of allergies should consult a medical specialist before giving peanut-containing foods to the children. It's always important to discuss when to introduce new foods to your baby with the infant's health care provider.

People who have food intolerances experience negative side effects after they consume specific foods, such as milk, aged cheese, or wheat products. Unlike a food allergy, a **food intolerance** doesn't involve the immune system. Such nonallergic responses to food can mimic the signs and symptoms of food allergies. Lactose intolerance (see Unit 5) is a common type of food intolerance.

Some individuals experience negative reactions when they consume **sulfites,** a food additive. Sulfites are a group of sulfur-containing compounds that can be found naturally in foods, but the compounds are often added to wines, potatoes, and shrimp as a preservative. People who have asthma often develop breathing difficulties after consuming food treated with sulfites. Other sulfite-sensitive people report skin flushing (redness and warmth), hives, difficulty swallowing, vomiting, diarrhea, and dizziness after consuming foods that contain the compounds. People who have food intolerances often must learn which foods to avoid eating.

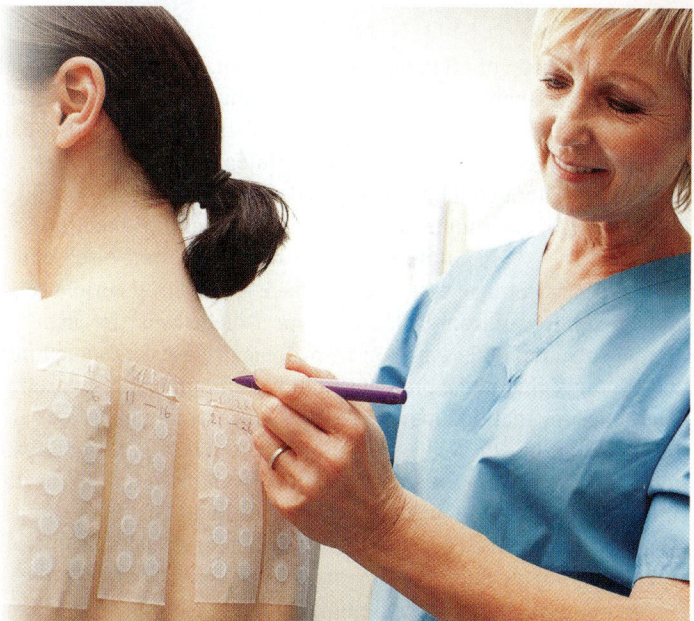

Skin patch testing for allergies

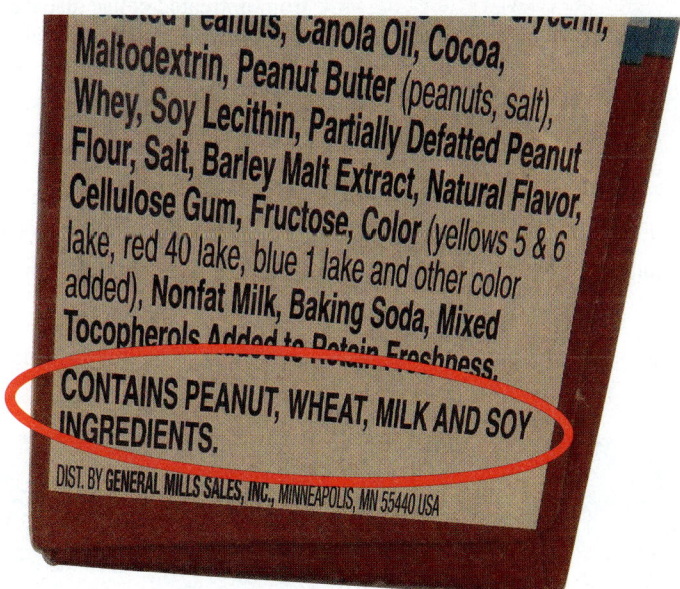

Figure 7.7 Allergen labeling.

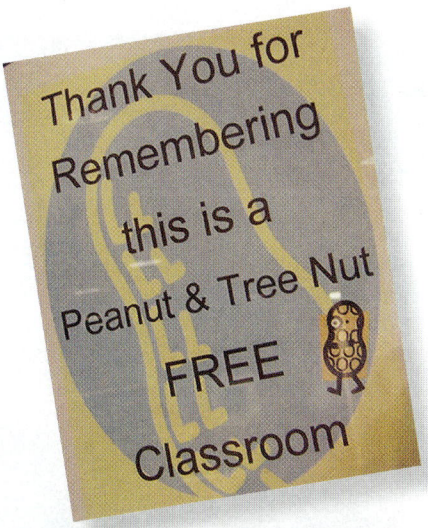

This sign on the door of an elementary school classroom lets people know to avoid bringing anything containing peanuts and tree nuts into the room.

food intolerance negative physical reactions to eating a food that don't involve the immune system

sulfites group of sulfur-containing compounds in foods and often added to wines, potatoes, and shrimp as a preservative

Allergen information label, Classroom door sign: Wendy Schiff; Allergy patch test: Science Photo Library/Getty Images

7.5d What's Gluten?

Gluten is a group of related proteins in wheat, barley, and rye. In the United States, about 1 in 141 people has **celiac** (*see'-lee-ak*) **disease** (see Unit 4's opener that features Karlin West).[19] People with the disease cannot tolerate foods that contain gluten, a protein in wheat, rye, and barley. Although the tendency to develop celiac disease is probably inherited, environmental factors may trigger the condition.

Celiac disease is an **autoimmune disease,** a chronic disease in which certain immune system cells attack and destroy normal cells in the body. Recall from Unit 5 that type 1 diabetes is also an autoimmune disease. After a person with celiac disease eats something that contains gluten, the protein stimulates an immune response in the small intestine that inflames or destroys villi (see Figure 4.5 for an illustration of healthy villi). This inflammation results in poor absorption of nutrients from the small intestine. Even though people with celiac disease may follow a nutritionally adequate diet, they often become malnourished because their intestinal tract lacks healthy villi.

The signs and symptoms of celiac disease vary from person to person but usually include abdominal bloating, chronic diarrhea, and weight loss. In some cases, people with celiac disease don't have the usual signs and symptoms, but their long-term health is negatively affected. Serious health problems such as anemia (a blood disorder), osteoporosis, infertility, liver disease, and intestinal cancer can result from untreated celiac disease.

To provide a definite diagnosis, a physician usually orders a blood test and an intestinal biopsy. The blood test detects and measures certain immune system factors that are present in people with celiac disease. The biopsy involves removing tiny pieces of tissue from the small intestine. The tissue samples undergo microscopic examination to evaluate the condition of the villi. The presence of damaged villi can help confirm the diagnosis of celiac disease.

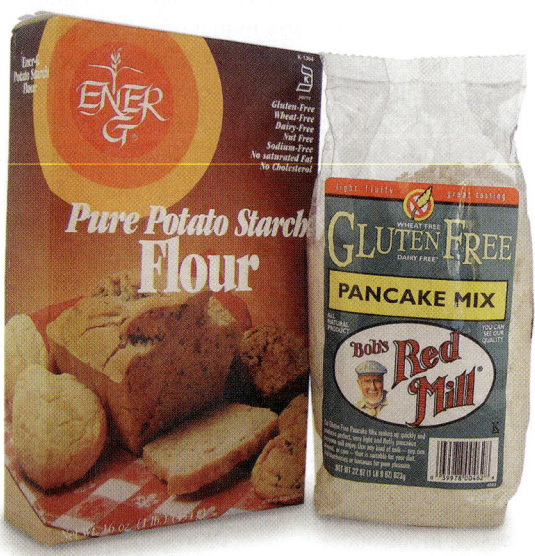

There is no cure for celiac disease, but persons with the condition can achieve and maintain good health by carefully following a special gluten-free diet for the rest of their lives. Many supermarkets carry a variety of gluten-free foods. **Table 7.4** lists foods that people with celiac disease must avoid as well as those that are generally safe for them to consume.

People who have intestinal discomfort, especially pain and diarrhea, after eating gluten-containing foods, may have *non-celiac gluten sensitivity*. Non-celiac gluten sensitivity (gluten sensitivity) is difficult to diagnose. However, the treatment for gluten sensitivity is the same as for celiac disease—avoiding gluten-containing foods and products.[20]

Many Americans have adopted gluten-free diets because they think the diets are healthier than the typical diet. Some people even claim that gluten-free diets helped them lose weight. At this point, there's no evidence that gluten-free diets are useful for healthy people or persons who need to lose weight.[19] Unless you have celiac disease or non-celiac gluten sensitivity, you probably don't need to avoid gluten, and your health may actually benefit from keeping the protein in your diet.

gluten group of related proteins in wheat, barley, and rye

celiac disease chronic disease characterized by an autoimmune response in the small intestine to the protein gluten

autoimmune disease chronic disease in which certain immune system cells attack and destroy normal cells in the body

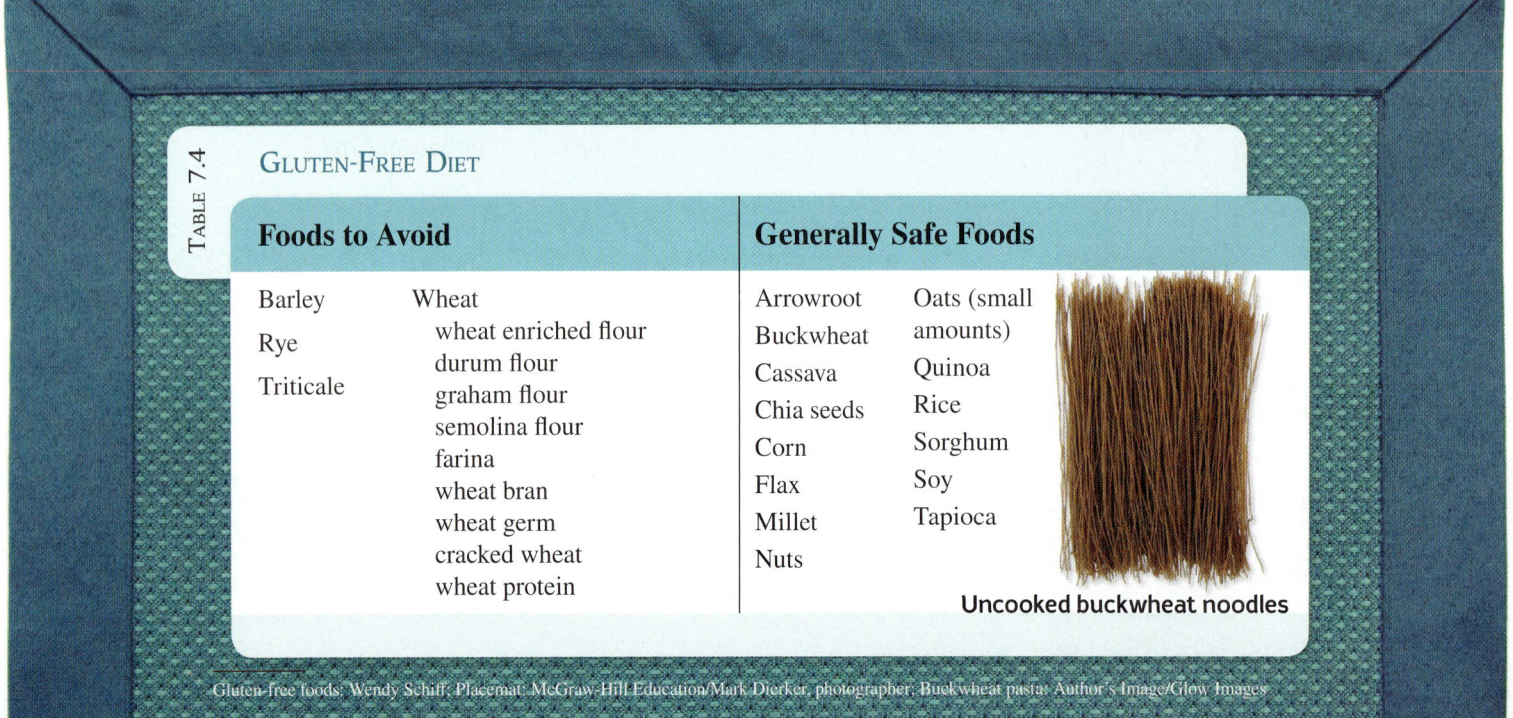

Table 7.4 Gluten-Free Diet

Foods to Avoid		Generally Safe Foods	
Barley	Wheat	Arrowroot	Oats (small amounts)
Rye	wheat enriched flour	Buckwheat	Quinoa
Triticale	durum flour	Cassava	Rice
	graham flour	Chia seeds	Sorghum
	semolina flour	Corn	Soy
	farina	Flax	Tapioca
	wheat bran	Millet	
	wheat germ	Nuts	
	cracked wheat		
	wheat protein		

Uncooked buckwheat noodles

Gluten-free foods: Wendy Schiff; Placemat: McGraw-Hill Education/Mark Dierker, photographer; Buckwheat pasta: Author's Image/Glow Images

Module 7.6

Stretching Your Food Dollars

7.6 - Learning Outcomes

After reading Module 7.6, you should be able to

1. List at least three ways you can reduce your weekly food costs.
2. Determine and compare unit costs of packaged foods.
3. Plan meatless meals that supply all essential amino acids.

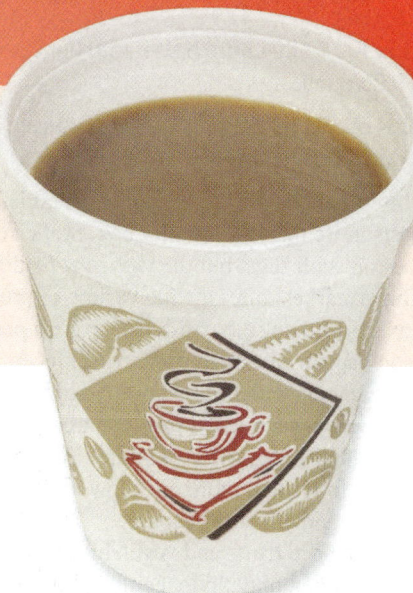

Hemera Technologies/PhotoObjects.net/Getty Images

How much money do you spend at coffee shops each week?

How can you lower your food costs and still have a nutritionally adequate diet? You can trim food costs, and even improve the nutritional quality of your diet, by evaluating your food buying practices and making a few changes. You can eat well for less!

7.6a Where and What You Buy

Where you buy foods and beverages and what you decide to purchase are major factors in determining your overall food costs. If you frequently purchase drinks, meals, and snacks from vending machines, food trucks, convenience stores, coffee shops, fast-food outlets, and other restaurants, you may be spending too much on foods and beverages. In general, the less time you spend preparing food, the more money you'll spend by having someone at a commercial outlet prepare the food for you. Even if a fast-food outlet's hamburger seems like a bargain because it's "only $3.00," you're likely paying a premium for the French fries and soft drink that you purchase to accompany the sandwich. From a nutrition standpoint, fast foods and beverages are often energy dense—high in saturated fat and added sugars—and low in fiber, phytochemicals, and micronutrients (except sodium).

Bulk Food Stores

A good way to save money is to buy foods in large quantities at "bulk" food stores or at smaller, "no frills," cash-only grocery stores. Although shopping at these places can reduce your food costs, food choices are usually more limited than the selection in supermarkets. It's important to recognize that buying food in bulk is a bargain only if you can use or safely store the item before it spoils.

Support Your Local Farmers

Produce that's grown in the United States is usually less expensive when it's in season and more plentiful. For example, berries are plentiful in the spring and early summer, tomatoes and melons in late summer, and apples in the fall. Consider buying fresh produce directly from local farmers, if possible. Although you still need to compare prices of farmers' market items with those of fresh produce sold in supermarkets, you may be able to find reasonably priced produce that's grown within 100 miles of your home at farmers' markets. Buying produce from local farmers helps support your community's economy, too.

How to Shop Wisely in Supermarkets

To lower your food costs, plan your meals and snacks before you shop for food. Prepare a shopping list to help avoid needless or impulse purchases and having to return to the store to buy forgotten items. Keep the grocery list in a convenient place, such as on or next to the refrigerator, and jot down items as they become depleted.

When shopping for groceries, you'll need to compare *unit* (pound, ounce, or other measure) costs of similar food products. Using a calculator to compare prices can be helpful. For example, a box of one brand of shredded wheat cereal contains 15.0 ounces of cereal and costs $3.89; a box of a different brand of shredded wheat that contains 11.5 ounces of cereal costs $3.69. Which box contains cereal that's lower in cost? To answer this question, determine the unit price of the cereal in each box by dividing the cost of the entire package by the number of units of food it contains.

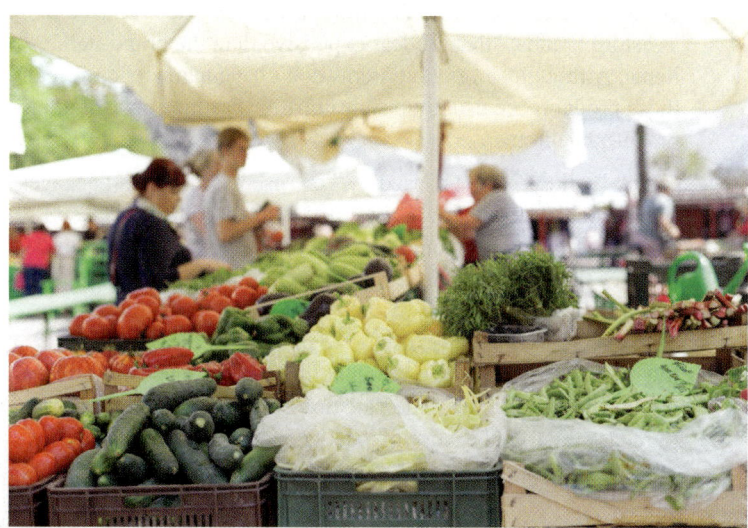

kasto/123RF

Farmers' markets can be a source of fresh foods that are often reasonably priced.

Box #1: $3.89 entire box ÷ 15.0 ounces = approximately $0.26/ounce

Box #2: $3.69 entire box ÷ 11.5 ounces = approximately $0.32/ounce

In this situation, the larger box of cereal is a better buy, even though it costs more than the smaller box. Some supermarkets indicate unit prices on shelf tags, but the tags may be difficult to read or confusing.

Supermarkets offer a wide variety of prepared foods, including deli items, cooked entrées, fresh cut-up fruit packaged in single-serving plastic bags or bins, and rotisserie chicken. Although these "fast foods" are convenient, food preparation and packaging add to the cost of food. Plus, such foods may contain unhealthy amounts of salt, solid fat, or added sugar. To save money and improve your diet, rely less on prepared foods and more on "slow foods"—foods that require some of your time and effort to prepare.

Eating more fruits and vegetables is the natural way to add micronutrients, fiber, and phytochemicals to your diet. Many supermarkets offer fresh fruit and vegetables that have been trimmed, cut up, and packed into containers. Before you reach for one of these items, compare its price with that of its raw counterpart. For example, a 2.2-oz, single-serving package of sliced apples sells for $1.25, and a pound of raw apples is priced at $1.99. In this case, buying the raw apples and slicing them yourself is a money-saving practice. An ounce of the packaged apples costs about $0.57 ($1.25 divided by 2.2 oz/package). A pound of apples equals 16 ounces, so an ounce of these apples costs about $0.12 ($1.99 divided by 16). Although there's no waste (apple cores), the prepackaged sliced apples cost more than the bulk raw apples.

Practical Grocery Shopping Tips The following practices can help you save money when shopping for food:

- Be wary of appealing offers that aren't really bargains. For example, oranges marked "5 for $10" can be confusing. A grocery store usually doesn't require you to buy the entire quantity. However, paying $2 for an orange isn't a bargain! The same store may be selling a bag of 10 oranges for $10. At that price, each orange costs $1.

- Use coupons when purchasing brand-name items. However, be aware that many stores offer similar products, often referred to as "store brands," that are less expensive than the brand-name items. Although store brand items don't have name recognition, these products are usually just as nutritious as the corresponding brand-name items.

- Check "sell by," "best if used by," or "use by" dates on packages of perishable foods such as eggs and dairy products. The "sell by" date informs store employees about the length of time the product should be displayed for sale. Obviously, it's best to buy foods well before the sell-by date so you have time to use them. The "best if used by" or "use by" date indicates the last day for the consumer to use the product before it loses its best flavor and other sensory qualities. The date doesn't indicate the last day to purchase the food because of safety concerns.

- Be wary when you're standing in line to pay for groceries. Checkout lanes are usually lined with small, expensive containers of unhealthy, energy-dense foods such as candy bars, energy drinks, and salty snacks ("impulse buys").

- Be wary of food items ("specials") that are displayed at the ends of aisles. They may be overpriced compared to the same foods that you missed while shopping in the main aisles of the store.

- Limit your carbonated soft drink, energy drink, and bottled water purchases. Before you leave home, fill a small thermos with water and ice cubes and take the bottle with you. When you're thirsty, locate the nearest water fountain and have a drink for free!

- If you drink coffee, buy a small coffeemaker, a can of ground coffee, and coffee filters to make the beverage. Consider carrying a small thermos of coffee in your backpack. It's much less expensive to make a cup of your own coffee than to buy one from a coffee shop.

7.6b Where's the Meat?

Meat may be among the most expensive items on your grocery list. The following tips can help you keep your food budget under control without sacrificing essential protein intakes:

- Include only one animal source of protein in a meal and reduce its serving size.

- Several times a week, replace meals that feature large portions of red meat with meals that contain other high-quality protein sources. Eggs, chicken, fat-free milk, canned sardines and tuna, reduced-fat cheese, and low-fat yogurt are animal sources of high-quality protein that you can substitute for the more expensive meat items in your diet.

- Prepare meals that contain more plant than animal proteins. Most animal foods contain enough essential amino acids to "beef up" the lower-quality proteins in peas, beans, cereals, and other grain products (see Module 7.3). Examples include

  - Cereal with milk, pancakes, and waffles;
  - Asian dishes that mix small amounts of chicken, beef, or seafood with large portions of rice;
  - Italian dishes that combine small amounts of cheese or meat sauce with large amounts of pasta;
  - Macaroni and cheese;
  - Chili con carne;
  - Tuna-noodle casserole; and
  - Tacos or burritos filled with black beans and grated cheddar cheese.

In a Nutshell

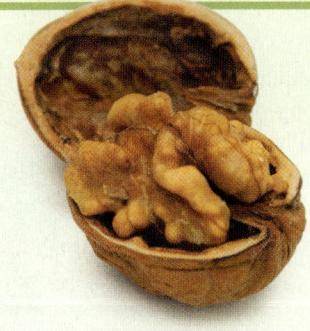

Module 7.1 What Are Proteins?
- Proteins are organic nutrients that contain nitrogen. Proteins have numerous functions in the body. They're needed for growth, maintenance, and repair of tissues.
- The typical amino acid has a nitrogen-containing or amino group, an acid group, and the R-group.
- Human proteins are comprised of 20 different amino acids arranged in various combinations.
- The diet must supply 9 of the amino acids because the body cannot make these essential amino acids or make enough of them to meet its needs. Under normal conditions, cells can produce the remaining amino acids if the raw materials are available.

Module 7.2 What Happens to the Protein You Eat?
- Protein digestion begins in the stomach, where pepsin breaks proteins into shorter polypeptides. In the small intestine, enzymes secreted by the pancreas and absorptive cells digest the polypeptides primarily into peptides with two or three amino acids. The border of the absorptive cell contains enzymes that complete the digestion of the simple polypeptides, converting them into amino acids. The absorptive cells remove the free amino acids from the digestive tract.
- The end products of protein digestion, amino acids, travel to the liver. The liver uses the amino acids or releases them into the general circulation.
- Cells use amino acids to make proteins. Each protein can differ in the kinds of amino acids it contains, the order in which the amino acids are strung, and the number of them that are used. The wide variety of proteins in your body reflects the numerous ways your cells can connect amino acids to form proteins.
- The body conserves nitrogen by recycling amino acids, but each day it loses some protein and nitrogen, primarily in urine. Amino acids from food replace the lost nitrogen.
- The protein requirement increases during pregnancy, breastfeeding, periods of growth, and recovery from serious illnesses, blood losses, and burns.
- The adult RDA for protein (healthy adults who aren't athletes) is 0.8 g/kg of body weight daily.
- The AMDR for adults is 10 to 35% of energy intake from protein. Excess amino acids are metabolized for energy or converted into body fat.

Module 7.3 Proteins in Foods
- Legumes are plants that produce pods that have a single row of seeds, such as soybeans, peas, peanuts, lentils, and beans.
- Animal foods generally provide more protein than do similar quantities of plant foods.
- High-quality protein is well digested and contains all essential amino acids in amounts that will support protein deposition and a young child's growth. In general, meat, fish, poultry, eggs, milk, and milk products contain high-quality proteins.
- Low-quality protein is low in one or more of the essential amino acids. When compared to animal foods, most plant foods provide low-quality protein.
- Quinoa and foods made from processed soybeans are good plant sources of essential amino acids.

Module 7.4 What's Vegetarianism?
- Vegetarian diets are based on plant foods and limit animal foods to some extent. Although vegetarians are generally healthier than people who eat Western diets, it's difficult to pinpoint diet as being solely responsible for vegetarians' better health.

- If not properly planned, plant-based diets may not contain enough omega-3 fatty acids, vitamins B-12 and D, iron, and calcium to meet a person's nutritional needs, especially children's needs.

Module 7.5 Proteins and Health

- An effective way to increase muscle mass safely is to combine a nutritionally adequate diet with a program of muscle-strengthening exercises. During high-intensity as well as long-duration physical training, an athlete's diet should supply enough calories to support good health and energy needs for increased physical activity. High-protein diets are generally safe for healthy people.

- Protein deficiency is rare in the United States. In impoverished developing countries, protein deficiency along with low-energy intake is a major cause of childhood deaths. Severely undernourished children don't grow properly and are very weak, irritable, and vulnerable to dehydration and life-threatening infections. Undernutrition during early childhood can cause permanent brain damage.

- A food allergy occurs when the body's immune system reacts to allergens in the food. Food allergens usually are proteins. The most allergenic proteins are in cow's milk, eggs, peanuts and other nuts, wheat, soybeans, fish, and shellfish. A food intolerance isn't the same condition as a food allergy. People with celiac disease and gluten sensitivity must avoid foods that contain gluten.

Pixtal/agefotostock

Module 7.6 Stretching Your Food Dollars

- Where you buy foods and beverages and what you decide to purchase are major factors in determining your overall food costs. Generally, the less time you spend preparing food, the more money you'll spend by having someone at a commercial outlet prepare the food for you.

- Fast foods and beverages are often energy dense—high in saturated fat and added sugars—and low in fiber, phytochemicals, and micronutrients (except sodium).

- Tips for reducing your food costs include planning your meals and snacks, preparing a shopping list, comparing unit prices of similar food products, avoiding "impulse" purchases, and preparing more meatless meals.

What's in Your Diet?!

1. Refer to the 3-day food log from the "What's in Your Diet?!" feature in Unit 3. Calculate your average protein intake by adding the grams of protein eaten each day, dividing the total by 3, and rounding the figure to the nearest whole number.

Sample Calculation:

Day 1	76 g
Day 2	55 g
Day 3	103 g
Total grams	234 g ÷ 3 days = 78 g of protein/day

Your Calculation:

Day 1	_____ g
Day 2	_____ g
Day 3	_____ g
Total grams	_____ ÷ 3 days = _____ g/day

My average daily protein intake was _____ g.

2. The RDA for protein is based on body weight. Using the RDA of 0.8 g of protein/kg of body weight, calculate the amount of protein that you need to consume daily to meet the recommendation. To determine your body weight in kilograms, divide your weight (pounds) by 2.2, then multiply this number by 0.8 to obtain your RDA for protein. Then round the figure to the nearest whole number.

   My weight in pounds _____ ÷ 2.2 = _____ kg

   My weight in kg _____ × 0.8 = _____ g   My RDA for protein = _____ g

   a. Did your average intake of protein meet or exceed your RDA level that was calculated in step 1?
      _____ yes _____ no

   b. If your answer to 2a is "yes," which foods contributed the most to your protein intake?

3. Review the log of your 3-day food intake. Calculate the average number of kilocalories that protein contributed to your diet each day during the 3-day period.

   a. Each gram of protein provides about 4 kcal; therefore, you must multiply the average number of grams of protein obtained in step 1 by 4 kcal to obtain the average number of kcal from protein.

   ### Sample Calculation:

   78 g/day × 4 kcal/g = 312 kcal from protein

   ### Your Calculation:

   _____ g/day × 4 kcal/g = _____ average number of kcal from protein

4. Determine your average energy intake over the 3-day period by adding the kilocalories for each day and dividing the sum by 3, and round to the nearest whole number.

   ### Sample Calculation:

Day 1	2500 kcal
Day 2	3200 kcal
Day 3	2750 kcal
Total kcal	8450 ÷ 3 days = 2817 kcal/day (average kcal intake)

   ### Your Calculation:

Day 1	_____ kcal
Day 2	_____ kcal
Day 3	_____ kcal
Total kcal	_____ ÷ 3 days = _____ kcal/day (average)

5. Determine the average percentage of energy that protein contributed to your diet by dividing the average kilocalories from protein obtained in step 3 by the average total daily energy intake obtained in step 4. Then round this figure to the nearest one-hundredth. Multiply this value by 100, move the decimal point two places to the right, drop the decimal point, and add a percent symbol.

   ### Sample Calculation:

   312 kcal from protein ÷ 2817 kcal intake = 0.11 (rounded)

   0.11 × 100 = 11%

   ### Your Calculation:

   _____ kcal from protein ÷ _____ kcal intake = _____

   _____ × 100 = _____ %

6. Did your average intake of protein meet the recommendation of 10 to 35% of total kilocalories? If your average protein intake was below 10%, list at least five foods you could eat that would boost your intake.

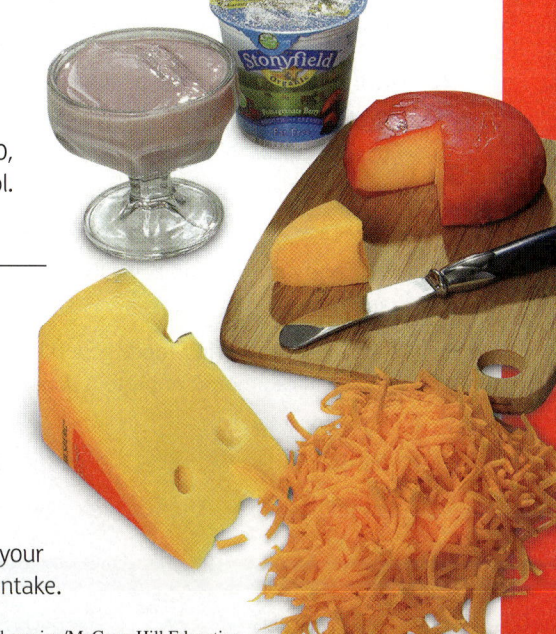

John Thoeming/McGraw-Hill Education

Consider This...

1. A recipe for bean salad has the following main ingredients:

    1 cup kidney beans

    1 cup green beans

    1 cup lima beans

    1 cup black beans

    1½ cups wine vinegar

    ⅓ cup canola oil

    ¼ cup chopped onion

    Explain why this recipe isn't a complementary mixture of plant proteins. What plant foods could you add to the recipe to make it a complementary mixture?

2. A recipe mixes cereals made from wheat, rice, and corn. What plant foods could you add to this combination of cereals to make the recipe a source of high-quality protein?

3. Are you a vegetarian? If so, describe your dietary practices (e.g., vegan or semivegetarian) and explain why you decided to become vegetarian. If you're not a vegetarian, explain why you would or would not consider this lifestyle.

4. Using only plant foods, plan a day's meals and snacks for a healthy 154-pound (70 kg) adult vegan male. The menu should supply at least 2200 kcal, follow the recommendations of the MyPlate plan, and include foods from the major food groups (except for the dairy group, unless calcium-fortified soy milk is used).

5. Does a recipe that combines apples, grapes, peaches, and oranges with pecans provide a complementary mixture of amino acids? Explain why or why not.

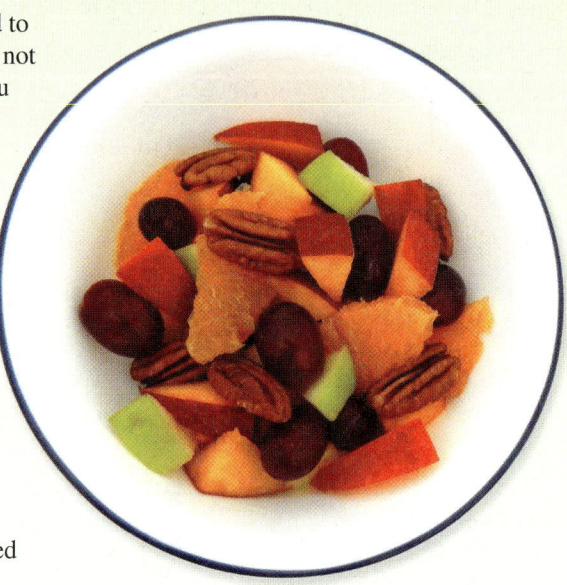
Wendy Schiff

Test Yourself

Select the best answer.

1. Which of the following nutrients has nitrogen in its chemical structure?
    a. Protein
    b. Cholesterol
    c. Glucose
    d. Glycogen

2. Which of the following statements is false?
    a. Proteins are the building blocks of triglycerides.
    b. Nearly all enzymes are proteins.
    c. Cells use amino acids to make proteins.
    d. The body uses amino acids to make antibodies.

3. Which of the following foods generally provides the least amount of protein per serving?
    a. Sunflower seeds
    b. Fat-free milk
    c. Almonds
    d. Apples

4. Which of the following foods is not a source of high-quality protein?
    a. Milk
    b. Broccoli
    c. Fish
    d. Eggs

5. What's the RDA for protein of a healthy adult woman who isn't an athlete and weighs 71 kg?
    a. 36.8 g
    b. 46.8 g
    c. 56.8 g
    d. 66.8 g

6. Which of the following foods isn't a source of complementary protein?
    a. Red beans and rice
    b. Macaroni and cheese
    c. Soy nut butter on a bagel
    d. Split pea soup with noodles

7. A person following a lacto-ovovegetarian diet wouldn't eat
   a. eggs.
   b. cheese.
   c. nuts.
   d. fish.

8. Which of the following nutrients is most likely to be lacking in a vegan's diet?
   a. Magnesium
   b. Fiber
   c. Iron
   d. Vitamin C

9. People with celiac disease should
   a. take amino acid supplements.
   b. limit their protein intake to 20 g per day.
   c. avoid foods that contain wheat.
   d. eliminate protein from plant sources.

10. Which of the following substances is needed to digest proteins?
    a. Bile
    b. Pepsin
    c. Sucrase
    d. Alanine

11. Annie experiences diarrhea and abdominal discomfort a few hours after she eats wheat bread, barley cereal, and rye crackers. Based on this information, she should obtain medical testing that can diagnose
    a. lactose intolerance.
    b. gallstones.
    c. protein toxicity.
    d. celiac disease.

12. A can of frozen orange juice that costs $2.00 makes 48 fl oz of juice, when the proper amount of water is added to it. A 59-fl oz container of 100% fresh orange juice costs $3.79. The unit price of the reconstituted frozen juice is about ____ cents/fl oz, and the unit price of the 100% juice is about ____ cents/fl oz.
    a. 2; 8
    b. 5; 4
    c. 6; 9
    d. 4; 6

Answers: 1. a 2. a 3. d 4. b 5. c 6. b 7. d 8. c 9. c 10. b 11. d 12. d

Answer This (Module 7.2d)

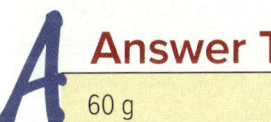

60 g

References → See Appendix D.

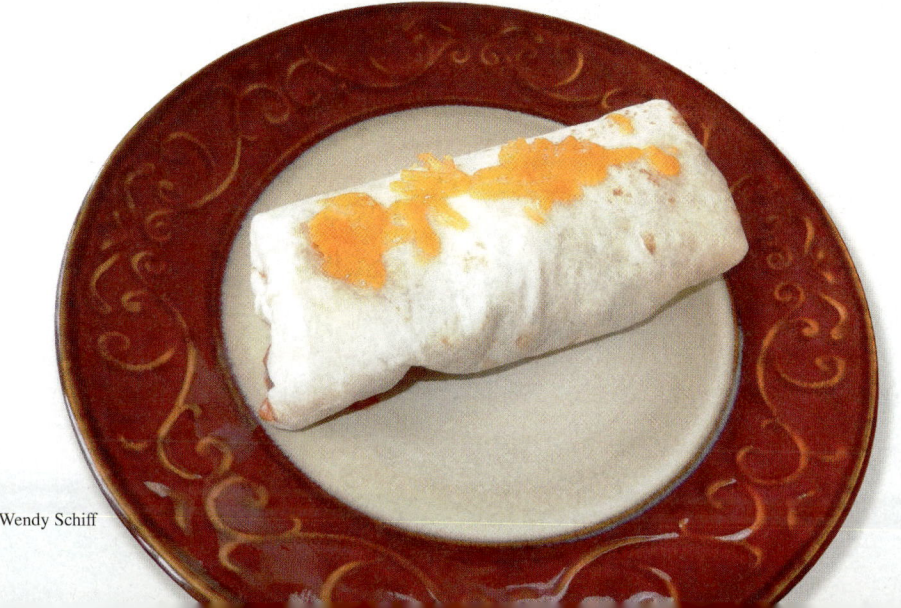

Wendy Schiff

Design elements: Spiral notebook paper background, Stacked paper with clip background, Marginal note clip, and Culture & Cuisine globe icon: ©McGraw-Hill Education; In a Nutshell walnut: ©McGraw-Hill Education/Mark A. Dierker, photographer; Test Yourself red pepper: Iconotec/Glow Images

Unit 8
Vitamins
NUTRIENTS THAT MULTITASK

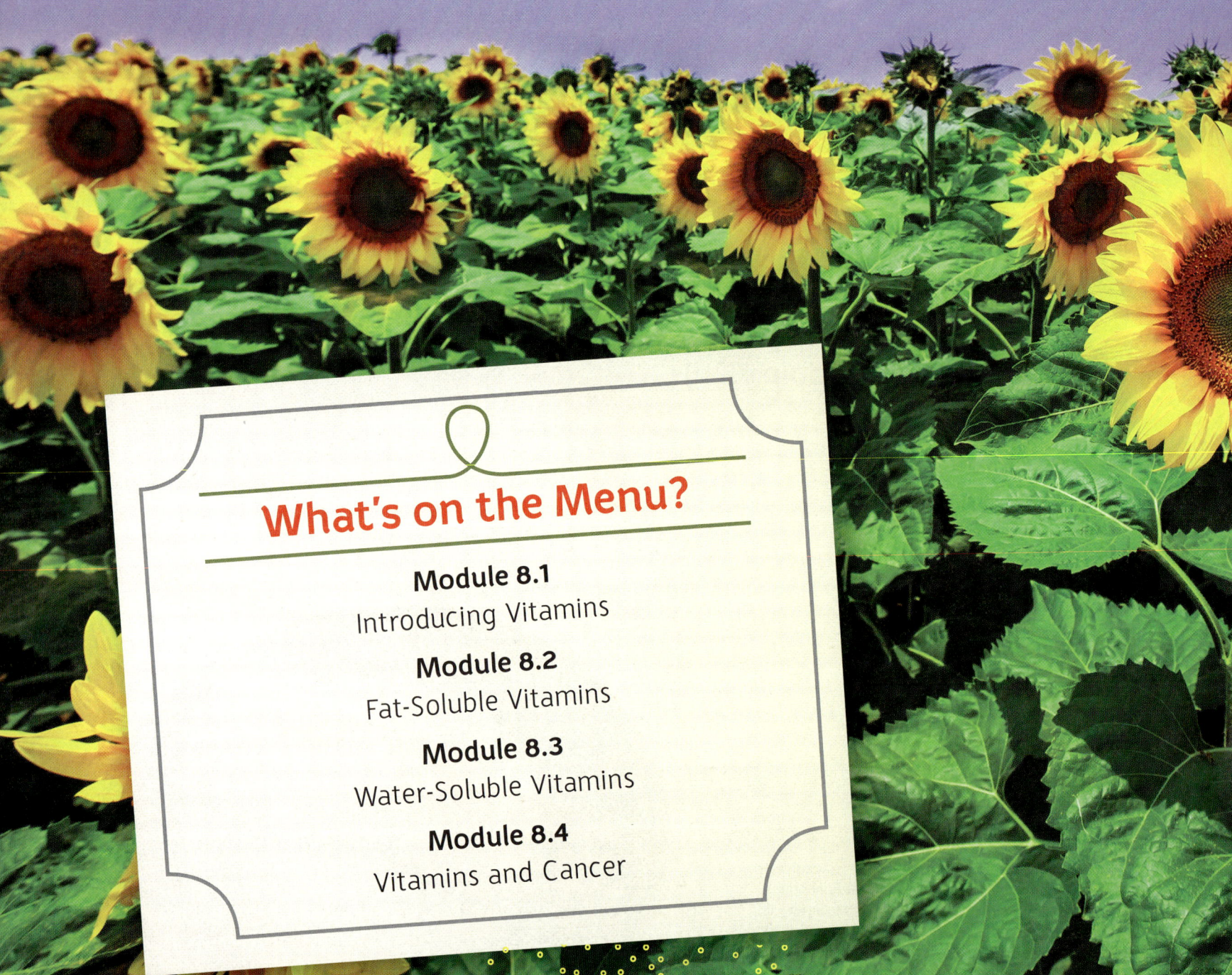

What's on the Menu?

Module 8.1
Introducing Vitamins

Module 8.2
Fat-Soluble Vitamins

Module 8.3
Water-Soluble Vitamins

Module 8.4
Vitamins and Cancer

"I'm taking a prescription dose of vitamin D because my family doctor tested my blood and found out that I didn't have enough of the vitamin in my body. She told me that people need sunlight to make vitamin D, but she said she wasn't surprised that I'm deficient, since I have red hair. I told her that I try to avoid being out in the sun for more than 30 minutes, because I 'crisp' when I get exposed to sun. My skin is so light, I even got a sunburn in Kansas in the middle of October because I was outside for a couple hours! Anyway, I don't notice that much of a difference now that I'm on the medication."

Amanda Croker

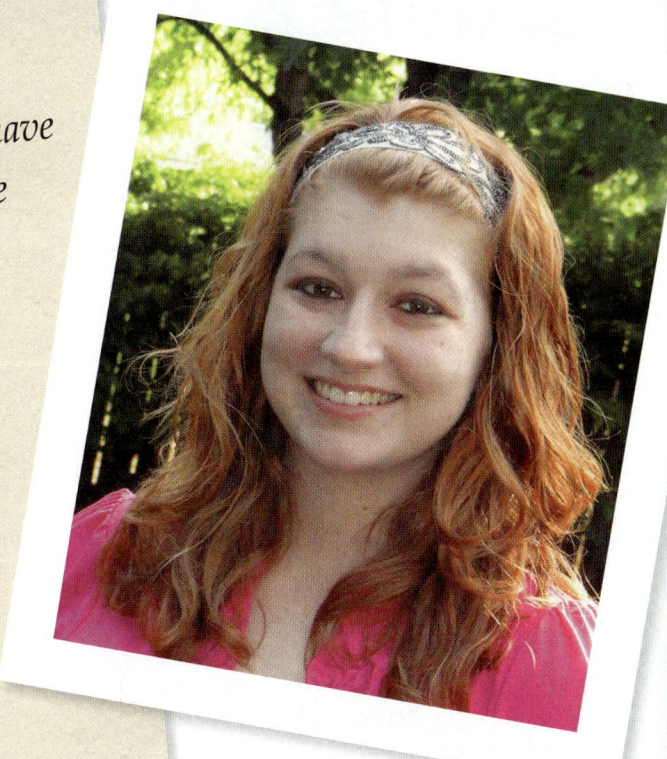
Alicia Croker

Amanda Croker, a recent graduate of the University of Kansas, routinely tried to limit her sun exposure to avoid sunburn and the possibility of skin cancer in the future. She was unaware that her efforts to protect her skin were also limiting her body's ability to make vitamin D, "the sunshine vitamin." If her doctor hadn't discovered that Amanda was vitamin D–deficient and treated her with the nutrient, her bones eventually may have become soft and weak.

Rickets, the vitamin D deficiency disease in children, is characterized by weak and deformed bones. Several decades before vitamin D's discovery in the early 1920s, scientists knew that exposure to sunlight could cure as well as prevent rickets, but they didn't know why. They also learned that cod liver oil contained a factor that prevented and cured the disease. In the mid-1930s, scientists extracted vitamin D from the oil and confirmed that it was the factor that prevented rickets. By the 1950s, scientists had determined the role that sunlight plays in the body's ability to form the vitamin. In this unit, you will learn about vitamin D and its functions in your body.

This unit provides information about vitamin D, the 12 other vitamins, and the vitamin-like nutrient choline. By reading this unit, you'll learn what can happen when your intake of vitamins is too low or too high. The last section of this unit focuses on cancer, including the role of diet in the development of the disease and whether vitamin supplements can prevent cancer.

Sunflowers are the state flower of Kansas.

Module 8.1
Introducing Vitamins

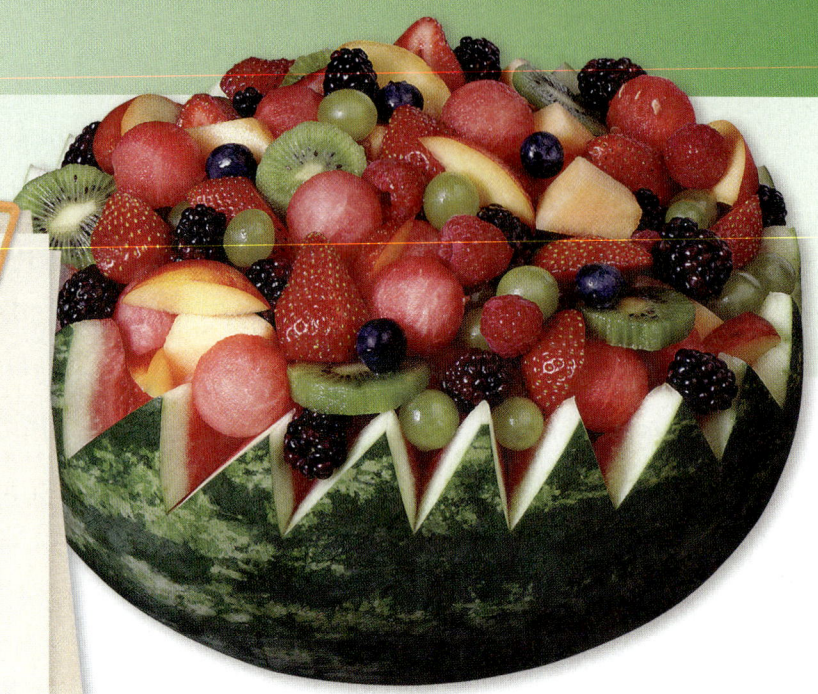
Brand X Pictures/PunchStock

8.1 - Learning Outcomes

After reading Module 8.1, you should be able to

1. Define all of the **key terms** in this module.
2. Describe the basic features that distinguish a vitamin from other naturally occurring substances in foods.
3. Classify vitamins according to their solubility in fat or water.
4. Discuss conditions or factors that affect the absorption of vitamins in your digestive tract.
5. Explain how an antioxidant can protect your body against free radical damage.
6. Discuss at least five ways to conserve the vitamin content of fruits and vegetables during food preparation and storage.

8.1a What's a Vitamin?

A **vitamin** is an organic micronutrient that

- regulates certain processes in your body;
- isn't made by your body, or it's not made in amounts your body needs for good health;
- occurs naturally in commonly eaten foods; and
- prevents a specific deficiency disorder when consumed in adequate amounts.

Foods generally contain much smaller amounts of vitamins than of macronutrients. Furthermore, your body requires vitamins in very small amounts (milligram or microgram quantities), but it needs grams of macronutrients.

A few vitamins have **precursors (provitamins, previtamins).** These are substances in foods or your body that don't function as vitamins until your cells convert them into the active forms.

Vitamin Deficiencies

You're at risk of a vitamin deficiency disorder when your diet doesn't supply enough of the micronutrient to meet your needs. Additionally, diseases that reduce your intestinal tract's ability to absorb nutrients can increase your body's losses of vitamins and result in deficiencies of these micronutrients.

If your usual diet is nutritionally adequate but you occasionally have low intakes of vitamins, you're unlikely to develop most vitamin deficiency diseases. Why? Your cells store vitamins to some extent. However, the likelihood of developing a deficiency disease increases when your diet consistently lacks a particular vitamin. When this happens, your body's tissue levels of the vitamin become depleted, and the signs and symptoms of the nutrient's deficiency disease begin to occur. To estimate your intakes of certain vitamins, complete the "What's in Your Diet?!" activity at the end of this unit.

vitamin organic micronutrient that can have a variety of functions in the body

vitamin precursors (provitamins, previtamins) substances in food or the body that cells can convert into active vitamins

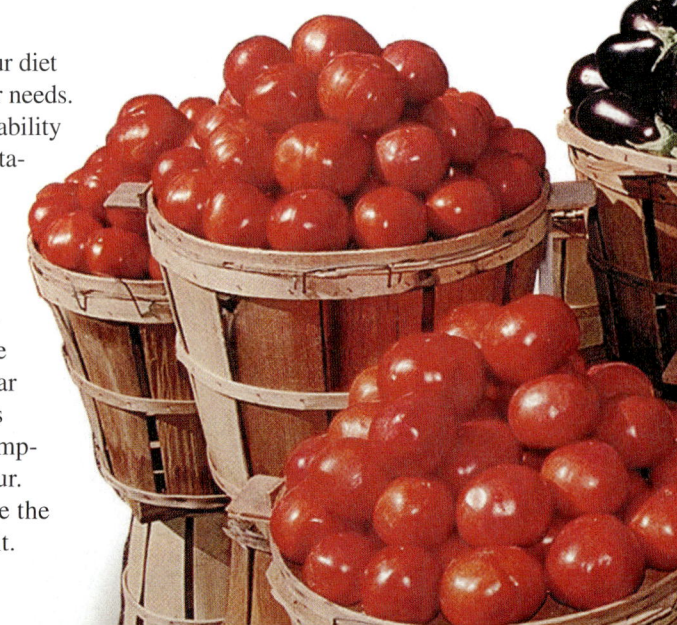

Vitamin Toxicities

When your cells have enough vitamins to meet their needs, you're more likely to experience good health. However, supplying your body with amounts of vitamins that are much higher than required doesn't mean you'll become super healthy as a result. Vitamin excesses can lead to toxicity signs and symptoms. This is because vitamins can have druglike or toxic effects on your body when you take them in large amounts.

Most commonly eaten foods don't contain toxic levels of vitamins. Vitamin toxicity is most likely to occur in people who take megadoses of vitamin supplements or consume large amounts of vitamin-fortified foods regularly. Recall from Unit 3 that a megadose of a vitamin is an amount that greatly exceeds the recommended amount of the nutrient.

8.1b Classifying Vitamins

Vitamins A, D, E, and K are **fat-soluble vitamins.** These vitamins are fat soluble because they dissolve in fats, oils, and the fatty portions of foods. Such vitamins tend to associate with fats in your body. Vitamin C and the "B vitamins" (thiamin, riboflavin, niacin, vitamin B-6, pantothenic acid, folate, biotin, and vitamin B-12) are **water-soluble vitamins.** Water-soluble vitamins dissolve in the watery components of food and your body. The vitamin-like nutrient choline has water-soluble and fat-soluble forms. **Table 8.1** presents the vitamins and provides some other names that are sometimes used to identify them.

Table 8.1 Classifying Vitamins

Fat-Soluble Vitamins	Water-Soluble Vitamins	Vitamin-Like
A (retinol)	Thiamin (thiamine, B-1)	Choline
D	Riboflavin (B-2)	
E (alpha-tocopherol)	Niacin (B-3, nicotinamide, nicotinic acid)	
K	B-6 (pyridoxine)	
	B-12 (cobalamin, cobalamine)	
	Biotin (H)	
	Pantothenic acid (B-5)	
	Folate, folic acid	
	C (ascorbic acid)	

Placemat: McGraw-Hill Education/Mark A Dierker, photographer

Why is it important to know the difference between fat- and water-soluble vitamins? Your body stores excess fat-soluble vitamins because these nutrients don't dissolve in watery substances such as urine. Over time, these vitamins can accumulate in body fat or the liver and cause toxicity. Water-soluble vitamins are generally not as toxic as fat-soluble vitamins. Why? Your body stores only limited amounts of most water-soluble vitamins. Furthermore, your kidneys can remove excess water-soluble vitamins from your bloodstream and eliminate them in urine.

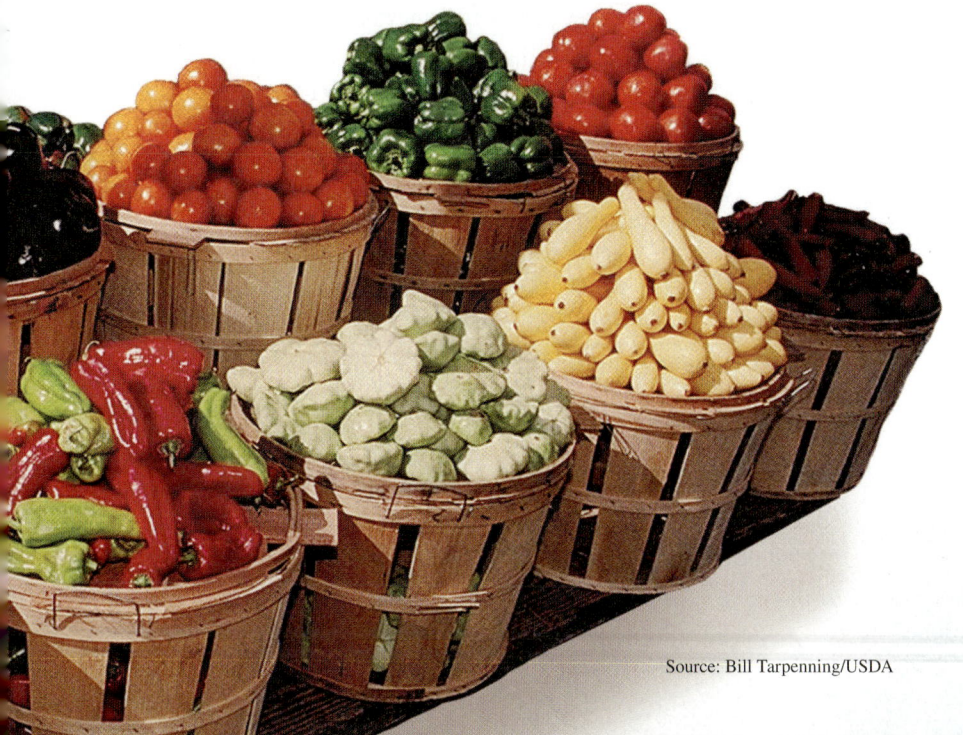

To maximize your vitamin intakes from fresh produce, consider buying locally grown fruits and vegetables.

Source: Bill Tarpenning/USDA

fat-soluble vitamins vitamins A, D, E, and K

water-soluble vitamins thiamin, riboflavin, niacin, vitamin B-6, pantothenic acid, folate, biotin, vitamin B-12, and vitamin C

8.1c Vitamins: Digestion and Absorption

Vitamins don't undergo digestion because they would lose their ability to function as a result. The small intestine absorbs vitamins, but it doesn't absorb 100% of the vitamins in food. Vitamin absorption tends to increase when needs for the micronutrients increase, such as during periods of growth and pregnancy.

Bile enhances lipid as well as fat-soluble vitamin absorption (see Unit 6). Therefore, adding a small amount of fat to low-fat foods, such as tossing raw vegetables with some salad dressing, adding a pat of soft margarine to steamed carrots, or stir-frying green beans in peanut oil, can enhance your intestinal tract's ability to absorb the fat-soluble vitamins in these foods. Diseases that interfere with fat absorption, such as cystic fibrosis, can lead to deficiencies of fat-soluble vitamins.

People who are unable to absorb vitamins may need to take large oral doses of vitamin supplements just to enable small amounts of the vitamins to be absorbed. In other cases, physicians inject vitamins into their patients' bodies, completely bypassing the need for the intestine to absorb the micronutrients. To review lipid digestion, see Unit 6.

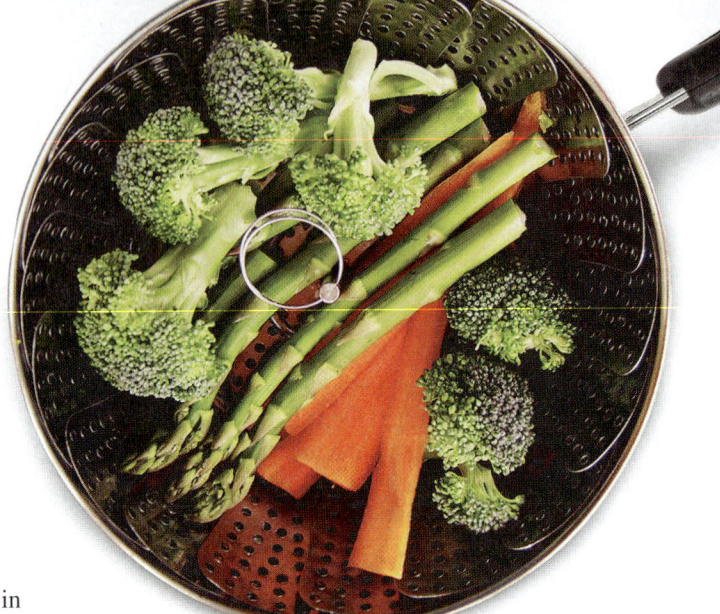

Steaming vegetables can preserve their vitamin content.

8.1d Retaining the Vitamin Content of Foods

Exposure to air, excessive heat, alkaline conditions, and light can destroy certain vitamins. The following tips can help you conserve much of the vitamins in your food.

- Purchase fresh produce when it's in season or at local farmers' markets. Fresh produce loses some vitamin content, especially if it has to be shipped hundreds of miles to reach your supermarket.
- Eat fruits and vegetables when they are fresh—cooking can reduce their vitamin content.
- Cook fresh or frozen vegetables by microwaving, steaming, or stir-frying. Cooking them in water increases the loss of water-soluble vitamins. Vegetables generally have high water content; therefore, add no water or just a small amount when microwaving vegetables.
- Don't overcook vegetables, and minimize reheating—prolonged heating can reduce vitamin content.
- When cooking vegetables in water, don't add baking soda. Baking soda makes the water more alkaline, which destroys certain vitamins.
- Don't add fat to vegetables during cooking. Fat-soluble vitamins and phytochemicals in the food may enter the fat and be discarded when the vegetables are drained before serving. Add some fat, such as olive oil or liquid margarine, to vegetables after they're cooked.
- Store canned foods in a cool place. Canned foods can vary in the amount of nutrients they contain, largely because of differences in storage times and temperatures. If the can has been on the shelf for a year or more, the food's vitamin content may be reduced. To get maximal nutritive value from canned vegetables, drain the liquid that's packed with the food and use it as a base for soups, sauces, or gravies. If the liquid is too salty, discard it.

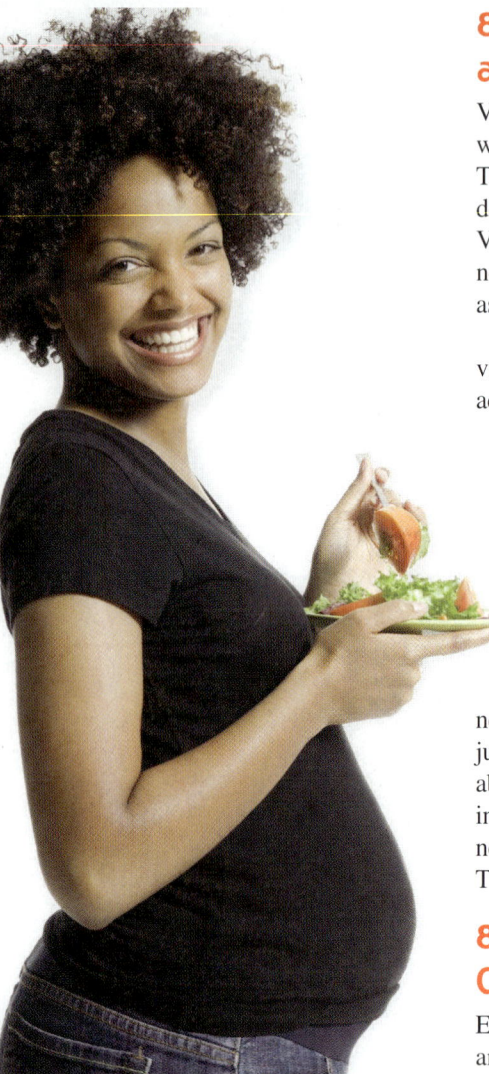

Vitamin needs generally increase during periods of growth, such as pregnancy.

Adding some healthy fats, such as olive oil, to foods enhances the absorption of the fat-soluble vitamins in them.

Steaming vegetables, Salad with dressing: Wendy Schiff; Pregnant woman: rubberball/Getty Images

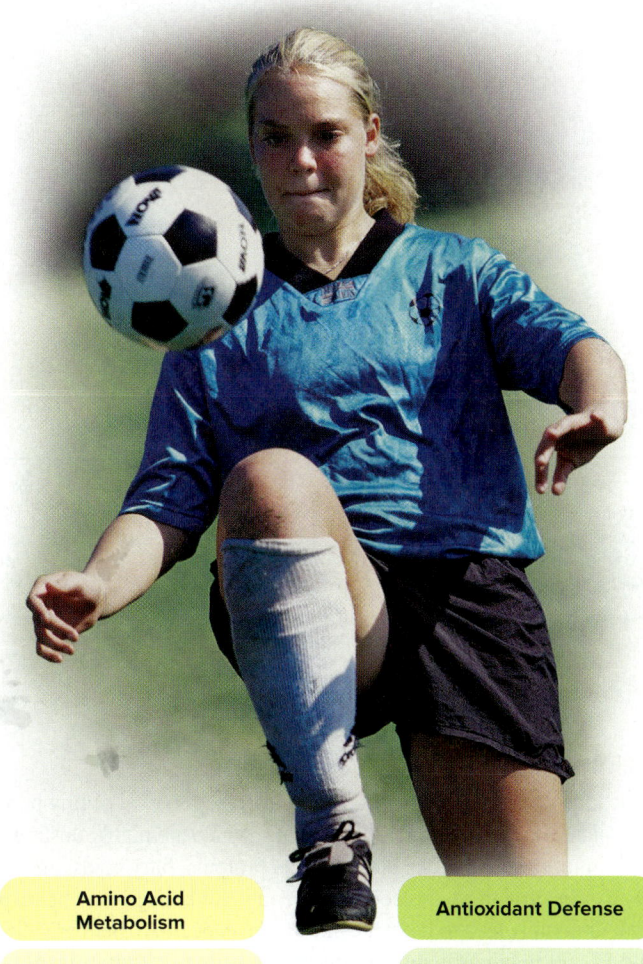

Bone Health
- Vitamin A
- Vitamin D
- Vitamin K
- Vitamin C

Energy Metabolism
- Thiamin
- Riboflavin
- Niacin
- Pantothenic acid
- Biotin
- Vitamin B-12
- Vitamin B-6

Blood Clotting
- Vitamin K

Amino Acid Metabolism
- Vitamin B-6
- Folate
- Vitamin B-12
- Vitamin C
- Choline

Growth and Development
- Vitamin A
- Vitamin D
- Choline

Red Blood Cell Formation
- Vitamin B-6
- Vitamin B-12
- Folate
- Riboflavin (indirect)

Immune Function
- Vitamin A
- Vitamin C
- Vitamin D
- Vitamin E

Antioxidant Defense
- Vitamin E
- Vitamin C (likely)
- Certain carotenoids

Figure 8.1 Major functions of vitamins and related compounds.

8.1e General Roles of Vitamins

Vitamins play numerous roles in your body, and each of these micronutrients generally has more than one function (**Fig. 8.1**). Advertisements for vitamin supplements often promote the notion that the micronutrients can "give" you energy. Vitamins, however, aren't a source of energy because cells don't metabolize them for energy. Although your body doesn't use vitamins directly for energy, certain B vitamins, including niacin, participate in the chemical reactions that release energy from glucose, fatty acids, and amino acids.

Girl: Purestock/SuperStock; Blue corn kernels, Blue corn chips: Wendy Schiff

Culture & Cuisine

Corn contains niacin, but the vitamin is tightly bound to a protein that resists digestion. Thus, people who eat corn as their staple food are likely to develop pellagra. The Mexican practice of soaking corn kernels in water that contains calcium hydroxide (slaked lime) before using them to prepare tortillas helps free the niacin, enhancing its ability to be absorbed. In the United States, corn products such as hominy and grits are sources of niacin because the corn used to make them has been treated with calcium hydroxide before cooking.

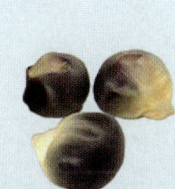
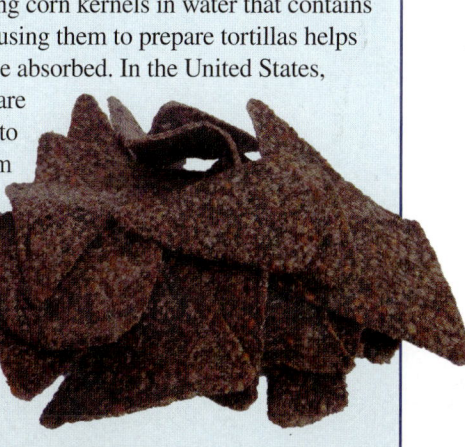

Blue corn kernels are used to make blue corn chips.

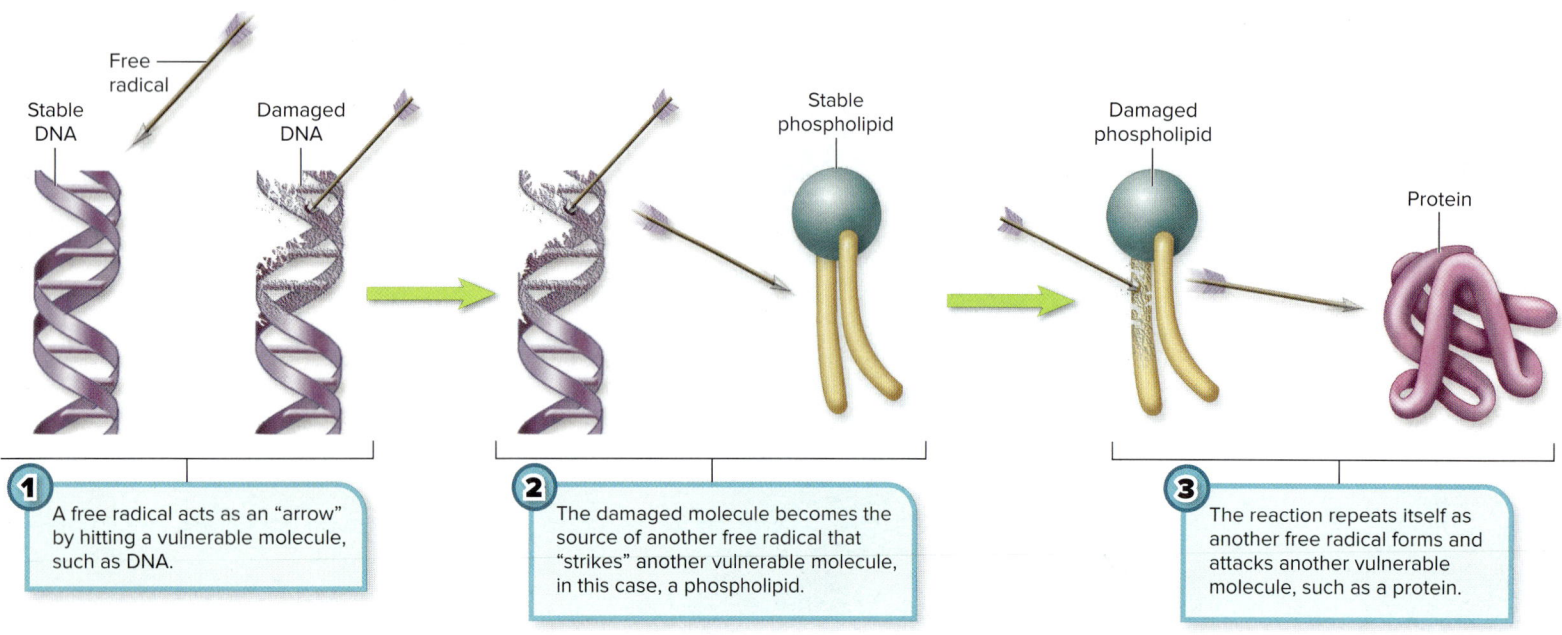

Figure 8.2 Free radical damage.

■ *Why is it important to reduce the damaging effects of free radicals?*

What's an Antioxidant?

Many chemical reactions that occur in your body result in the removal of tiny particles (*electrons*) from atoms or molecules. This chemical change can form free radicals, which are highly unstable substances. Free radicals can remove electrons from more stable molecules, such as proteins, fatty acids, and DNA (**Fig. 8.2**). As a result, free radicals can damage or destroy these molecules. Free radical damage may be responsible for promoting chemical changes in cells that ultimately lead to heart attack, stroke, cancer, Alzheimer's disease, and even the aging process.

Vitamins C and E, and beta-carotene, a plant pigment that is a vitamin A precursor, function as antioxidants. Antioxidants protect cells by giving up electrons to free radicals. When the chemically unstable substance accepts an electron, it can form a more stable structure that doesn't pull an electron away from another compound. By sacrificing electrons, antioxidants protect molecules such as polyunsaturated fatty acids or DNA from being damaged by free radicals (**Fig. 8.3**).

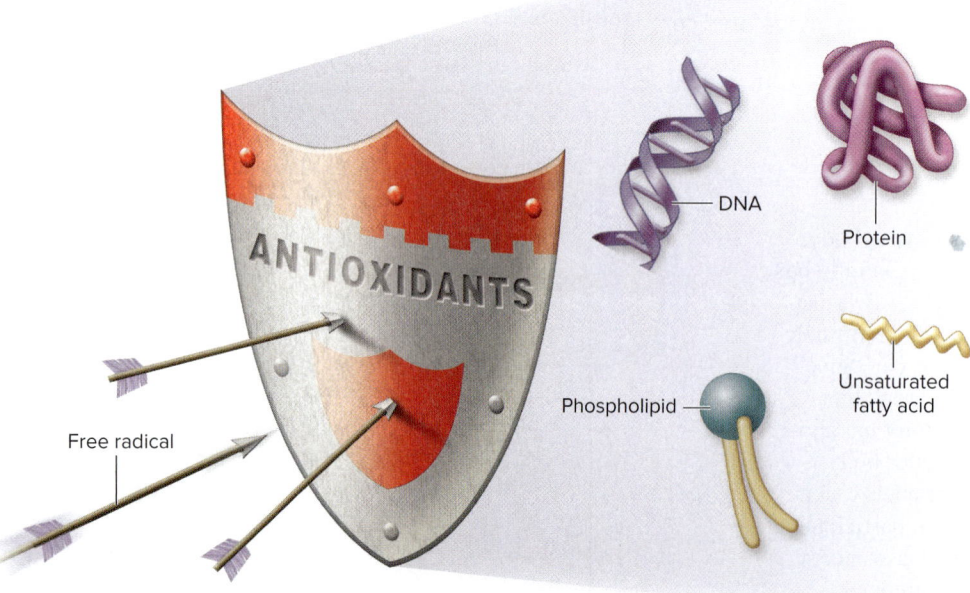

Figure 8.3 Antioxidants protect DNA and other body compounds from being harmed by free radicals.

■ *How do antioxidants reduce the damaging effects of free radicals?*

Module 8.2
Fat-Soluble Vitamins

8.2 - Learning Outcomes

After reading Module 8.2, you should be able to

1. Define all of the **key terms** in this module.
2. Identify the fat-soluble vitamins and foods that are rich sources of these micronutrients.
3. Explain a major function of each fat-soluble vitamin in the body.
4. Describe major deficiency and/or toxicity signs and symptoms for each fat-soluble vitamin.

This module of Unit 8 focuses on fat-soluble vitamins. At the end of each section that discusses a particular vitamin, you'll find a table that summarizes the information about the vitamin. **Figure 8.4** indicates food groups of MyPlate that are good sources of fat-soluble vitamins.

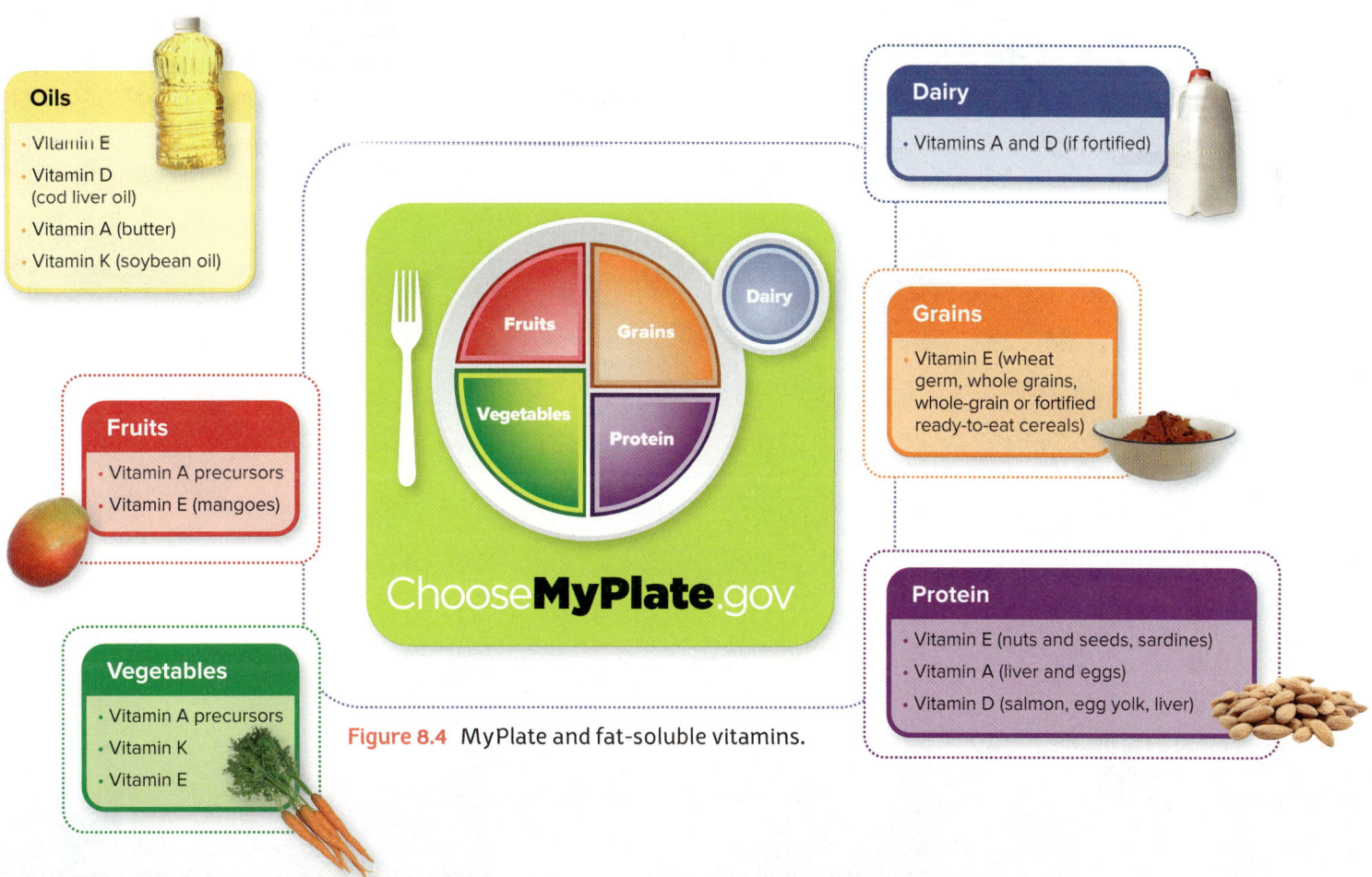

Oils
- Vitamin E
- Vitamin D (cod liver oil)
- Vitamin A (butter)
- Vitamin K (soybean oil)

Fruits
- Vitamin A precursors
- Vitamin E (mangoes)

Vegetables
- Vitamin A precursors
- Vitamin K
- Vitamin E

Dairy
- Vitamins A and D (if fortified)

Grains
- Vitamin E (wheat germ, whole grains, whole-grain or fortified ready-to-eat cereals)

Protein
- Vitamin E (nuts and seeds, sardines)
- Vitamin A (liver and eggs)
- Vitamin D (salmon, egg yolk, liver)

Figure 8.4 MyPlate and fat-soluble vitamins.

Choose MyPlate: Source: ChooseMyPlate.gov; Pumpkin, Carrots: Ingram Publishing/Alamy; Cooking oil: D. Hurst/Alamy; Milk, Almonds: Judith Collins/Alamy; Mango, Bowl of cereal: Wendy Schiff

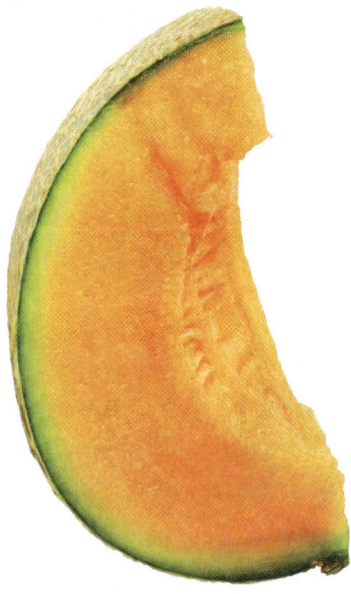

8.2a Vitamin A

Vitamin A is actually a family of compounds that includes **retinol,** which may be called **preformed vitamin A.** Although retinol is only in animal foods, plants contain yellow, orange, and red pigments called **carotenoids.** The body can convert a few kinds of carotenoids, particularly **beta-carotene,** into retinol. We sometimes refer to these carotenoids as **"provitamin A."**

Why Does My Body Need Vitamin A?

Do you associate vitamin A with eating carrots and good vision? It's true that vitamin A is involved in the visual process and carrots contain lots of beta-carotene. However, vitamin A can multitask, that is, the micronutrient has numerous functions in the body. Vitamin A participates in the processes of cell production, growth, and development. Vitamin A is also needed for building strong bones, regulating immune system activity, and maintaining epithelial cells. **Epithelial cells** form protective tissues that include your skin and linings of the respiratory, reproductive, and intestinal tracts. Some epithelial cells secrete mucus. Mucus keeps tissues moist and forms a sticky barrier against many environmental pollutants and infectious agents.

Food Sources of Vitamin A

Animal foods such as liver, butter, fish liver oils, and eggs are good sources of preformed vitamin A. Other important sources of the vitamin include vitamin A–fortified milk, yogurt, margarine, and cereals. A fruit or vegetable's color is usually an indication of its provitamin A content. To maximize your provitamin A intake, choose produce with dark green, orange, red, or yellow colors.

In addition to the antioxidant beta-carotene, common carotenoids include lutein (*loo'-tee-en*), zeaxanthin (*zee-ah-zan'-thin*), and lycopene (*lie'-ko-peen*). Green, leafy vegetables, such as spinach and kale, have high concentrations of lutein and zeaxanthin. Tomato juice and other tomato products, including pizza sauce, contain considerable amounts of lycopene. Although lutein, zeaxanthin, and lycopene are carotenoids, the body doesn't convert them to vitamin A. Nevertheless, these plant pigments may function as beneficial antioxidants in the body.

retinol (preformed vitamin A) form of vitamin A that's in animal sources of food

carotenoids yellow, orange, and red pigments in fruits and vegetables

beta-carotene carotenoid that the body can convert to vitamin A

provitamin A carotenoids that the body converts to vitamin A

epithelial cells cells that form protective linings of the body

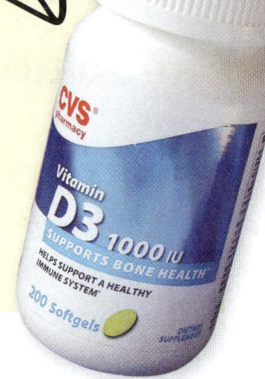

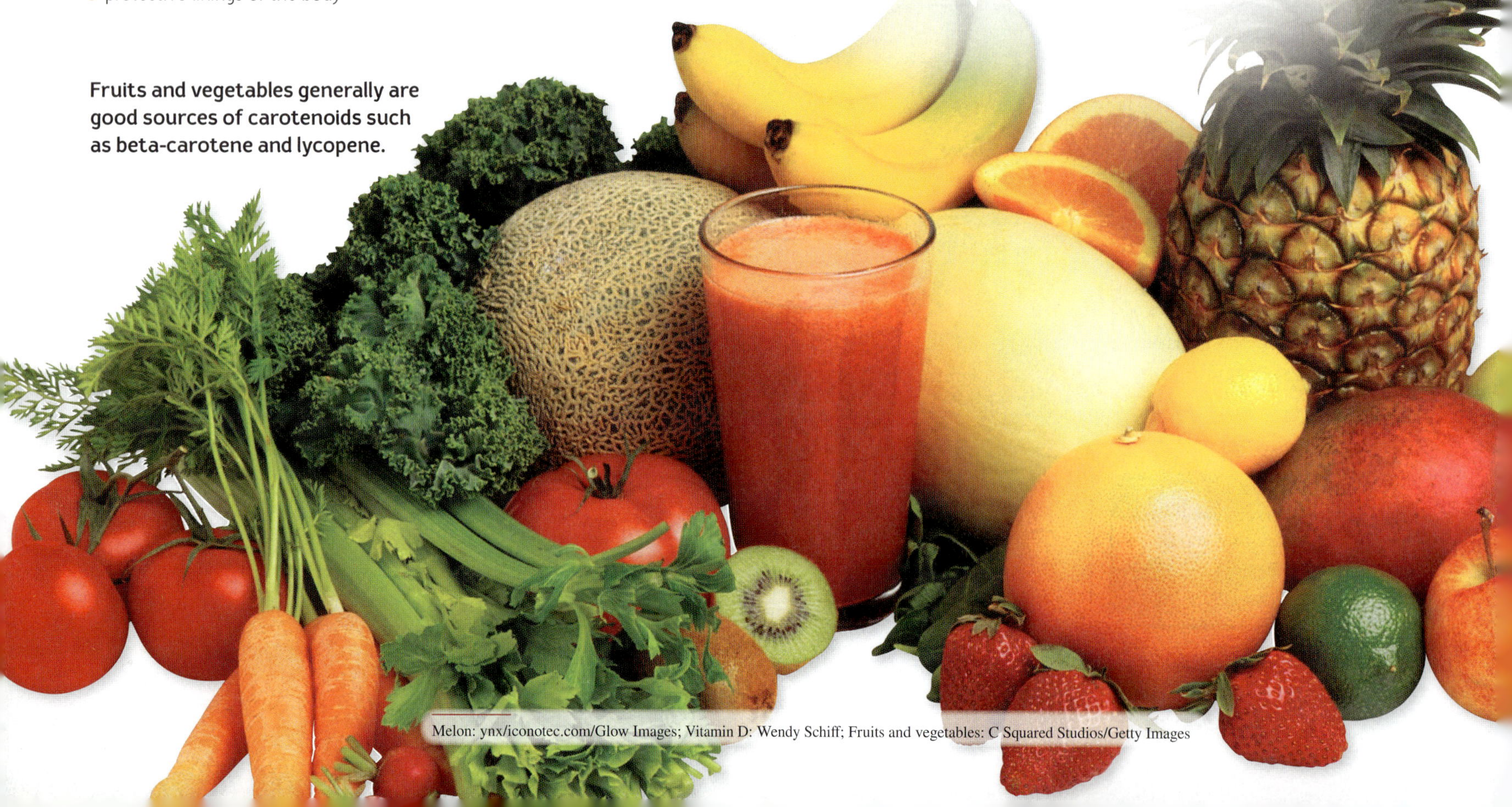

TASTY Tidbits

In the past, amounts of fat-soluble vitamins in foods were often indicated as *International Units* (IUs). Today, IUs have largely been replaced with more precise milligram and microgram measures.

Fruits and vegetables generally are good sources of carotenoids such as beta-carotene and lycopene.

Melon: ynx/iconotec.com/Glow Images; Vitamin D: Wendy Schiff; Fruits and vegetables: C Squared Studios/Getty Images

What IS That?

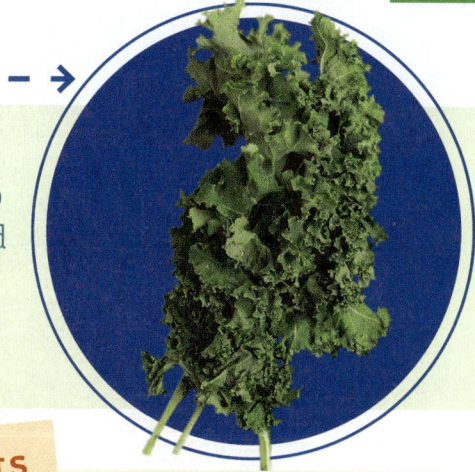

Kale is a leafy, green, cruciferous (*krew-siff'-er-rus*) vegetable that's related to cabbage and broccoli. Cruciferous vegetables contain antioxidants that may protect against cancer. Kale is a rich source of beta-carotene, fiber, and vitamins B-6 and C. The raw vegetable has a strong flavor, so tear raw kale leaves into small pieces and add them to salad greens. Cooking small pieces of the leaves in soups or stews adds nutrients and fiber to the meals.

Table 8.2 lists some foods that are sources of vitamin A or provitamin A carotenoids. Amounts of vitamin A in food are often reported as micrograms of *retinol activity equivalents* (*RAEs*). One RAE is approximately 1 mcg of retinol. Americans who are 2 years of age and older consume diets that provide, on average, a little less than the RDA for vitamin A.[1]

Vitamin A Deficiency

Epithelial cells are among the first to become affected by a deficiency of vitamin A. When mucus-secreting epithelial cells lack the vitamin, they no longer produce mucus, and the cells lose their effectiveness in preventing infections. Thus, vitamin A–deficient people are at greater risk of infections than are those with adequate levels of the vitamin in their bodies.

TASTY Tidbits

Dark yellow, red, and orange fruits and vegetables usually contain more beta-carotene and other provitamin A carotenoids than does lightly colored produce. Dark green fruits and vegetables also contain provitamin A, but their green pigment hides the yellow, orange, and red pigments. So, don't discard the dark green leaves of cabbage, lettuce, or broccoli when preparing food. Use them in salads and soups or on sandwiches.

Table 8.2 — Vitamin A Content of Selected Foods (Approximate)

Food	mcg RAE
Beef liver, braised, 3 oz	8026
Sweet potato, baked, ½ cup	961
Pumpkin, canned, ½ cup	953
Butternut squash, cooked, cubed, ½ cup	572
Carrots, raw, chopped, ½ cup	534
Mustard greens, frozen, boiled, drained, ½ cup	266
Mixed vegetables, frozen, boiled, drained, ½ cup	195
Fat-free milk with vitamin A, 1 cup	149
Cantaloupe, cubed, ½ cup	135
Butter, 1 Tbsp	97
Egg, hard-cooked, large, 1	74
Spinach, raw, ½ cup	70
Green peas, cooked, drained, ½ cup	32

RDA for adult women = 700 mcg/day
RDA for adult men = 900 mcg/day

Source: U.S. Department of Agriculture, Agricultural Research Service: *USDA National Nutrient Database for Standard Reference Legacy Release,* April 2018. https://ndb.nal.usda.gov/ndb/search/list?home=true Accessed: September 2018

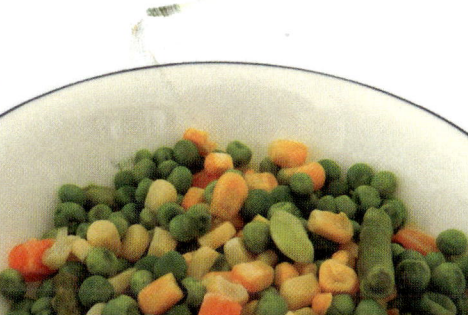

Kale: Stockdisc/PunchStock; Green cabbage: Burke Triolo Productions/Getty Images; Sweet potato, Mixed cooked vegetables: Wendy Schiff

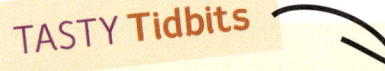

Figure 8.5 Vitamin A and vision. Rods and cones need vitamin A to function properly.

What Is Night Blindness? Have you ever walked from a brightly lit theater lobby into the darkened movie auditorium and felt blinded for a few seconds? This is a normal visual response to the sudden and dramatic reduction in light intensity. The *retina*, the light-sensitive area inside each eye, contains rods and cones, which are specialized nerve cells that are essential for vision **(Fig. 8.5)**. Rods and cones need vitamin A, particularly retinol, to function properly. *Night blindness*, the inability to see in dim light, occurs if retinol is unavailable. Night blindness is an early sign of vitamin A deficiency.

What Is Dry Eye? The **cornea** is the clear covering that enables light to enter your eye, which is necessary for vision (see Figure 8.5). The epithelial cells that line the inner eyelids secrete mucus, which helps keep the cornea moist and clean. In a person suffering from vitamin A deficiency, these cells harden and stop producing mucus. This condition causes the corneas to become dry and easily damaged by dirt and bacteria. Unless the affected person receives vitamin A, he or she will become blind.

Each year, an estimated 250,000 to 500,000 children in developing nations become blind because of severe vitamin A deficiency.[2] Worldwide, vitamin A deficiency is the primary cause of preventable blindness among children. Vitamin A deficiency also reduces the effectiveness of the immune system, so many vitamin A–deficient children die from infections such as measles. In developing countries, efforts to improve people's health and prevent blindness include

- promoting the production of foods that are rich in beta-carotene,
- fortifying foods with vitamin A, and
- providing dietary supplements that contain vitamin A to members of the population who are most at risk.[2]

TASTY Tidbits

Tomatoes are a good source of certain carotenoids, particularly beta-carotene and lycopene. Exposure to heat can break down plant cells, and as a result, the cells release carotenoids. Thus, cooking tomatoes can improve the intestinal tract's ability to absorb carotenoids in the food.

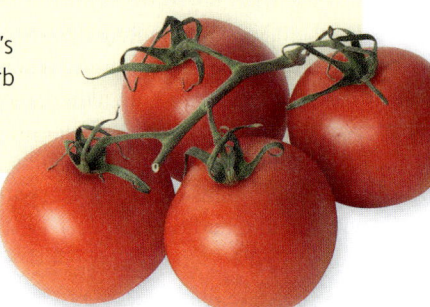

Ingram Publishing/Alamy

cornea clear covering over the front of eyeball

carotenodermia yellowish-orange discoloration of the skin that results from excess beta-carotene in the body

teratogen agent that causes birth defects

TASTY Tidbits

Carotenodermia (*kar'-o-tee-no-derm'-e-ah*) is a condition characterized by skin that becomes yellowish-orange as a result of eating too much beta-carotene-rich produce. This condition occasionally develops in infants who eat a lot of baby foods that contain carrots, apricots, winter squash, or green beans. Carotenodermia is harmless.[3] The skin's natural color eventually returns when the carotenoid-rich foods are no longer eaten.

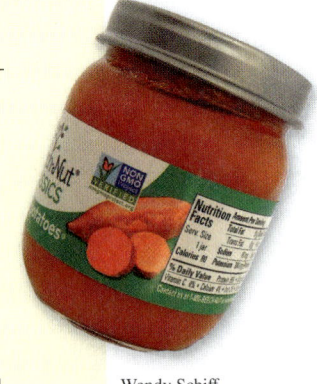

Wendy Schiff

Can Vitamin A Be Toxic?

Compared to other vitamins, vitamin A is very toxic. Toxicity signs and symptoms include

- headache,
- nausea and vomiting,
- visual disturbances,
- hair loss, and
- bone pain and fractures.

When taken during pregnancy, excess vitamin A is a **teratogen**, an agent that causes birth defects. Medications that are chemically similar to vitamin A, such as tretinoin (Retin-A), may be prescribed to treat severe acne. Although these medications are less toxic than natural vitamin A, there's a lack of information concerning whether they're safe to use during pregnancy. If you're using such medications, check with your physician if you're planning a pregnancy.

Answer This

A young man who's been a vegan for several years doesn't take a dietary supplement that contains vitamin A. Why doesn't he have night blindness or become blind? You can find the answer on the last page of this unit.

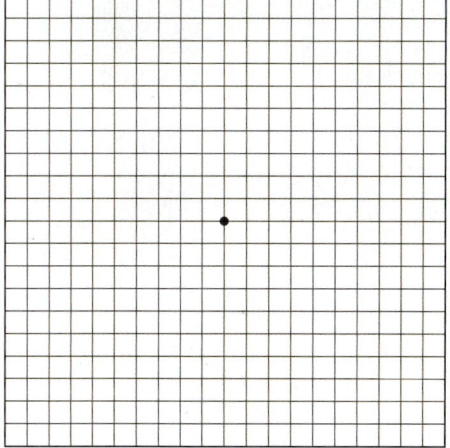
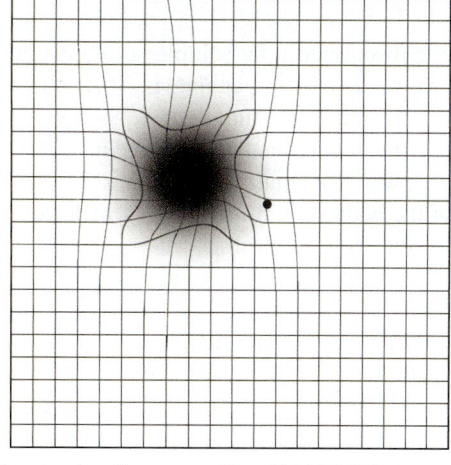
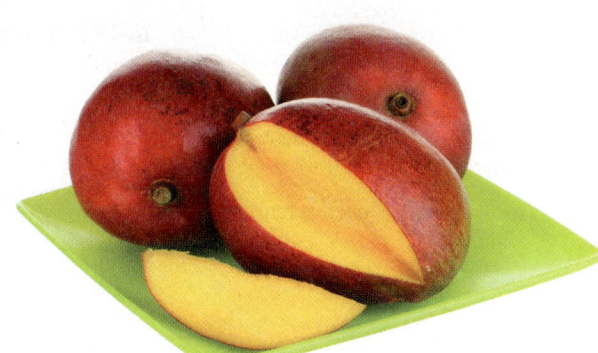

Mango is a rich source of beta-carotene.

Figure 8.6 Simple screening test for age-related macular degeneration (AMD). When people who don't have AMD look at the center of the grid on the left, they will see straight grid lines. If people who have AMD look at the center of that grid, they will see a distorted image, such as the grid on the right.

What's Age-Related Macular Degeneration?

Results of studies suggest an association between eating diets that are rich in fruits and vegetables and lower risk of *age-related macular degeneration (AMD)*. Such diets provide plenty of beta-carotene and other antioxidant carotenoids. Should you take dietary supplements that contain carotenoids to prevent AMD?

AMD is a leading cause of blindness in the United States. People with AMD have damaged maculas. The macula is the region within the eye that provides the most detailed central vision (see Figure 8.5). When the macula is damaged, objects appear to be distorted, as in the grid shown in **Figure 8.6** (right side). Major risk factors for AMD are genetics, smoking, and advanced age, but diet also plays a role in the development of the condition.

In the Age-Related Eye Disease Study (AREDS), patients who already had AMD took dietary supplements that contained relatively high amounts of beta-carotene, vitamins C and E, and the minerals zinc and copper. The combination of these substances appeared to slow the progression of vision loss associated with macular degeneration. Scientists, however, later determined that it wasn't necessary to include beta-carotene with the other nutrients because it wasn't effective.[5]

Vitamin A: Reviewing the Basics

Table 8.3 provides a summary of basic information about vitamin A, including Dietary Reference Intake (DRI) recommendations, and major signs and symptoms of the vitamin's deficiency and toxicity disorders.

TABLE 8.3 VITAMIN A SUMMARY

Major Functions in the Body	Adult RDA	Major Dietary Sources	Major Deficiency Signs and Symptoms	Major Toxicity Signs and Symptoms
Normal vision and reproduction, cellular growth, and immune system function	700–900 mcg RAE	Preformed: liver, milk, fortified cereals Provitamin: yellow, red, orange, and dark green fruits and vegetables	Night blindness, dry eye, poor growth, dry skin, reduced immune system functioning	Adult Upper Level (UL) = 3,000 mcg/day Nausea and vomiting, headaches, bone pain and fractures, hair loss, liver damage, interference with vitamin K absorption

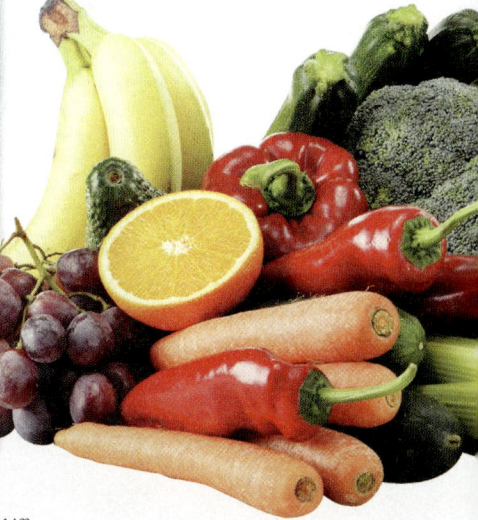

Mangoes: Shutterstock/Africa Studio; Fruits and vegetables: Getty Images/iStockphoto; Squash: Wendy Schiff

8.2b Vitamin D

In 1922, scientists discovered a fat-soluble substance in cod liver oil that people needed for proper bone health and to prevent rickets. As mentioned in the unit opener, children with **rickets** have bones that are soft and can become misshapen. Leg bones, for example, bow under the weight of carrying the upper part of the body **(Fig. 8.7)**. Children with rickets can also develop other bone deformities and may complain of muscle pain. The scientists named the substance that cured rickets *vitamin D*.

Today, the fat-soluble substance that cured rickets is still called a vitamin because rickets can be prevented or treated by taking vitamin D supplements or eating vitamin D–rich foods. Vitamin D, however, is a hormone as well as a nutrient. **Essential Concept 8.1** shows how your body can make vitamin D when your skin is exposed to sunlight.

rickets vitamin D deficiency disorder in children

previtamin D inactive form of vitamin D

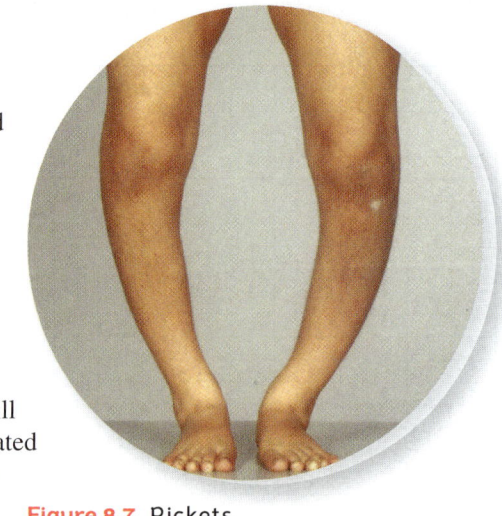

Figure 8.7 Rickets.

■ *Why does a child with rickets have weak leg bones?*

Clinical Photography, Central Manchester University Hospitals NHS Foundation Trust, UK/Science Source

Essential Concept

8.1 How Your Body Makes Vitamin D

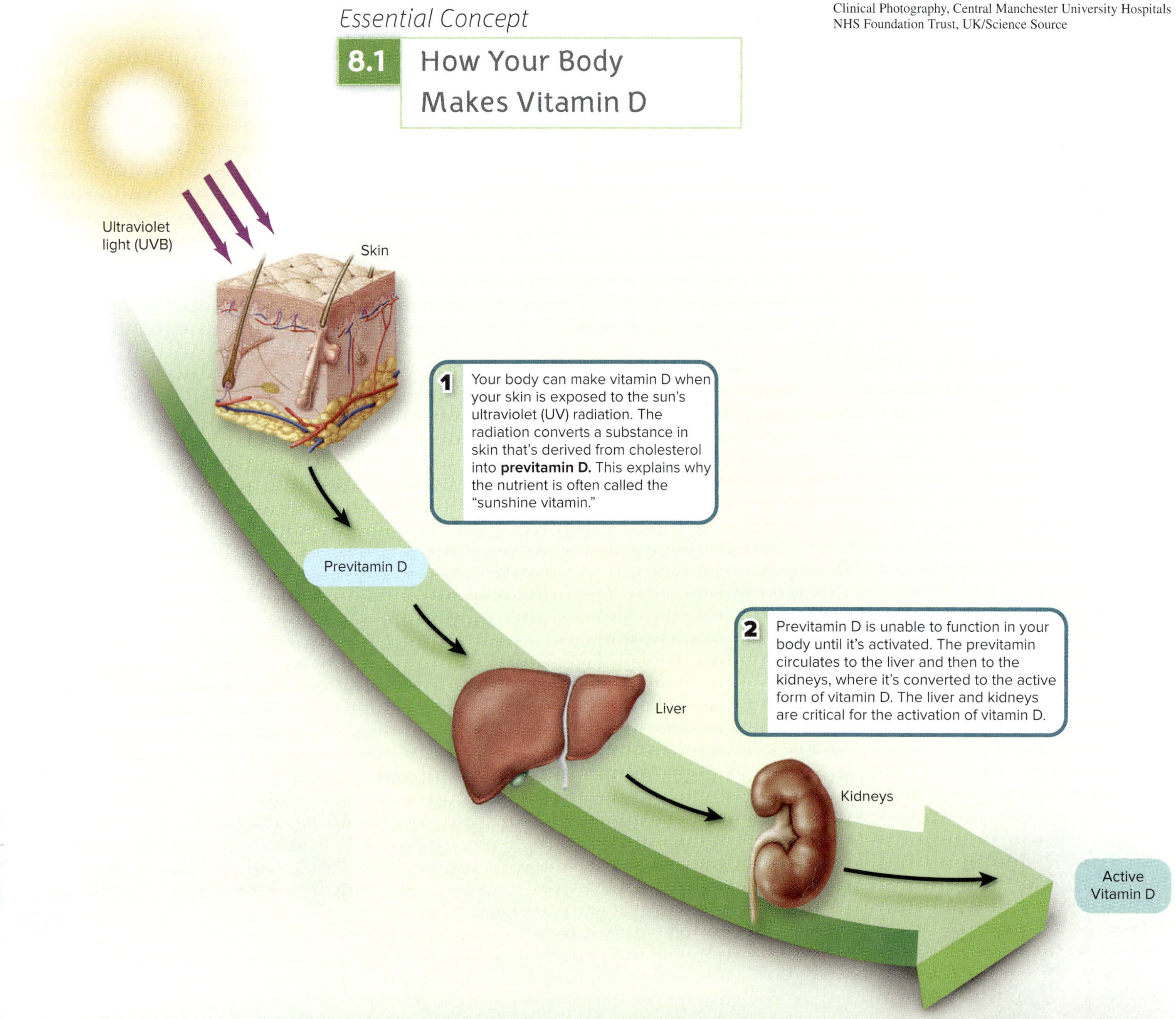

Ultraviolet light (UVB)

Skin

1 Your body can make vitamin D when your skin is exposed to the sun's ultraviolet (UV) radiation. The radiation converts a substance in skin that's derived from cholesterol into **previtamin D**. This explains why the nutrient is often called the "sunshine vitamin."

Previtamin D

Liver

2 Previtamin D is unable to function in your body until it's activated. The previtamin circulates to the liver and then to the kidneys, where it's converted to the active form of vitamin D. The liver and kidneys are critical for the activation of vitamin D.

Kidneys

Active Vitamin D

Why Does My Body Need Vitamin D?

Vitamin D's most well-known role is in the production and maintenance of healthy bones. The minerals calcium and phosphorus are essential for strong bones. Vitamin D stimulates bone cells to form *calcium phosphate,* the hard major mineral compound in bone tissue. Without adequate vitamin D, bone cells can't deposit enough calcium phosphate to produce strong bones (**Fig. 8.8**). The vitamin also enhances the absorption of calcium and phosphorus by the small intestine and reduces the elimination of calcium by the kidneys.

Vitamin D has other roles in the body, including regulating neuromuscular and immune function and reducing inflammation.[4] Vitamin D is also involved in controlling cell growth and, as a result, the micronutrient may reduce the risk of certain cancers. However, more research is needed to clarify the vitamin's role in immune function and chronic disease prevention.

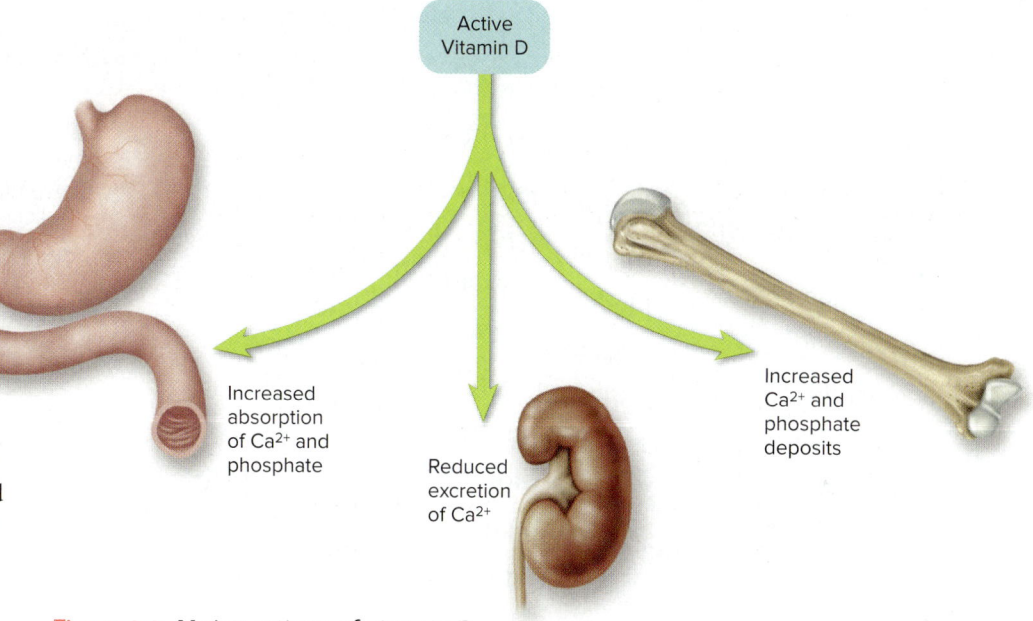

Figure 8.8 Major actions of vitamin D.

Food Sources of Vitamin D

Fish liver oils and fatty fish, especially salmon, sardines, and tuna, are among the few foods that naturally contain vitamin D. Milk is routinely fortified with vitamin D, and some brands of ready-to-eat cereals, orange juice, and margarine also have the vitamin added to them. **Table 8.4** lists some food sources of vitamin D. Food composition tables often list the vitamin D content of foods in International Units; 1 mcg of vitamin D equals 40 IU.

TASTY Tidbits

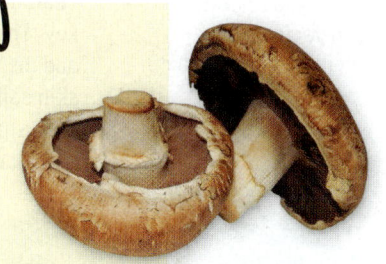

Vitamin D has two major forms—D_2 and D_3. Some kinds of mushrooms produce vitamin D_2; animals make vitamin D_3. Your body generally uses both forms of the vitamin effectively.[4]

TABLE 8.4 — VITAMIN D CONTENT OF SELECTED FOODS (APPROXIMATE)

Food	Vitamin D (mcg)
Cod liver oil, 1 Tbsp	34
Salmon, pink, canned, 3 oz	12
Sardines, Atlantic, canned in oil, drained, 3 oz	4
Milk, fat-free, vitamin D–fortified, 1 cup	3
Tuna, canned in water, drained, 3 oz	2
Egg, whole, hard-cooked, 1 large	1

RDA for adults = 15–20 mcg/day

Source: U.S. Department of Agriculture, Agricultural Research Service: *USDA National Nutrient Database for Standard Reference Legacy Release, April 2018.* https://ndb.nal.usda.gov/ndb/search/list?home=true Accessed: September 2018

Placemat: Mark Dierker/McGraw-Hill Education; Mushrooms: Wendy Schiff; Milk: McGraw-Hill Education; Fish: Digital Vision/Getty Images

Amanda, the student featured in the opener of this unit, took a high-dose supplement of vitamin D that was prescribed by her doctor. As a result of the treatment, her blood level of the vitamin became normal within a few weeks. Because few foods are good sources of vitamin D, she'll need to take a daily supplement of the micronutrient that's available without a prescription for the rest of her life. By taking the supplement, she should be able to maintain a healthy blood level of vitamin D.

TASTY Tidbits

Too much sun exposure may lead to skin cancer. Therefore, physicians who treat skin disorders often advise people to apply sunscreens consistently before going outdoors. When properly applied, a sunscreen with a sun protection factor (SPF) of 8 or more blocks sunlight that's needed to form vitamin D.[4] To allow your body to make some vitamin D, some health experts suggest exposing skin to the sun for 5 to 30 minutes twice a week *before* applying a commercial sunscreen.

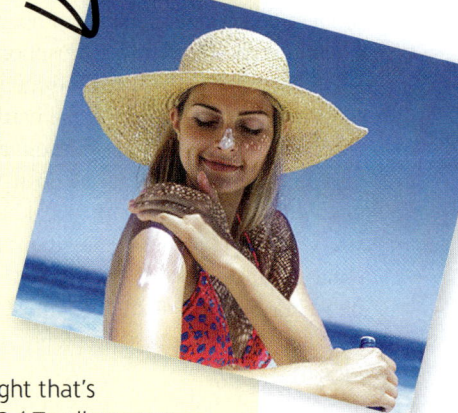

Purestock/SuperStock

osteomalacia adult rickets; condition characterized by poorly mineralized (soft) bones

Vitamin D and Sunlight Because vitamin D isn't widespread in food, you can't count on eating enough vitamin D–rich foods to meet your needs. Therefore, your body must make up the difference, and sunlight is the key. The amount of vitamin D your body makes depends on many factors, including your age, skin color, location, and the time of year.[5] Older adults don't make as much vitamin D as they did when they were younger. Darker skin contains higher amounts of the pigment *melanin,* which may reduce the skin's ability to produce vitamin D from sunlight. Clouds, shade, window glass, air pollution, and clothing are environmental factors that can limit the amount of UV radiation that reaches your skin.

If you live in the Northern Hemisphere, north of the 33rd parallel, the angle of the winter sun is such that the sun's rays must pass through more of the atmosphere than at other times of the year **(Fig. 8.9).** As a result, your skin may not make sufficient amounts of vitamin D during the winter.[5] Therefore, you may need to take a supplement that contains 100% of the adult Daily Value for vitamin D (600 IU or 15 mcg), especially from November through February.

Vitamin D Deficiency

Many Americans don't consume enough vitamin D to meet the RDA.[1] Although rickets isn't a widespread health problem among children in the United States, some medical experts are concerned that many Americans don't have enough vitamin D in their bodies for optimal health. Thus, vitamin D is a nutrient of public health concern, according to the *Dietary Guidelines for Americans.*

Breast milk doesn't contain enough vitamin D to prevent rickets. Infants who are most likely to develop rickets are breastfed, and they have dark skin, minimal sunlight exposure, and little or no vitamin D intake.[4] Therefore, most breastfed infants should consume a daily vitamin D supplement soon after birth.

The adult form of rickets is called **osteomalacia** (*ahs'-tee-o-mah-lay'-she-a*). The bones of people with osteomalacia are soft and break easily because they contain less-than-normal amounts of calcium. Bone pain and muscle weakness are symptoms of osteomalacia.

Osteomalacia is rare in the United States. The following people, however, are at risk of osteomalacia and may need to take a vitamin D supplement:

- Older adults: As a person ages, production of previtamin D in skin declines.
- People who have liver or intestinal diseases because these conditions may reduce both vitamin D production and calcium absorption.
- Adults who stay indoors or are almost fully covered during the day.[4]

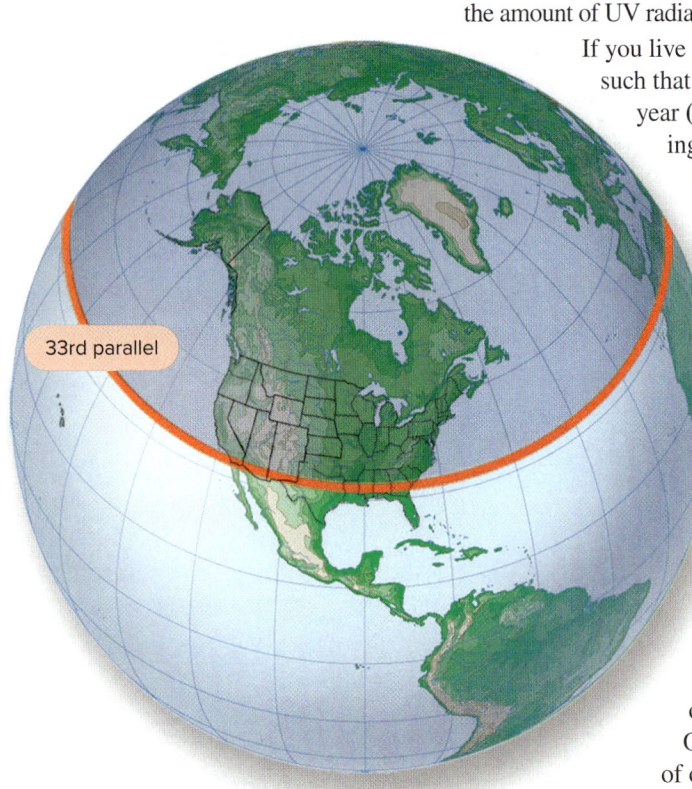

Figure 8.9 Vitamin D and geography.

■ *To form the most vitamin D throughout the year, where would be the best place in the United States for you to live?*

TABLE 8.5 VITAMIN D SUMMARY

Major Functions in the Body	Adult RDA	Major Dietary Sources	Major Deficiency Signs and Symptoms	Major Toxicity Signs and Symptoms
Absorption of calcium and phosphorus, maintenance of normal blood calcium, calcification of bone	15–20 mcg (600–800 IU)	Vitamin D–fortified milk, fortified cereals, fish liver oils, fatty fish, such as salmon	Rickets in children, osteomalacia in adults: soft bones, muscular weakness	Adult UL = 100 mcg/day (4000 IU) Loss of appetite, calcium deposits in soft tissues

People (adults) with osteomalacia may also have *osteoporosis,* a condition characterized by loss of bone mass that usually occurs with aging. Although osteoporosis is usually associated with low calcium intakes, a long-term vitamin D deficiency contributes to the condition because lack of the vitamin reduces calcium absorption.[4] The calcium section of Unit 9 provides more information about osteoporosis.

Can Vitamin D Be Toxic?

Your body stores vitamin D. Taking vitamin D supplements that supply 10,000 to 40,000 IU/day over a long period of time can cause the vitamin to accumulate in your body and produce toxicity.[4] The excess vitamin D stimulates your small intestine to absorb too much calcium from foods. When this occurs, calcium deposits form in your soft tissues, including the kidneys, heart, and blood vessels. The calcium deposits can interfere with cells' ability to function and cause their death. Other signs and symptoms of vitamin D toxicity include kidney stones. You don't have to be concerned about your body making toxic levels of vitamin D when exposed to sunlight because skin limits its production of previtamin D.

Vitamin D: Reviewing the Basics

Table 8.5 provides a summary of basic information about vitamin D, including Dietary Reference Intake (DRI) recommendations, and major signs and symptoms of the vitamin's deficiency and toxicity disorders.

8.2c Vitamin E

There are different forms of vitamin E, but your body uses only the **alpha-tocopherol** (*al'-fah toe-kof'-eh-roll*) form.[6] Alpha-tocopherol is an antioxidant that protects polyunsaturated fatty acids in cell membranes from being damaged by free radicals (**Fig. 8.10**). Preventing free radical damage may lower your risk of atherosclerosis, cancer, and premature cellular aging and death. Other roles for vitamin E include maintaining healthy nervous tissue and immune system function.

Salmon is a good source of vitamin D. — Wendy Schiff

alpha-tocopherol vitamin E

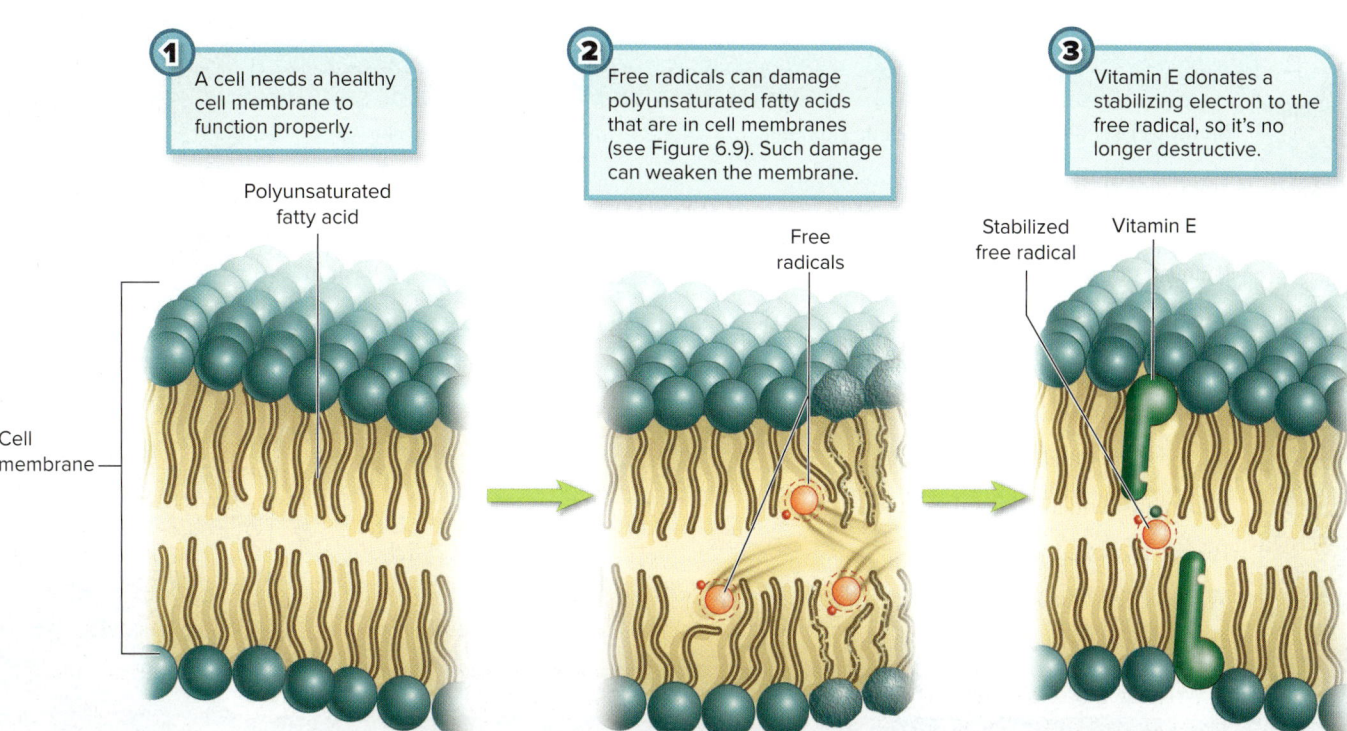

1. A cell needs a healthy cell membrane to function properly.
   Polyunsaturated fatty acid
   Cell membrane

2. Free radicals can damage polyunsaturated fatty acids that are in cell membranes (see Figure 6.9). Such damage can weaken the membrane.
   Free radicals

3. Vitamin E donates a stabilizing electron to the free radical, so it's no longer destructive.
   Stabilized free radical
   Vitamin E

Figure 8.10 Vitamin E's antioxidant activity.

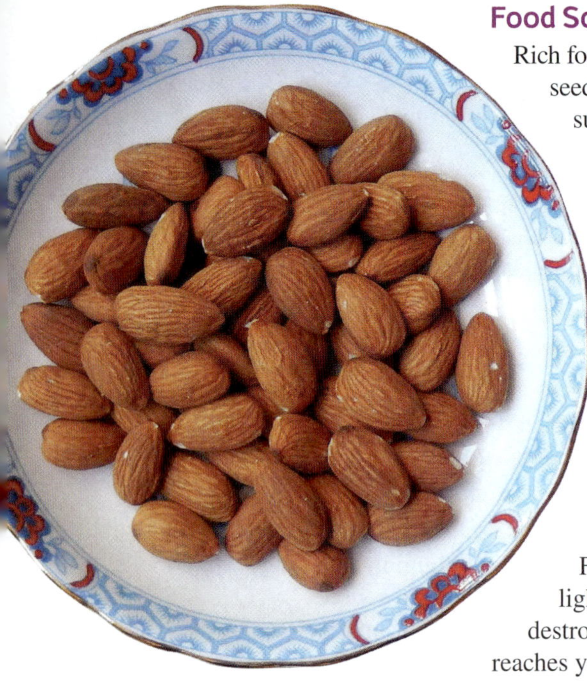

Food Sources of Vitamin E

Rich food sources of vitamin E include sunflower seeds, almonds, and plant oils, especially sunflower, safflower, and olive oils. Products made from vitamin E–rich plant oils—margarine and salad dressings—also supply the micronutrient. Meats, processed grain products, and dairy products generally don't contain much vitamin E.

Table 8.6 lists some common foods that are sources of vitamin E.

Harvesting, processing, storage, and cooking methods can reduce amounts of vitamin E in food. During the milling process, most of the vitamin E that's in whole grains is lost, and it's not restored by grain enrichment. Furthermore, exposure to oxygen, metals, light, and high cooking temperatures can destroy much of the vitamin E in food before it reaches your table.

Vitamin E Deficiency

Americans, on average, don't consume enough vitamin E to meet the RDA for the nutrient.[1] However, vitamin E deficiency rarely occurs in healthy adults.[6] High-risk populations include people who have intestinal diseases that interfere with vitamin E absorption. Common signs and symptoms of the deficiency are nerve damage, difficulty walking, and reduced immune function.

Can Vitamin E Be Toxic?

Unlike vitamins A and D, vitamin E has low toxicity.[6] However, taking dietary supplements that supply excessive amounts of vitamin E may interfere with vitamin K's role in blood clotting and lead to uncontrolled bleeding. Therefore, people who take medications that interfere with blood clotting ("blood thinners") should check with their physicians before using vitamin E supplements.

Vitamin E Supplements and Chronic Diseases

According to the results of several large population studies, taking vitamin E supplements is not likely to reduce your risk of cardiovascular diseases, including heart disease and cancer.[6]

Furthermore, studies generally don't provide evidence that vitamin E supplements help people with signs of *mild cognitive impairment,* a condition characterized by declining thought-processing abilities that can progress to Alzheimer's disease.[6] Despite these findings, scientists continue to conduct research to determine whether taking vitamin E alone or with other antioxidant nutrients can reduce the risk of heart disease, cancer, and AMD.

Table 8.6 — Vitamin E Content of Selected Foods (Approximate)

Food	Alpha-tocopherol (mg)
Sunflower seed kernels, dry-roasted, 1 oz	7.4
Vegetable oil (safflower), 1 Tbsp	4.6
Mango, 1 raw	3.0
Peanuts, dry roasted, 1 oz (approx. 28)	2.2
Olive oil, 1 Tbsp	2.0
Spinach, frozen, cooked, drained, ½ cup	1.9
Sardines, canned in oil, drained, 3 oz	1.7
Red pepper, sweet, raw, sliced, 1 cup	1.4
Asparagus, boiled, drained, ½ cup	1.4
Broccoli, cooked, chopped, ½ cup	1.1
Whole-grain bread, 1 slice	0.1

RDA for adults = 15 mg/day

Source: U.S. Department of Agriculture, Agricultural Research Service: *USDA National Nutrient Database for Standard Reference Legacy Release, April 2018.* https://ndb.nal.usda.gov/ndb/search/list?home=true Accessed: September 2018

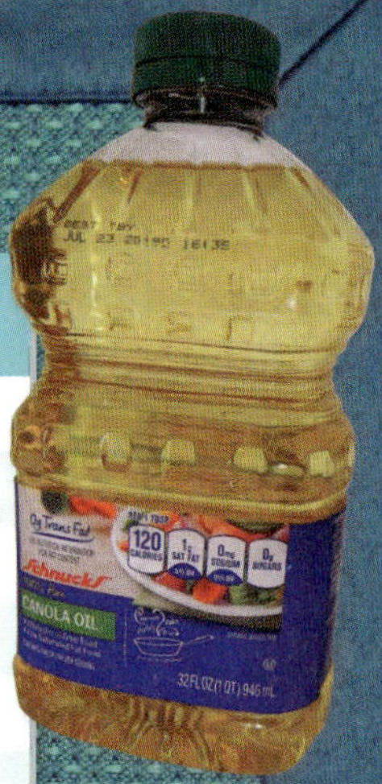

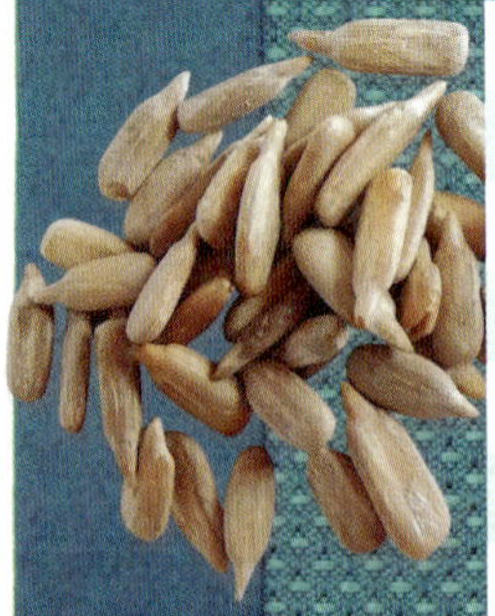

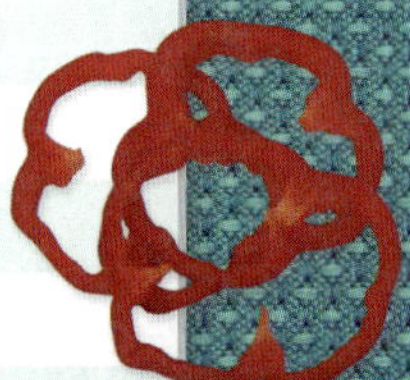

Almonds, Sunflower seeds, Canola oil, Red pepper slices: Wendy Schiff; Placemat: McGraw-Hill Education/Mark A Dierker, photographer

TABLE 8.7 VITAMIN E SUMMARY

Major Functions in the Body	Adult RDA	Major Dietary Sources	Major Deficiency Signs and Symptoms	Major Toxicity Signs and Symptoms
Antioxidant	15 mg (22.5 IU)	Vegetable oils and products made from these oils, certain fruits and vegetables, nuts and seeds, fortified cereals	Loss of muscular coordination, reduced immune function	Adult UL = 1000 mg/day Excessive bleeding as a result of interfering with vitamin K

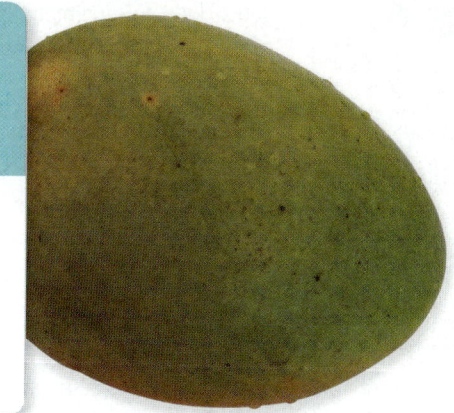

Mangoes are rich sources of vitamin E.

Vitamin E: Reviewing the Basics

Table 8.7 provides a summary of basic information about vitamin E, including Dietary Reference Intake (DRI) recommendations, and major signs and symptoms of the vitamin's deficiency and toxicity disorders.

8.2d Vitamin K

Your liver needs vitamin K to produce four blood-clotting factors. When a blood vessel is cut, the blood in the area of the injury needs to form a clot to stop the bleeding **(Essential Concept 8.2)**. If your body lacks vitamin K, you may experience excessive bleeding because all the blood-clotting factors aren't available. Some people take the prescribed medication *warfarin* because their blood clots too easily. Warfarin decreases vitamin K's ability to form blood clots. Vitamin K can interfere with warfarin's "blood-thinning" activity, so people who take the medication should not use vitamin K supplements.

Vitamin K also helps bone-building cells produce a protein that's needed for healthy bones. Low blood levels of vitamin K are associated with the risk of the bone disorder osteoporosis, but more research is needed to clarify the vitamin's role in bone health.

Essential Concept

8.2 Vitamin K and Blood Clotting

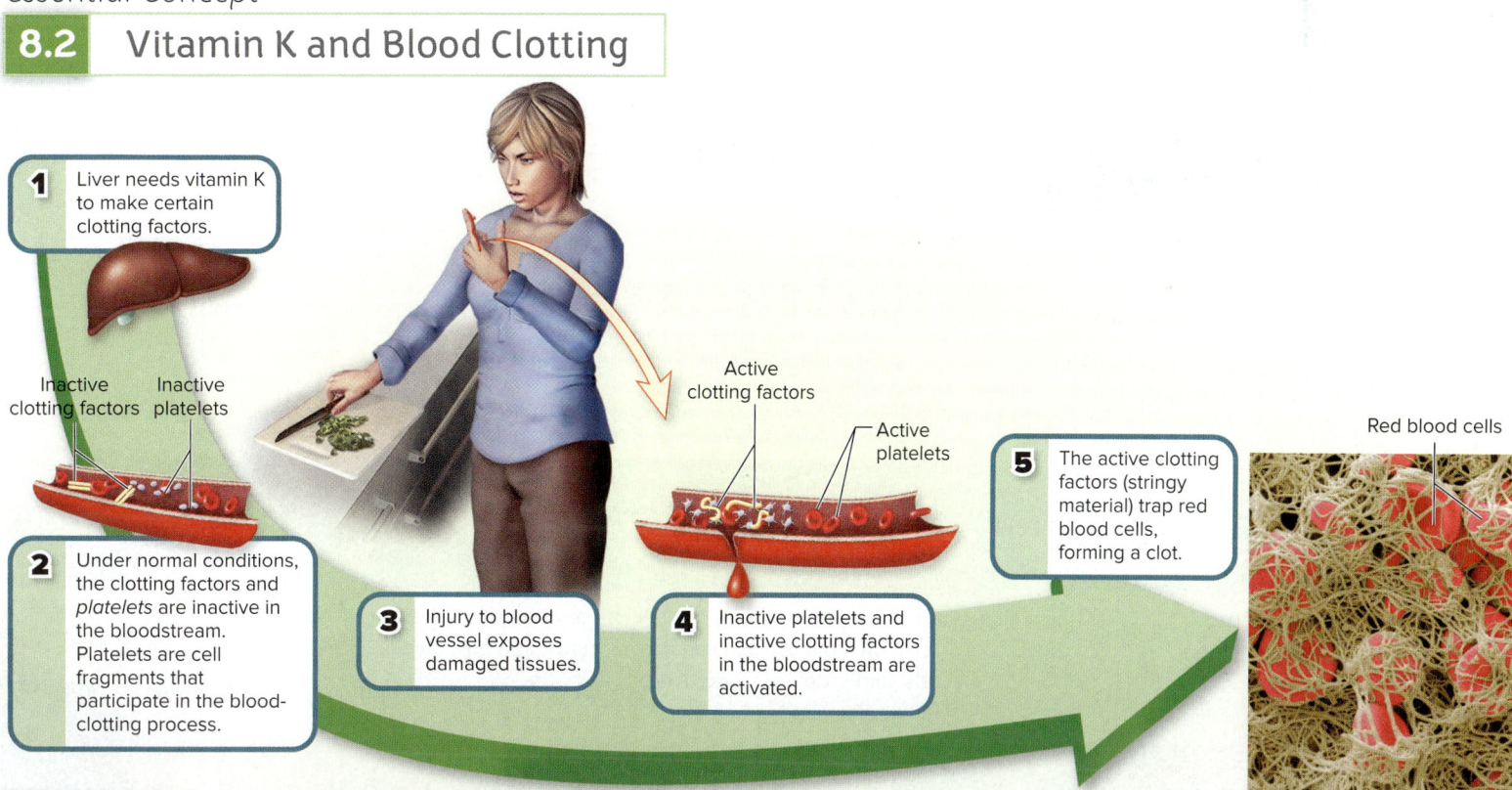

1. Liver needs vitamin K to make certain clotting factors.
2. Under normal conditions, the clotting factors and *platelets* are inactive in the bloodstream. Platelets are cell fragments that participate in the blood-clotting process.
3. Injury to blood vessel exposes damaged tissues.
4. Inactive platelets and inactive clotting factors in the bloodstream are activated.
5. The active clotting factors (stringy material) trap red blood cells, forming a clot.

Peanuts, Mango: Wendy Schiff; Blood clot: Science Photo Library/Alamy

Sources of Vitamin K

Major food sources of vitamin K are green leafy vegetables such as kale, turnip greens, salad greens, cabbage, and spinach. Other reliable sources of the vitamin are soybean and canola oils, and products made from these oils, such as some salad dressings.

Table 8.8 lists some foods that are sources of the vitamin. Vitamin K is very stable and resists being destroyed by usual cooking methods.

Vitamin K Deficiency

Your body stores very little vitamin K, but you're unlikely to become vitamin K–deficient because bacteria that normally live in your large intestine make vitamin K. The intestine may absorb some of the vitamin.[7] Vitamin K deficiency, however, can develop in people who have liver diseases or conditions that impair fat absorption, such as cystic fibrosis. Additionally, long-term antibiotic therapy can reduce the number of bacteria that make vitamin K and, as a result, contribute to a deficiency of the nutrient. The most reliable sign of vitamin K deficiency is an increase in the time it takes for blood to clot.

Infants are born with low amounts of vitamin K in their bodies. Therefore, babies can develop a deficiency of the vitamin soon after birth. Vitamin K–deficient infants are at risk of serious bleeding that can be deadly. To prevent vitamin K deficiency from developing during infancy, newborns generally receive a single injection of vitamin K.

Vitamin K: Reviewing the Basics

Table 8.9 provides a summary of basic information about vitamin K, including Dietary Reference Intake (DRI) recommendations, and major signs and symptoms of the vitamin's deficiency and toxicity disorders.

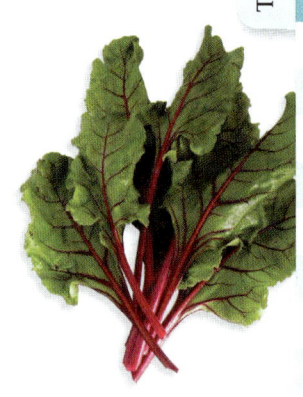

Table 8.8 Vitamin K Content of Selected Foods (Approximate)

Food	Vitamin K (mcg)
Spinach, boiled, drained, ½ cup	444
Beet greens, boiled, drained, ½ cup	348
Turnip greens, boiled, drained, ½ cup	265
Kale, boiled, drained, ½ cup	247
Brussels sprouts, boiled, drained, ½ cup	109
Broccoli, spears, frozen, boiled, drained, ½ cup	92
Spinach, raw, ½ cup	72
Asparagus, frozen, boiled, ½ cup	72
Green beans, frozen, microwaved, ½ cup	32
Cabbage, raw, shredded, ½ cup	27
Soybean oil, 1 Tbsp	25
Lettuce, romaine, shredded, ½ cup	24
Blueberries, raw, ½ cup	14

AI for adult men = 120 mcg/day
AI for adult women = 90 mcg/day

Source: U.S. Department of Agriculture, Agricultural Research Service: *USDA National Nutrient Database for Standard Reference Legacy Release, April 2018.* https://ndb.nal.usda.gov/ndb/search/list?home=true Accessed: September 2018

Table 8.9 Vitamin K

Major Functions in the Body	Adult AI	Major Dietary Sources	Major Deficiency Signs and Symptoms	Major Toxicity Signs and Symptoms
Production of active blood-clotting factors, bone growth	90–120 mcg	Green leafy vegetables, broccoli, soybean and canola oils, and products made from these oils	Easy bruising, bleeding gums, and nosebleeds Excessive bleeding from wounds	Adult UL = undetermined Unknown

Salad greens, Broccoli: Ingram Publishing; Beet greens, Blueberries: Wendy Schiff

Module 8.3

Water-Soluble Vitamins

8.3 - Learning Outcomes

After reading Module 8.3, you should be able to

1. Define all of the **key terms** in this module.
2. Explain how most B vitamins function as coenzymes.
3. List major functions and food sources for each water-soluble vitamin.
4. Describe major deficiency and/or toxicity signs and symptoms for each water-soluble vitamin.

BROWNBERRY
Whole Grains
100% WHOLE WHEAT

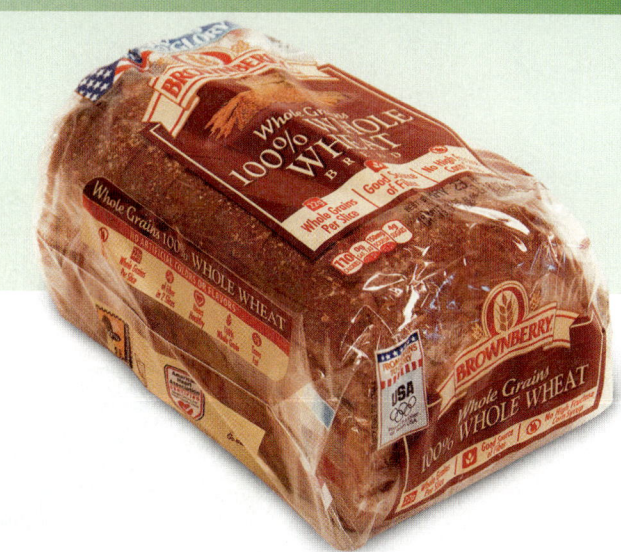

McGraw-Hill Education/Mark A Dierker, photographer

Recall that the water-soluble vitamins are thiamin, riboflavin, niacin, folate, B-6, B-12, pantothenic acid, biotin, and vitamin C. Most water-soluble vitamins have no function unless they're in a coenzyme. **Essential Concept 8.3** describes a coenzyme and how it activates an enzyme.

coenzyme small molecule that interacts with an enzyme, enabling the enzyme to function

Essential Concept

8.3 What's a Coenzyme, and How Does It Function?

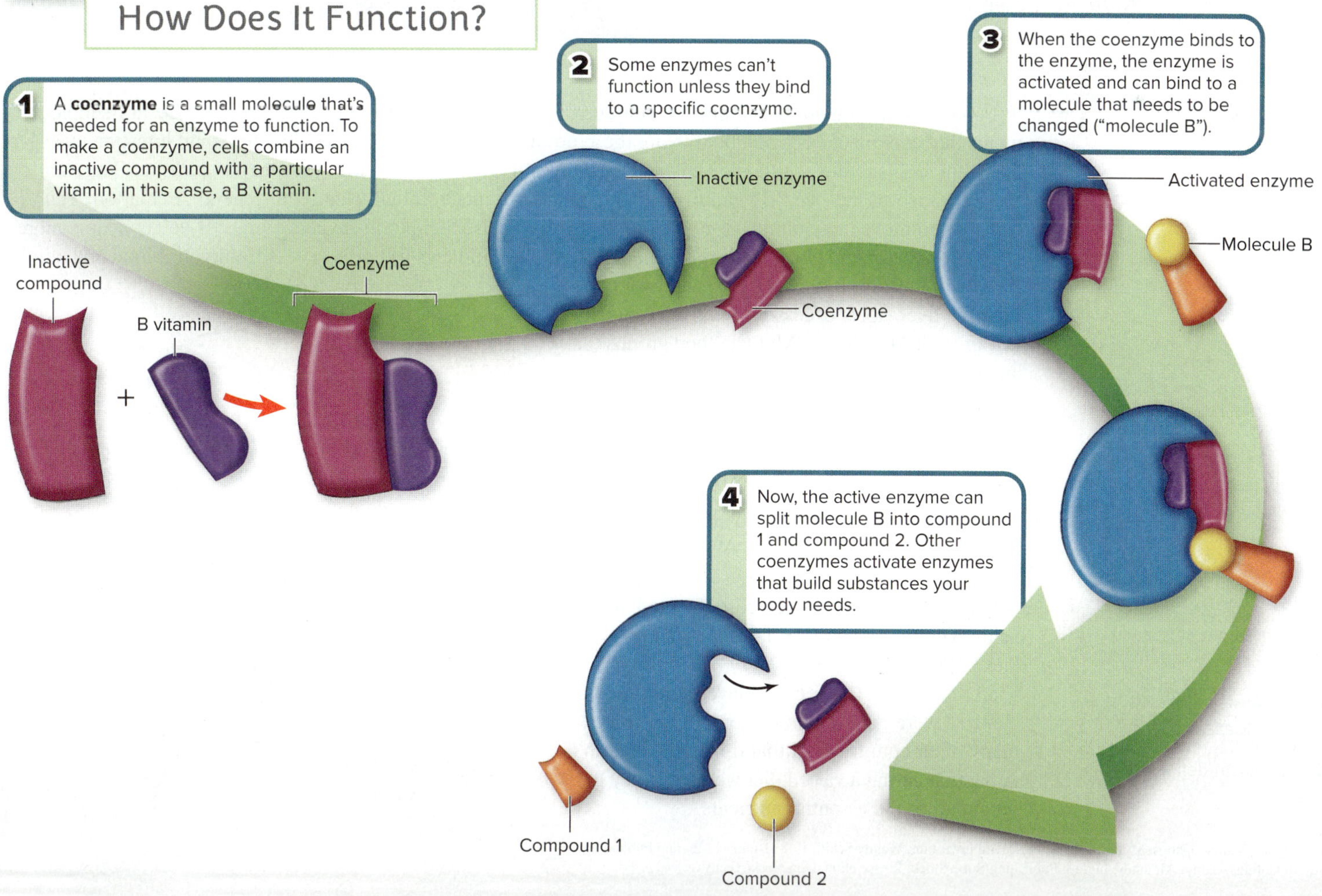

1 A **coenzyme** is a small molecule that's needed for an enzyme to function. To make a coenzyme, cells combine an inactive compound with a particular vitamin, in this case, a B vitamin.
Inactive compound
B vitamin
Coenzyme
2 Some enzymes can't function unless they bind to a specific coenzyme.
Inactive enzyme
Coenzyme
3 When the coenzyme binds to the enzyme, the enzyme is activated and can bind to a molecule that needs to be changed ("molecule B").
Activated enzyme
Molecule B
4 Now, the active enzyme can split molecule B into compound 1 and compound 2. Other coenzymes activate enzymes that build substances your body needs.
Compound 1
Compound 2

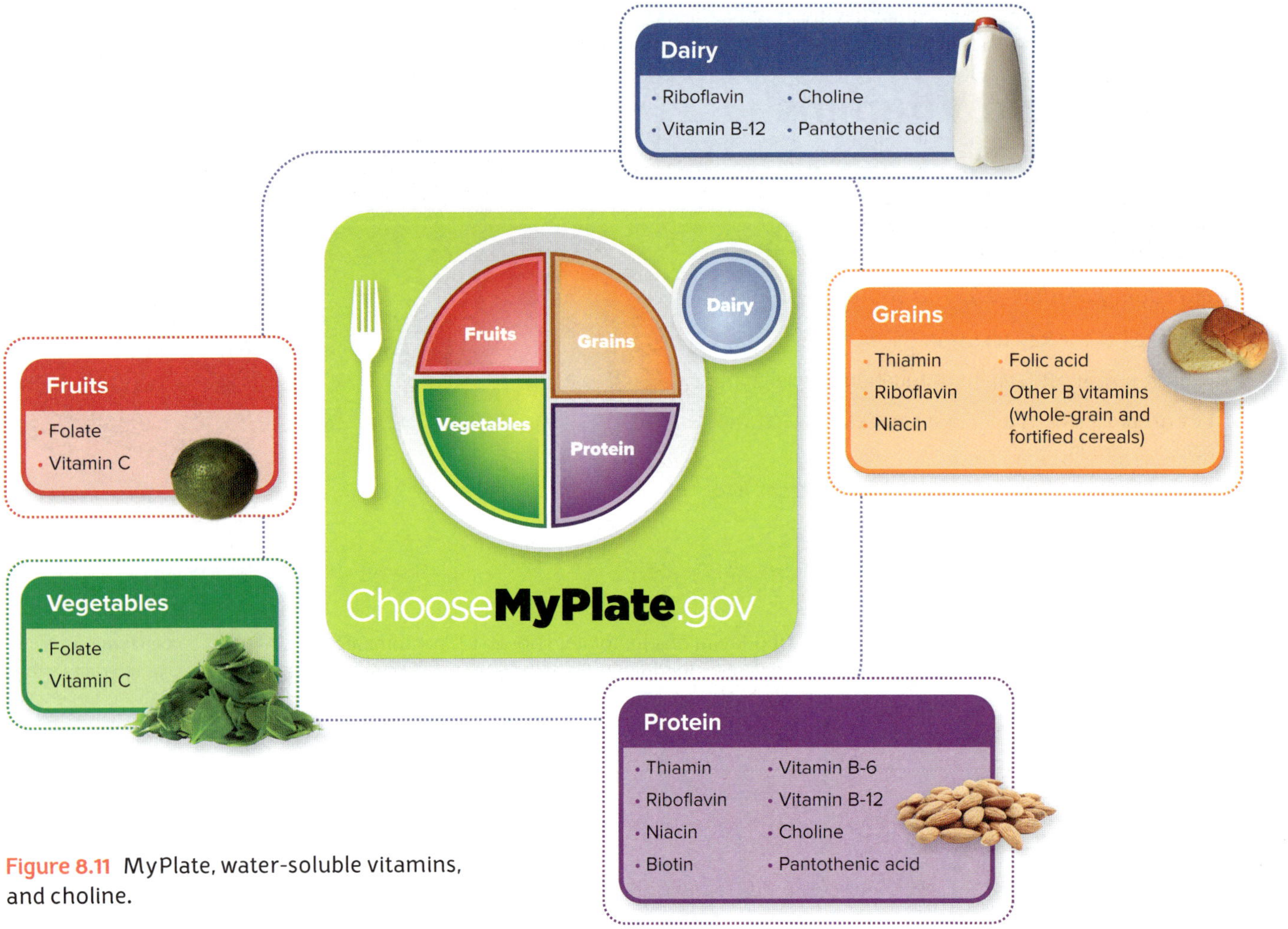

Unit 8 Vitamins: Nutrients That Multitask

Figure 8.11 MyPlate, water-soluble vitamins, and choline.

Dairy
- Riboflavin
- Vitamin B-12
- Choline
- Pantothenic acid

Fruits
- Folate
- Vitamin C

Vegetables
- Folate
- Vitamin C

Grains
- Thiamin
- Riboflavin
- Niacin
- Folic acid
- Other B vitamins (whole-grain and fortified cereals)

Protein
- Thiamin
- Riboflavin
- Niacin
- Biotin
- Vitamin B-6
- Vitamin B-12
- Choline
- Pantothenic acid

Foods usually contain B vitamins in their coenzyme forms. Health-food stores often sell dietary supplements that contain coenzymes, but buying these products is a waste of money. In your small intestine, coenzymes in food and dietary supplements undergo digestion to release their B-vitamin components. The small intestine absorbs the freed B vitamins, and the micronutrients eventually enter the general circulation. Your cells then remove the vitamins from the bloodstream and use them to make coenzymes. If you consume more coenzymes or water-soluble vitamins than you need, your kidneys filter the excess from your blood and eliminate them in urine. Vitamin B-12 is a major exception; the liver stores excesses of this micronutrient.

Figure 8.11 indicates MyPlate food groups that are good sources of water-soluble vitamins. This section of Unit 8 focuses on the eight water-soluble vitamins and the vitamin-like nutrient choline.

8.3a The Power Player Vitamins

Thiamin, riboflavin, and niacin are B vitamins that we refer to as "power players." Why? Your cells need these micronutrients to make coenzymes that help release energy from glucose, fat, and amino acids. Therefore, you'll feel tired if your body lacks the power players.

In the early 1900s, power player vitamin deficiencies were common in the United States and many other countries. At that time, people didn't know that eating a varied diet was necessary to obtain all of the essential nutrients.

beriberi thiamin deficiency disease

ariboflavinosis riboflavin deficiency disease

pellagra niacin deficiency disease

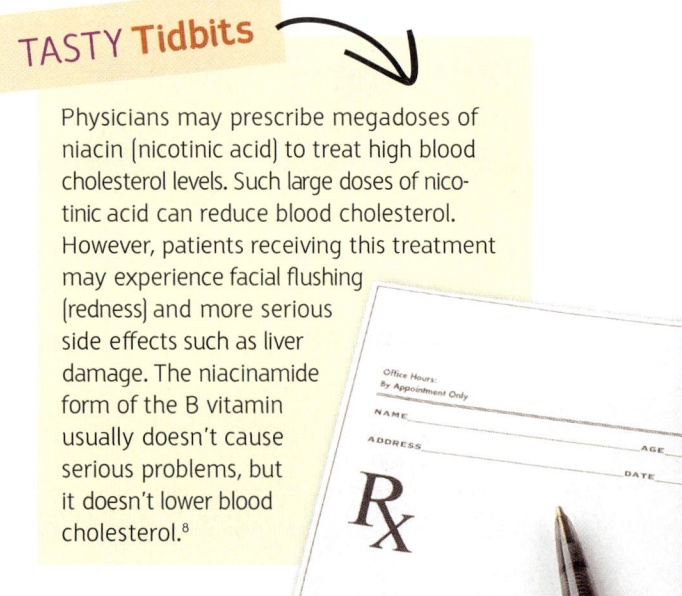

TASTY Tidbits

Physicians may prescribe megadoses of niacin (nicotinic acid) to treat high blood cholesterol levels. Such large doses of nicotinic acid can reduce blood cholesterol. However, patients receiving this treatment may experience facial flushing (redness) and more serious side effects such as liver damage. The niacinamide form of the B vitamin usually doesn't cause serious problems, but it doesn't lower blood cholesterol.[8]

Choose MyPlate: Source: ChooseMyPlate.gov; Lime, Hamburger bun: Wendy Schiff; Pile of spinach: Ingram Publishing; Milk: Judith Collins/Alamy; Almonds: Ingram Publishing/SuperStock; Prescription: Comstock/Alamy

The thiamin deficiency disease is called **beriberi**; **ariboflavinosis** is the riboflavin deficiency disorder; the niacin deficiency disease is **pellagra** (*peh-lah'-gra* or *peh-lay'-gra*).

People suffering from beriberi are very weak, and they have poor muscular coordination. Ariboflavinosis causes muscle weakness and inflamed eyes and mouth. The classic signs and symptoms of severe pellagra are *dermatitis* (scaly, reddened skin), *diarrhea, dementia* (loss of normal thinking abilities), and *death*—the "4 Ds of pellagra" (**Fig. 8.12**). In the 1940s, the introduction of the enrichment program, which added these vitamins to grains, greatly reduced the number of people suffering from beriberi, ariboflavinosis, and pellagra in the United States. Today, Americans generally consume adequate amounts of thiamin, riboflavin, and niacin.[1]

Food Sources of Power Player Vitamins

Whole-grain and enriched breads and cereals are among the best sources of the power player vitamins. Milk, yogurt, and other milk products are among the best sources of riboflavin. Exposure to light causes the vitamin to break down rapidly. Therefore, riboflavin-rich foods, such as milk and milk products, shouldn't be kept in clear glass containers. Niacin is very heat stable, so food retains much of its niacin content during usual preparation and cooking methods. **Tables 8.10, 8.11,** and **8.12** list rich sources of thiamin, riboflavin, and niacin, respectively.

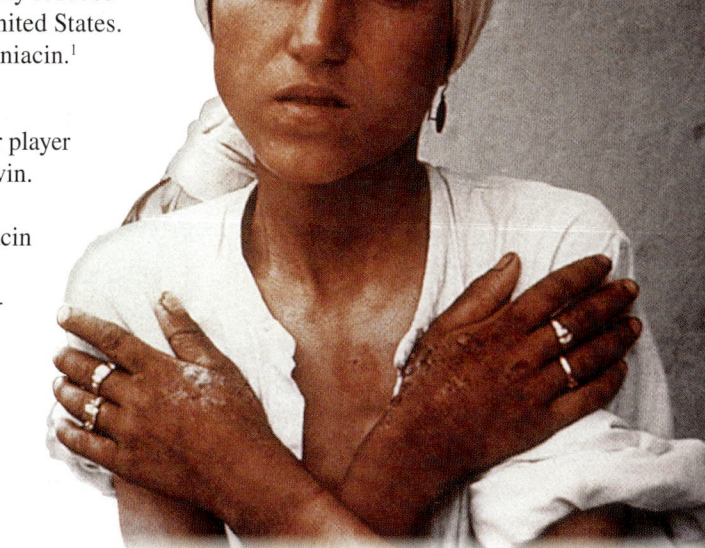

Figure 8.12 Pellagra.

■ *What are the "4 Ds of pellagra"?*

Table 8.10 — Thiamin Content of Selected Foods (Approximate)

Food	Thiamin (mg)
Pork blade steak, grilled, 3 oz	.59
Ham, deli slices, 3 oz	.53
Flour tortilla, 10" diameter, 1	.36
White bread, enriched, 1 slice	.28
Cooked green peas, frozen, boiled, drained, ½ cup	.27
Wheat germ, toasted, 1 Tbsp	.15
Whole-wheat bread, 1 slice	.13
Baked beans, canned, ½ cup	.12
Orange juice, frozen, unsweetened, diluted, ½ cup	.07

RDA for adult women = 1.1 mg/day
RDA for adult men = 1.2 mg/day

Source: U.S. Department of Agriculture, Agricultural Research Service: *USDA National Nutrient Database for Standard Reference Legacy Release, April 2018.* https://ndb.nal.usda.gov/ndb/search/list?home=true Accessed: September 2018

Woman with pellagra: Centers for Disease Control and Prevention; Ham slices, Tortilla: Wendy Schiff; Peas: Ingram Publishing/SuperStock

Table 8.11 Riboflavin Content of Selected Foods (Approximate)

Food	Riboflavin (mg)
Beef liver, braised, 3 oz	2.9
Wheaties™ cereal, 3 oz	2.4
Chicken liver, pan fried, 3 oz	2.0
All-Bran® wheat flakes cereal, ¾ cup	1.7
Cottage cheese, 2% fat, 1 cup	0.6
Yogurt, plain, low-fat, 6 oz	0.4
Milk, fat-free, 1 cup	0.4
Almonds, dry roasted, 1 oz	0.3
Mushrooms, large, white, raw, 3	0.3
Spinach, boiled and drained, ½ cup	0.2
Chicken, meat only, roasted, diced, 1 cup	0.2

RDA for adult women = 1.1 mg/day
RDA for adult men = 1.3 mg/day

Source: U.S. Department of Agriculture, Agricultural Research Service: *USDA National Nutrient Database for Standard Reference Legacy Release, April 2018.* https://ndb.nal.usda.gov/ndb/search/list?home=true Accessed: September 2018

Table 8.12 Niacin Content of Selected Foods (Approximate)

Food	Niacin (mg)
Beef liver, braised, 3 oz	14.9
Chicken, breast meat, roasted, 3 oz	11.6
Turkey, meat only, roasted, 3 oz	8.10
Pork loin, roasted, 3 oz	6.18
Quaker Oat Life®, plain, ready-to-eat cereal, ¾ cup	5.50
Peanuts, dry roasted, ¼ cup	5.24
Raisin bran, ready-to-eat cereal, 1 cup	5.00
Tuna, canned in water, drained, 3 oz	4.93
Potato, baked with skin, 6 oz	2.60
White rice, enriched, cooked, ½ cup	1.17
Macaroni, enriched, elbow, cooked, ½ cup	1.01

RDA for adult women = 14 mg/day, RDA for adult men = 16 mg/day
Source: U.S. Department of Agriculture, Agricultural Research Service: *USDA National Nutrient Database for Standard Reference Legacy Release, April 2018.* https://ndb.nal.usda.gov/ndb/search/list?home=true Accessed: September 2018

Bowl of cereal flakes, Chicken, Cottage cheese, Tuna, Bowl of cereal squares: Wendy Schiff

Nutrition Fact or Fiction?

When it comes to taking niacin, more is better.

High doses of vitamin supplements or medications, particularly those that contain niacin, can be quite toxic. In rare cases, liver damage, and even liver failure, can result from niacin toxicity.[9] In one reported case, a 17-year-old male followed advice that he obtained on the Internet concerning a nonnutritional use of niacin supplements. According to the Internet sources, high doses of niacin interfere with the reliability of urine testing to detect recent marijuana use. The teenager took very high doses of niacin prior to having his urine screened for the presence of illegal drugs. As a result, he experienced abnormal liver function that was serious enough to require hospitalization.[10] Fortunately, the young man recovered without the need for a liver transplant. It is important to note that there's no reliable scientific evidence that supports taking niacin to hide drug use during urine testing.

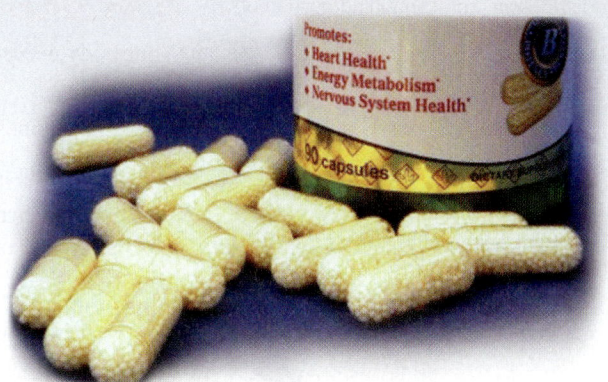

Wendy Schiff

Reviewing the Basics: Power Player Vitamins

Table 8.13 summarizes information about the power player vitamins. The table includes Dietary Reference Intake (DRI) recommendations and major signs and symptoms of the vitamins' deficiency and toxicity disorders.

TABLE 8.13 — THIAMIN, RIBOFLAVIN, AND NIACIN: THE POWER PLAYER VITAMINS

Vitamin	Major Functions in the Body	Adult RDA	Major Dietary Sources	Major Deficiency Signs and Symptoms	Major Toxicity Signs and Symptoms
Thiamin	Part of a coenzyme needed for energy metabolism	1.1–1.2 mg	Pork, wheat germ, enriched breads and cereals	Beriberi	None (Upper Level [UL] not determined)
Riboflavin	Part of coenzymes needed for energy metabolism	1.1–1.3 mg	Milk and other milk products, enriched breads and cereals, liver	Ariboflavinosis	None (UL not determined)
Niacin	Part of coenzymes needed for energy metabolism	14–16 mg	Enriched breads and cereals, beef, liver, tuna, poultry, pork, mushrooms	Pellagra	Adult UL = 35 mg/day. Flushing of facial skin, liver damage

McGraw-Hill Education/Mark A Dierker, photographer

heme iron-containing portion of hemoglobin

hemoglobin protein in red blood cells that transports oxygen

homocysteine a toxic amino acid

8.3b Vitamin B-6: Amino Acid Manager

Your body needs vitamin B-6 to make a coenzyme that's involved in amino acid metabolism. The coenzyme is needed to

- make nonessential amino acids;
- make glucose from certain amino acids;
- produce **heme,** the iron-containing portion of hemoglobin. **Hemoglobin** is the protein in red blood cells that transports oxygen;
- make proteins that transmit messages between nerves; and
- convert a toxic amino acid **homocysteine** to a nonessential amino acid. If the body lacks vitamin B-6, homocysteine can accumulate in blood. High homocysteine levels may contribute to cardiovascular disease.

TASTY Tidbits

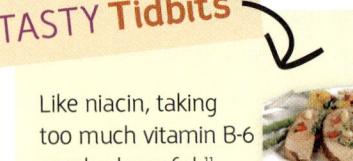

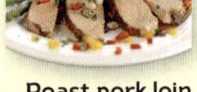

Roast pork loin

Like niacin, taking too much vitamin B-6 can be harmful.[11] Vitamin B-6 causes severe nerve damage when taken in doses that exceed the UL (100 mg/day) for extended periods. Signs and symptoms of vitamin B-6 toxicity include walking difficulties and numbness of the hands and feet. The nerve damage usually resolves when the affected person stops taking vitamin B-6 supplements. The foods shown in Table 8.14, including pork loin, supply safe amounts of vitamin B-6.

Food Sources of Vitamin B-6

Liver, meat, fish, and poultry are among the best dietary sources of vitamin B-6. Additionally, potatoes and bananas are good sources of the vitamin. During the refining process, the vitamin B-6 that's naturally in grains is lost, and the nutrient isn't added back to the grain products during enrichment. However, many ready-to-eat and cooked cereals have been fortified with the vitamin. **Table 8.14** lists some foods that supply vitamin B-6. During cooking, excessive heat can cause major losses of the vitamin. Nevertheless, most Americans consume adequate amounts of vitamin B-6.[1]

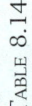

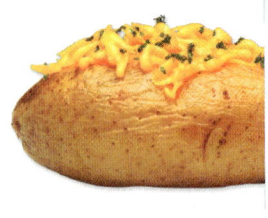

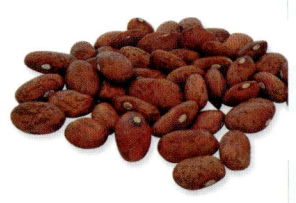

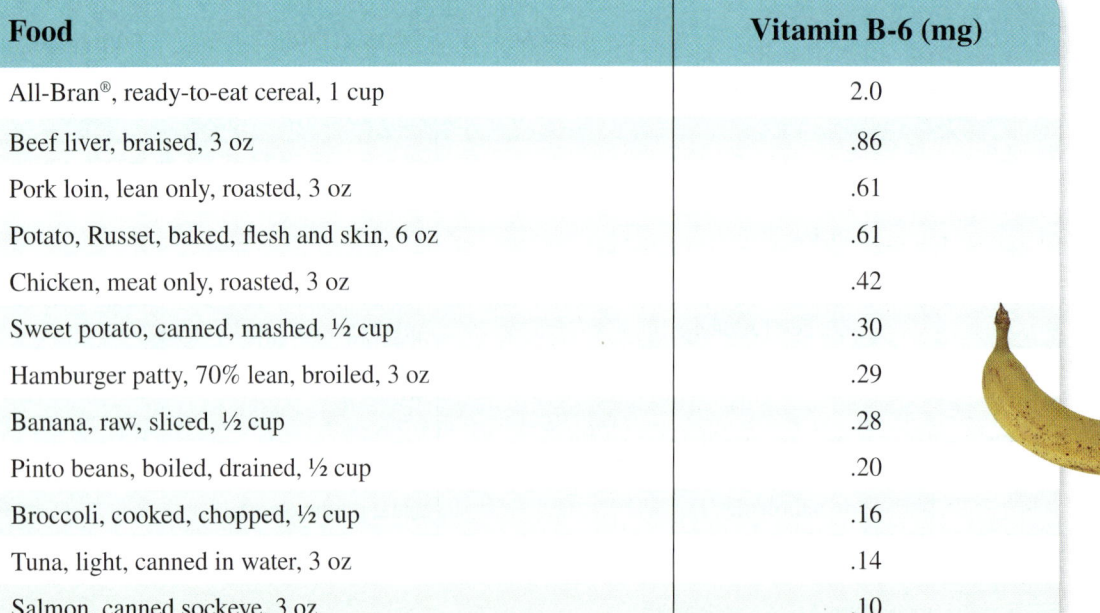

TABLE 8.14 VITAMIN B-6 CONTENT OF SELECTED FOODS (APPROXIMATE)

Food	Vitamin B-6 (mg)
All-Bran®, ready-to-eat cereal, 1 cup	2.0
Beef liver, braised, 3 oz	.86
Pork loin, lean only, roasted, 3 oz	.61
Potato, Russet, baked, flesh and skin, 6 oz	.61
Chicken, meat only, roasted, 3 oz	.42
Sweet potato, canned, mashed, ½ cup	.30
Hamburger patty, 70% lean, broiled, 3 oz	.29
Banana, raw, sliced, ½ cup	.28
Pinto beans, boiled, drained, ½ cup	.20
Broccoli, cooked, chopped, ½ cup	.16
Tuna, light, canned in water, 3 oz	.14
Salmon, canned sockeye, 3 oz	.10

RDA for adult women = 1.3 mg/day, RDA for adult men = 1.7 mg/day

Source: U.S. Department of Agriculture, Agricultural Research Service: *USDA National Nutrient Database for Standard Reference Legacy Release, April 2018.* https://ndb.nal.usda.gov/ndb/search/list?home=true Accessed: September 2018

Banana, Beans, Mixed meats: Wendy Schiff; Baked potato with cheese: Ingram Publishing/Alamy; Pork loins: Ingram Publishing/SuperStock

Table 8.15 Vitamin B-6

Major Functions in the Body	Adult RDA	Major Dietary Sources	Major Deficiency Signs and Symptoms	Major Toxicity Signs and Symptoms
Part of coenzyme needed for amino acid metabolism and production of heme and chemicals that nerves use to transmit information	1.3–1.7 mg	Beef, pork, fish, and poultry; potatoes, bananas, broccoli, fortified cereals	Dermatitis, anemia, depression and confusion, swollen tongue	Adult UL = 100 mg/day; Nerve destruction, skin sores, nausea, and heartburn

Reviewing the Basics: Vitamin B-6

Table 8.15 summarizes information about vitamin B-6. The table includes Dietary Reference Intake (DRI) recommendations, major food sources, and major signs and symptoms of the vitamin's deficiency and toxicity disorders.

8.3c Folate and Vitamin B-12: DNA Duo

Certain roles of folate and vitamin B-12 are interrelated, but these B vitamins also have unique functions in your body. *Folate* refers to a family of related compounds that includes **folic acid** and naturally occurring **food folate.** Folic acid is the form of folate that's in dietary supplements, and it's used to fortify foods.

Your cells need folate to make coenzymes involved in DNA production. Vitamin B-12 is needed to make a coenzyme involved in folate metabolism. Most of a cell's DNA is in the nucleus. Before a cell can divide, its nucleus needs to make enough DNA for the two new cells that are produced. Thus, a person's requirements for folate and vitamin B-12 are high during periods of rapid growth, such as before birth, and in pregnancy, infancy, and childhood.

Initially, folate and vitamin B-12 deficiencies affect cells that rapidly divide, such as red blood cells (RBCs). Mature RBCs don't have nuclei, and they live for only about 4 months. Thus, your body must replace old or worn-out RBCs constantly. To keep up with their rapid rate of cell division, the cells that mature into RBCs (RBC precursors) must make DNA. Without vitamin B-12 and folate, RBC precursor cells that are in your bone marrow enlarge, but they cannot divide normally because they're unable to form new DNA. The bone marrow releases some of the abnormal RBCs into your bloodstream before they mature (**Essential Concept 8.4**). This condition, called **megaloblastic** (*mega* = large; *blast* = immature cell) **anemia,** is characterized by large, immature RBCs (megaloblasts) that still have nuclei and don't carry normal amounts of oxygen (see Essential Concept 8.4).

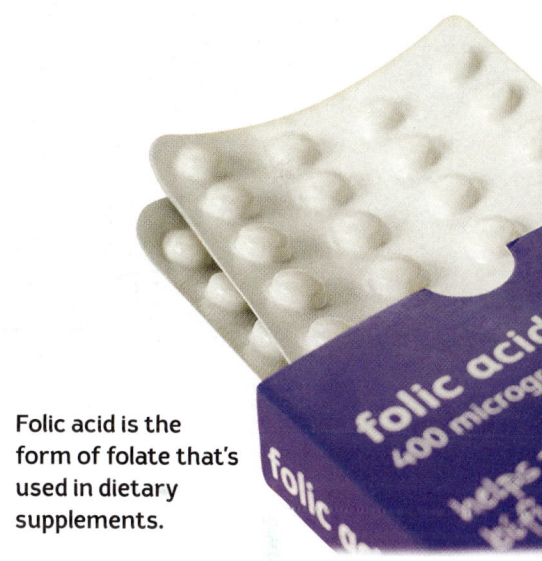

Folic acid is the form of folate that's used in dietary supplements.

Banana Stock/PunchStock

Another important function of folate and vitamin B-12 is related to amino acid metabolism. The two B vitamins work together to make the amino acid methionine from the toxic amino acid homocysteine. Recall that vitamin B-6 also helps convert homocysteine to methionine.

Cells need vitamin B-12 to protect the covering over many nerves. When cells lack the vitamin, the nerves become damaged. Such damage may result in the loss of ability to walk properly.[12]

folic acid and **food folate** forms of folate

megaloblastic anemia condition characterized by fewer and abnormal red blood cells

Essential Concept

8.4 Red Blood Cell Production Needs Folate and B-12

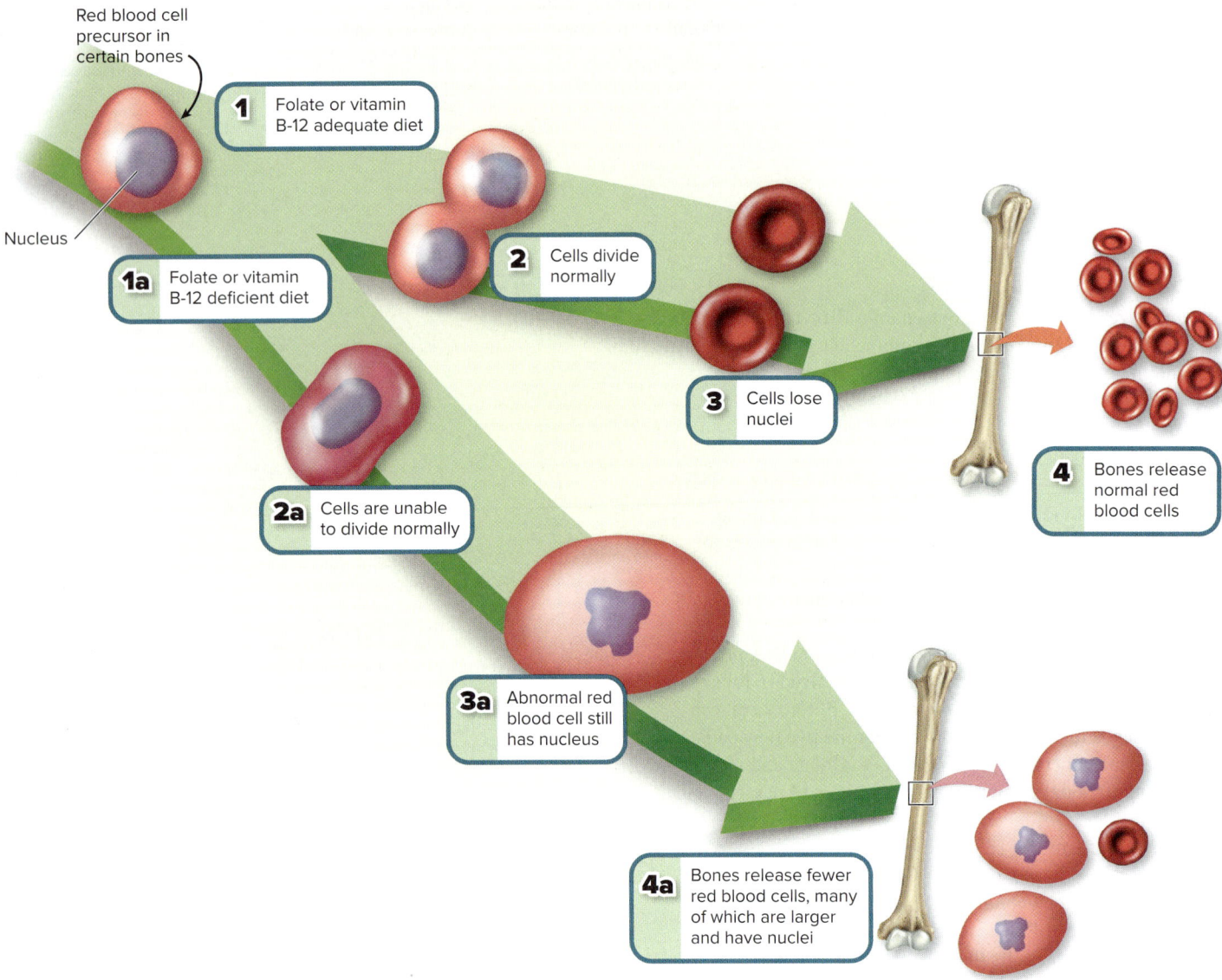

Food Sources of Folate and Vitamin B-12

Green leafy vegetables, enriched grain products, and fortified cereals are among the richest sources of folate in the American diet. **Table 8.16** lists some foods and their folate contents, which are reported as micrograms of dietary folate equivalents (DFEs).

Plants don't make vitamin B-12, so we rely almost entirely on animal foods to supply the vitamin naturally. Major sources of vitamin B-12 in the typical American's diet are meat, milk and milk products, poultry, fish, shellfish, and eggs. Although liver isn't a popular food, it's one of the richest sources of vitamin B-12. Many soy products, such as soy milk, and ready-to-eat cereals are fortified with vitamin B-12. **Table 8.17** lists some foods that are good sources of this micronutrient.

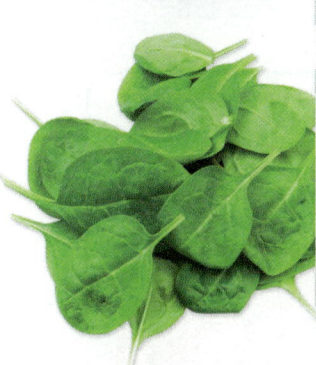

Table 8.16 Folate Content of Selected Foods (Approximate)

Food	Folate (mcg DFE)
Chicken liver, pan fried, 3 oz	476
Special K™, ready-to-eat cereal, ¾ cup	300
Asparagus (frozen), cooked, drained, ½ cup	122
Turnip greens, boiled, drained, chopped, ½ cup	85
White rice, long-grain, cooked, enriched, ½ cup	77
Spinach, raw, 1 cup	58
English muffin, plain, toasted, enriched, 1	57
Kidney beans, cooked, ½ cup	46
Papaya, raw, mashed, ½ cup	43
Orange sections, 1 cup	31
Broccoli, raw, chopped, ½ cup	29

RDA for adults = 400 mcg (DFE)/day; RDA for pregnant women = 600 mcg (DFE)/day
Source: U.S. Department of Agriculture, Agricultural Research Service: *USDA National Nutrient Database for Standard Reference Legacy Release, April 2018.* https://ndb.nal.usda.gov/ndb/search/list?home=true Accessed: September 2018

Table 8.17 Vitamin B-12 Content of Selected Foods (Approximate)

Food	Vitamin B-12 (mcg)
Beef liver, cooked, 3 oz	60.0
Chicken liver, cooked, 3 oz	14.3
Sardines, canned in oil, drained, 3 oz	7.60
Salmon, sockeye, canned, 3 oz	4.67
Special K™, ready-to-eat cereal, ¾ cup	4.51
Ground beef patty, 80% lean, cooked, 3 oz	2.32
Raisin bran, ready-to-eat cereal, ¾ cup	1.11
Tuna, light, canned in water, drained, 3 oz	0.99
Milk, fat-free, 1 cup	0.96
Egg, scrambled, 1 large	0.46

RDA for adults = 2.4 mcg/day
Source: U.S. Department of Agriculture, Agricultural Research Service: *USDA National Nutrient Database for Standard Reference Legacy Release, April 2018.* https://ndb.nal.usda.gov/ndb/search/list?home=true Accessed: September 2018

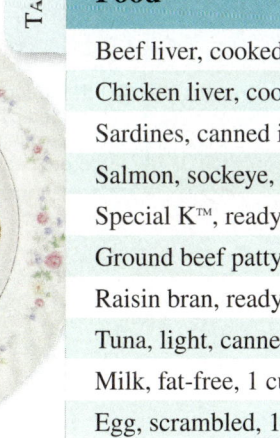

Beef liver

Absorbing Vitamin B-12

Absorbing the vitamin B-12 that's naturally in foods requires a complex series of steps that are unique for a vitamin (see **Essential Concept 8.5**).

Bowl of cereal, Asparagus, Beef liver: Wendy Schiff; Baby spinach leaves: daniel vincek/123RF

Essential Concept

8.5 Absorbing the Vitamin B-12 in Your Food

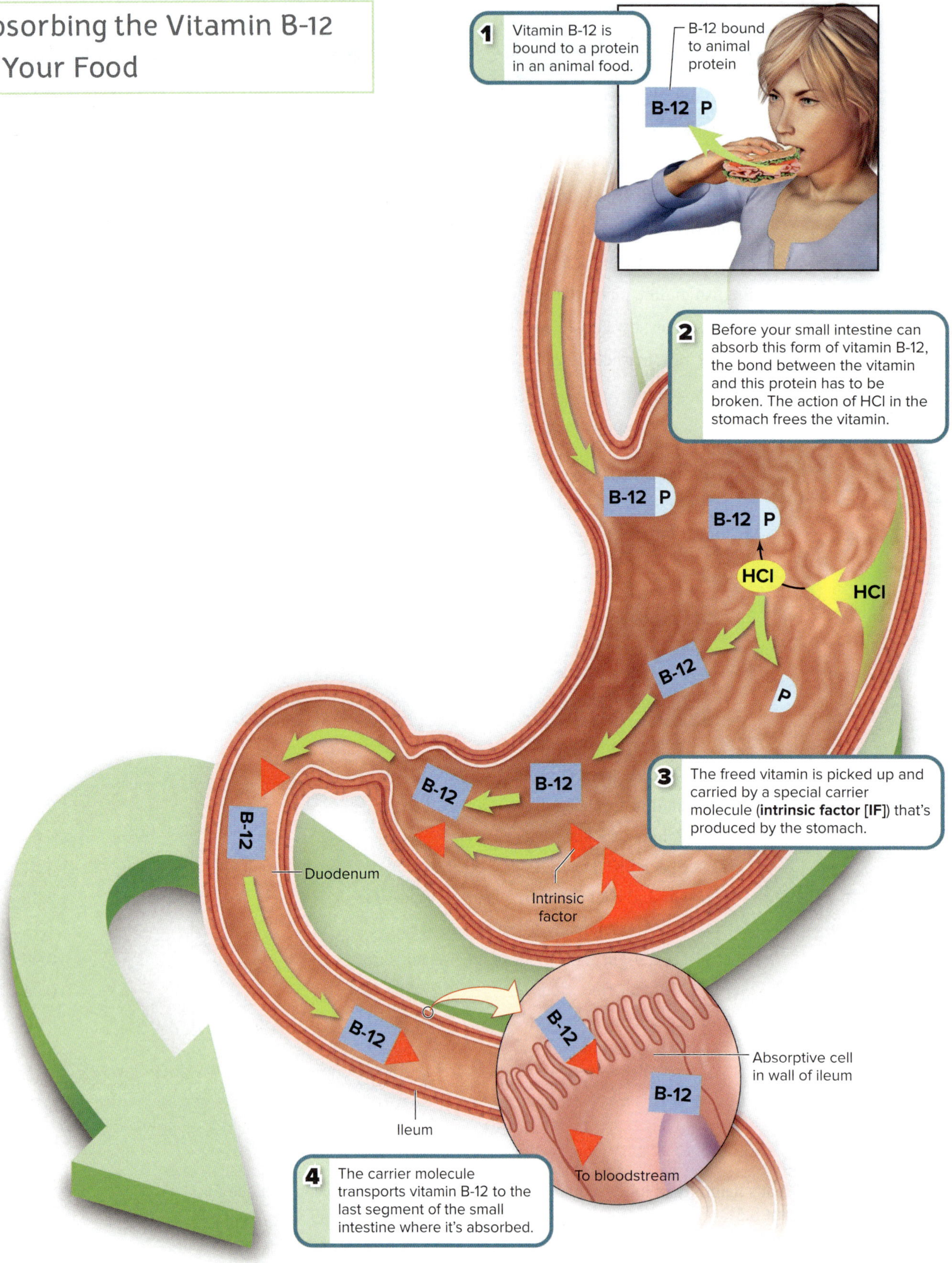
1 Vitamin B-12 is bound to a protein in an animal food.
B-12 bound to animal protein
B-12 P
2 Before your small intestine can absorb this form of vitamin B-12, the bond between the vitamin and this protein has to be broken. The action of HCl in the stomach frees the vitamin.
B-12 P
B-12 P
HCl
HCl
B-12
P
B-12
B-12
B-12
Duodenum
Intrinsic factor
3 The freed vitamin is picked up and carried by a special carrier molecule (**intrinsic factor [IF]**) that's produced by the stomach.
B-12
B-12
B-12
Absorptive cell in wall of ileum
Ileum
To bloodstream
4 The carrier molecule transports vitamin B-12 to the last segment of the small intestine where it's absorbed.

intrinsic factor (IF) substance produced in the stomach that helps vitamin B-12 absorption

Unlike the other B vitamins, the liver stores excesses of vitamin B-12. A healthy liver has enough vitamin B-12 reserves to last 5 to 10 years.[13] Therefore, a person who follows a diet that completely lacks vitamin B-12 may not develop the vitamin's deficiency disorder for as long as 10 years.

Folate and Vitamin B-12 Deficiencies

If you develop megaloblastic anemia, it's important to determine whether you have a deficiency of folate or B-12. Taking folic acid supplements for a vitamin B-12 deficiency doesn't help protect your nerves.

What Are Neural Tube Defects? For pregnant women, the RDA is 600 mcg (DFE), which is 50% higher than the RDA for women who aren't pregnant. However, it's very important for a woman to have adequate folate in her body when she *becomes* pregnant. An embryo undergoes extremely rapid cell division, so it has a very high need for folate.

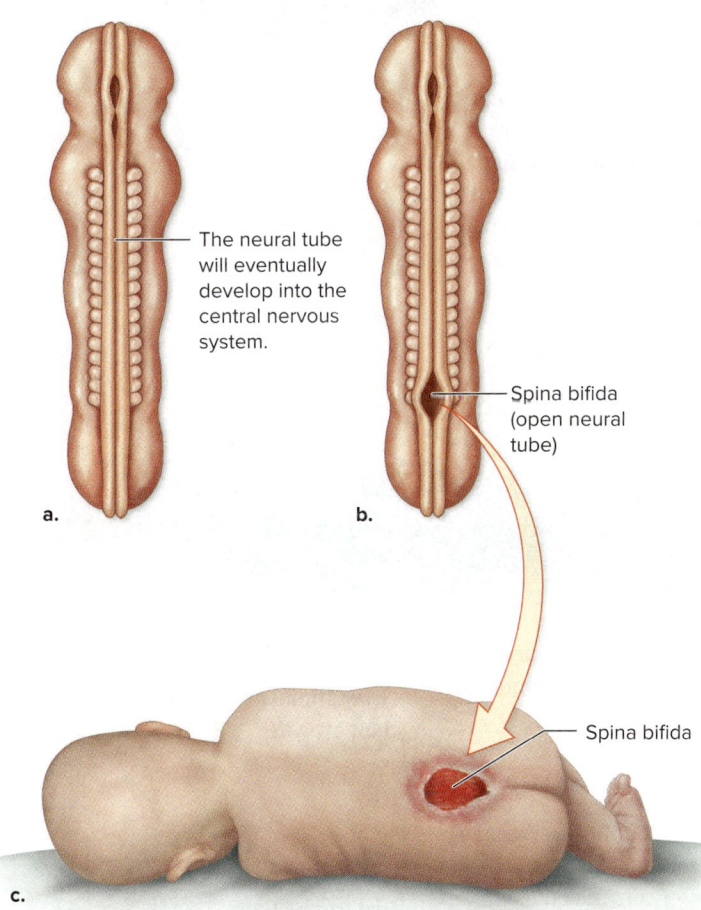

Figure 8.13 Neural tube formation. (a) Normal neural tube in a human embryo. (b) Open neural tube. (c) Newborn with severe spina bifida.

neural tube embryonic structure that eventually develops into the brain and spinal cord

spina bifida type of neural tube defect in which the spine doesn't form properly before birth and it fails to enclose the spinal cord

pernicious anemia condition caused by the lack of intrinsic factor

During the first few weeks after conception, the **neural tube** forms in the embryo **(Fig. 8.13)**. The neural tube develops into the brain and spinal cord. Pregnant women who are deficient in folate have a high risk of giving birth to infants with neural tube defects, such as **spina bifida** (spy'-na bif'-eh-dah). Spina bifida occurs when the embryo's spine doesn't form properly and the bones fail to enclose the spinal cord. Infants with severe spina bifida can have a section of their spinal cord bulging through an opening in their backs (see Figure 8.13). Often, people with severe spina bifida are unable to walk independently. Each year, over 1600 babies are born with spina bifida in the United States.[14] The good news: Cases of spina bifida have declined sharply since enrichment of foods with folic acid began in 1999.

Because women of childbearing age may become pregnant at some point, they need to be aware of the link between neural tube defects and the lack of folate. In addition to including folate-rich foods in their diets, women can prepare for pregnancy by taking a daily multivitamin supplement that contains 400 mcg of synthetic folic acid.

Megaloblastic Anemia Your body replaces old red blood cells (RBCs) constantly. Therefore, the cells that divide to form red blood cells have high folate and vitamin B-12 needs. Without these B vitamins, the body produces large, immature RBCs that don't carry oxygen properly (see Essential Concept 8.4).

Megaloblastic anemia is a sign of both folate and vitamin B-12 deficiencies. Common signs and symptoms of vitamin B-12 deficiency include

- muscle weakness,
- sore mouth,
- smooth and shiny tongue,
- memory loss and confusion,
- difficulty walking and maintaining balance, and
- numbness and tingling sensations, particularly in legs and feet.

What's Pernicious Anemia? Approximately 2% of people who are over 60 years of age have an *autoimmune* disorder that causes inflammation and destruction of the cells in the stomach that produce intrinsic factor, the special vitamin B-12 carrier molecule.[12] (An autoimmune disorder results when a person's immune system attacks his or her own cells.) In these cases, diets may supply adequate amounts of vitamin B-12, but there's no carrier molecule to help the intestine absorb the micronutrient. Eventually, a person with this condition develops **pernicious** ("deadly") **anemia,** a form of anemia that features megaloblastic red blood cells and nerve damage. As its name implies, pernicious anemia can be deadly. Treatment involves bypassing the need for intestinal absorption, usually by providing routine vitamin B-12 injections.

Family history is a risk factor for pernicious anemia. Therefore, consider having your blood tested for signs of vitamin B-12 deficiency as you grow older, especially if you have a close relative with pernicious anemia.

Vitamin B-12 Deficiency in Older Adults Vitamin B-12 deficiency usually occurs in older adults and results from conditions that interfere with intestinal absorption of the vitamin in foods and not from inadequate intakes.[12] As people age, the production of hydrochloric acid (HCl) in the stomach declines. Thus, many older adults are unable to release vitamin B-12 from the protein to which it's bound in food. People with this condition develop vitamin B-12 deficiency despite consuming diets that contain the vitamin. In addition to advanced age, alcoholism, gastric bypass surgeries for weight reduction, and medications that reduce stomach acid production can contribute to a deficiency of the vitamin. Older adults with reduced stomach acid can take dietary supplements that contain synthetic vitamin B-12 because this form of the vitamin doesn't require the action of stomach acid. Vegans should also be concerned about the need for vitamin B-12 because plant foods aren't natural sources of the vitamin. For more information about vitamin B-12 and vegetarians, see the "What's Vegetarianism?" section of Unit 7.

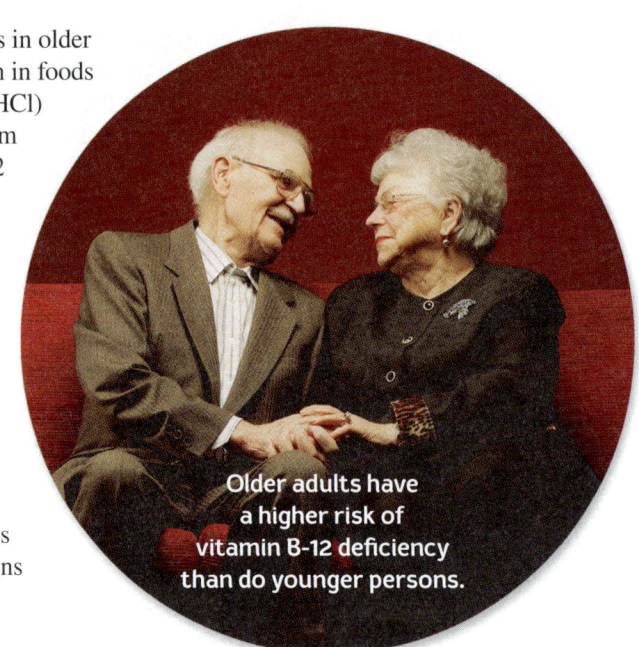

Older adults have a higher risk of vitamin B-12 deficiency than do younger persons.

Reviewing the Basics: DNA Duo

Table 8.18 summarizes information about folate and vitamin B-12. The table includes Dietary Reference Intake (DRI) recommendations, major food sources, and major signs and symptoms of the vitamins' deficiency and toxicity disorders.

8.3d Pantothenic Acid, Biotin, and Choline

Pantothenic acid, biotin, and the vitamin-like nutrient choline are in a wide variety of foods. Therefore, deficiencies of these micronutrients are uncommon, especially among healthy adults who eat items from all food groups regularly. Furthermore, bacteria that normally live in the human large intestine make biotin, and the intestine may absorb some of the vitamin. It is important to note that pregnant women who don't consume enough choline during pregnancy have a high risk of delivering babies with birth defects, such as neural tube defects. For more information about neural tube defects, see section 8.3c. **Table 8.19** summarizes basic information about pantothenic acid, biotin, and choline.

TABLE 8.18 FOLATE AND VITAMIN B-12

Major Functions in the Body	Adult RDA	Major Dietary Sources	Major Deficiency Signs and Symptoms	Major Toxicity Signs and Symptoms
Folate Part of coenzyme needed for DNA metabolism, preventing homocysteine accumulation	400 mcg DFE	Green leafy vegetables, liver, legumes, asparagus, broccoli, orange juice, enriched breads and cereals (folic acid)	Megaloblastic anemia, neural tube defects in embryos	Adult UL = 1000 mcg/day May stimulate cancer cell growth
Vitamin B-12 Part of coenzymes needed for various cellular processes, including folate metabolism and maintenance of healthy nerves	2.4 mcg	Animal foods, fortified cereals, fortified soy milk	Pernicious anemia: megaloblastic anemia and nerve damage resulting in paralysis and death	None (UL not determined)

Liverwurst (liver sausage)

Older adult couple: Kelly Redinger/Design Pics; Peas and pea pod: C Squared Studios/Getty Images; Liver sausage: Wendy Schiff; Orange juice: Stockbyte/Getty Images

TABLE 8.19 PANTOTHENIC ACID, BIOTIN, AND CHOLINE

Vitamin and Vitamin-Like	Major Functions in the Body	Adult RDA/AI	Major Dietary Sources	Major Deficiency Signs and Symptoms	Major Toxicity Signs and Symptoms
Pantothenic Acid	Part of the coenzyme needed for making fat and releasing energy from macronutrients	5 mg	Beef and chicken liver, sunflower seeds, mushrooms, yogurt, soy milk, fortified cereals	Rarely occurs	Unknown (UL not determined)
Biotin	Needed for enzymes involved in glucose and fatty acid production	30 mcg	Liver, eggs, peanuts, salmon, and pork	Rarely occurs: skin rash, hair loss, convulsions, developmental delays in infants	Unknown (UL not determined)
Choline	Cellular growth and maintenance; Production of phospholipids and chemicals that transmit messages between nerves	425–550 mg	Liver, meat, poultry, fish, and eggs	Rarely occurs: liver damage in adults; deficiencies during pregnancy may result in certain birth defects	Fishy body odor and reduced blood pressure

TASTY Tidbits

Avidin is a protein in raw egg whites that binds to biotin, making the vitamin resist digestion. If you eat raw eggs regularly, you may develop a skin rash and other signs of biotin deficiency. Cooking eggs destroys avidin, making biotin available for absorption.

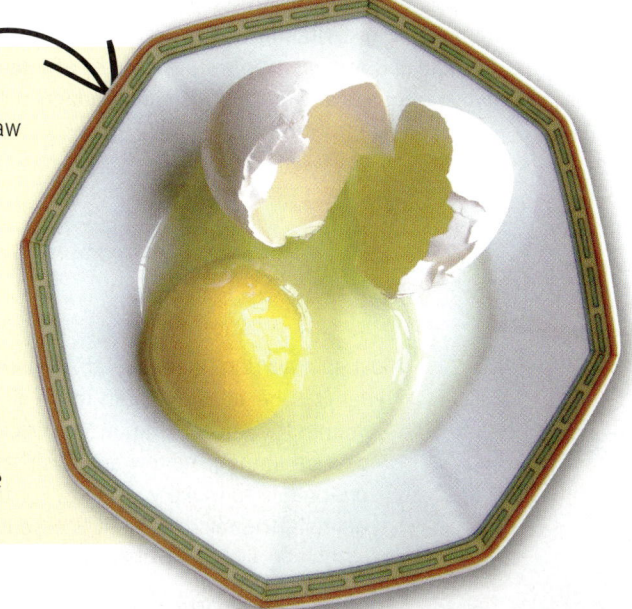

Striped placemat: McGraw-Hill Education/Mark A Dierker, photographer; Mushrooms: Purestock/SuperStock; Broken egg: Wendy Schiff

Nutrition Fact or Fiction?

Taking vitamin C protects you against infection by cold viruses.

Results of several scientific studies indicate that routine vitamin C supplementation (200 mg or more of the vitamin daily) doesn't prevent colds in the general population.[15] However, taking such large doses of the vitamin may reduce the duration of cold symptoms by a day or so. Although vitamin C manufacturers may promote different forms of the vitamin, there's no medical advantage to taking less costly supplements that just contain ascorbic acid.[16]

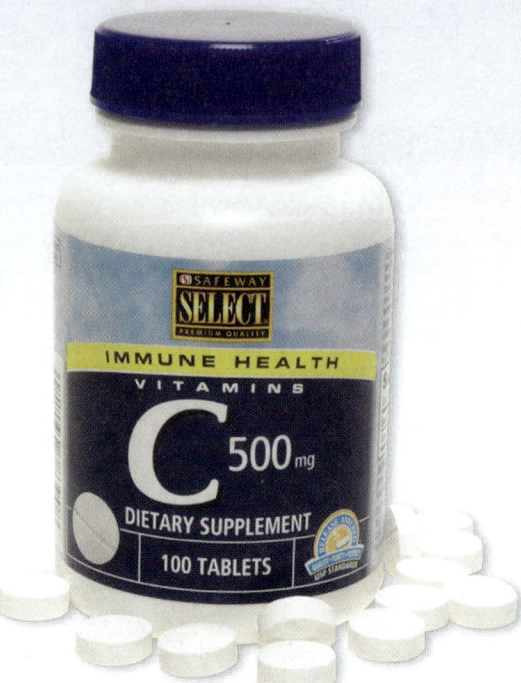

John Flournoy/McGraw-Hill Education

8.3e Vitamin C: Collagen Connector

Vitamin C (**ascorbic acid**) enables many enzymes to work, but the vitamin doesn't function as part of a coenzyme as do most B vitamins. Your body uses vitamin C to form and maintain **collagen,** the protein that gives strength to connective tissue. Connective tissues, such as bone, cartilage, and tendons, connect and support other structures in your body. If vitamin C is unavailable, your body forms weak connective tissue and is unable to maintain existing collagen. Weak collagen can allow teeth to loosen and fall out of their sockets and scars to break down.

In addition to forming and maintaining collagen, your body needs vitamin C to

- maintain the immune system,
- produce bile,
- make certain chemicals that transmit messages between nerves, and
- produce various hormones, including the "stress hormone" cortisol.

Vitamin C also serves as an antioxidant by donating electrons to stabilize free radicals. Vitamin C can give an electron to another antioxidant—vitamin E. Thus, vitamin C recycles vitamin E, enabling it to regain its antioxidant function. *Calcium ascorbate* and *sodium ascorbate* are forms of vitamin C that are often added to packaged foods to protect against free radical damage. Such antioxidants increase a food's shelf life.

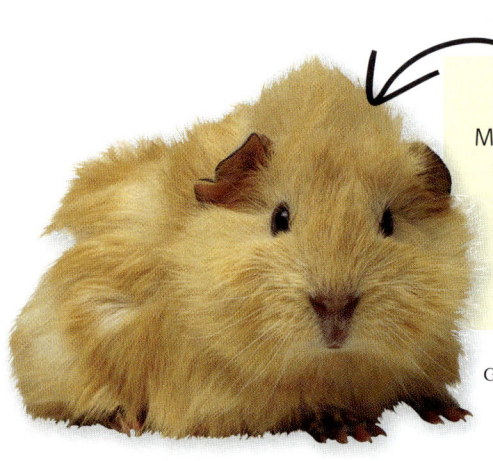

TASTY Tidbits

Most animals don't need dietary sources of vitamin C because they can make all the vitamin they need. Humans and guinea pigs are among the few animals that are unable to make vitamin C. For these animals, the micronutrient is essential.

G.K. & Vikki Hart/Getty Images

ascorbic acid vitamin C

collagen fibrous protein that gives strength to connective tissue

What IS That?

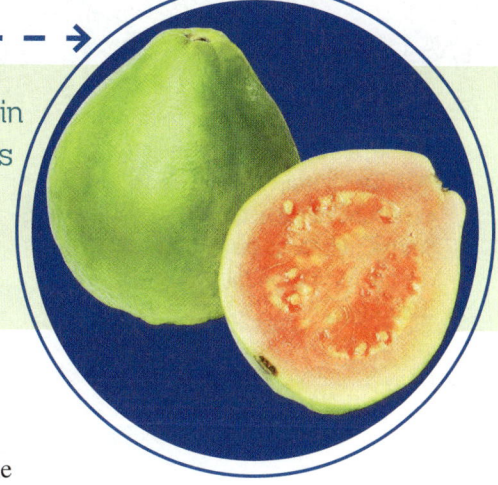

Guava is a tropical fruit that's available in many varieties. Although guavas can be eaten fresh, the fruit is often used to make sauces, jellies, and juices. Guavas are an excellent source of fiber and vitamin C.

Three ounces of the fruit contain about 125 g of vitamin C, which is almost four times the vitamin C that's in the same amount of fresh orange slices.

Food Sources of Vitamin C

Table 8.20 lists some common foods and their vitamin C contents. Note that plant foods are among the best dietary sources of vitamin C. Most animal foods aren't sources of the micronutrient. By including vitamin C–rich fruits and vegetables in your diet each day, you can obtain adequate amounts of vitamin C.

Vitamin C is very unstable in the presence of heat, oxygen, light, alkaline conditions, and the minerals iron and copper. Storing vitamin C–rich foods in cool conditions, such as in the refrigerator, will help preserve the micronutrient. Because vitamin C is water soluble and destroyed by heat, it's easily lost when you use large amounts of water and high heat to cook foods. Therefore, avoid overcooking vegetables, use a minimum amount of cooking water, and eat raw fruits and vegetables whenever possible.

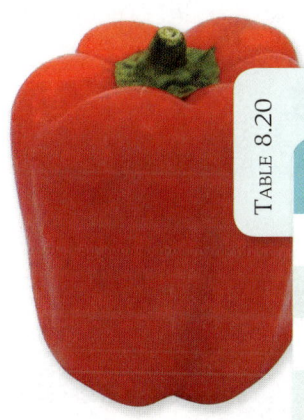

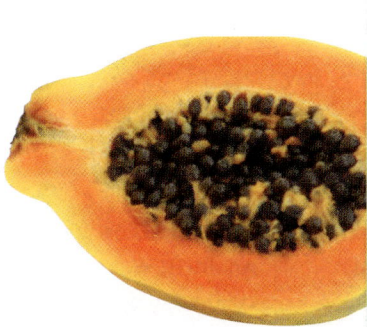

Table 8.20: Vitamin C Content of Selected Foods (Approximate)

Food	Vitamin C (mg)
Red peppers, sweet, raw, chopped, ½ cup	95
Kiwifruit, raw, green, 1	64
Green pepper, sweet, raw, chopped, ½ cup	60
Broccoli, cooked, drained, chopped, ½ cup	51
Strawberries, raw, sliced, ½ cup	49
Brussels sprouts, cooked, drained, ½ cup	48
Papaya, pieces, ½ cup	44
Orange juice, from concentrate, ½ cup	42
Peas, edible pods, boiled, drained, ½ cup	38
Cantaloupe, raw, cubed, ½ cup	29
Potato, Russet, baked with skin, approx. 6 oz	14
Cabbage, shredded, ½ cup	13
French fries, fast food, large, 6 oz	7

RDA for adult women (nonsmokers) = 75 mg/day; RDA for adult men (nonsmokers) = 90 mg/day
Source: U.S. Department of Agriculture, Agricultural Research Service: *USDA National Nutrient Database for Standard Reference Legacy Release, April 2018.* https://ndb.nal.usda.gov/ndb/search/list?home=true Accessed: September 2018

Guava: Glass frog/Shutterstock; Pepper: Wendy Schiff; Papaya: Rosemary Calvert/Photographer's Choice RF/Getty Images; Strawberries: Burke/Triolo Productions/Getty Images

TASTY Tidbits

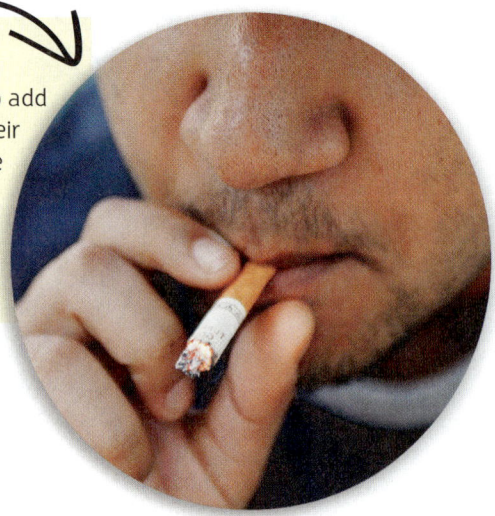

Cigarette smokers need to add an extra 35 mg/day to their RDA for vitamin C because exposure to tobacco smoke increases free radical formation in their lungs.[16]

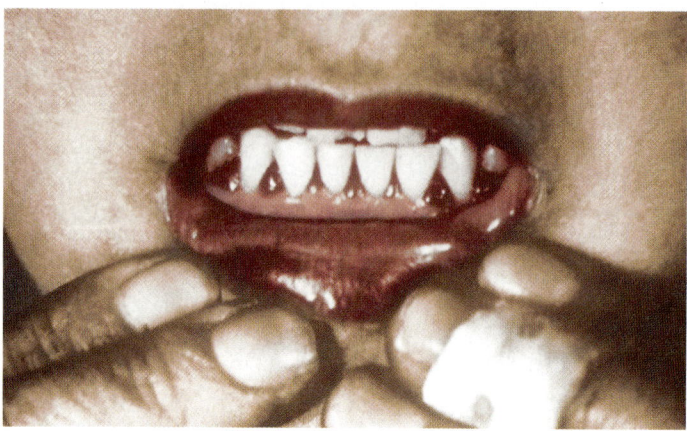

Figure 8.14 Bleeding gums are a sign of scurvy.

What's Scurvy?

Scurvy is the vitamin C deficiency disease. Signs of scurvy include swollen gums that bleed easily, teeth that loosen and fall out, skin that bruises easily, and old scars that open. These signs result from poorly formed and maintained collagen (**Fig. 8.14**).

Even if you don't regularly eat foods that contain the vitamin or take a vitamin C supplement, you're unlikely to develop scurvy. Why? Most people require less than 10 mg of the vitamin daily to prevent scurvy.[16] A 6-ounce serving of fresh orange juice provides about 60 mg of vitamin C—well beyond the requirement. Additionally, Americans rarely develop scurvy because vitamin C is added to many popular processed foods, including fruit and sports drinks, ready-to-eat cereals, and nutrition or power bars.

scurvy vitamin C deficiency disease

Can Vitamin C Be Toxic?

When adults exceed the UL of the vitamin (2000 mg/day), gastrointestinal upsets, including diarrhea, often occur.[16] Taking megadoses of vitamin C supplements is wasteful because your small intestine reduces absorption of the micronutrient when intakes of the vitamin are more than 200 mg/day. Furthermore, when your cells contain all the vitamin C they can hold, the excess vitamin and *oxalate,* a by-product of breaking down vitamin C, circulate in your bloodstream. Your kidneys filter and eliminate these unnecessary substances in urine. Excess oxalate in the kidneys may raise the risk of kidney stones, particularly in people who are at high risk of developing the stones.[16] Therefore, consider avoiding vitamin C supplements, especially if you have a history of kidney stones.

Reviewing the Basics: Vitamin C

Table 8.21 summarizes information about vitamin C. The table includes Dietary Reference Intake (DRI) recommendations, and major signs and symptoms of the vitamin's deficiency and toxicity disorders.

Table 8.21 Vitamin C

Major Functions in the Body	Adult RDA	Major Dietary Sources	Major Deficiency Signs and Symptoms	Major Toxicity Signs and Symptoms
Antioxidant; connective tissue production and maintenance; production of chemicals that transmit messages between nerves; production of certain hormones; immune system functioning	75–90 mg (nonsmokers) 110–125 mg (smokers)	Peppers, citrus fruits, papaya, broccoli, cabbage, berries	Scurvy: Poor wound healing, pinpoint bleeding, bleeding gums, bruises, depression	Adult UL = 2000 mg/day Diarrhea and GI tract discomfort

Person smoking: Gary He/McGraw-Hill Education; Fruits and vegetables: Wendy Schiff; Sign of scurvy: Centers for Disease Control and Prevention

Module 8.4
Vitamins and Cancer

8.4 - Learning Outcomes

After reading Module 8.4, you should be able to

1. Define all of the **key terms** in this module.
2. Identify lifestyle practices and other factors that are associated with increased risk of certain cancers.
3. Identify foods that may reduce your risk of cancer.
4. Explain why it may not be useful to take dietary supplements for cancer prevention.

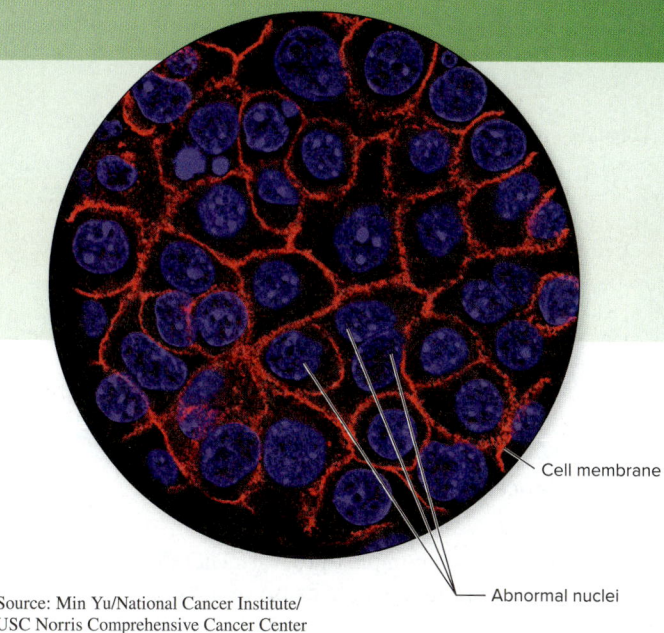

Source: Min Yu/National Cancer Institute/ USC Norris Comprehensive Cancer Center

Pancreatic cancer cells

Are you among the millions of Americans who take vitamin supplements? If your answer is "yes," why do you use them? Vitamin supplements are effective for treating people with specific vitamin deficiency diseases, disorders that increase vitamin requirements, and a few other medical conditions. However, scientific evidence generally doesn't support claims that megadoses of vitamins can prevent or treat serious chronic diseases, including cancer. This module of Unit 8 takes a closer look at cancer and the role that diet may play in the prevention and treatment of the disease.

8.4a What's Cancer?

As mentioned in Unit 7, DNA is the material in cells that contains the instructions for protein production. Sometimes, the parts of DNA (genes) that regulate a cell's growth, reproduction, and death become damaged. In many cases, a specific **carcinogen** such as a virus or toxic chemical harms the DNA. When the damage leads to rapid cell growth and unchecked cell division, cancer can result. **Cancer** refers to a group of chronic diseases characterized by abnormal cells that are "out of control."

Cancer cells are *malignant* because they divide repeatedly and frequently, and they don't die **(Fig. 8.15)**. When a cell becomes malignant, it doesn't perform the specialized functions of the cells from which it was derived. A cancerous liver cell, for example, doesn't remove toxins from the bloodstream or store nutrients properly.

As a result of their rapid growth rate, many types of cancer cells form masses, called malignant tumors. Malignant cells often break away from the tumor. These cells can move to and invade other parts of the body. When cancer spreads to other tissues, the disease has *metastasized* (*meh-tass'-tah-sized*).

Because of their rapid growth and frequent cell divisions, malignant cells require more nutrients than do normal cells. To supply enough nutrients to meet their needs, cancerous tumors stimulate the body to form blood vessels that divert blood away from healthy cells and into the tumor (see Figure 8.15). Eventually, healthy tissues are unable to obtain adequate supplies of nutrients, and they die.

What Are Risk Factors for Cancer?

In the United States, the most common kinds of cancer (excluding skin cancers) are breast, lung, prostate, and colorectal cancers.[17] Medical researchers have discovered several risk factors for many forms of cancer. These factors include

- age (older adults),
- family history of cancer,
- tobacco use,
- exposure to some forms of radiation,
- exposure to certain environmental substances,
- chronic inflammation,
- history of certain viral or bacterial infections,
- high levels of certain hormones,
- diet,
- alcohol use, and
- excess body fat.[18]

carcinogen agent that causes cancer

cancer group of diseases characterized by abnormal cell behavior

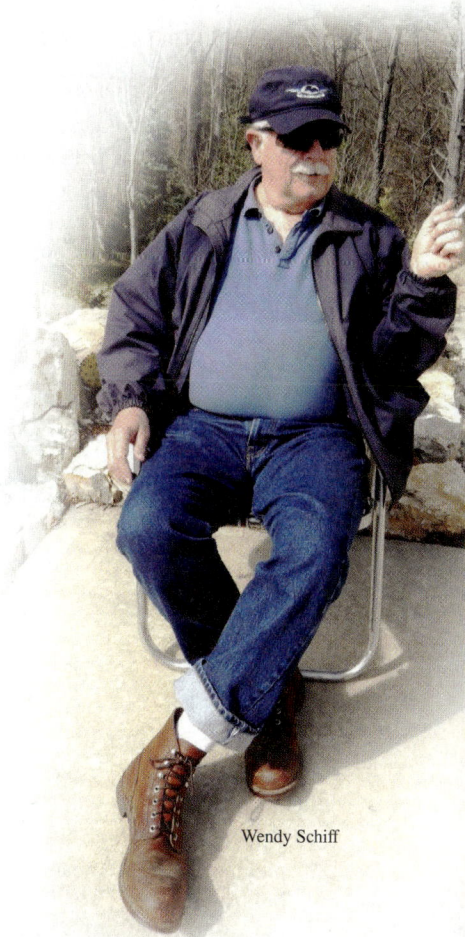

Wendy Schiff

Smoking, advanced age, obesity, and physical inactivity are risk factors for cancer.

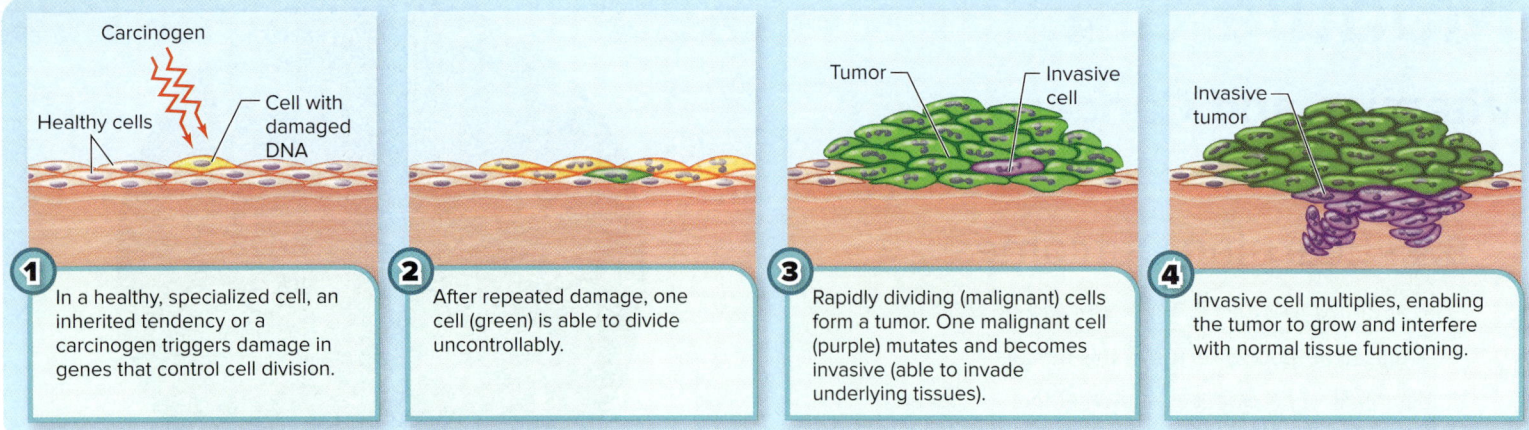

Figure 8.15 Cancer progression.

Cancer causation is a complex process. Therefore, it may be impossible to pinpoint a single cause of a patient's cancer. Individuals differ widely in their genetic makeups, lifestyle practices, environmental exposures, and nutritional states. Some medical experts estimate that over 50% of cancer deaths among Americans can be prevented if people adopt healthier lifestyles, including their diets.[19]

8.4b The Role of Obesity and Diet in Cancer Development

Obesity is a risk factor for certain cancers, particularly breast cancer (after menopause) and cancers of the esophagus, lining of the uterus, colon and rectum, kidney, pancreas, thyroid, and gallbladder.[20] Medical researchers don't fully understand why obesity increases the risk of these forms of cancer. One possible explanation has to do with fat tissue's production of the female hormone estrogen. High levels of estrogen are associated with the risk of breast, uterine, and some other types of cancer. Obesity can also increase blood insulin levels, which may promote cancer development.

Some foods and beverages contain carcinogens. Alcohol, for example, is a carcinogen.[21] People who consume alcohol regularly have higher risks of cancers of the head and neck, esophagus, liver, colon, rectum, and breast.[21] In general, the higher the alcohol intake, the greater the risk of these cancers. Furthermore, the chances of developing cancers of the mouth, throat, or voice box increase sharply when cigarette smoking is combined with drinking. To reduce your risk of cancer, it's wise to limit your consumption of alcohol or avoid the drug altogether. If you drink, do so in moderation—no more than one standard drink per day for women and no more than two standard drinks per day for men. (A standard alcoholic drink is 1.5 oz of liquor, 12 oz of regular beer, or 5 oz of wine.)

Table 8.22 lists dietary factors that may be associated with increased risk of various cancers. Currently, there's no scientific

Table 8.22 Possible Diet-Related Carcinogens

Possibly Carcinogenic	Common Dietary Sources	Possible or Known Action
Aflatoxin	Moldy nuts and grains	Increases risk of liver cancer
Alcohol	Alcoholic beverages	Unclear, but may increase certain hormone levels or the body's breakdown of alcohol may result in carcinogens
Arsenic	Natural contaminant in drinking water	May increase risk of bladder cancer
Benzene	Contaminated water	Known carcinogen
Fried, grilled, smoked, pickled, or salted meat and poultry	Foods exposed to salt or high temperatures, especially grilled meat that has charred areas	May increase risk of throat, stomach, and colorectal cancers
Processed meat	Deli meats	Increased risk of colorectal cancer
Salted fish	Chinese-style fish; pickled herring	Increased risk of stomach cancer

Fatty meats, Mug of beer, Pretzel: Wendy Schiff

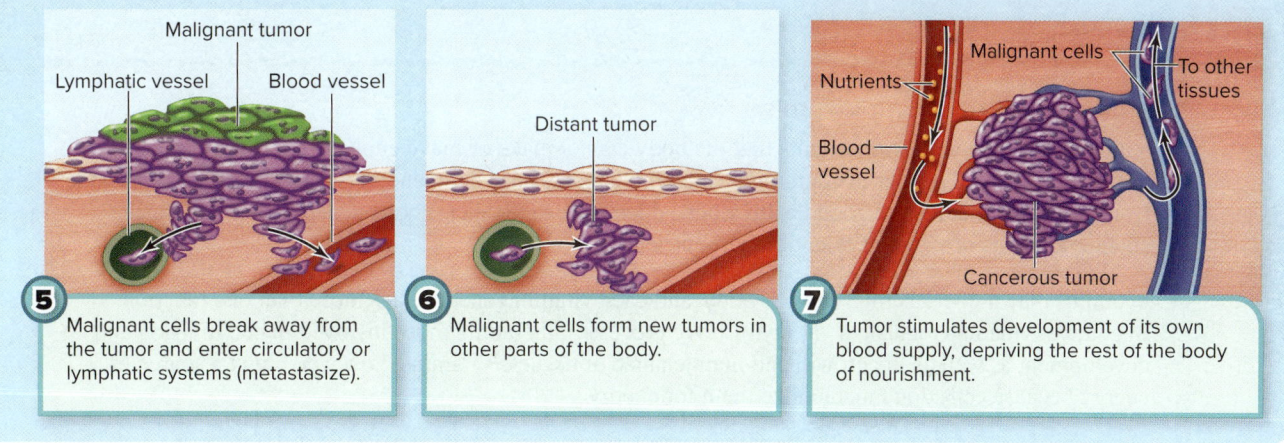

5 Malignant cells break away from the tumor and enter circulatory or lymphatic systems (metastasize).

6 Malignant cells form new tumors in other parts of the body.

7 Tumor stimulates development of its own blood supply, depriving the rest of the body of nourishment.

evidence that consuming artificial sweeteners such as aspartame, coffee, bioengineered foods, or foods preserved by radiation causes cancer.[22]

Diet and Cancer Risk Reduction

You can reduce your risk of cancer by

- avoiding exposure to tobacco smoke,
- achieving and maintaining a healthy weight,
- adopting a physically active lifestyle, and
- eating a healthy diet that limits intakes of alcohol and red and processed meat; and emphasizes intakes of plant foods, including fruits, vegetables, and whole grains.

Although research is ongoing, results of scientific studies generally don't provide evidence that taking dietary supplements that contain antioxidants reduces the risk of cancer.[22]

Consuming a wide variety of vitamins and phytochemicals in their natural states and concentrations (in foods) may be the most effective way to lower your risk of developing cancer and many other serious chronic diseases. Why? These substances probably work together to enhance health, and isolating them from their natural sources and making them into supplements may reduce their usefulness and increase their risk of toxicity. Therefore, registered dietitian nutritionists recommend that healthy adults eat a variety of fruits and vegetables each day rather than take antioxidant or phytochemical supplements.

TASTY Tidbits

High temperatures used to cook meat may cause charring of the meat and the formation of a group of possible human carcinogens called heterocyclic (het'-eh-ro-si'-klic) amines. Therefore, you may be able to reduce your risk of certain cancers by limiting your intake of grilled meats and avoiding charred parts of charcoal-grilled meats.[23] Also, covering the grate with aluminum foil, poking a few holes in the foil, and placing the meat on top of it will reduce charring of the meat.

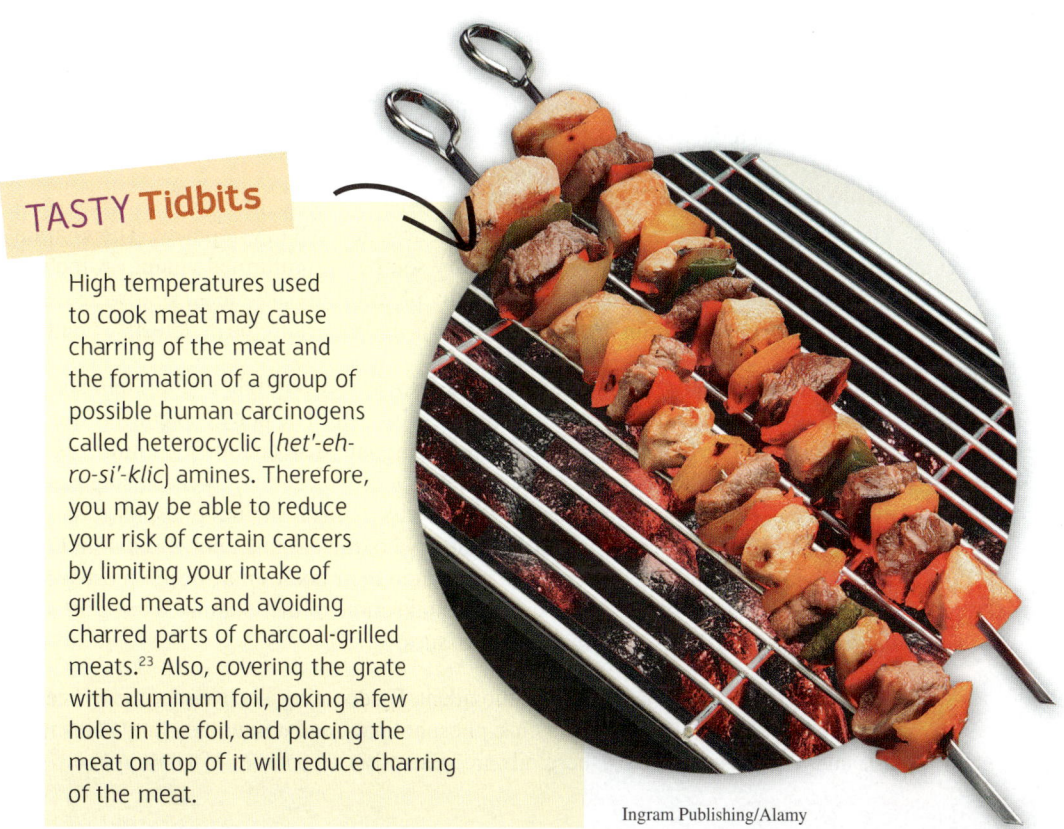

Ingram Publishing/Alamy

In a Nutshell

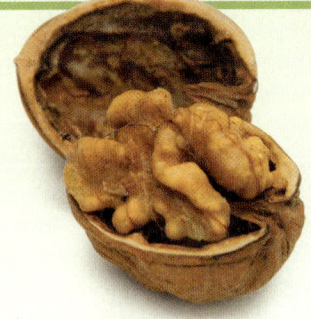

Module 8.1 Introducing Vitamins

- Vitamins are organic micronutrients that the body cannot make or make enough of to maintain good health; that naturally occur in commonly eaten foods; that cause deficiency disease when they're missing from diets; and that restore good health when added back to the diet. Foods generally contain much smaller amounts of vitamins than of macronutrients.

- Vitamins play numerous roles in your body, and each vitamin generally has more than one function. In general, vitamins regulate a variety of body processes, including those involved in cell division and development as well as the growth and maintenance of tissues. Vitamins, however, aren't a source of energy because cells don't metabolize them for energy.

- Certain chemical reactions can form free radicals. A free radical is a chemically unstable substance because it is missing an electron. Free radicals can damage or destroy molecules by removing electrons from them. Many medical researchers suspect excess free radical damage in the body ultimately leads to heart attack, stroke, cancer, Alzheimer's disease, and even the aging process. Cells normally regulate free radical formation by using antioxidants such as vitamin E.

- Vitamins A, D, E, and K are fat-soluble vitamins; thiamin, riboflavin, niacin, vitamin B-6, pantothenic acid, folate, biotin, vitamin B-12, and vitamin C are water-soluble vitamins. (The vitamin-like substance choline is water soluble.) Your body has more difficulty eliminating excess fat-soluble vitamins than water-soluble vitamins. As a result, your body stores extra fat-soluble vitamins. Over time, these vitamins can accumulate and cause toxicity. Water-soluble vitamins are generally not as toxic as fat-soluble vitamins.

- Exposure to air, excessive heat, alkaline conditions, and light can destroy certain vitamins. Eat produce when it's fresh. Cooking vegetables in water can cause losses of water-soluble vitamins.

- Vitamin needs generally increase during periods of growth and pregnancy. Vitamin deficiency disorders generally result from inadequate diets or conditions that increase the body's requirements for vitamins or reduce the intestinal tract's ability to absorb nutrients. Your chances of developing a vitamin deficiency disease increase when your diet consistently lacks the micronutrient and levels of the nutrient in your body become too low.

- Most commonly eaten foods don't contain toxic levels of vitamins. Vitamin toxicity is most likely to occur in people who take megadoses of vitamin supplements or consume large amounts of vitamin-fortified foods regularly.

Module 8.2 Fat-Soluble Vitamins

- Vitamin A is involved in vision, immune function, and cell development. The vitamin A provitamin, beta-carotene, functions as an antioxidant. Dietary sources of preformed vitamin A include liver and fortified milk; provitamin A carotenoids are especially plentiful in dark green, yellow, red, and orange fruits and vegetables. Excess vitamin A can be quite toxic and can cause birth defects when taken during pregnancy.

- Vitamin D is both a hormone and a vitamin. Exposure to sunlight enables human skin to make a previtamin vitamin D from a cholesterol-like substance. The body can convert this substance to the active form of the vitamin. A few foods, including fatty fish and fortified milk, are dietary sources of the vitamin. Vitamin D helps regulate the level of blood calcium by increasing calcium absorption from the intestine. Vitamin D also stimulates bone cells to form calcium phosphate, the hard major mineral compound in bone tissue. Infants and children who don't obtain enough vitamin D may develop rickets. Adults with inadequate amounts of the vitamin in their bodies may develop osteomalacia. Older adults and breastfed infants often need a supplemental source of the vitamin. Excess intakes of vitamin D can cause the body to deposit calcium in soft tissues.

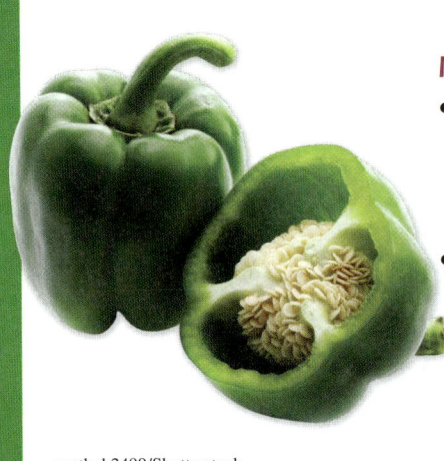
matkub2499/Shutterstock

- Vitamin E functions primarily as an antioxidant. By donating electrons to free radicals, vitamin E stabilizes them. This effect shields DNA, proteins, phospholipids, and unsaturated fatty acids from destruction. Plant oils and products made from these oils are generally rich sources of vitamin E.

Module 8.3 Water-Soluble Vitamins

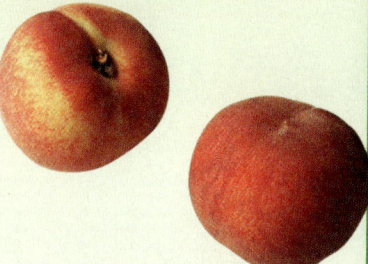

- Most B vitamins function as a part of coenzymes. Thiamin, riboflavin, and niacin play key roles as part of coenzymes in energy-yielding reactions. These water-soluble vitamins help cells metabolize carbohydrates, fats, and proteins. Whole-grain and enriched grain products are common sources of all three of the vitamins. Beriberi is the severe thiamin deficiency disease; ariboflavinosis results from the lack of riboflavin; pellagra results from a severe lack of niacin. Excess intakes of niacin can cause toxicity.

- Vitamin B-6 is involved in the production of nonessential amino acids. The vitamin is also needed to produce chemicals that transmit messages between nerves and metabolize homocysteine. High doses of vitamin B-6 may cause nerve damage.

- Folate plays important roles in DNA production and homocysteine metabolism. Rich food sources of folate are leafy vegetables, organ meats, and orange juice. Signs of folate deficiency include megaloblastic anemia. Pregnancy increases the body's needs for folate; a deficiency during the first month of pregnancy can result in neural tube defects in offspring. Women of childbearing age can meet the RDA for the vitamin by taking dietary supplements that contain folic acid, which is the form of folate used in supplements.

- The body needs vitamin B-12 to metabolize folate and homocysteine, and maintain nerves. Although vitamin B-12 doesn't occur naturally in plant foods, the vitamin is in animal foods and products that have been fortified with the micronutrient. Vitamin B-12 deficiency is more common in older adults. As people age, their stomachs produce less HCl. This condition can result in vitamin B-12 deficiency even though adequate amounts of the micronutrient are consumed in foods. Furthermore, a vitamin B-12 deficiency and a condition called pernicious anemia result if the stomach is unable to produce the vitamin B-12 carrier protein.

- The body uses vitamin C to make and maintain collagen, a major protein in connective tissue. Vitamin C also functions as an antioxidant. Fresh fruits and vegetables, especially citrus fruits, are generally good sources of the micronutrient. Because vitamin C is easily lost in cooking, diets should emphasize raw or lightly cooked fruits and vegetables. Smoking increases the body's requirement for vitamin C. Scurvy is the vitamin C deficiency disease. Excess vitamin C may cause diarrhea and increase the risk of kidney stones in some people.

Module 8.4 Vitamins and Cancer

- Cancer occurs when DNA undergoes changes that affect a cell's growth, reproduction, and death. Such changes result in abnormal cell development, rapid cell growth, and unchecked cell division.

- Maintaining a healthy body weight, exercising regularly, consuming diets that supply plenty of fruits and vegetables, limiting intakes of red and/or processed meat, and avoiding tobacco smoke and excess alcohol may reduce the risk of cancer.

What's in Your Diet?!

Using the DRIs: Vitamins

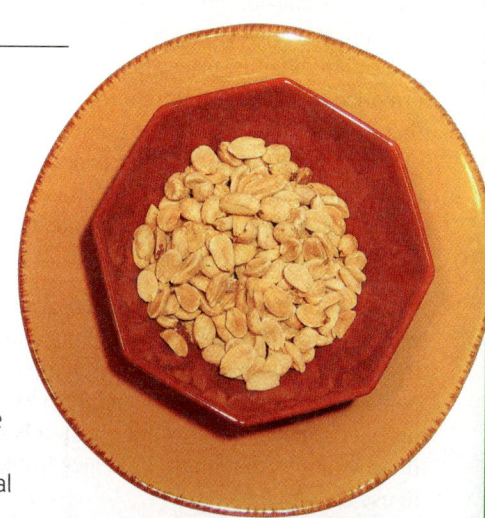

1. Refer to your 1- or 3-day food log from the "What's in Your Diet?!" feature in Unit 3.

   a. Find the RDA values for vitamins under your life stage/sex group category in the DRI tables (see **Appendix E**). Write those values under the "My RDA" column in the table at the end of this activity.

   b. Review your personal dietary assessment. Find your 3-day average intakes of vitamins A, E, C, D, folate, B-12, thiamin, riboflavin, and niacin. Write those values under the "My Average Intake" column of the table.

   c. Calculate the percentage of the RDA you consumed for each vitamin by dividing your intake by the RDA amount and multiplying the figure you obtain by 100. For example, if your average intake of vitamin C was 100 mg/day and your RDA for the vitamin was 75 mg/day, you would divide 100 mg by 75 mg to obtain 1.25. To multiply this figure by 100, simply move the decimal

Peaches: I. Rozenbaum & F. Cirou/PhotoAlto; Whole-grain bread: Ingram Publishing/Alamy; Bowl of peanuts: Wendy Schiff

point two places to the right, and replace the decimal point with a percentage sign (125%). Thus, your average daily intake of vitamin C was 125% of the RDA. Place the percentages for each vitamin under the "% of My RDA" column.

d. Under the ">, <, or =" column, indicate whether your average daily intake was greater than (>), less than (<), or equal to (=) the RDA.

2. Use the information you calculated in the first part of this activity to answer the following questions:

a. Which of your average vitamin intakes equaled or exceeded the RDA value?

b. Which of your average vitamin intakes was below the RDA value?

c. What foods would you eat to increase your intake of the vitamins that were less than the RDA levels? (Review food sources of the vitamins in Unit 8.)

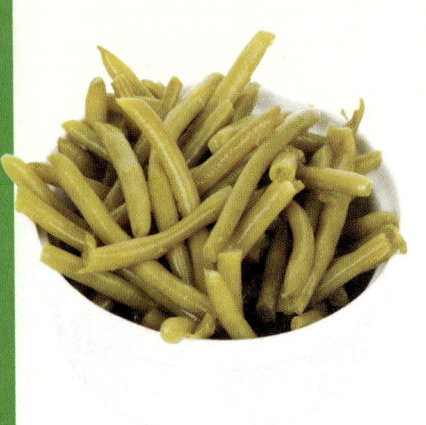
ncognet0/iStock/Getty Images Plus

Vitamin	My RDA	My Average Intake	% of My RDA	>, <, or =
A				
E				
C				
D				
Folate				
B-12				
Thiamin				
Riboflavin				

Consider This...

1. Choose a vitamin and type the nutrient's name in the search box of an Internet browser. Locate three sites that sell products containing the vitamin. Review the pages of each site, making notes about claims, prices, and the kinds of links provided. Then write a three- to five-page report that describes and compares the information you found at the sites. In your paper, discuss any claims made on behalf of these products that you consider false or misleading. Include the URLs for the sites in your report.

2. Nick complains of having no energy and feeling tired most of the time. He's thinking about taking high doses of dietary supplements that contain thiamin, riboflavin, and niacin to boost his energy level. What would you tell Nick about these vitamins that might influence his decision to use the supplements?

3. While at a popular video-sharing website, you watch a man, who refers to himself as a "nutrition expert," claim to have discovered a new vitamin in chickpeas. If you had the opportunity, what questions would you ask the expert to ascertain whether the substance truly is a vitamin?

4. One of your friends takes megadoses of vitamins A, C, B-6, and E because she thinks they help her stay healthy. What would you tell her about taking such large doses of these vitamins?

5. Consider your current lifestyle and the recommendations for reducing cancer risk that are provided in this unit. Which recommendations are you unlikely to follow? Explain why you are not likely to follow those recommendations.

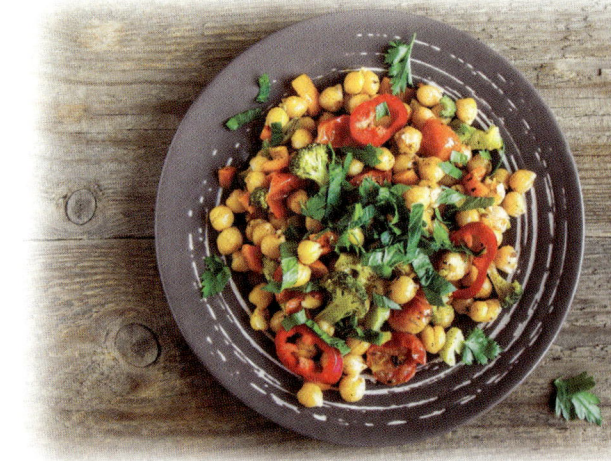

Chickpeas are a good source of folate.
Mizina/Getty Images

Test Yourself

Select the best answer.

1. Vitamin toxicities generally occur as a result of
   a. eating enriched breads and cereal products.
   b. consuming a wide variety of foods.
   c. taking megadoses of dietary supplements.
   d. having diseases that interfere with intestinal absorption.

2. Vitamins
   a. occur in gram amounts in foods.
   b. don't provide any calories.
   c. aren't organic molecules.
   d. are macronutrients.

3. People who are unable to absorb fat are likely to develop a _____ deficiency.
   a. vitamin B-12   c. vitamin D
   b. folate   d. riboflavin

4. Enriched grain products have specific amounts of _____ added during processing.
   a. pantothenic acid
   b. riboflavin
   c. biotin
   d. vitamin D

5. Which of the following foods is not a rich source of provitamin A?
   a. Fish   c. Broccoli
   b. Carrots   d. Sweet potato

6. During pregnancy, excess _____ intake is known to be teratogenic.
   a. pantothenic acid
   b. vitamin A
   c. vitamin K
   d. choline

7. Vitamin K can be produced by
   a. skin exposure to ultraviolet radiation.
   b. hydrolysis of seawater.
   c. red blood cell synthesis.
   d. intestinal bacteria.

8. To reduce the likelihood of giving birth to babies with neural tube defects, women of childbearing age should obtain adequate
   a. vitamin K.   c. folate.
   b. biotin.   d. niacin.

9. Major food sources of vitamin B-12 include
   a. enriched grain products.
   b. meat and dairy products.
   c. fruit and vegetables.
   d. nuts and seeds.

10. Which of the following statements is true?
    a. The stomach can easily absorb vitamin B-12.
    b. Vitamin B-12 deficiency is common among older adults.
    c. Patients with pernicious anemia are treated with high doses of folic acid.
    d. Vitamin B-12 is absorbed in the lower segment of the large intestine.

11. Which of the following foods is a rich source of vitamin C?
    a. Whole milk   c. Guava
    b. Egg white   d. Egg yolk

12. Which of the following practices may reduce your risk of cancer?
    a. Consuming salted fish
    b. Eating grilled meats regularly
    c. Smoking no more than 10 cigarettes daily
    d. Eating fruits and vegetables

Answers: 1.c 2.b 3.c 4.b 5.a 6.b 7.d 8.c 9.b 10.b 11.c 12.d

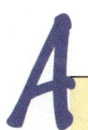

Answer This (Module 8.2a)

The young man consumes plenty of vitamin A precursors in plant foods.

References ➡ See Appendix D.

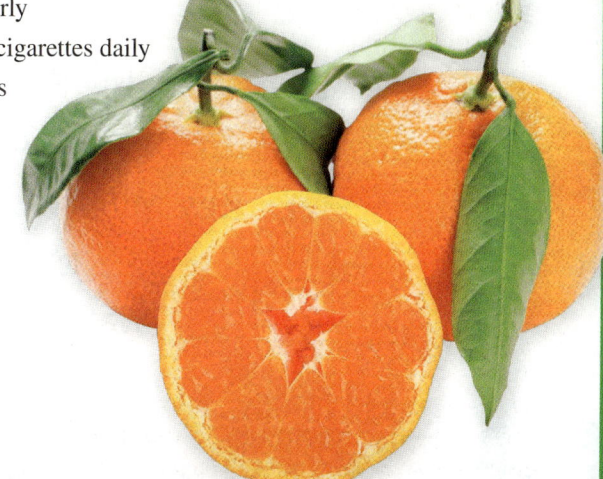

sanmai/Getty Images

Design elements: Spiral notebook paper background, Stacked paper with clip background, Marginal note clip, and Culture & Cuisine globe icon: ©McGraw-Hill Education; In a Nutshell walnut: ©McGraw-Hill Education/Mark A. Dierker, photographer; Test Yourself red pepper: Iconotec/Glow Images

Unit 9

Key Minerals, Water, and the Nonnutrient Alcohol

What's on the Menu?

Module 9.1
Minerals for Life

Module 9.2
Key Minerals and Your Health

Module 9.3
Water: Liquid of Life

Module 9.4
Drink to Your Health?

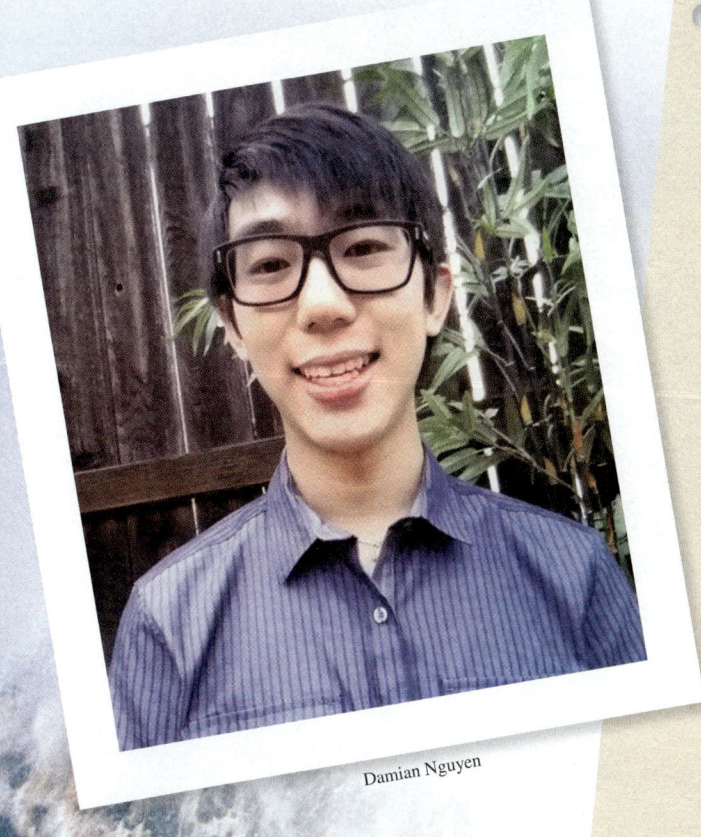
Damian Nguyen

"When I was in middle school, I found out that I developed lactose intolerance. I could drink small amounts of milk and eat a little ice cream, though I'd find myself with stomach problems later if I ate as much as my friends. I tried taking [lactase] tablets when I consumed dairy products, but I got tired of using them. They seemed to become less effective over time as well. For a little while, I tried other kinds of milk, like coconut milk. I couldn't get used to the taste. I also have soy, nut, and fish allergies, so soy and almond milk aren't viable alternatives. Now, I eat cheese and drink Lactaid® milk, so hopefully I get enough calcium in my diet."

Damian Nguyen

Damian Nguyen is majoring in music composition and instrumental music education at the Bob Cole Conservatory of Music, California State University–Long Beach. Should Damian be concerned about his calcium intake? Yes, because men as well as women can develop weak bones as a result of low intakes of the mineral.

Minerals, such as calcium, are elements in Earth's rocks, soils, and natural water sources, especially the ocean. Plants, animals, and other living things cannot make minerals. Plants obtain the minerals they need to grow and survive from soil or fertilizer. You obtain the minerals that you require when you eat plants and animals or substances that contain these elements.

The functions of many minerals in your body involve water. Although alcohol isn't a nutrient, the chemical affects your body's contents of water, minerals, and other nutrients. This unit focuses on some key mineral nutrients, water, and the nonnutrient alcohol.

minerals elements in the Earth's rocks, soils, and natural water sources

Module 9.1
Minerals for Life

9.1 - Learning Outcomes

After reading Module 9.1, you should be able to

1. Define all of the **key terms** in this module.
2. Classify a mineral nutrient as a major, trace, or possible essential mineral.
3. Describe general functions of mineral nutrients.
4. Discuss practical ways of retaining the mineral contents of foods.
5. Discuss factors that influence the body's ability to absorb and use minerals.

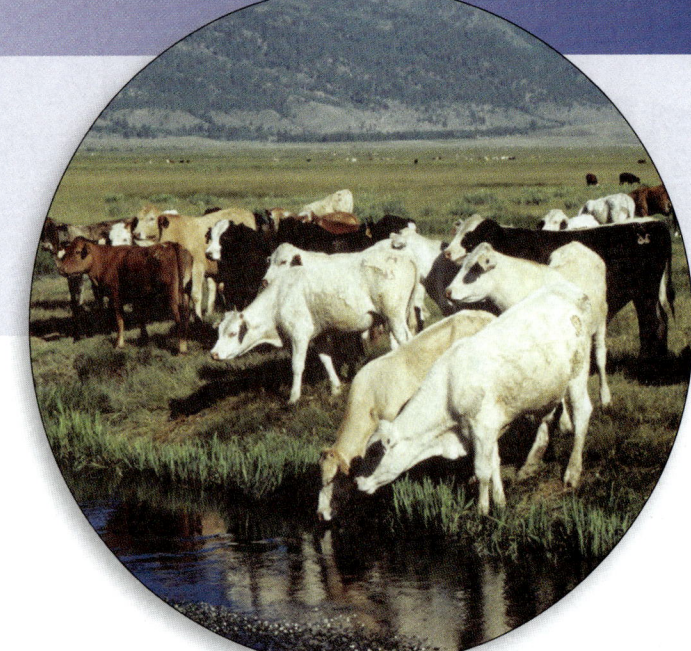

Minerals are naturally in your environment.

In their natural state, most foods contain small amounts of minerals. **Figure 9.1** indicates food groups from MyPlate that are generally rich sources of various minerals.

Figure 9.1 MyPlate major food sources of mineral nutrients.

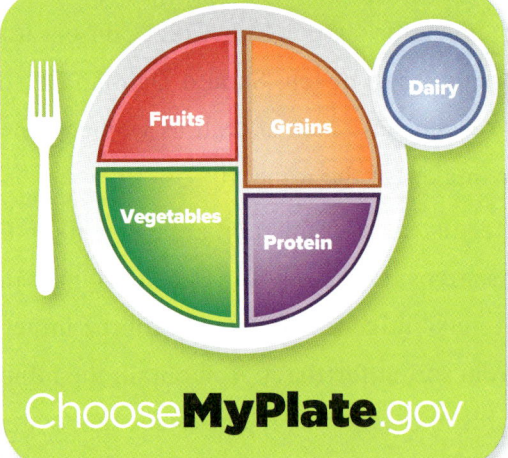

Dairy
- Calcium
- Phosphorus
- Zinc
- Magnesium
- Sodium (cheese)
- Iodine

Grains
- Processed foods
  - Sodium chloride
- Whole-grain, enriched, and/or fortified
  - Calcium
  - Phosphorus
  - Magnesium
  - Iron
  - Zinc
  - Copper
  - Selenium
  - Chromium

Fruits
- Potassium
- Magnesium
- Boron

Vegetables
- Potassium
- Magnesium
- Calcium (kale, leafy greens)
- Sodium chloride (processed foods)

Protein
- Sodium chloride (processed foods)
- Potassium
- Phosphorus
- Magnesium
- Selenium
- Iron
- Zinc
- Copper
- Calcium (fish with small bones)
- Iodine (seafood)

Choose MyPlate: Source: ChooseMyPlate.gov; Cattle: Image Source/Getty Images; Kale: Stockdisc/PunchStock; Milk: Jonelle Weaver/Getty Images; Bowl of cornflakes: Keith Leighton/Alamy; Banana, Sardines: Wendy Schiff

9.1a Major Mineral or Trace Mineral?

About 15 mineral elements have known functions in your body and are necessary for health **(Table 9.1).** Your body requires mineral nutrients in milligram or microgram amounts. The essential minerals are classified into two groups: major minerals and trace minerals. If a person requires 100 mg or more of a mineral per day, the mineral is classified as a **major mineral;** otherwise, the micronutrient is a **trace mineral.**

Your body also contains very small amounts of other minerals, such as nickel and arsenic. This particular group of minerals may have roles in the body that have yet to be determined (see "Possible Essential Mineral" column in Table 9.1). Some minerals, including lead, cadmium, and mercury, may be in the human body, but they're environmental contaminants that have no known functions and are toxic.

As with vitamins, cells don't obtain any calories from minerals. Unlike vitamins, minerals cannot be destroyed. Thus, heating a food or exposing it to most other environmental conditions will not affect the food's mineral content. However, minerals are water soluble, and they can leach out of a food and into cooking water. By using the cooking water to make soups or sauces, you can obtain minerals from the food that would otherwise be discarded.

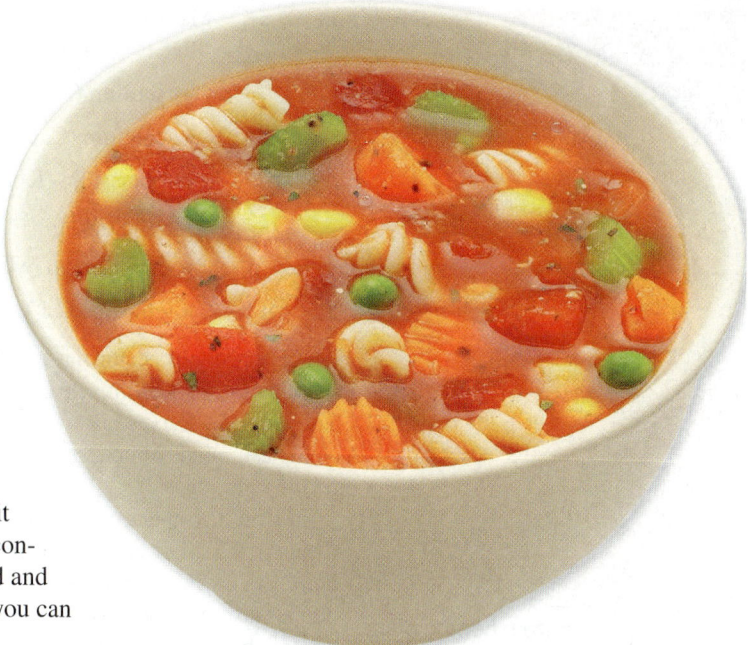

Minerals are water soluble, so they can leach out of foods, such as vegetables, and into the cooking water.

9.1b Why Are Minerals Necessary?

Most mineral nutrients have more than one function in your body **(Fig. 9.2).** Some minerals form inorganic structural components of tissues, such as calcium and phosphorus in your bones and teeth. Many minerals are components of various substances, including enzymes, hormones, or other organic molecules. For example, cobalt is in vitamin B-12, iron is in the hemoglobin of red blood cells (RBCs), and sulfur is in the amino acids methionine and cysteine. Although cells cannot metabolize minerals for energy, certain minerals are involved in chemical reactions that release energy from macronutrients.

TABLE 9.1 CLASSIFYING MINERALS WITH KNOWN OR POSSIBLE ROLES IN THE BODY*

Major Mineral	Trace Mineral	Possible Essential Mineral
Calcium (Ca)	Chromium (Cr)	Arsenic (As)
Chloride (Cl$^-$)	Copper (Cu)	Boron (B)
Magnesium (Mg)	Fluoride (F$^-$)**	Lithium (Li)
Phosphorus (P)	Iodine (I)	Nickel (Ni)
Potassium (K)	Iron (Fe)	Silicon (Si)
Sodium (Na)	Manganese (Mn)	Vanadium (V)
Sulfur (S)	Molybdenum (Mo)	
	Selenium (Se)	
	Zinc (Zn)	

*Chemical symbol is shown in parentheses next to mineral's name.
**Although your body can use trace amounts of fluoride, the mineral generally isn't considered to be essential.[1]

major minerals essential mineral elements required in amounts of 100 mg or more per day

trace minerals essential mineral elements required in amounts that are less than 100 mg per day

Vegetable soup: Getty Images/iStockphoto/Lew Robertson; Placemat: McGraw-Hill Education/Mark A. Dierker, photographer; Cheese: Wendy Schiff

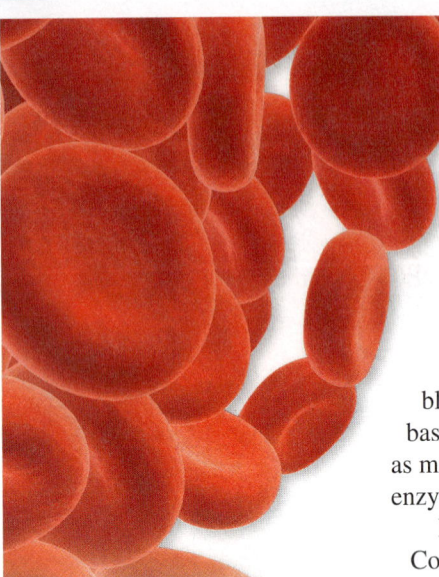

Red blood cells contain hemoglobin.
Ingram Publishing/SuperStock

Many minerals also function as electrolytes (*ions*). **Electrolytes** are minerals that have positive (+) or negative (−) electrical charges when they're dissolved in water. Electrolytes include

- sodium (Na^+),
- calcium (Ca^{2+}),
- potassium (K^+),
- zinc (Zn^{2+}),
- magnesium (Mg^{2+}), and
- chloride (Cl^-).

Electrolytes perform a variety of functions in your body. Calcium ions, for example, are needed for blood clotting and muscle contraction. Sodium, potassium, and chloride ions participate in fluid and acid-base balance. Nerves also use sodium and chloride ions to send messages to other cells. Certain ions, such as magnesium and copper, are cofactors. A **cofactor** is an ion or small, nonprotein molecule that helps an enzyme function.

In Unit 8, you learned about coenzymes, which are needed to activate certain enzymes (see Essential Concept 8.3). The enzymes won't be able to enable chemical reactions to occur without the coenzyme's help. Coenzymes are associated with B vitamins (organic substances). Ions such as magnesium, zinc, and copper also participate in a variety of chemical reactions in the body, but they don't need to be part of an organic molecule to function.

electrolytes minerals that have electrical charges when dissolved in water; ions

cofactor ion or small, nonprotein molecule that helps an enzyme function

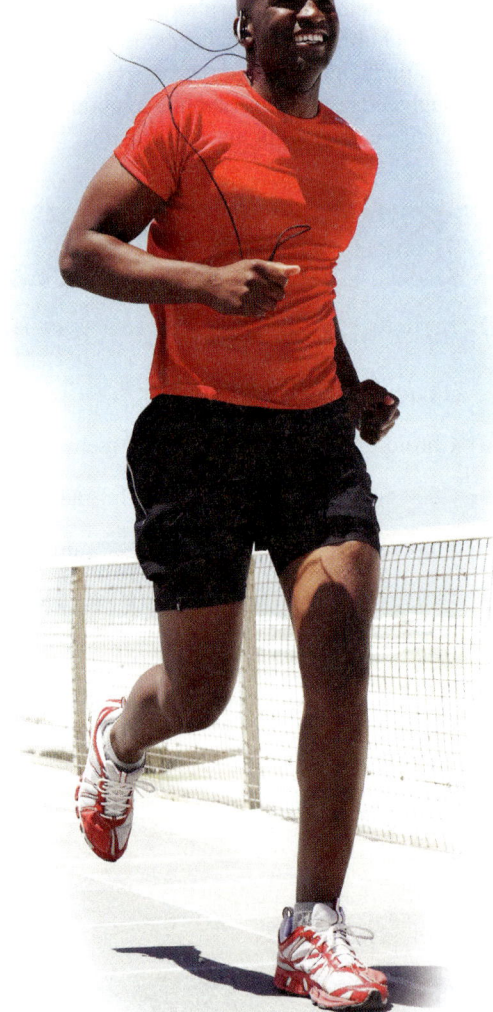

Bone Health
- Calcium
- Phosphorus
- Iron
- Zinc
- Copper
- Manganese
- Fluoride
- Magnesium

Fluid Balance
- Sodium
- Potassium
- Chloride
- Phosphorus
- Magnesium

Blood Clotting
- Calcium

Transmission of Nerve Impulses
- Sodium
- Potassium
- Chloride
- Calcium

Red Blood Cell Formation
- Iron
- Copper

Muscle Contraction and Relaxation
- Sodium
- Potassium
- Calcium
- Magnesium

Cellular Metabolism
- Iron
- Calcium
- Phosphorus
- Magnesium
- Zinc
- Chromium
- Iodine
- Copper
- Manganese

Antioxidant Defense
- Selenium
- Zinc
- Copper
- Manganese

Growth and Development
- Calcium
- Phosphorus
- Zinc

Figure 9.2 Major functions of minerals in your body.

Matthew Leete/Getty Images

9.1c Factors That Affect Mineral Absorption and Use

Your digestive tract doesn't absorb 100% of the minerals in foods or dietary supplements. The tract's ability to absorb and use mineral nutrients (**bioavailability**) depends on many factors.

- *Need for the mineral:* In general, mineral requirements increase during periods of growth, such as during infancy, puberty, and pregnancy, and when producing milk for breastfeeding. Furthermore, you're likely to absorb more of a mineral nutrient if your body lacks it.

- *Sources of minerals:* Compared to plant foods, animal foods tend to be more bioavailable sources of minerals, such as iron and calcium. Why? Animal products often have higher concentrations of these minerals. Additionally, plant foods can contain substances that reduce the intestinal tract's ability to absorb certain minerals, particularly calcium, zinc, and iron. On the other hand, plant foods supply more magnesium and manganese than do animal foods. By eating a balanced diet that includes a variety of plant and animal foods, you can enhance your body's ability to absorb minerals.

- *Food processing:* In general, the more processing a plant food undergoes, the lower its natural mineral content. Cereal grains, for example, naturally contain selenium, zinc, copper, and some other minerals. When grains are refined, they can lose a lot of their natural mineral contents. Iron is the only mineral added to grains if they undergo enrichment.

If your digestive tract absorbs more minerals than your body needs, the excess is excreted, primarily in urine or feces. In some instances, however, your body stores the extra minerals in the liver, bones, or other tissues. When the need arises, your body releases minerals from storage so they can be used by all cells. Toxicity signs and symptoms occur when minerals accumulate in the body to such an extent that they interfere with the functioning of cells. The summary table for each mineral that's featured in this unit and Table 9.18 provide signs and symptoms of mineral toxicity disorders.

Should You Take Mineral Supplements?

A daily multiple vitamin and mineral supplement is generally safe for healthy people because a dose of this type of supplement doesn't provide high amounts of minerals. However, you need to be careful when taking dietary supplements that contain individual minerals, such as iron or selenium. Many minerals have a narrow range of safe intake; therefore, it's easy to consume a toxic amount, especially by taking supplements that contain only a particular mineral. Additionally, an excess of one mineral can interfere with your body's ability to absorb and use other minerals. For example, having high amounts of zinc in your intestinal tract decreases copper absorption. Single-mineral supplements are usually unnecessary unless they're prescribed to treat a specific medical condition, such as iron deficiency.

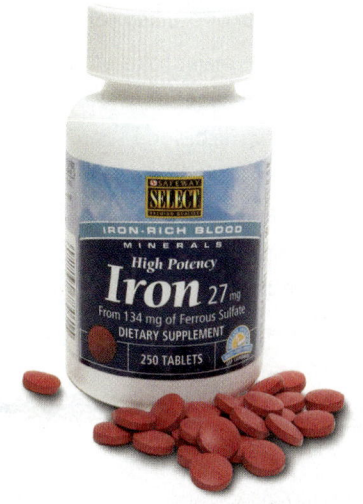

bioavailability body's ability to absorb and use a nutrient

Culture & Cuisine

Throughout the world, especially in India and Pakistan, millions of people consume plant-based diets. In these regions, red meat may be culturally unacceptable or too costly to eat. In addition to grains (especially wheat, corn, and rice), plant-based diets often include protein-rich nuts and legumes, such as beans, dry (split) peas, lentils, and chickpeas (see Unit 7). You may see the term *pulses* used to refer to dry peas, lentils, and chickpeas.

Although legumes are good sources of iron, calcium, zinc, copper, and magnesium, these plant foods also contain substances that interfere with your digestive tract's ability to absorb the minerals. *Oxalic (awk-sal'-ik) acid* and *phytic (feye'-tik) acid* are among the naturally occurring substances in plant foods that can bind to certain minerals, reducing their absorption. Soaking dry beans and peas in water and discarding the soaking water before cooking them reduces their oxalic acid contents. Soaking and cooking lentils, however, appears to have little effect on their phytic acid contents.

The human intestinal tract lacks the enzyme that can digest phytic acid. As a result, minerals in food can bind to the phytic acid, and the minerals are eliminated from the body in feces. Plant scientists are trying to develop new varieties of legumes that will naturally have less phytic acid. If successful, such bioengineering efforts could improve the bioavailability of minerals in the legumes.

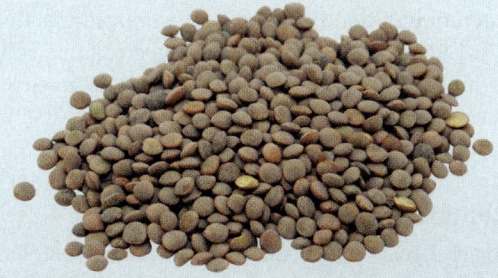
Lentils

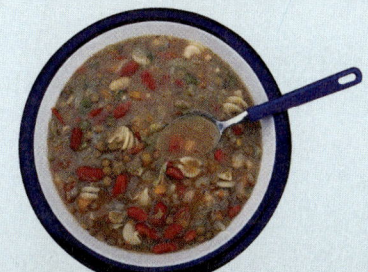
Vegetable soup with lentils

Iron pills: John Flournoy/McGraw-Hill Education; Soup: IngramPublishing/Alamy; Lentils: asterix0597/Getty Images

Module 9.2

Key Minerals and Your Health

9.2 – Learning Outcomes

After reading Module 9.2, you should be able to

1. Define all of the **key terms** in this module.
2. Describe major roles of key minerals in achieving and maintaining good health.
3. Identify major food sources of key minerals.
4. Identify signs and symptoms associated with deficiencies and excesses of the key minerals.
5. Identify major risk factors for osteoporosis and hypertension.

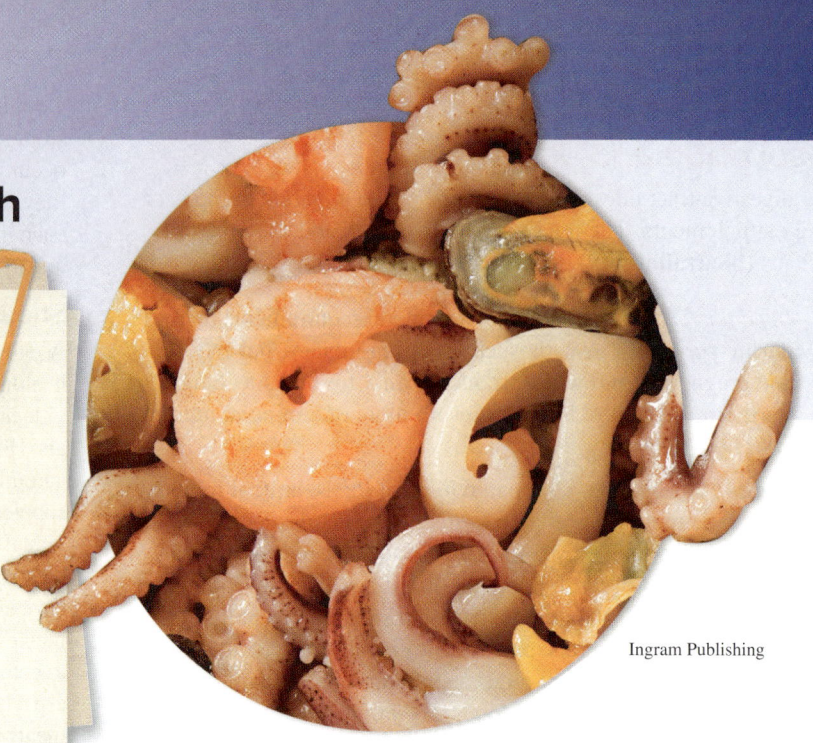

Ingram Publishing

Seafood, including shrimp and octopus, is a rich source of many minerals.

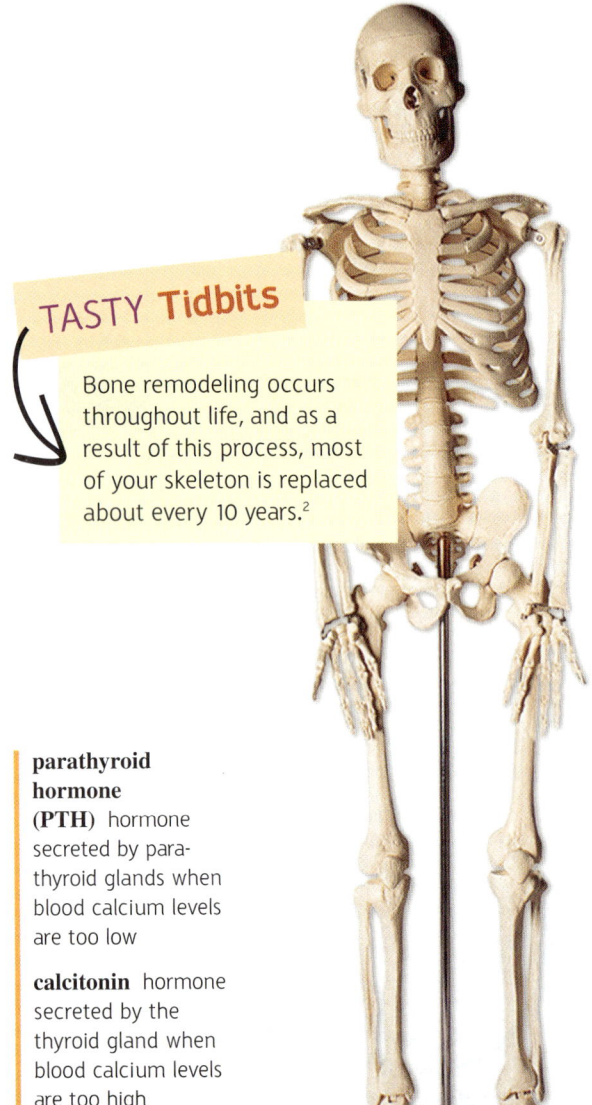

TASTY Tidbits

Bone remodeling occurs throughout life, and as a result of this process, most of your skeleton is replaced about every 10 years.[2]

Comstock/Alamy

parathyroid hormone (PTH) hormone secreted by parathyroid glands when blood calcium levels are too low

calcitonin hormone secreted by the thyroid gland when blood calcium levels are too high

This module focuses primarily on calcium, fluoride, potassium, sodium, iron, magnesium, selenium, copper, iodine, zinc, and chromium. For basic information about some other mineral nutrients, see Table 9.18 at the end of this module.

9.2a Hard Tissue Builders: Calcium and Fluoride

The major mineral calcium (Ca) is the most plentiful mineral element in the human body. Your body needs calcium to build and maintain strong bones and teeth. The mineral is also needed for other important functions, including blood clotting, blood vessel function, and muscle contraction.

Regulating Your Blood's Calcium Level

In addition to vitamin D, two other hormones are involved in regulating your body's calcium level. These hormones are **parathyroid hormone (PTH),** which is made by the four tiny parathyroid glands on the back side of your thyroid gland, and **calcitonin,** a hormone that's made by your thyroid gland. In response to falling blood calcium levels, the parathyroid glands secrete PTH. This hormone signals special bone cells to tear down bone tissue **(Fig. 9.3).** As a result, bones release calcium into the bloodstream, raising its calcium level. PTH also works with vitamin D to increase intestinal calcium absorption and reduce calcium elimination in urine. When the level of calcium in blood is too high, the thyroid gland secretes calcitonin (*cal'-sih-toe'-nin*). Calcitonin signals another type of bone cell to stop tearing down bone tissue, which allows the blood's calcium level to become normal. As a result of these hormonal responses, your body maintains its blood calcium level within the normal range.

Dietary Sources of Calcium

On average, Americans who are 2 years of age and over consume about 950 mg of calcium daily.[3] This amount is less than the RDAs for some groups of people (see the DRI tables in **Appendix E**). In the United States, calcium deficiency is rare.[4]

234

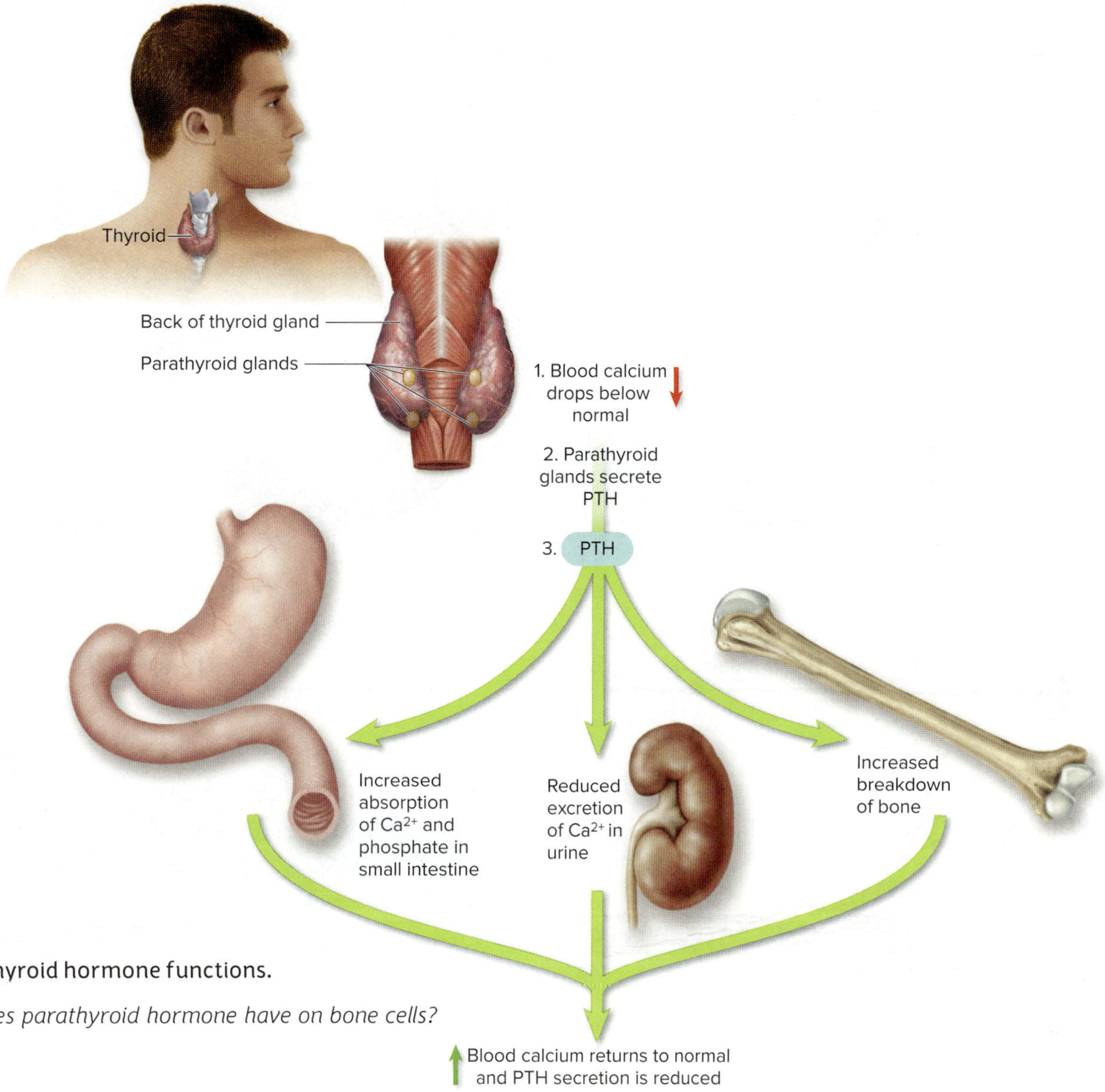

Figure 9.3 Parathyroid hormone functions.

■ *What effect does parathyroid hormone have on bone cells?*

Nevertheless, calcium is a nutrient of public health concern, because many Americans have low intakes of the mineral.

Healthy adults absorb about 30% of the calcium in foods, but this percentage can be higher or lower, depending on the type of food.[4] During early stages of life when the body needs extra calcium—such as infancy and childhood—absorption can be as high as 60%. Older people, especially aging women, don't absorb calcium as well as do younger people. Other factors that reduce calcium absorption include being deficient in vitamin D and taking too many dietary supplements that contain calcium at one time.

Dairy foods are reliable sources of calcium. Each of the foods shown in **Figure 9.4** contains approximately the same amount of calcium that's in 1 cup of fat-free milk (approximately 300 mg):

- 1¼ cups low-fat (2% milk) cottage cheese;
- 1 oz processed cheese (American cheese);
- ⅔ cup plain, fat-free yogurt;
- 1.5 oz natural cheese (e.g., Cheddar or Swiss); and
- 1 cup calcium-fortified soy milk (soy beverage).

TASTY Tidbits

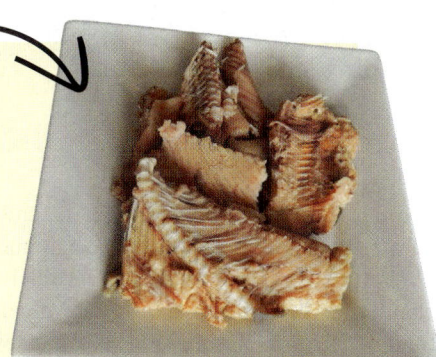

Canned fish with edible soft bones, such as salmon and sardines, are good calcium sources. When making salmon patties using canned fish, for example, mash up the bones along with the salmon. The bones are so soft, you won't notice them in the cooked product.

Canned pink salmon with edible bones

Wendy Schiff

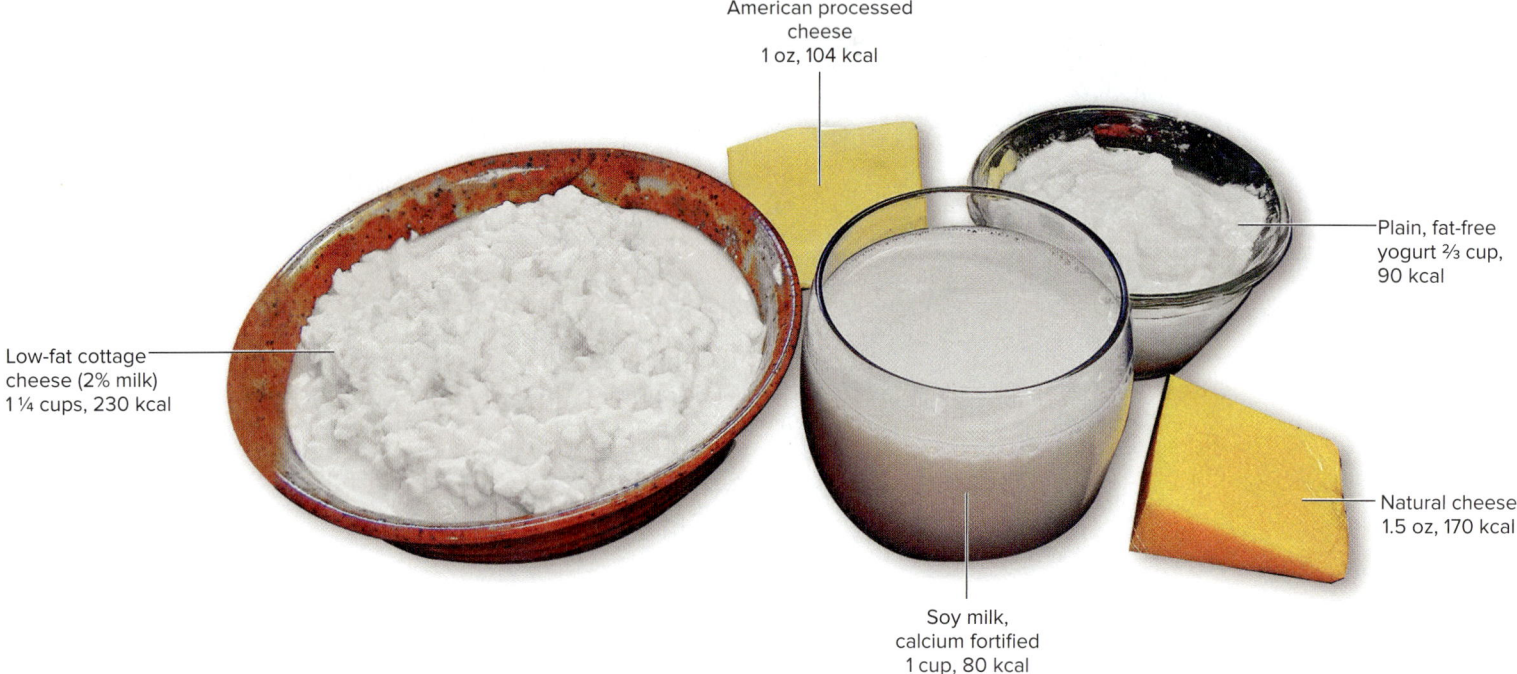

Figure 9.4 Calcium-rich food equivalents from dairy foods group.

Wendy Schiff

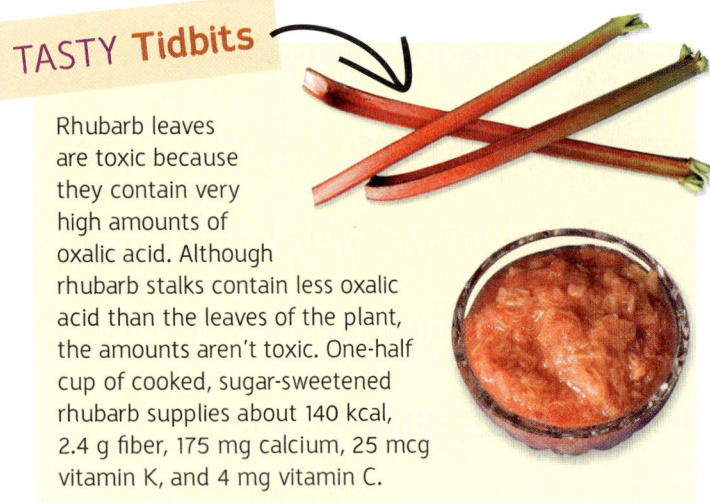

TASTY Tidbits

Rhubarb leaves are toxic because they contain very high amounts of oxalic acid. Although rhubarb stalks contain less oxalic acid than the leaves of the plant, the amounts aren't toxic. One-half cup of cooked, sugar-sweetened rhubarb supplies about 140 kcal, 2.4 g fiber, 175 mg calcium, 25 mcg vitamin K, and 4 mg vitamin C.

Table 9.2 CALCIUM CONTENT OF SELECTED FOODS (APPROXIMATE)

Food	Calcium (mg)
Tofu, made with calcium sulfate, ½ cup	861
Milk, 1%, 1 cup	314
American cheese, pasteurized process, 1 oz	296
Yogurt, plain, low-fat, 1 cup	287
Swiss cheese, 1 oz	252
Cottage cheese, 2% fat, 1 cup	250
Salmon, canned, with bones, 3 oz	241
Kale, frozen, boiled, drained, 1 cup	177
Bok choy, raw, shredded, 1 cup	158
Baked beans, canned, plain, 1 cup	134
Ice cream, vanilla, light, ½ cup	115

RDA for adults = 1000–1200 mg/day

Source: U.S. Department of Agriculture, Agricultural Research Service: *USDA National Nutrient Database for Standard Reference Legacy Release, April 2018.* https://ndb.nal.usda.gov/ndb/search/list?home=true Accessed: September 2018

Chinese cabbage (bok choy), kale, and broccoli are good plant sources of calcium. However, the calcium in other plant foods is generally not as bioavailable as the calcium in dairy foods. Why? Plant foods such as spinach, collard greens, and sweet potatoes contain calcium, but the foods also contain oxalic acid. Oxalic acid binds to calcium, interfering with its absorption as a result. If you eat foods that contain oxalic acid as part of a varied diet and meet the RDA for calcium, you're unlikely to become deficient in the mineral.[4]

Calcium is added to a variety of foods, including many ready-to-eat breakfast cereals, fortified orange juice, margarine, soy milk, and breakfast bars. Another source of calcium is soybean curd (tofu) that's made with calcium sulfate. **Table 9.2** includes some foods that often supply calcium in American diets. **Figure 9.5** indicates food groups from MyPlate that are good sources of calcium.

Calcium-rich foods, Rhubarb stems, Cooked rhubarb: Wendy Schiff

What *IS* That?

Bok choy is a vegetable that's related to cabbage and broccoli. The leaves and stalks are steamed or sautéed with other vegetables. The vegetable can also be shredded and added to salads. One cup of raw, shredded bok choy provides 74 mg calcium, 176 mg potassium, 32 mg vitamin C, 32 mcg vitamin K, and only 9 kcal.

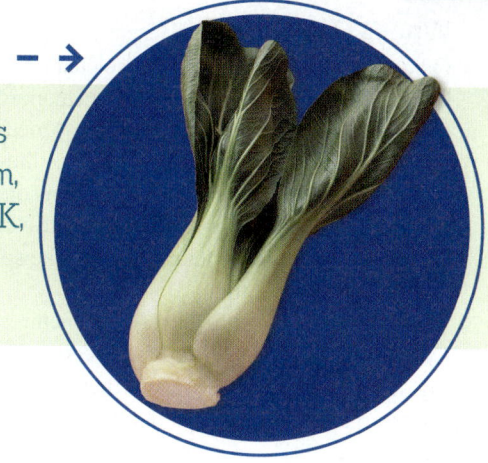

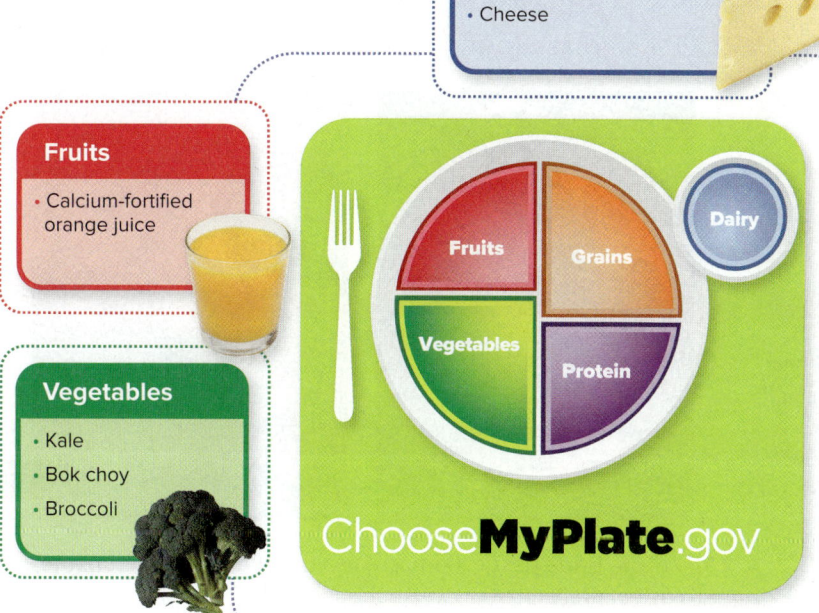

Dairy
- Milk
- Yogurt
- Cheese
- Calcium-fortified soy milk

Fruits
- Calcium-fortified orange juice

Vegetables
- Kale
- Bok choy
- Broccoli

Grains
- Calcium-fortified flour tortillas
- Calcium-fortified ready-to-eat cereals

Protein
- Tofu, made with calcium sulfate
- Almonds
- Soy milk
- Canned sardines and salmon, with bones

Figure 9.5 MyPlate: Good food sources of calcium.

The following tips can help add more calcium to your diet.

- Sprinkle grated low-fat cheeses on top of salads, bean or pasta dishes, and cooked vegetables.
- Add shredded bok choy to salads or soups.
- If you don't like the taste of plain fat-free milk or plain yogurt, try blending it with one-half of a banana, raspberries, mango, or some strawberries.
- For a snack, melt a slice of low-fat cheese on half a whole-wheat bagel, whole-wheat crackers, or a slice of rye bread.
- If a recipe calls for water, substitute fat-free milk for water if it's appropriate. For example, use fat-free milk or plain soy milk when making cooked oatmeal or pancake batter.
- Add ¼ cup nonfat milk powder to 1 pound of raw ground meat when preparing hamburgers, meatballs, or meatloaf.
- Make homemade smoothies by blending plain low-fat yogurt with fresh or frozen fruit and fat-reduced ice cream or sherbet.

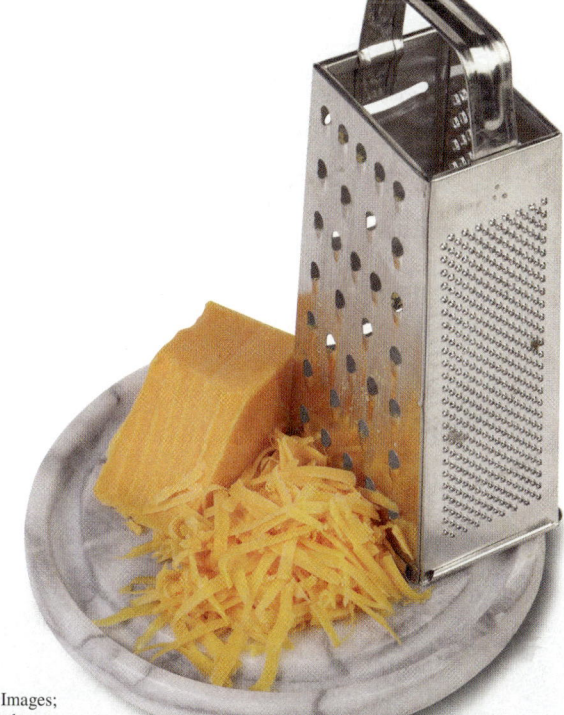

Choose MyPlate: Source: ChooseMyPlate.gov; Broccoli: Burke Triolo Productions/Getty Images; Orange juice: Stockbyte/Getty Images; Swiss cheese: Comstock/Jupiter Images; Bowl of cereal, Almonds: Wendy Schiff; Cheese and grater: Ingram Publishing/SuperStock; Bok choy: Image100/SuperStock

What's Osteoporosis?

Osteoporosis is a chronic disease characterized by a loss of normal bone mass **(Fig. 9.6)**. People with osteoporosis have weak bones that fracture easily. More than 40 million Americans either have osteoporosis or a high risk of the disease because they have reduced bone mass.[4] About half of all women and as many as one in four men older than 50 years of age will break a bone because of osteoporosis.[5] Fractures of the hip, wrist, or vertebra (bone of the spine) are common among people in this age group.

Among older adults, most bone fractures are the result of falling. Older adults who receive proper treatment for hip fractures, including surgery, often recover from their injuries. Many of these persons, however, are unable to live independently and require costly long-term health care.

Osteoporosis-related fractures often involve the upper spine. In severe cases, bones in the upper spine fracture and then heal in an abnormally curved position, giving the obvious "widow's (dowager's) hump" appearance associated with osteoporosis **(Fig. 9.7)**. Osteoporosis is a major cause of pain and disability among older adults.

What Causes Osteoporosis?

You're more likely to develop osteoporosis if you didn't reach optimal peak bone mass by the end of your bone-building years. During your childhood and teenage years, your body added new bone tissue faster than it removed old bone tissue. As a result, your bones became larger and denser. Girls achieve as much as 90% of their total bone mass by the time they're 18 years of age; boys reach up to 90% of their "peak" bone mass when they're 20 years of age.[6] By around 30 years of age, a person has maximized his or her bone mass. Bone loss is slow and steady beginning around age 30. In women, however, the rate of bone loss increases significantly after *menopause*—that is, after menstrual cycles have ceased. At this time of life, women have the highest risk of osteoporosis. Why? The hormone estrogen is needed for normal bone development and maintenance.

After menopause, a woman's ovaries produce considerably less estrogen than when she was in her childbearing years. Eventually, her ovaries stop making the hormone. As a result, her rate of bone loss exceeds the rate of bone replacement during this stage of life.

Damian, the young man featured in the unit opener, has lactose intolerance. He now drinks lactase-treated milk, a rich source of calcium and vitamin D, micronutrients that can help keep his bones healthy. While he's young, he should consider adding foods to his diet that have been fortified with the calcium, such as certain brands of orange juice and ready-to-eat cereals.

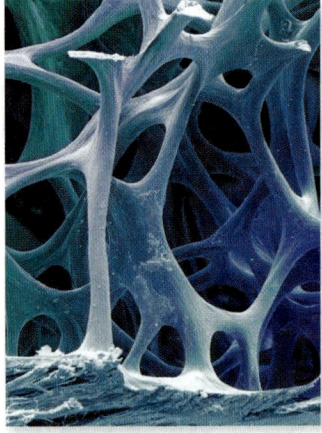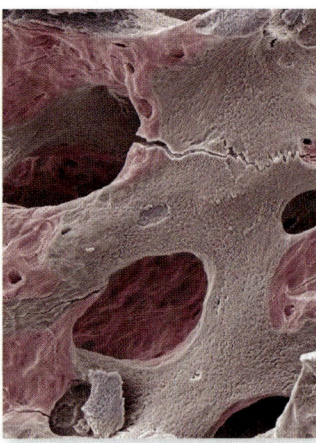

Figure 9.6 Bone tissue. Compare healthy bone tissue (left photo) with osteoporotic bone tissue (right photo).

■ *What is osteoporosis?*

Several factors contribute to bone loss and osteoporosis. Major risk factors are

- growing older and being a *postmenopausal* woman,
- having white or Asian ancestry,
- having a family history of osteoporosis,
- having a small body frame,
- having low estrogen levels in women and low testosterone levels in men,
- following diets that contain inadequate amounts of calcium and vitamin D,
- being physically inactive,
- smoking cigarettes,
- consuming excessive alcohol, and
- having anorexia nervosa (an eating disorder).[7]

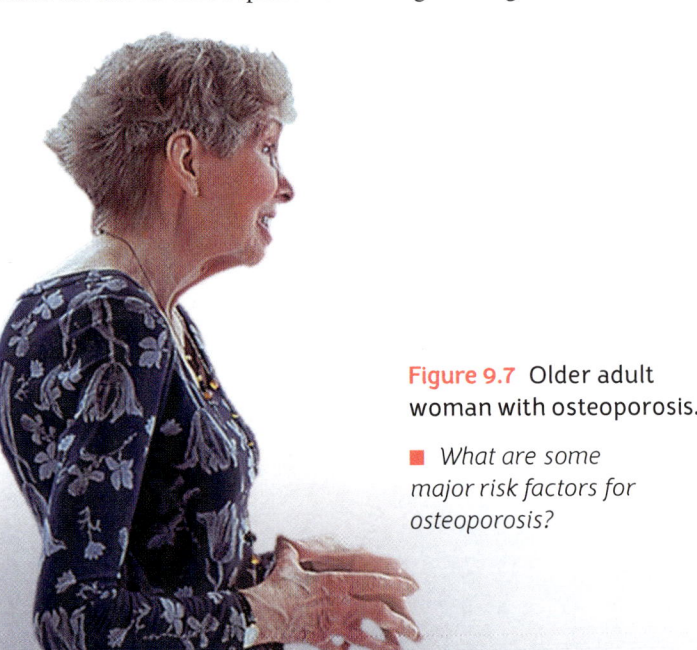

Figure 9.7 Older adult woman with osteoporosis.

■ *What are some major risk factors for osteoporosis?*

osteoporosis chronic disease characterized by bones with low mass and reduced structure

Healthy bone: Science Photo Library/Alamy Stock Photo; Osteoporotic bone: Steve Gschmeissner/Science Photo Library/ Science/Source; Woman: Yoav Levy/Phototake.com

Efforts to reduce the risk of osteoporosis should begin early in life. Proper diet and regular exercise are especially important from early childhood through late adolescence because the body actively builds bone during these life stages. By following the recommendations of MyPlate, you can obtain adequate amounts of calcium from foods. Exposing skin to sunlight can stimulate your body's ability to form vitamin D, but you may need to take vitamin D supplements.

Exercise, especially weight-bearing activities, increases bone mass because contracting muscles keep tension on bones.[7] Such tension stimulates bones to become stronger. Weight-bearing activities include

- dancing;
- playing basketball;
- walking, jogging, and hiking;
- jumping rope;
- stair climbing; and
- strength training with weights.

Should You Take a Calcium Supplement? Dietary supplements that contain calcium generally provide calcium carbonate or calcium citrate.[4] Calcium carbonate is 40% elemental calcium by weight, whereas calcium citrate is 21% elemental calcium by weight. (Check the Supplement Facts panel on the product's label for information about the milligrams of elemental calcium in each pill.) The calcium in calcium carbonate is absorbed most efficiently when taken with food because this form of the mineral relies on stomach acid for absorption. Calcium citrate can be taken with or without food.

The long-term safety and effectiveness of taking calcium supplements hasn't been established. Results of some studies found that taking supplements containing high amounts of calcium (more than 1000 mg) increased the risk of dying from cardiovascular disease (CVD). Results of other studies, however, didn't find that calcium supplementation increased the risk of dying from CVD. More research is needed to determine whether calcium supplementation poses serious risks to health. It's always a good idea to check with your physician before taking any dietary supplement, and if you do use a calcium supplement, don't exceed the Upper Level (UL).[4]

Consider improving your intake of foods that are naturally rich sources of calcium before using a dietary supplement to boost your intake of the mineral. **Table 9.3** summarizes basic information about calcium. RDA values are for adults, excluding pregnant or breastfeeding women.

Fluoride and Health

Although fluoride (F^-) generally isn't considered to be an essential nutrient, the mineral strengthens bones and teeth when ingested in small amounts. In some parts of the United States, well water contains high amounts of the trace mineral. To ensure that people living in other sections of the country obtain healthful amounts of fluoride, the mineral is often added to public water supplies (fluoridation), toothpastes, and dental rinses. Tea naturally contains fluoride.

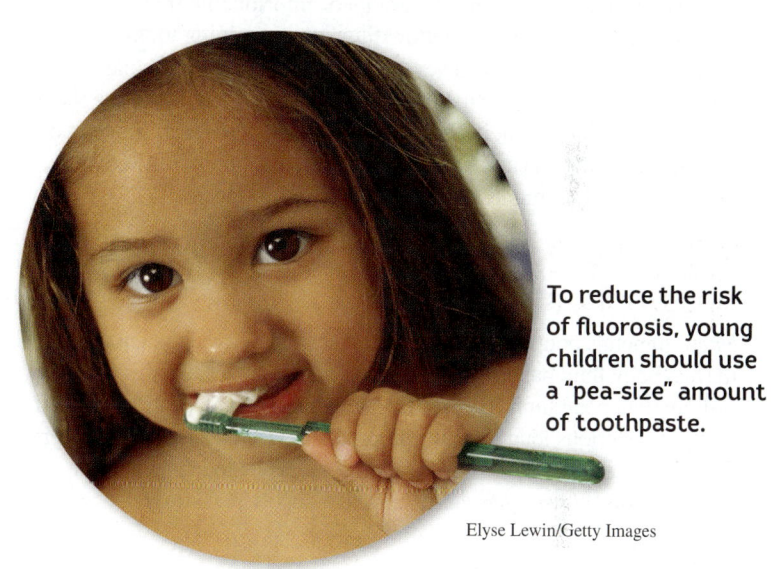

To reduce the risk of fluorosis, young children should use a "pea-size" amount of toothpaste.

Elyse Lewin/Getty Images

TABLE 9.3 CALCIUM AND FLUORIDE: SUMMARY OF BASIC NUTRITION INFORMATION

Mineral	Major Functions in the Body	Adult RDA/AI	Major Dietary Sources	Major Deficiency Signs and Symptoms	Major Toxicity Signs and Symptoms
Calcium (Ca)	Structural component of bones and teeth Blood clotting Transmission of nerve impulses Muscle contraction Regulation of metabolism	1000–1200 mg	Dairy foods, canned fish, tofu made with calcium sulfate, leafy vegetables, calcium-fortified foods such as orange juice	Increased risk of osteoporosis May increase risk of hypertension	UL = 2.0 to 2.5 g/day Intakes > 2.5 g/day: Bone pain, headaches, constipation, abdominal discomfort; kidney stones (excess dietary supplements)
Fluoride (F^-)	Increased resistance of tooth enamel to cavity formation Bone formation stimulation	Men: 4 mg Women: 3 mg	Fluoridated water, tea, seaweed	No true deficiency but increased risk of tooth decay	UL = 10 mg/day Stomach upset, fluorosis, bone deterioration

McGraw-Hill Education

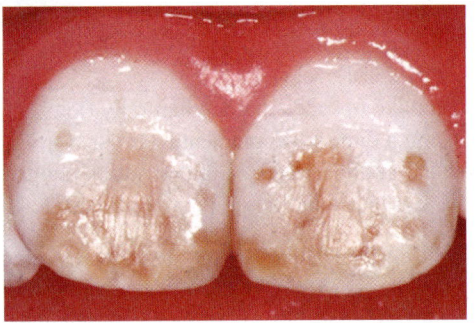

Figure 9.8 Stained teeth due to dental fluorosis.

Diets that lack fluoride don't cause a deficiency disease. However, long-term consumption of too much fluoride can cause *fluorosis*. In cases of skeletal fluorosis, excess fluoride builds up in bones, causing joint stiffness and bone pain. Skeletal fluorosis rarely occurs in the United States. Dental fluorosis often affects young children who drink well water that contains high amounts of fluoride, but it also can occur in children who routinely swallow fluoride-containing toothpaste and dental rinses. Children with severe fluorosis develop permanently stained teeth that don't resist decay as do healthy teeth (**Figure 9.8**). Parents should teach their children to place a "pea-sized" amount of toothpaste on their brush, rinse with water, and spit out the excess fluid. Table 9.3 summarizes information about fluoride.

9.2b The Fluid Balancers: Potassium and Sodium

Major minerals potassium and sodium play a vital role in maintaining normal body fluid balance. The typical American diet supplies far more sodium than potassium. This mineral imbalance may lead to high blood pressure, a serious long-term health problem. However, you may lower the risk that excess sodium poses to your health by reducing your intake of sodium and consuming more foods that supply potassium.[9]

Potassium

Potassium (K) is the major positively charged ion in the fluid that's inside cells. Fresh fruits, fruit juice, and vegetables are good dietary sources of potassium. Milk, whole grains, dried beans, and meats are also major contributors of potassium to American diets.

Many Americans, particularly adult men, don't consume recommended amounts of potassium.[3] According to the *Dietary Guidelines for Americans,* potassium is a nutrient of public health concern. You can raise your potassium intake by eating more fruits, vegetables, whole-grain breads and cereals, and low-fat and fat-free dairy foods. **Table 9.4** provides information about the potassium content of a few selected foods. **Figure 9.9** indicates food groups that are naturally good sources of potassium.

People who experience excessive body fluid losses through sweating, vomiting, or diarrhea are at risk for electrolyte depletion. Symptoms of low blood potassium levels generally include muscle cramps, confusion, and constipation. In severe cases, the lack of potassium causes muscular weakness and abnormal heartbeat. Therefore, it's important to seek medical treatment when potassium depletion is suspected.

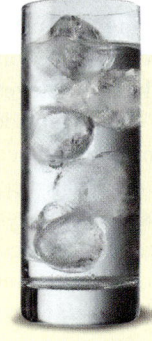

TASTY Tidbits

The majority of the U.S. population served by community water systems has access to drinking water that contains optimal fluoride levels.[8] Some Americans oppose fluoridation for a variety of reasons, including the belief that the practice is a form of involuntary medication. Other people oppose fluoridation because they're concerned about long-term risks of drinking the treated water. For more information about fluoridation, visit www.cdc.gov/fluoridation/index.html

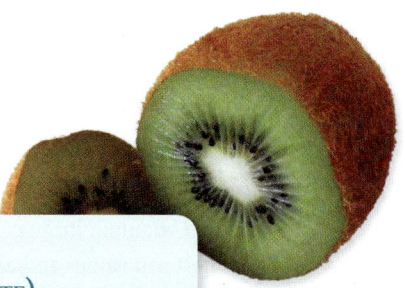

TABLE 9.4 POTASSIUM CONTENT OF SELECTED FOODS (APPROXIMATE)

Food	Potassium (mg)
Beet greens, boiled, drained, 1 cup	1309
Baked potato, including skin, 6 oz	952
Spinach, cooked, drained, 1 cup	839
Coconut water, 1 cup	600
Kiwi, sliced, 1 cup	562
Banana, sliced, 1 cup	537
Sweet potato, canned, mashed, 1 cup	536
Orange juice, frozen, reconstituted, 1 cup	443
Yogurt, non-fat, plain, 6 oz	434
Cantaloupe, cubes, 1 cup	427
Milk, fluid, 1% fat, 1 cup	397
Corn, canned, yellow, 1 cup	389
Peaches, raw, sliced, 1 cup	293
Salmon, pink, canned, 3 oz	292
Grapes, raw, red, 1 cup	288
Papaya, raw, 1" pieces, 1 cup	264
Tuna, white, canned in water, drained, 3 oz	201

AI for adults = 2600 mg/day for women; 3400 mg/day for men
Source: U.S. Department of Agriculture, Agricultural Research Service: *USDA National Nutrient Database for Standard Reference Legacy Release,* April 2018. https://ndb.nal.usda.gov/ndb/search/list?home=true Accessed: September 2018

Teeth: Centers for Disease Control and Prevention; Glass of iced water: 81a/age fotostock; Kiwi fruit, Coconut water: Wendy Schiff

Figure 9.9 MyPlate: Good food sources of potassium.

Dairy
- Milk
- Yogurt

Fruits
- Pears
- Prunes
- Peaches
- Avocados
- Cantaloupes
- Bananas

Grains
- Whole-wheat bread
- Whole-grain products

Vegetables
- Spinach
- Squash
- Potatoes
- Tomatoes
- Lettuce
- Lima beans

Protein
- Meat
- Chicken
- Fish
- Shrimp
- Beans

Sodium

Sodium (Na) is the major positively charged ion in the fluid that surrounds cells. Most uncooked vegetables, raw meats, and grain products are naturally low in sodium. Table salt is sodium chloride, a compound comprised of two minerals, sodium and chloride.

Manufacturers often add salt to food during processing, and you may add more salt when you prepare or eat the food. Processed foods, however, are the primary sources of sodium in American diets. Salted snack foods, French fries, canned and dried soups, sauces and gravies, hot dogs and "deli" meats, cottage cheese, and pickled foods are high in sodium. **Table 9.5** lists some selected foods and their sodium contents.

TASTY Tidbits

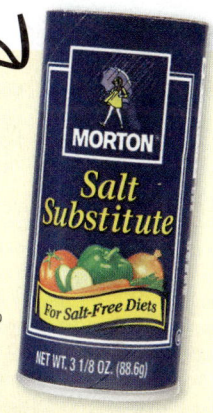

Salt substitutes often contain a type of salt called potassium chloride. People who have kidney disease may accumulate toxic levels of potassium in their blood. Therefore, kidney disease patients should consult their physicians before using salt substitutes made with potassium chloride.[10] To increase your potassium intake safely, consider adding more fruits, vegetables, whole grains, and low-fat dairy foods to your diet.

TABLE 9.5 SODIUM CONTENT OF SELECTED FOODS (APPROXIMATE)

Food	Sodium (mg)
Fast food: biscuit with egg, cheese, and bacon	1183
Chicken soup, chunky, canned, prepared, 1 cup	867
Ham, honey, smoked, 3 oz	765
Cottage cheese, 2% milk, 1 cup	696
Miso (soybean paste), 1 Tbsp	634
Hot dog, pork, one link	620
Tomato sauce, canned, ½ cup	581
Sauerkraut, canned, solids and liquid, ½ cup	469
Sliced turkey breast, packaged, 3 slices	431
Soy sauce, 1 tsp	335
Dill pickle, 1 spear, approx. 1 oz	283
Tortilla chips, nacho cheese, 1 oz	196

AI for adults = 1500 mg/day

Source: U.S. Department of Agriculture, Agricultural Research Service: *USDA National Nutrient Database for Standard Reference Legacy Release, April 2018.* https://ndb.nal.usda.gov/ndb/search/list?home=true Accessed: September 2018

Pickle: Kevin Sanchez/Cole Group/Getty Images; Salt substitute: David A. Tietz/Editorial Image, LLC; Choose MyPlate: Source: ChooseMyPlate.gov; Acorn squash: Burke/Triolo Productions/Getty Images; Pear Stockbyte/Getty Images; Yogurt: Ingram Publishing/SuperStock; Bread, Shrimp: Wendy Schiff

What's Hypertension? **Hypertension** is a condition characterized by chronic high blood pressure. Compared to people with normal blood pressure, hypertensive individuals have greater risk of CVD, especially heart disease and stroke, as well as kidney failure and damage to other organs. In the United States, hypertension is a widespread disease. Approximately 50% of adult Americans have hypertension.[11]

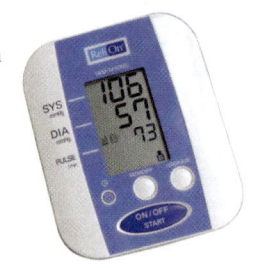
Ilene MacDonald/Alamy

Hypertension is often called the "silent killer" because high blood pressure generally doesn't cause symptoms until the affected person's organs and blood vessels have been damaged. The best way to detect hypertension is to have regular blood pressure screenings. When you have your blood pressure determined, two measurements are actually taken. The first measurement is the **systolic pressure,** which is the maximum blood pressure within an artery. This value occurs when the heart's pumping chambers contract. The second measurement is the **diastolic pressure,** which measures the pressure in an artery when the heart relaxes between contractions. The systolic value, which is reported first, is always higher than the diastolic value. Taking your own blood pressure at home is easy if you have a blood pressure measuring device. **Figure 9.10** provides basic tips for measuring blood pressures at home or in clinical settings.

Table 9.6 presents four categories for blood pressure levels in adults. For adults, healthy blood pressure readings are less than 120/80 millimeters of mercury (mm Hg). If someone's blood pressure measures 180 over 120 (180/120) mm Hg or more, it's critical to obtain immediate medical help for the affected person.

Even if your blood pressure is normal now, it's important to have regular blood pressure checks as you grow older because the risk of hypertension increases with age. In the United States, approximately 90% of the population will develop hypertension during their lifetime.[12] When

hypertension condition characterized by persistently elevated blood pressure

systolic pressure maximum blood pressure within an artery that occurs when the heart contracts

diastolic pressure pressure in an artery that occurs when the heart relaxes between contractions

TASTY Tidbits

Try using garlic, citrus juice, and herbs and spices instead of salt to enhance the taste of foods. Furthermore, consider avoiding seasonings with added salt, such as "garlic salt" or "onion salt." Check the ingredients list to purchase seasonings without added salt (garlic powder or onion powder) instead.

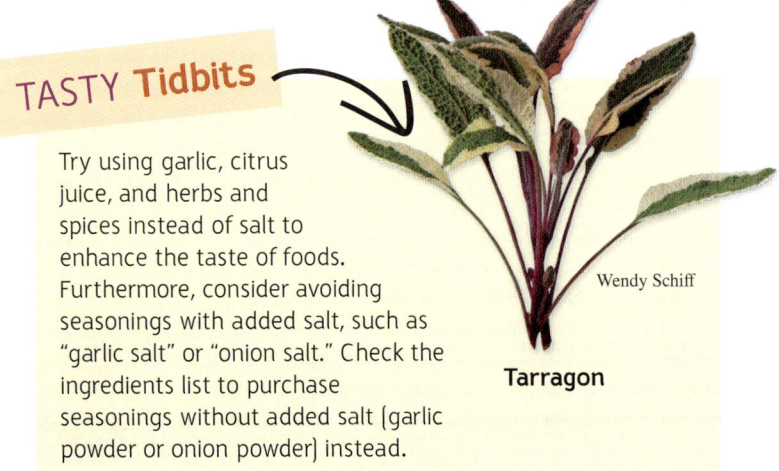
Wendy Schiff
Tarragon

TABLE 9.6 CLASSIFYING BLOOD PRESSURE LEVELS (ADULTS)*

Blood Pressure Classification	Systolic mm Hg	And/Or	Diastolic mm Hg
Normal	< 120	and	< 80
Elevated	120–129	and	< 80
Hypertension: Stage 1	130–139	or	80–89
Hypertension: Stage 2	≥ 140	or	≥ 90

*Key: < is "less than"; ≥ is "more than or equal to."
Source: American Heart Association: *Monitoring your blood pressure at home.* 2017. www.heart.org/en/health-topics/high-blood-pressure/understanding-blood-pressure-readings/monitoring-your-blood-pressure-at-home Accessed: July 6, 2019

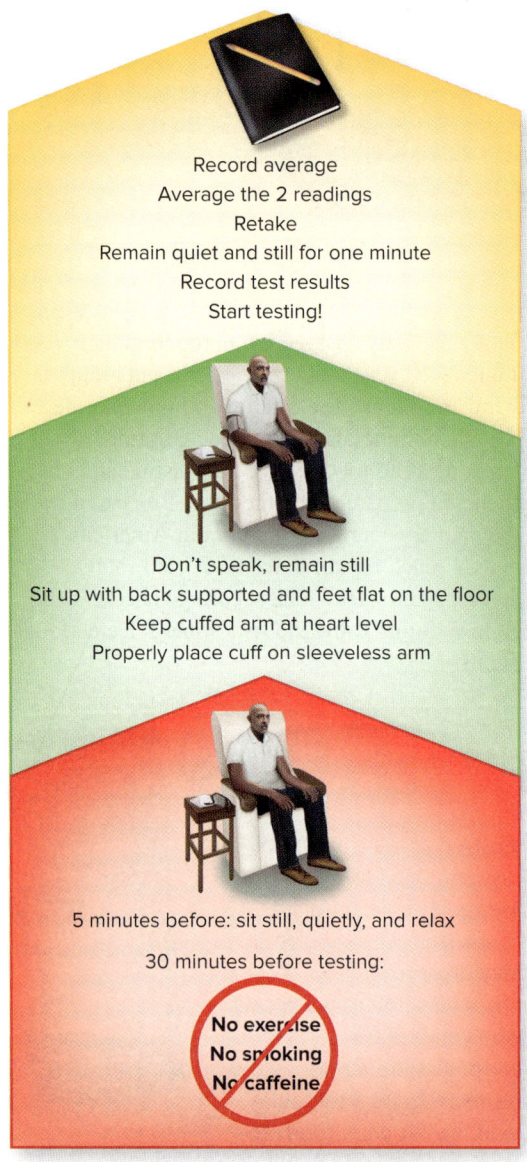

Figure 9.10 Tips for taking your blood pressure.

Source: Adapted from: American Heart Association (www.heart.org/en/news/2018/10/05/how-many-at-home-checks-does-it-take-to-diagnose-high-blood-pressure)

was the last time you had your blood pressure measured? What were the systolic and diastolic values? Every time you have your blood pressure measured, ask the clinician for your systolic and diastolic readings and keep a record of the values.

What Causes Hypertension? Most cases of hypertension don't have simple causes, but major risk factors for the condition are

- family history,
- advanced age,
- African-American ancestry,
- obesity and physical inactivity,
- consumption of excess sodium and not enough potassium,
- use of tobacco and excess alcohol, and
- type 2 diabetes.[12]

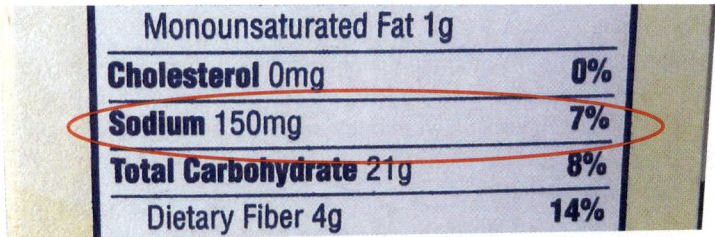
Wendy Schiff

Sodium Intake and Hypertension Risk High sodium intakes are strongly associated with the development of hypertension.[13] On average, Americans who were 2 years of age or older consumed more than 3400 mg of sodium per day in 2015–2016.[3] According to the *Dietary Guidelines for Americans,* healthy people should consume less than 2300 mg of sodium daily.[13] That's the amount of sodium in about 1 teaspoon of table salt. Experts with the American Heart Association set 1500 mg per day as the upper limit for most Americans' sodium intake.[14]

Treating the "Silent Killer" Treatment for hypertension usually includes taking certain medications, following dietary modifications, and making some other lifestyle changes. Research indicates that you may be able to lower your blood pressure and risk of CVD by losing excess body fat, increasing physical activity, and following a diet that is low in sodium and high in fruits, vegetables, and low-fat dairy foods. The DASH diet is a healthy eating plan that includes more fruits and vegetables than the typical American diet. For more information about the DASH diet, visit www.nhlbi.nih.gov/health-topics/dash-eating-plan.

To reduce your sodium intake, consider taking these actions:

- Limit your intake of processed foods. Processed foods are the leading source of sodium in our diets.[15] Therefore, read the Nutrition Facts panel and choose foods with low sodium contents.
- Don't add salt while preparing foods, even though instructions tell you to "add salt."
- Taste your food before salting it and don't keep a salt shaker on your table.
- When ordering items in restaurants, request that no salt be added to your food while it's being prepared.

You can learn more about your sodium-related dietary habits by taking the Sodium Intake Assessment that's near the end of the unit. **Table 9.7** summarizes basic information about potassium and sodium, including major food sources of the minerals.

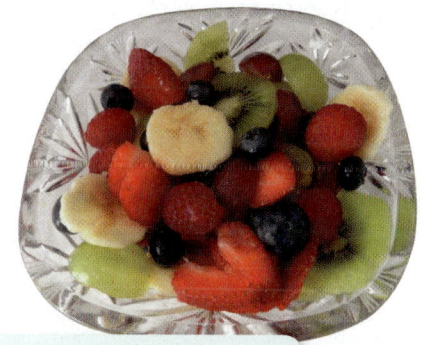
Wendy Schiff

TABLE 9.7 POTASSIUM AND SODIUM: SUMMARY OF BASIC NUTRITION INFORMATION

Mineral	Major Functions in the Body	Adult AI	Major Dietary Sources	Major Deficiency Signs and Symptoms	Major Toxicity Signs and Symptoms
Potassium (K)	Maintenance of proper fluid balance Transmission of nerve impulses Maintenance of acid-base balance	4700 mg	Fruits, vegetables, milk, meat, legumes, whole grains	Irregular heartbeat Muscle cramps Muscle weakness	No UL has been determined. Slowing of heart rate that can result in death
Sodium (Na)	Maintenance of proper fluid balance Transmission of nerve impulses Muscle contraction Transport of certain substances into cells	1500 mg (19–50 years of age)	Processed foods, luncheon meat; pretzels, chips, and other snack foods; condiments; sauces	Muscle cramps	No UL has been determined. Contributes to hypertension in susceptible individuals Increases urinary calcium losses

Nutrition Fact or Fiction?

Children should eat spinach because it's a rich source of iron.

The cartoon character Popeye may have inspired some children to eat spinach, especially those hoping to become instantly strong. Spinach does contain iron, but it's not as bioavailable as the iron in meat. Naturally occurring substances in spinach bind to iron, reducing the intestinal tract's ability to absorb the mineral.[16] Although spinach isn't a good source of iron, the leafy green vegetable is a rich source of folate, beta-carotene, potassium, and dietary fiber.

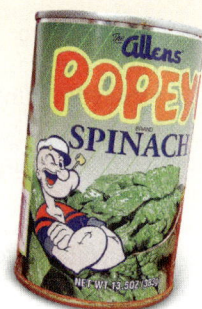

Wendy Schiff

9.2c Iron and Magnesium: Power Minerals

Although minerals don't provide any calories (energy), magnesium and iron are involved in chemical reactions that release energy from macronutrients. The major mineral magnesium is a cofactor that helps regulate energy metabolism. The trace mineral iron helps release energy from macronutrients and transport oxygen in red blood cells (RBCs). Oxygen is critical for energy metabolism. Without a source of oxygen, cells can't obtain much energy and die.

Iron

Iron (Fe) is a component of hemoglobin and myoglobin (*my'-o-glow-bin*). **Hemoglobin** is the iron-containing protein in RBCs that transports oxygen to tissues. **Myoglobin** is the iron-containing protein in muscle cells that controls their removal of oxygen from RBCs. Cells also have a group of iron-containing proteins that are necessary for the release of energy from macronutrients. If the body doesn't have enough iron to make hemoglobin, myoglobin, and the energy-releasing proteins, muscle and other cells cannot obtain the energy they need to perform work. Thus, feeling tired is a major symptom of iron deficiency. Iron also plays roles in immune system function and brain development.

Dietary Sources On average, American males who are 2 years of age and older obtained adequate amounts of iron in 2015–2016.[3] However, the typical diet of American females, especially those who were of childbearing age, provided less than recommended amounts of the mineral. Meat is the major source of iron in the typical American diet. Other important sources of iron are fortified cereals and products made from enriched flour, such as breads and rolls. Dairy foods are poor sources of iron.

The two major forms of iron in food are heme and nonheme iron. Your body absorbs more **heme iron** than **nonheme iron**. Beef, fish, and poultry ("meat") contain heme and nonheme iron. However, plant foods and eggs contain only nonheme iron.

Consuming foods that contain vitamin C (ascorbic acid) can boost your body's absorption of nonheme iron.[16] For example, adding orange slices or lemon juice to a spinach salad can enhance the absorption of the iron in the leafy vegetable. You can also drink orange juice with an iron-fortified breakfast cereal to improve the absorption of iron in the cereal. Another way to increase your body's ability to absorb the nonheme iron in foods is by adding some sources of heme iron to menu items. For example, add cooked chicken cubes to a salad that contains spinach and raisins or eat a hamburger with baked beans to increase your body's absorption of the nonheme iron in the plant foods.

Figure 9.11 indicates MyPlate food groups that are good sources of iron. **Table 9.8** lists some foods that are sources of iron.

> **hemoglobin** iron-containing protein in red blood cells that transports oxygen to tissues
>
> **myoglobin** iron-containing protein in muscle cells that controls oxygen uptake from red blood cells
>
> **heme iron** form of iron that's well absorbed
>
> **nonheme iron** form of iron in vegetables, grains, meats, and supplements

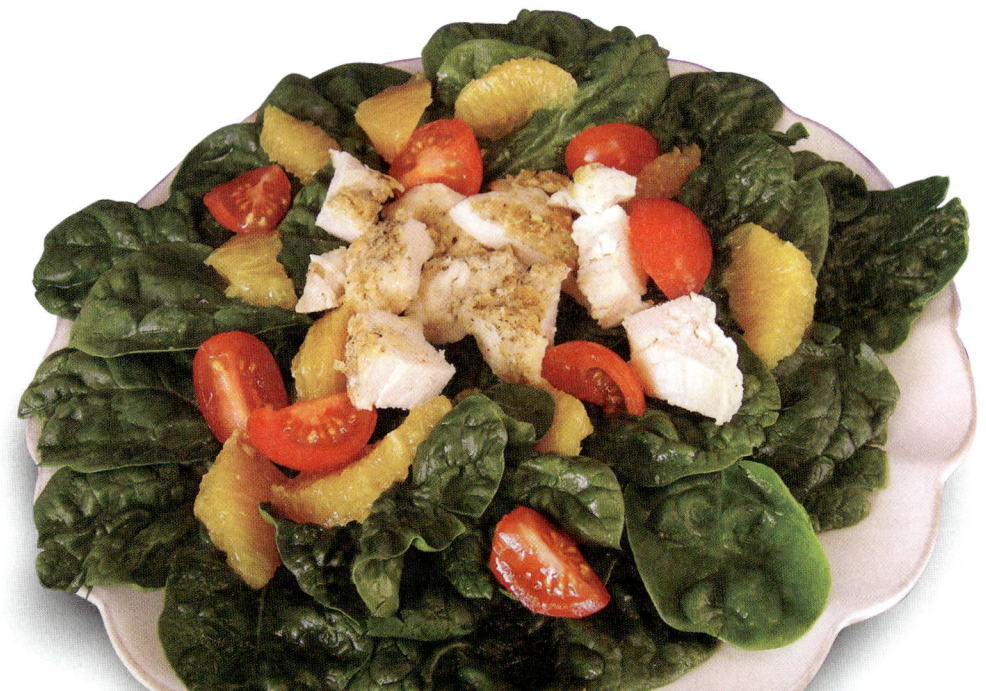

Adding sources of vitamin C to a vegetable salad can boost your body's absorption of nonheme iron.

Wendy Schiff

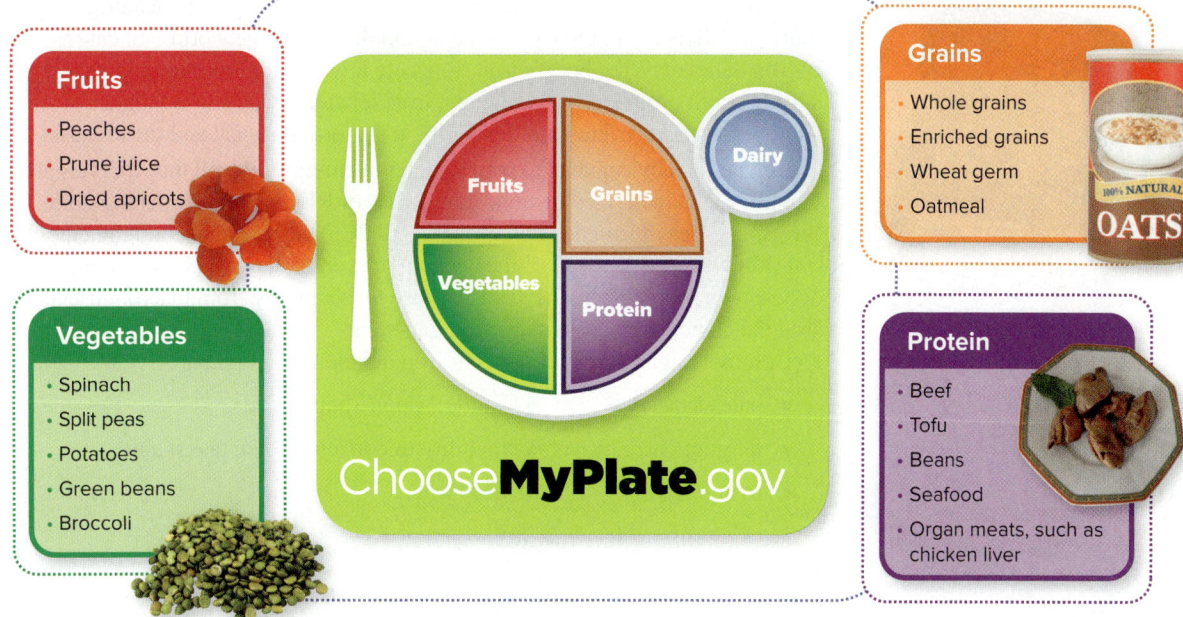

Figure 9.11 MyPlate: Good food sources of iron.

Table 9.8 Iron Content of Selected Foods (Approximate)

Food	Iron (mg)
Quick cooking oats, with iron, ½ cup	19.8
Oatmeal squares, with iron, 1 cup	16.4
Chicken liver, cooked, 3 oz	11.0
Liver sausage, 3 oz	8.9
Split peas, green, raw, ½ cup	4.6
Baked beans, canned, plain, ½ cup	4.0
Cocoa, dry powder, ¼ cup	3.0
Beef round, cooked, 3 oz	2.3
Clams, canned, drained, 3 oz	2.28
Kidney beans, canned, drained, ½ cup	2.00
Turkey, roasted, 3 oz	1.60
Peas, edible pods, frozen, boiled, drained, ½ cup	1.58
White enriched rice, cooked, ½ cup	0.95
Raisins, seedless, ¼ cup	0.78

RDA for women 19–50 years of age = 18 mg/day; >50 years of age = 8 mg/day
RDA for adult men = 8 mg/day
Source: U.S. Department of Agriculture, Agricultural Research Service: *USDA National Nutrient Database for Standard Reference Legacy Release, April 2018.* https://ndb.nal.usda.gov/ndb/search/list?home=true Accessed: September 2018

Iron Deficiency–Related Disorders

Iron deficiency is the leading nutrient deficiency in the United States and the rest of the world.[17] In cases of iron deficiency, the body's iron stores are low but not low enough to cause severe health problems. Nevertheless, iron deficiency can cause fatigue (tiredness) and interfere with the ability to perform physical and mental tasks.

Iron deficiency can lead to **iron deficiency anemia.** Recall that anemias are conditions characterized by unhealthy RBCs or RBCs with low hemoglobin levels. In cases of iron deficiency anemia, RBCs don't contain enough hemoglobin (**Fig. 9.12**). As a result of the anemia, oxygen transport in blood is impaired. When cells lack oxygen, they can't release much energy from macronutrients. Iron deficiency is the leading cause of anemia.[17]

Common signs and symptoms of iron deficiency anemia are

- pale skin;
- fatigue;
- irritability;
- sore tongue;
- brittle, spoon-shaped nails;
- inability to concentrate on tasks; and
- headache.[18]

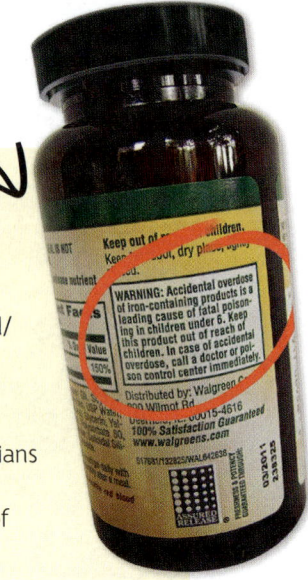

TASTY Tidbits

Accidental ingestion of iron supplements is a leading cause of poisoning among preschool children.[16] Children's vitamin and/or mineral supplements often look and taste like candy, which makes them very appealing to preschoolers. Parents and guardians should keep iron-containing and other dietary supplements out of young children's reach.

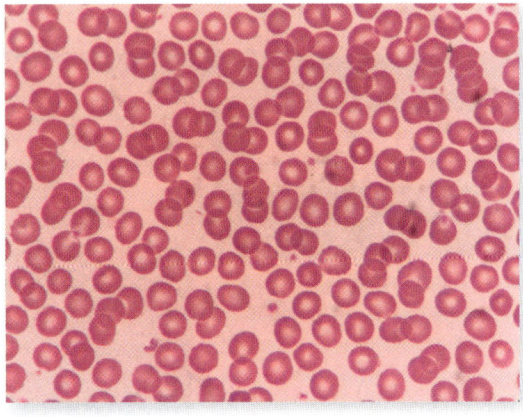
a.

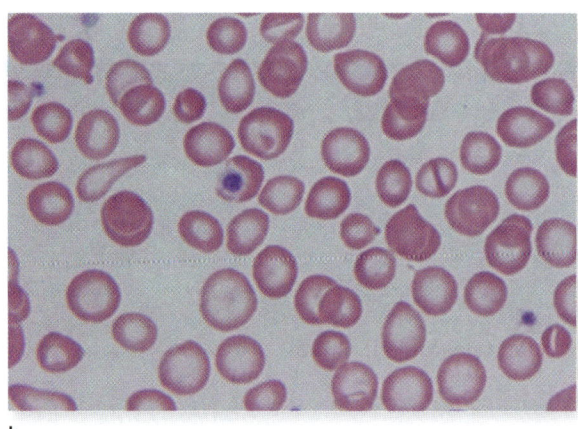
b.

Figure 9.12 Red blood cells. (a) Normal red blood cells; (b) red blood cells of a person with iron deficiency anemia.

■ What is the connection between iron and red blood cells?

TASTY Tidbits

Anemia doesn't always develop as a result of iron deficiency. Vitamin B-12, folate, and vitamin B-6 deficiencies also cause types of anemias. Furthermore, some people have inherited conditions, such as sickle cell anemia or thalassemia (*thal-ah-see'-me-ah*), that result in abnormal hemoglobin formation and anemia. Chronic infection and inflammation, as well as diseases of the blood-forming tissues, can cause anemia.

Abnormal red blood cells in a person with sickle cell anemia.

iron deficiency anemia
condition characterized by red blood cells that don't contain enough hemoglobin

Diets that don't contain adequate amounts of iron and blood loss are major causes of iron deficiency anemia. Women with heavy menstrual blood losses are especially prone to iron deficiency anemia. Although pregnant women don't experience menstrual blood losses, they still should be concerned about their iron intake. A woman's RDA for iron increases dramatically during pregnancy. She requires the extra iron to meet her body's needs as well as those of her developing fetus. Iron deficiency during pregnancy can result in giving birth to a low-birth-weight baby or a baby that's born too early (premature birth). According to the *Dietary Guidelines for Americans*, iron is a nutrient of public health concern for pregnant women.

Children with anemia often experience poor physical growth and abnormal mental functioning. Treatment for iron deficiency anemia generally includes iron supplements and the addition of iron-rich foods to the diet.

Increasing Your Iron Intake To add more iron to your diet or increase your body's ability to absorb iron, consider

- eating lean meat, poultry, or fish with plant sources of iron;
- combining soybeans with tomatoes or tomato sauce;
- adding orange segments or chopped tomatoes to spinach salads or cooked spinach;
- adding chopped onions and green peppers to peas or beans;
- serving sweet potatoes with fresh orange segments or dried apricots;
- adding raspberries, strawberries, raisins, or dried apricots to cereal;
- drinking orange juice when eating peanut butter or soy nut butter sandwiches; and
- eating watermelon, dried plums, dried apricots, or raisins for snacks.

At the end of this section, **Table 9.10** summarizes basic information about iron. RDA values are for adults, excluding pregnant or breast-feeding women.

TASTY Tidbits

Donating 1 pint of blood represents a loss of approximately 200 to 250 mg of iron.[17] Your body generally needs several weeks to replace the iron that was in the donated blood. By taking an iron supplement, you may be able to replenish your body's iron stores more quickly.[16]

According to the American Red Cross, healthy people can give whole blood every 56 days.[19] Young women, however, may need to donate blood less often, especially if they have heavy menstrual losses of blood.

liquidlibrary/PictureQuest

TASTY Tidbits

Iron cookware may be a source of dietary iron. When you cook acidic foods, such as tomato sauce, in a cast-iron skillet, some iron leaves the cookware and enters the food. This unusual dietary source of iron can add to your overall iron intake. Replacing the iron cookware with lighter stainless steel and aluminum pots and pans can reduce the amount of iron in your diet.

Comstock/SuperStock

Magnesium

Your body needs magnesium (Mg) for energy metabolism, enzyme activity, and bone health. Magnesium also helps maintain normal blood sugar and blood pressure levels. More research is needed, but dietary supplements that contain the mineral may be useful in preventing or controlling hypertension and cardiovascular disease.[20]

Magnesium is in chlorophyll, the green pigment in plants. Therefore, plant foods, such as whole grains, beans, nuts, seeds, and chocolate, are among the richest sources of magnesium. Animal products, such as milk and meats, also supply some magnesium. Refined grains are generally low in magnesium because the magnesium-rich bran and germ are removed during processing. **Table 9.9** lists some commonly eaten foods that supply magnesium. **Figure 9.13** indicates MyPlate food groups that are naturally good sources of magnesium.

In 2015–2016, most Americans didn't consume recommended amounts of magnesium.[3] However, cases of magnesium deficiency rarely occur among healthy members of the population.[20] Alcoholics, people with poorly controlled diabetes, or persons who use certain medications that increase urinary losses of the mineral have high risk of magnesium deficiency. Older adults are also at risk of magnesium deficiency because their intake of the mineral is generally low. Furthermore, the body absorbs less of the mineral and urinary losses increase with advancing age. Magnesium toxicity rarely occurs in healthy people who don't use dietary supplements or medications that contain a lot of magnesium, such as milk of magnesia. At the end of this section, Table 9.10 summarizes basic information about magnesium, including signs and symptoms of magnesium deficiency and toxicity.

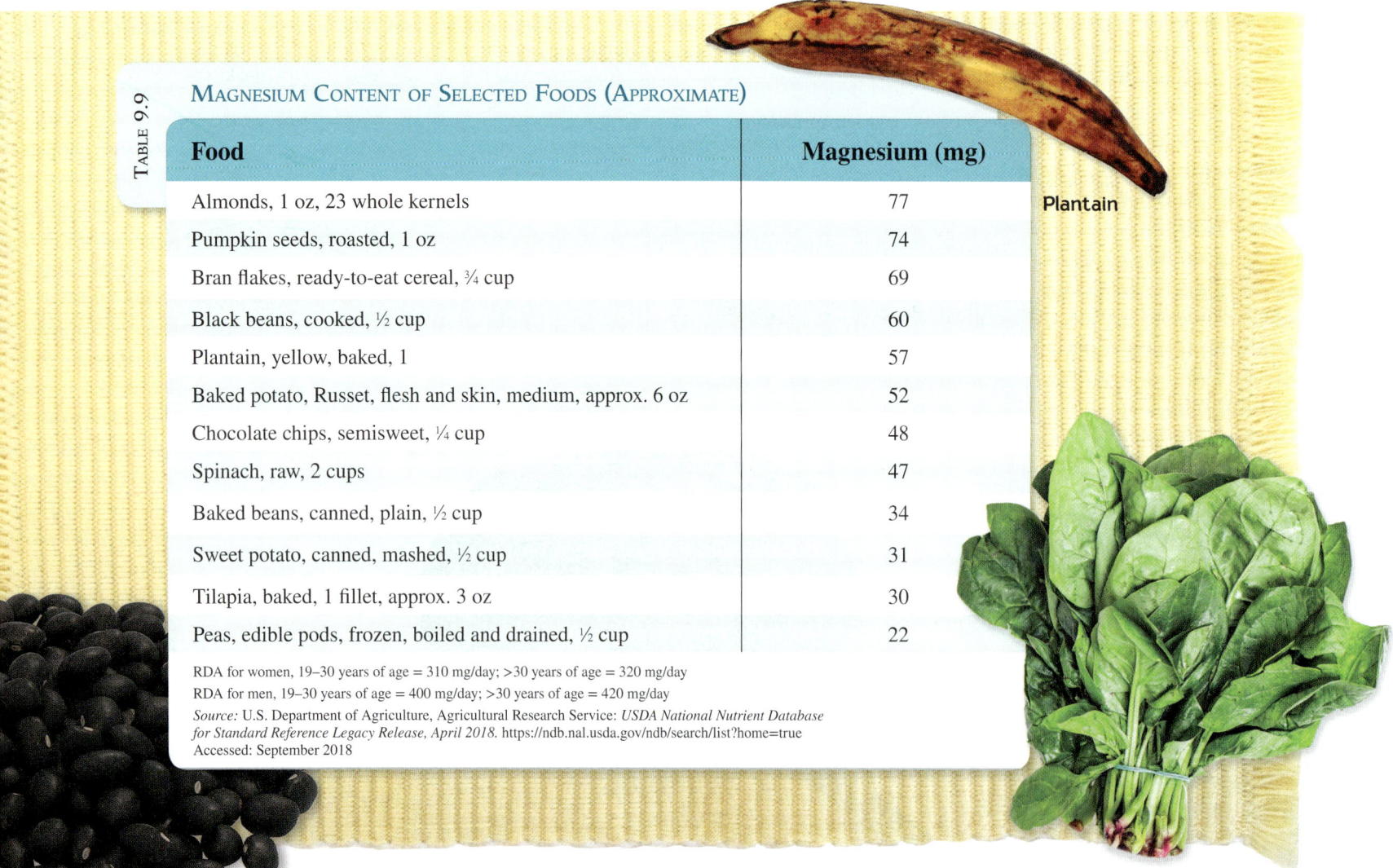

TABLE 9.9

MAGNESIUM CONTENT OF SELECTED FOODS (APPROXIMATE)

Food	Magnesium (mg)
Almonds, 1 oz, 23 whole kernels	77
Pumpkin seeds, roasted, 1 oz	74
Bran flakes, ready-to-eat cereal, ¾ cup	69
Black beans, cooked, ½ cup	60
Plantain, yellow, baked, 1	57
Baked potato, Russet, flesh and skin, medium, approx. 6 oz	52
Chocolate chips, semisweet, ¼ cup	48
Spinach, raw, 2 cups	47
Baked beans, canned, plain, ½ cup	34
Sweet potato, canned, mashed, ½ cup	31
Tilapia, baked, 1 fillet, approx. 3 oz	30
Peas, edible pods, frozen, boiled and drained, ½ cup	22

RDA for women, 19–30 years of age = 310 mg/day; >30 years of age = 320 mg/day
RDA for men, 19–30 years of age = 400 mg/day; >30 years of age = 420 mg/day
Source: U.S. Department of Agriculture, Agricultural Research Service: *USDA National Nutrient Database for Standard Reference Legacy Release, April 2018.* https://ndb.nal.usda.gov/ndb/search/list?home=true Accessed: September 2018

Plantain: Wendy Schiff; Placemat: McGraw-Hill Education/Mark A. Dierker, photographer; Black beans: Jacques Cornell/McGraw-Hill Education; Spinach: vvoennyy/123RF

Key Minerals and Your Health

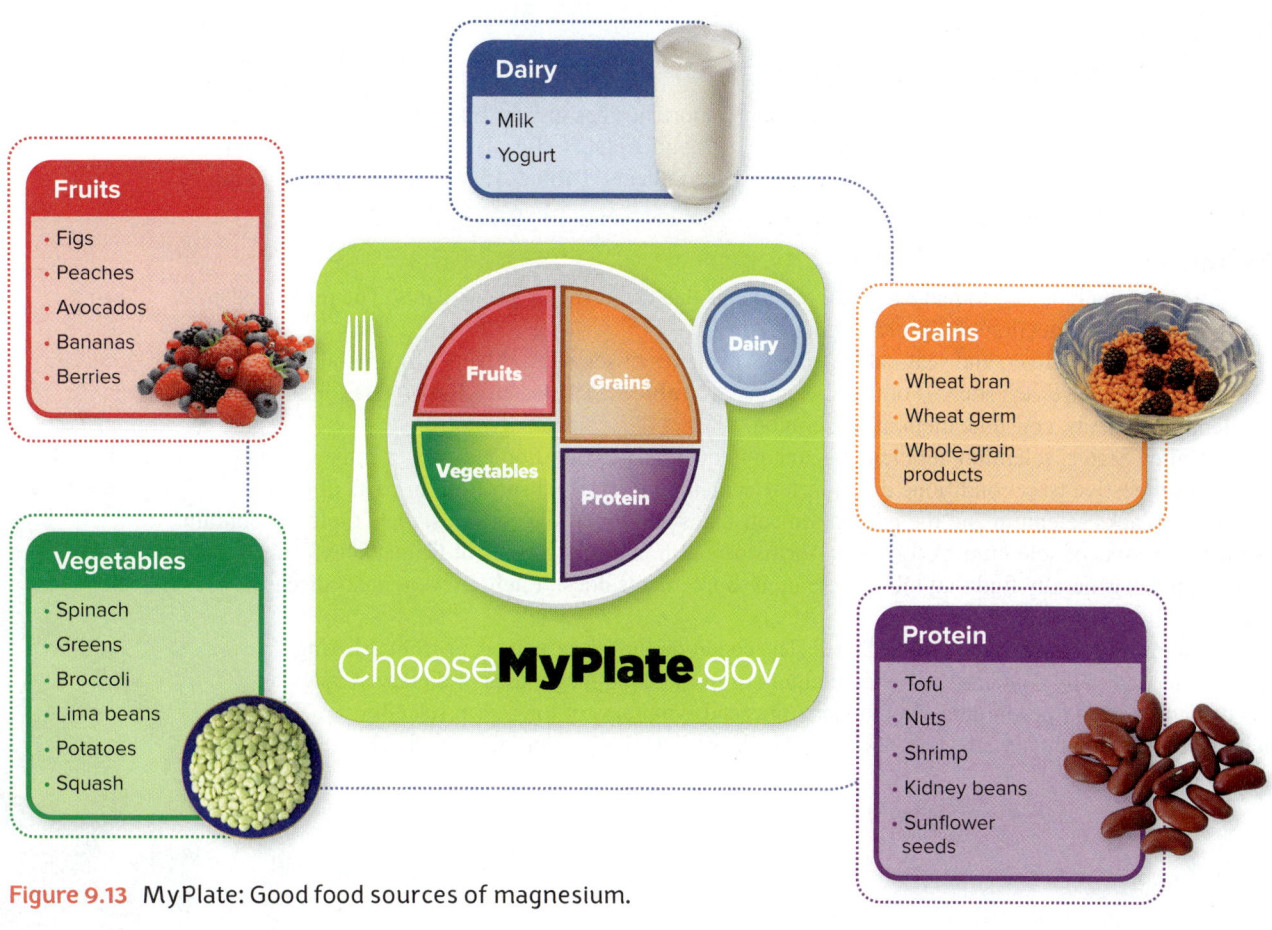

Figure 9.13 MyPlate: Good food sources of magnesium.

Table 9.10 Iron and Magnesium: Summary of Basic Nutrition Information

Mineral	Major Functions in the Body	Adult RDA	Major Dietary Sources	Major Deficiency Signs and Symptoms	Major Toxicity Signs and Symptoms
Iron (Fe)	Component of hemoglobin and myoglobin that carries oxygen; Energy generation; Immune system function	Women (of childbearing age): 18 mg; Men: 8 mg	Meat and other animal foods, except milk; whole-grain and enriched breads and cereals; fortified cereals	Fatigue upon exertion; Small, pale red blood cells; Low hemoglobin levels; Poor immune system function; Growth and developmental retardation in infants	UL = 45 mg/day; Intestinal upset; Organ damage; Death
Magnesium (Mg)	Bone strengthening; Cofactor for certain enzymes; Heart and nerve functioning	Men: 400–420 mg; Women: 310–320 mg	Wheat bran, green vegetables, nuts, chocolate, legumes	Muscle weakness and pain; Poor heart function	UL = 350 mg/day (when intake is from medications only); Diarrhea

Choose MyPlate: Source: ChooseMyPlate.gov; Lima beans: Brand Z Food/Alamy; Berries: David Cook/blueshiftstudios/Alamy; Milk: Ingram Publishing; Bowl of cereal, Kidney beans, Cashews: Wendy Schiff

9.2d Selenium and Copper: Free Radical Fighters

Selenium and copper are trace minerals that play many important roles in your body. These minerals are components of hundreds of enzymes, many of which act as antioxidants. Recall from Unit 8 that antioxidants protect your body's cells from being damaged by free radicals. **Table 9.13** summarizes the basic information about selenium and copper.

Selenium

Your body uses selenium (Se) to make a group of proteins that act as major antioxidants. The mineral also assists iodine in the production of thyroid hormone.

Organ meats, such as liver, and seafood are excellent sources of selenium.[21] Nuts, whole-grain products, turkey, and meat are also rich sources of the trace mineral **(Table 9.11)**. Because Brazil nuts can have very high selenium contents, consume them in moderation.

In the United States, selenium deficiency is uncommon, but the condition may occur in people who have serious digestive tract conditions that interfere with the mineral's absorption. In parts of China where the soil lacks selenium and the population consumes locally produced foods, diets typically contain inadequate amounts of selenium. A form of arthritis is common in these areas of China. The results of scientific studies generally find that taking selenium supplements doesn't help prevent heart disease or cancer.[21]

Selenium toxicity is rare in the United States. The condition, however, can occur from drinking well water that naturally contains too much selenium or from taking megadoses of dietary supplements that contain the trace mineral. In humans, signs and symptoms of long-term selenium toxicity include brittle fingernails, loss of hair and nails, garlicky body odor, nausea, diarrhea, and fatigue.

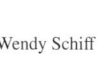

Brazil nuts are rich sources of selenium.

Wendy Schiff

TABLE 9.11 SELENIUM CONTENT OF SELECTED FOODS (APPROXIMATE)

Food	Selenium (mg)
Brazil nuts, 1 oz (6 nuts)	544
Oysters, Pacific, cooked, 5 medium	192
Fish, orange roughy, baked, 3 oz	75
Fish, tuna, white, canned in water, drained, 3 oz	56
Egg noodles, cooked, 1 cup	38
Sunflower seed kernels, roasted, ¼ cup	25
Hamburger patty, 80% lean, broiled, 3 oz	18

RDA = 55 mcg for adults

Source: U.S. Department of Agriculture, Agricultural Research Service: *USDA National Nutrient Database for Standard Reference Legacy Release, April 2018.* https://ndb.nal.usda.gov/ndb/search/list?home=true Accessed: September 2018

McGraw-Hill Education/Mark A. Dierker, photographer

Copper

Your body uses the trace mineral copper (Cu) to make several enzymes that act as antioxidants. The mineral is also involved in iron metabolism, immune function, and collagen production (see section 8.3e of Unit 8).

A wide variety of foods contain copper, but the foods listed in **Table 9.12** are among the richest sources of the micronutrient. Healthy people rarely develop copper deficiency or copper toxicity.[22] However, taking high doses of iron and zinc can interfere with the intestinal tract's ability to absorb copper, causing copper deficiency as a result. People with chronic digestive system diseases may also develop copper deficiency because their bodies' ability to absorb the mineral is reduced.

Table 9.12

Copper Content of Selected Foods (Approximate)

Food	Copper (mg)
Beef liver, braised, 3 oz	12.14
Chocolate, semisweet, mini chips, ¼ cup	0.70
Cashews, dry roasted, 1 oz	0.63
Crab meat, canned, ½ cup	0.55
Sunflower seeds, dry roasted, 1 oz	0.52
Mushrooms, white, cooked, drained, ½ cup	0.39
Soybeans, mature, boiled, drained, ½ cup	0.35
Baked beans, canned, with pork and tomato sauce, ½ cup	0.26

RDA adults = 0.9 mg/day

Source: U.S. Department of Agriculture, Agricultural Research Service: *USDA National Nutrient Database for Standard Reference Legacy Release, April 2018.* https://ndb.nal.usda.gov/ndb/search/list?home=true Accessed: September 2018

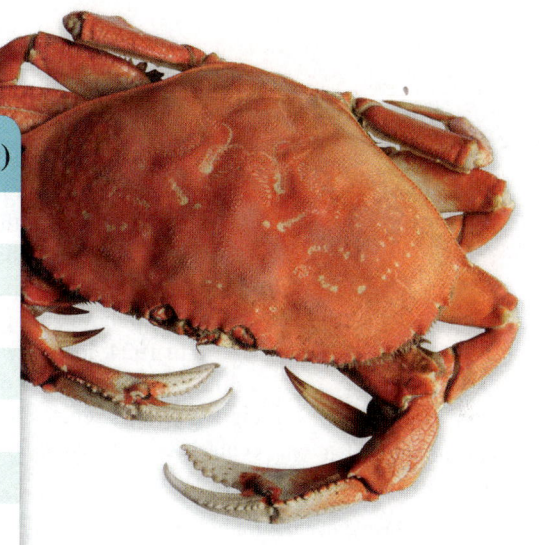

Alamy Stock Photo

Table 9.13

Selenium and Copper: Summary of Basic Nutrition Information

Mineral	Major Functions in the Body	Adult RDA	Major Dietary Sources	Major Deficiency Signs and Symptoms	Major Toxicity Signs and Symptoms
Selenium (Se)	Component of an antioxidant system	55 mcg	Meat, eggs, fish, seafood, whole grains	Joint pain; Form of heart disease	UL = 400 mcg/day; Nausea, diarrhea, hair loss, and weakness; Kidney failure, heart failure, and death
Copper (Cu)	Promotion of iron metabolism; Component of antioxidant enzymes; Component of enzymes involved in connective tissue formation	0.9 mg	Liver, cocoa, legumes, whole grains, shellfish	Anemia; Reduced immune system function; Poor growth and development	UL = 10 mg/day; Vomiting; Abnormal nervous system function; Liver damage

Wendy Schiff

9.2e Iodine, Zinc, and Chromium: Metabolism Regulators

Many minerals, including iodine, zinc, and chromium, are involved in the regulation of energy metabolism. This section provides some basic information about these trace minerals, including good food sources. **Table 9.17** summarizes the information about the three trace minerals.

Why Is Iodine Necessary?

Your thyroid gland traps iodine (in the form of *iodide*) from your bloodstream and uses the mineral for the production of **thyroid hormone** (see Figure 9.3). Thyroid hormone controls the rate of cell metabolism, that is, the rate at which your cells obtain energy. The lack of thyroid hormone can cause your thyroid gland to enlarge and metabolism rate to slow. It's important to note that an enlarged thyroid gland can also be a sign of an "overactive" thyroid gland that makes too much thyroid hormone and some conditions that aren't related to iodine intake.

During World War I, physicians noted that men drafted into the U.S. military from the Great Lakes region were far more likely to have **goiter** (*goy'-ter*) than men from some other areas of the country. Goiter is enlargement of the thyroid gland that's not the result of cancer (**Fig. 9.14**). Goiters often occur among populations living in areas that have iodine-depleted soil. In general, these regions are inland and far from an ocean. If people in these communities limit their diets to locally produced foods, they might not have enough iodine in their diets to prevent goiter.

In 1924, iodine was added to table salt in the United States, and as a result, cases of goiter caused by iodine deficiency rarely occur in this country. Today, the use of iodized salt is the major method of preventing iodine deficiencies in developed nations, but inadequate iodine intake and goiters are still common in central Asia and central Africa.

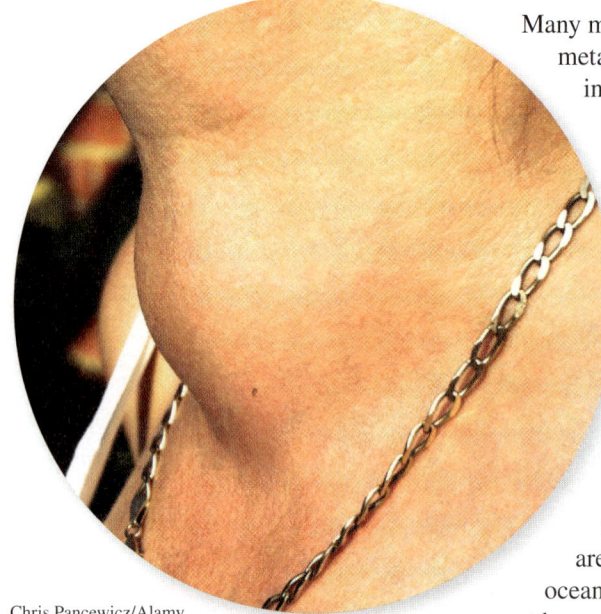
Chris Pancewicz/Alamy

Figure 9.14 Goiter.

thyroid hormone hormone that regulates the body's metabolic rate

goiter enlargement of thyroid gland

Food Sources of Iodine Major dietary sources of iodine include saltwater fish; seafood; seaweed; some plants, especially the leaves of plants grown near oceans; and iodized salt. Iodine fortification of salt is voluntary in the United States, so not all salt has the trace mineral added to it.[23] Other dietary sources of iodine include food additives that contain the mineral, such as certain dough conditioners and food dyes. **Table 9.14** lists some foods that are good sources of iodine.

Q Answer This

People who must restrict their sodium intake could have a higher-than-normal risk of _____ deficiency. You can find the answer on the last page of this unit.

Table 9.14 — Iodine Content of Selected Foods (Approximate)

Food	Iodine (mcg)
Seaweed, dried, ¼ oz	Varies but may be greater than 4500 mcg
Iodized salt, ½ tsp	231
Codfish, 3 oz	99
Milk (cow's), 8 fl oz	99
Potato, baked with peel, 1 medium	60
Shrimp, 3 oz	35
Egg, hard-cooked, 1 large	12

RDA = 150 mcg for adults

Source: Data from Higdon J: *Iodine.* Micronutrient Information Center, Linus Pauling Institute, Oregon State University, Updated 2015. https://lpi.oregonstate.edu/mic/minerals/iodine Accessed: October 6, 2018.

Dried seaweed
Wendy Schiff

Dietary Adequacy Most Americans have adequate iodine intakes.[23] As many Americans try to reduce their risk of hypertension by using less salt, iodine intakes may decline to marginal or inadequate levels.

Iodine-deficient people generally have low metabolic rates and elevated blood cholesterol levels. Other signs and symptoms of iodine deficiency include fatigue, difficulty concentrating on mental tasks, weight gain, intolerance of cold temperatures, constipation, and dry skin.

Throughout the world, millions of people are at risk of iodine deficiency. It's very important for pregnant women to have adequate iodine intakes. Pregnant women who are iodine deficient have a high risk of giving birth to a dead infant, a low-birth-weight baby, or a baby that has **cretinism** (*krē'-tin-ih-zim*). Babies with cretinism have permanent brain damage, reduced intellectual functioning, and growth retardation.

Worldwide, iodine deficiency is the most common cause of preventable brain damage.[23] Pregnant women can reduce the risk of giving birth to infants with cretinism by consuming adequate amounts of iodine throughout pregnancy.

Over time, consuming very high amounts of iodine can cause thyroid gland enlargement and reduced production of thyroid hormone. These side effects are the same as those that occur when diets are deficient in iodine. Excess iodine is also associated with an increased risk of a form of thyroid cancer.[23]

TASTY Tidbits

In the United States, manufacturers often add iodine to table salt to make "iodized salt." The sea salt that's usually sold in supermarkets isn't a good source of iodine because it hasn't been fortified with the mineral.[24] It's wise to avoid excess sodium from all sources, including sea salt.

cretinism condition that affects babies born to iodine-deficient women

Zinc

Zinc (Zn) is needed for a wide variety of functions in your body. The trace mineral is a component of about a hundred enzymes, many of which are involved in the metabolism of protein, carbohydrate, and fat.[25] Zinc is essential for growth and development during pregnancy, childhood, and adolescence. The micronutrient is also necessary for wound healing, the sense of taste and smell, DNA production, and proper functioning of the immune system.

Food Sources of Zinc Zinc is widespread in foods **(Table 9.15)**. Oysters are among the richest sources of zinc, but red meat, poultry products, and fortified cereals supply most of the zinc in the typical American's diet. **Figure 9.15** indicates MyPlate food groups that have foods that are good sources of zinc.

Table 9.15 — Zinc Content of Selected Foods (Approximate)

Food	Zinc (mg)
Oysters, eastern, farmed, cooked, dry heat, 6 medium	26.6
Beef, chuck, top blade, lean meat, broiled, 3 oz	7.6
Ground bison, 90% lean, broiled patty, 3 oz	4.5
Quaker Oat Life™, plain, ready-to-eat cereal, ¾ cup	4.4
Baked beans, canned, plain, ½ cup	2.9
Turkey, ground, cooked, 3 oz	2.6
Yogurt, plain, low-fat, 6 oz	1.5
Wild rice, cooked, ½ cup	1.1

RDA for women = 8 mg/day; RDA for men = 11 mg/day

Source: U.S. Department of Agriculture, Agricultural Research Service: *USDA National Nutrient Database for Standard Reference Legacy Release, April 2018.* https://ndb.nal.usda.gov/ndb/search/list?home=true Accessed: September 2018

Bison burger

Raw oyster

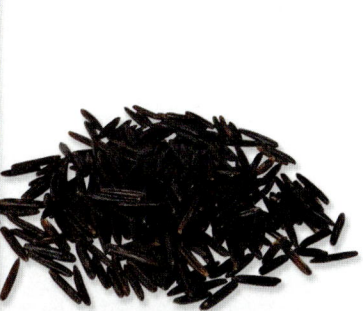

Wild rice

Sea salt, Raw oyster, Wild rice: Wendy Schiff; Bison burger: Purestock/SuperStock

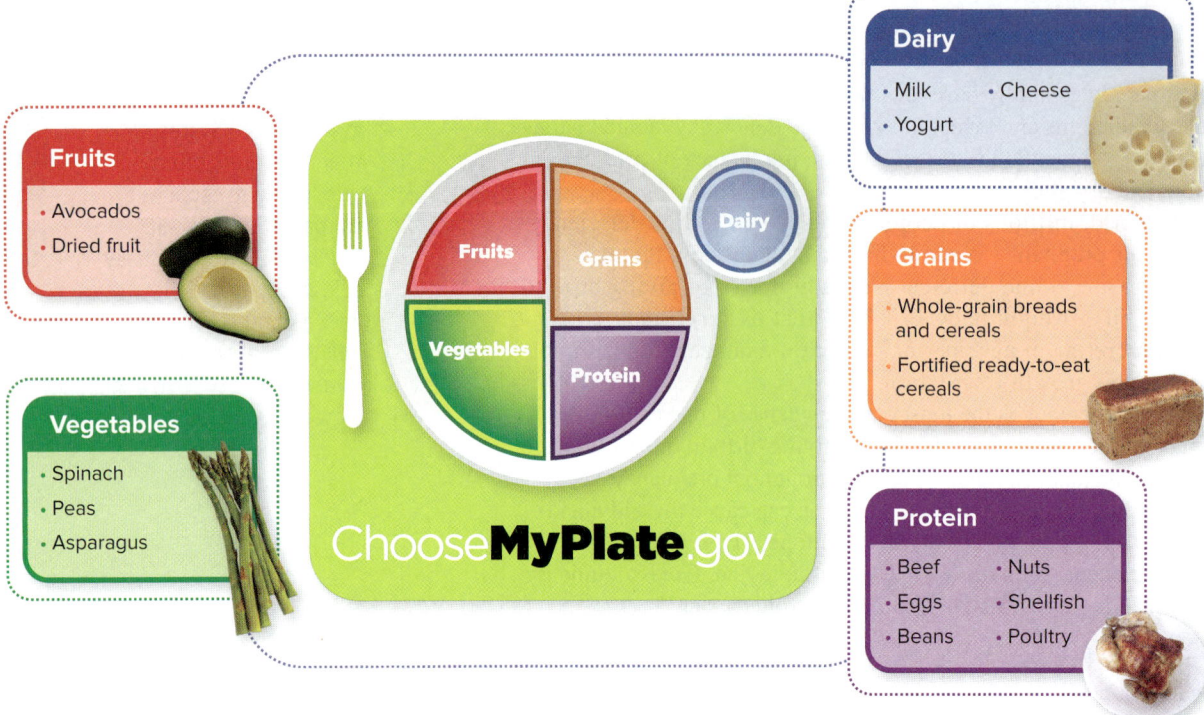

Figure 9.15 MyPlate: Good food sources of zinc.

The average adult American consumes adequate amounts of zinc.[3] Thus, zinc deficiency is not a widespread problem in the United States. However, alcoholics have a high risk of zinc deficiency because alcohol reduces zinc absorption and increases excretion of the mineral in urine. People with chronic diarrhea or digestive tract diseases can also develop zinc deficiency. Furthermore, vegetarians need more zinc than people who eat meat because the digestive tract does not absorb zinc from plant foods as well as from animal foods.[25] In children and adolescents, zinc deficiency can cause growth retardation and delayed sexual maturation. Other signs of zinc deficiency include loss of appetite, diarrhea, hair loss, dermatitis, poor wound healing, impaired sense of taste, and mental slowness.[25]

The UL (Upper Level) for zinc is 40 mg/day (adults). Ingesting amounts that are higher than the UL can cause diarrhea, nausea, vomiting, and depressed immune system functioning and can reduce beneficial HDL cholesterol levels.[25] Additionally, megadoses of zinc may interfere with copper absorption and metabolism. Therefore, you should avoid high intakes of zinc unless you are under a physician's supervision.

Chromium

The trace mineral chromium (Cr) plays an important role in maintaining proper carbohydrate and lipid metabolism. Chromium appears to promote energy metabolism by working with the hormone insulin to allow glucose to enter cells. Chromium may enhance insulin's action on cell membranes and, in a way, help to "hold the door open" for glucose's entry into the cells. Some people take chromium supplements to improve their blood glucose levels, but studies don't provide consistent evidence that the supplements are helpful for people with diabetes. Scientists continue to explore chromium's effects on metabolism.

Sources of Chromium Chromium is widely distributed in foods, but most foods contain less than 2 mcg of the mineral per serving.[26] In general, meat, whole-grain products, yeast, fruits, and vegetables are good sources of chromium (**Table 9.16**). The average American adult consumes a diet that provides adequate

Choose MyPlate: Source: ChooseMyPlate.gov; Avocado: Ingram Publishing/SuperStock; Swiss cheese: ballyscanlon/Photodisc/Getty Images; Bread: Everyday Images/Alamy; Asparagus, Roast chicken: Wendy Schiff

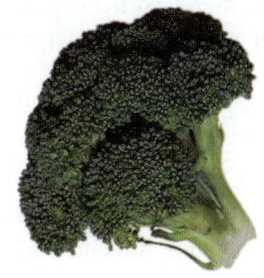

Table 9.16 Chromium Content of Selected Foods (Approximate)

Food	Chromium (mcg)
Broccoli, ½ cup	11
English muffin, whole-wheat, 1	4
Potatoes, mashed, 1 cup	3
Garlic powder, 1 tsp	3
Beef, 3 oz	2
Orange juice, 1 cup	2
Turkey breast, 3 oz	2
Whole-wheat bread, 1 slice	1

AI = 30–35 mcg for men; 20–25 mcg for women

Source: Data from Office of Dietary Supplements, National Institutes of Health: *Chromium.* Updated September 2018. https://ods.od.nih.gov/factsheets/Chromium-HealthProfessional/ Accessed: October 7, 2018

Table 9.17 Iodine, Zinc, and Chromium: Summary of Basic Nutrition Information

Mineral	Major Functions in the Body	Adult RDA/AI	Major Dietary Sources	Major Deficiency Signs and Symptoms	Major Toxicity Signs and Symptoms
Iodine (I)	Component of thyroid hormone	150 mcg	Iodized salt, saltwater fish, dairy foods	Enlargement of thyroid gland (goiter); Cretinism	UL = 1100 mcg/day; Reduced thyroid gland function
Zinc (Zn)	Component of numerous enzymes	Men: 11 mg; Women: 8 mg	Seafood, meat, whole grains	Skin rash; Diarrhea; Depressed sense of taste and smell; Hair loss; Poor growth and physical development	UL = 40 mg/day; Intestinal upset; Depressed immune system function; Supplement use can reduce copper absorption
Chromium (Cr)	Enhancement of insulin action	Men: 30–35 mcg; Women: 20–25 mcg	Egg yolks, whole grains, pork, nuts, mushrooms	Blood glucose level remains elevated after meals	Unknown but currently under scientific investigation; May interact with certain medications

Steamed mussels

Broccoli: Wendy Schiff; Mussels: Ingram Publishing

amounts of chromium.[26] In the past, a few cases of chromium deficiency were reported in people maintained on special-formula diets that did not contain chromium. The major sign of chromium deficiency is an elevated blood glucose level.

Amounts of chromium that are naturally in foods generally don't cause toxicity. However, the safety of taking various chromium supplements is unknown.[26] Until more is known about the safety of such products, consumers should check with their physician before taking them.

Other Important Minerals Table 9.18 provides basic information about some mineral nutrients that aren't covered in this unit because most Americans consume adequate amounts of them. It's important to note that most of these minerals can be toxic if taken in large amounts.

TABLE 9.18

SOME OTHER MINERAL NUTRIENTS: BASIC NUTRITION INFORMATION

Mineral	Major Functions in the Body	Adult RDA/AI	Major Dietary Sources	Major Deficiency Signs and Symptoms	Major Toxicity Signs and Symptoms
Phosphorus (P)	Structural component of bones and teeth Maintenance of acid-base balance Component of DNA, phospholipids, and other organic compounds	700 mg	Dairy foods, processed foods, soft drinks, fish, baked goods, meat	None reported	UL = 4 g/day Poor bone mineralization
Chloride (Cl⁻)	Maintenance of proper fluid balance Production of stomach acid Transmission of nerve impulses Maintenance of acid-base balance	2300 mg (19–50 years of age)	Processed foods, including salty snacks, table salt	Convulsions (observed in infants)	UL = 3600 mg/day Hypertension (because of the association with sodium in sodium chloride [table salt])
Manganese (Mn)	Component of several enzymes	AI = 1.8 mg for women; 2.3 mg for men	Tea, coffee, whole-grain cereals, nuts, legumes, blueberries	Not known	UL = 11 mg/day Irritability and lack of physical coordination

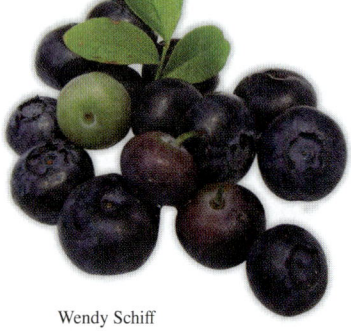

Wendy Schiff

Module 9.3
Water: Liquid of Life

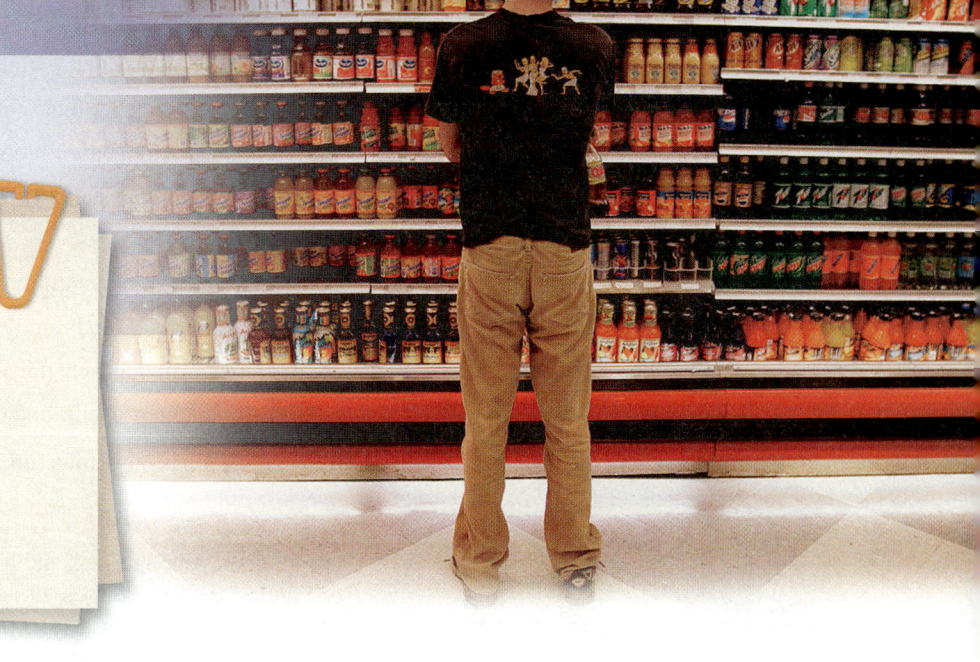

9.3 - Learning Outcomes

After reading Module 9.3, you should be able to

1. Define all of the **key terms** in this module.
2. List the primary functions of water in your body.
3. Identify typical sources of water intake and loss.
4. Explain how your body maintains its water balance.
5. Discuss the pros and cons of drinking bottled water.

Compared to other nutrients, water is so important, it's in a class of nutrients by itself. Your body has many kinds of watery fluids, including blood, lymph, and urine. Water is also a major component of many foods and beverages **(Table 9.19)**. Fat-free milk is about 90% water; bibb lettuce is almost 95% water; and a slice of whole-grain bread is about 39% water by weight. Water is such a simple molecule, it doesn't need to be digested before it's absorbed.

We often take water for granted, but this molecule is highly essential. You can survive for weeks, even months, if your diet lacks carbohydrates, lipids, proteins, and vitamins. But if you don't have any water from beverages and foods, your life will end within a few days or weeks, depending on your age, your state of health, and the temperature of your environment. This module focuses on the importance of water in your body.

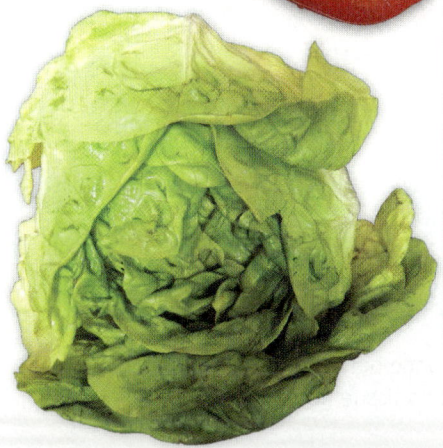

TABLE 9.19 — How Much Water Is in That Food or Beverage?

Food	Water % by Weight
Lettuce	95
Tomato	95
Watermelon	91
Milk, 1% fat	90
Apple, with skin	86
Avocado, Florida	79
Potato, Russet, baked with skin	74
Chicken, white meat, roasted	65
Bread, whole-wheat	39
Butter	16
Crackers, saltines	5
Canola oil	0

Source: U.S. Department of Agriculture, Agricultural Research Service: *USDA National Nutrient Database for Standard Reference Legacy Release, April 2018.* https://ndb.nal.usda.gov/ndb/search/list?home=true Accessed: September 2018

Man at supermarket: McGraw-Hill Education/Gary He; Tomato, Bibb lettuce, Watermelon: Wendy Schiff

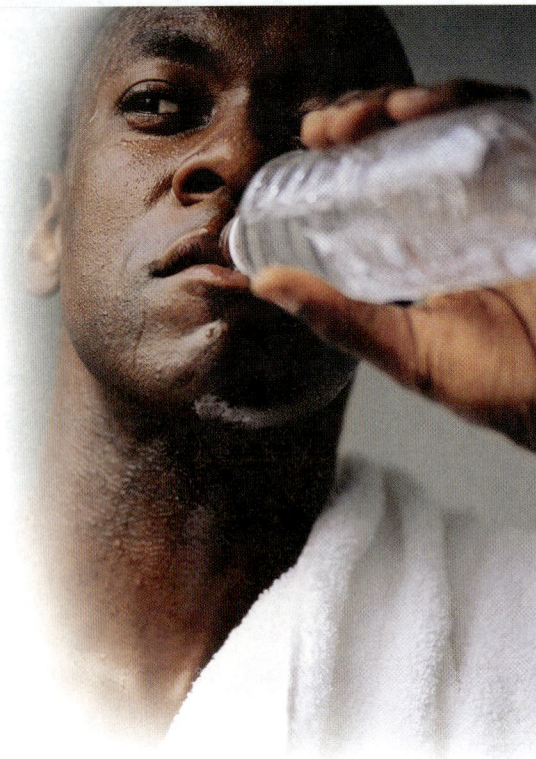

Fuse/Getty Images

9.3a What Water Does in Your Body

As a major component of body fluids, water has many functions in your body. Water

- is a **solvent** (water-soluble substances dissolve in it);
- is a major component of blood, saliva, sweat, tears, mucus, and joint fluid;
- helps transport substances;
- helps lubricate tissues;
- regulates body temperature;
- helps digest foods and remove wastes;
- participates in many chemical reactions; and
- helps maintain proper blood chemistry.

Although water has numerous functions in the body, this unique nutrient doesn't provide energy.

9.3b Your Body's Fluid Compartments

Depending on your age, sex, and body composition, 50 to 75% of your body is water weight (see Figure 1.3). Lean muscle tissue contains more water (about 73%) than is present in fat tissue (about 20%). On average, young adult men have more lean tissue than young women. Approximately 55 to 60% of an average young man's body weight is water. The average young adult woman's body has more fat and, therefore, slightly less water than an average young man's body. Your percentage of body weight that's water declines from birth to old age. Water may comprise only 45% of a typical older adult's weight.[27]

One reason why water is such a vital nutrient is its role in helping cells obtain materials from their environment and eliminate wastes. Each cell has a membrane that defines the area of the cell and controls the passage of material into and out of the cell.

To survive, your cells must maintain proper **hydration,** that is, adequate water status. Proper hydration requires a balance between the body's two major fluid compartments: **intracellular water** and **extracellular water (Fig. 9.16).** Intracellular water is the fluid inside cells. Extracellular water surrounds cells (tissue fluid) or is the fluid portion of blood (plasma).

solvent substance in which other substances dissolve

hydration water status

intracellular water fluid that's inside cells

extracellular water fluid that surrounds cells or is in blood

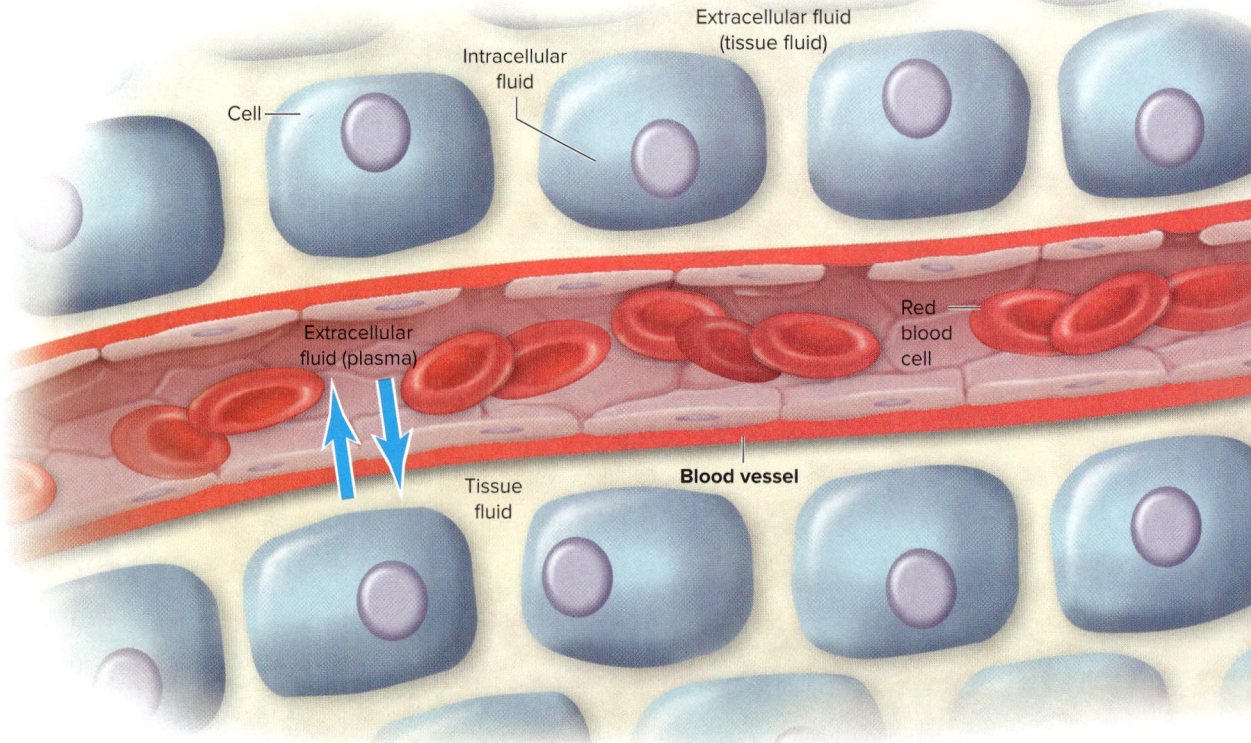

Figure 9.16 Fluid compartments. Your body must maintain a balance between the extracellular fluid and intracellular fluid. If too much plasma leaves a blood vessel and enters tissue fluid, the tissue swells (edema).

How Do Electrolytes Influence Hydration?

Cells maintain proper hydration primarily by controlling amounts of electrolytes in each compartment. Water is attracted to electrolytes. Overall, where these ions go, water follows. As a result, changes in normal electrolyte levels can cause water to shift out of one compartment and move into the other. Recall from Unit 7 that edema occurs when an excessive amount of water moves into the space surrounding cells (extracellular fluid). **Essential Concept 9.1** illustrates what can happen to your cells when there's an imbalance in the concentration of ions in intracellular fluid or extracellular fluid.

Essential Concept

9.1 Why Your Body Must Maintain Fluid Balance

1 Sodium (Na^+), for example, is a major extracellular ion. If extracellular fluid has fewer-than-normal sodium ions, water (H_2O) moves from the extracellular compartments into cells. When this occurs, the cells swell and can burst.

2 On the other hand, if extracellular fluid has an excess of sodium ions, water moves out of cells. As a result, the cells shrink and die because they lack enough intracellular fluid to function.

Dilute solution
Low concentration of Na^+

Concentrated solution
High concentration of Na^+

9.3c The Essential Balancing Act

An average healthy adult's water intake from foods and beverages is about 2.3 quarts per day.[27] Depending on your physical activity level, your body also forms about 1 cup of water daily as a result of energy metabolism. Such water (*metabolic water*) also contributes to the body's fluid balance. **Total water intake** refers to water obtained from all sources, including metabolic water, and amounts to about 2.5 quarts per day (**Fig. 9.17**).[27]

Your body loses about 2.5 quarts of water in urine, exhaled air, feces, and sweat (perspiration) each day (see Figure 9.17). Thus, your average daily total water intake is approximately equal to your average daily losses (output). To maintain good health, it's very important for your body to balance water intake with water output.

total water intake refers to water obtained from metabolic and external sources

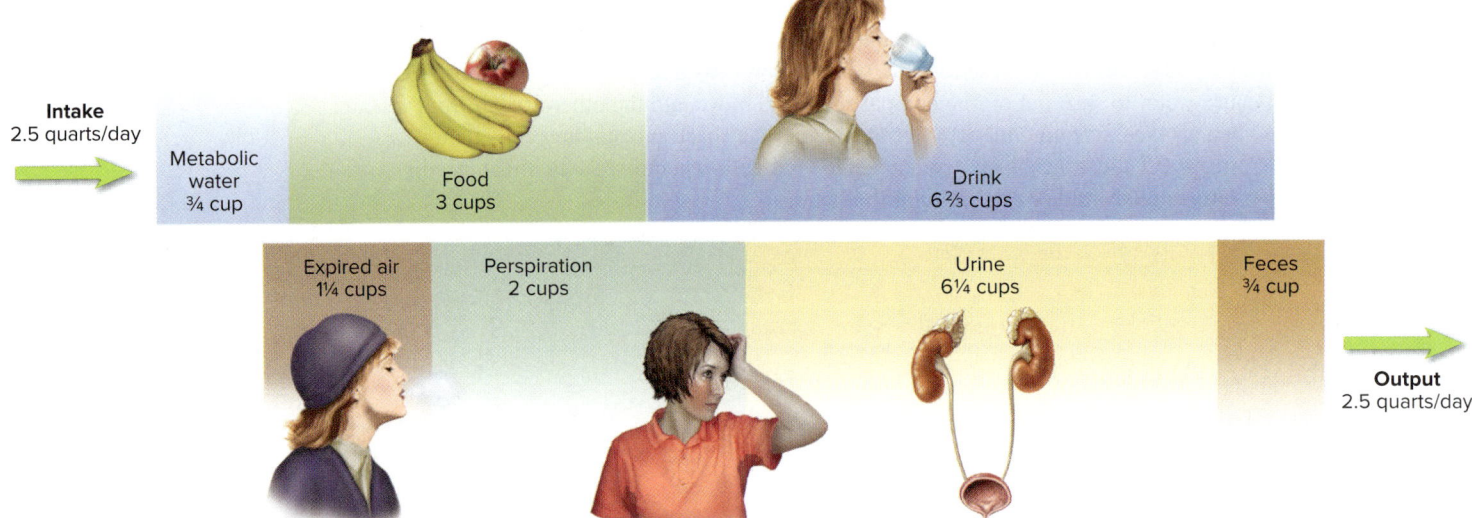

Figure 9.17 Daily water balance. To maintain proper hydration, your water intake should equal your water output.

■ *What happens to the excess water you drink?*

How Much Water Do You Need?

How much water is necessary to drink for good health? Contrary to popular belief, there's no "rule of thumb" recommendation for how many glasses of water you must consume each day.[28] The Adequate Intake (AI) for total water intake is approximately 11 cups for young women and approximately 15.5 cups for young men.[29] Factors such as environmental temperatures and your health, physical activities, and dietary choices influence your body's water requirements. Thus, total water intakes vary widely among individuals.

Water Losses

Your kidneys are the major regulator of your body's water content and ion concentrations. The kidneys remove excess ions from blood. When the kidneys remove ions such as sodium, water follows and becomes the main component of urine. The amount of urine you produce is determined primarily by your total water intake. A healthy person produces about 1.6 quarts of urine per day.[27] If you drink more watery fluids than your body needs, your kidneys excrete the excess water in urine.

Your body loses water and electrolytes, including sodium, potassium, and chloride, when you have vomiting, diarrhea, a fever, or a runny nose. That's why you're often reminded to drink plenty of fluids, such as clear soups or sports drinks, when you're sick. Environmental factors such as temperature, humidity, and altitude also affect body water losses. When you're in a hot environment, for example, you perspire heavily. Perspiration is body water that reaches the skin's surface and evaporates into the air. This process causes water losses, but it helps cool the body. Water is also lost when you breathe because warm, moist air leaves your lungs. Physical activity, especially when it's intense and performed in warm conditions, causes the body to sweat more heavily. Therefore, athletes and other people who work or exercise outdoors, especially in hot conditions, need to stay properly hydrated.

JGI/Blend Images LLC

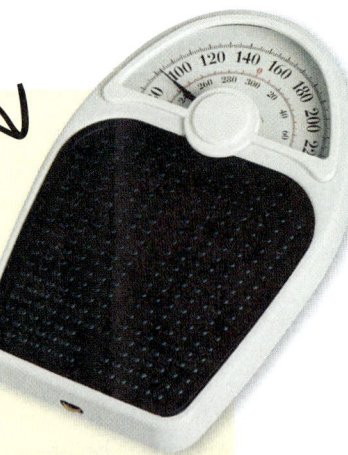

TASTY Tidbits

Have you ever noticed that your weight increases by a few pounds after you have eaten a lot of salty foods and then consumed beverages? The weight gain is due to a temporary increase in body water volume. If you resume eating foods that supply your usual intake of sodium, your kidneys will eliminate the excess sodium and water in urine within a day. As your body regains its normal fluid balance, your weight also returns to normal.

Comstock Images/Getty Images USA, Inc.

Dehydration When you're hot and sweating heavily, you become mildly dehydrated and your kidneys try to conserve water. Your mouth becomes dry and you feel uncomfortable. What do you do? You find something to drink! Most healthy, young people meet their AI for water by letting thirst be their guide.[29] Feeling thirsty is the brain's way of signaling you to drink watery fluids to avoid severe dehydration.

Dehydration occurs when your body's water content is too low. Dehydration can be a life-threatening condition. Rapid weight loss is a sign of dehydration. Every 16 ounces of water that the body loses represents a pound of body weight. If you lose 1 to 2% of your usual body weight in fluids, you will feel fatigued and thirsty. If you weigh 150 pounds, for example, and your weight drops 3 pounds after exercising in hot conditions, you've lost 2% of your body weight, primarily as water weight.

As the loss of body water approaches 4% of your weight, your muscles lose a lot of strength. By the time your body weight is reduced by 7 to 10% because of body fluid losses, severe weakness results. At a 20% reduction of body weight, you're likely to lose consciousness and die.

Older adults do not sense thirst as accurately as do younger adults.[30] Furthermore, older adults may be more susceptible to develop dehydration than younger persons because as kidneys age, they become less able to conserve water when fluid intakes are low. Therefore, it may be necessary to remind older adults to drink more watery fluids, especially when they're physically active or in warm conditions.

What Are Diuretics? A **diuretic** (*die'-uh-reh'-tic*) is a substance that stimulates kidneys to form urine. Caffeine is a mild diuretic. Coffee, tea, energy drinks, and soft drinks often contain caffeine or caffeine-related compounds. However, the water consumed in caffeinated beverages isn't completely lost in urine, so drinking these fluids still contributes to meeting your water needs.[31]

Alcohol is also a diuretic. Alcohol interferes with the kidneys' ability to conserve water, so the kidneys eliminate more urine than normal. Alcohol consumption actually results in urinary water losses that are greater than the volume of water consumed in the beverages. This explains why drinking alcohol increases the need to urinate and contributes to dehydration.

A "hangover" is the headache and overall discomfort that occurs a few hours after drinking too much alcohol. Dehydration, the body's immune response, a drop in blood glucose levels, and *congeners* may be responsible for a hangover.[32] Congeners are substances in alcoholic drinks that contribute to the taste and color of the beverages. Alcoholic drinks with high congener contents (brandy and whiskey, for example) tend to produce more severe hangovers than drinks with lower amounts of these substances, such as gin and vodka.

Can Too Much Water Be Toxic? There's no Upper Level for water. **Water intoxication,** however, can occur when an excessive amount of water is consumed in a short time period or when the kidneys have difficulty filtering water from blood. The excess water dilutes the sodium level of blood, upsetting the blood's water balance. As a result of the imbalance, too much water moves into cells, including brain cells. Signs and symptoms of water intoxication may include nausea and vomiting, headache, confusion, muscle spasms and weakness, and seizures.[33] If the condition isn't detected early and treated effectively, loss of consciousness and death can result.

Healthy people rarely drink enough water to become intoxicated. Water intoxication, however, can develop in people with disorders that interfere with the kidneys' ability to excrete water normally. Furthermore, marathon runners who consume large amounts of plain water in an effort to keep hydrated during competition may be at risk of water intoxication. Unit 10 provides more information about dehydration.

How Much Water Is Enough?

The simplest way to determine if you're consuming enough water is to note the volume of your urine. If you consume more fluid than needed, your kidneys will eliminate the excess, and you will produce plenty of urine. On the other hand, if you limit your fluid intake or have high fluid losses such as in sweat, you will produce small amounts of urine.

In addition to urine volume, the color of urine may be a useful sign of hydration status. Light yellow urine can indicate adequate hydration, whereas dark-colored urine may be a sign of dehydration. However, the color of urine isn't always a reliable guide for judging hydration status.[28] Having urinary tract infections or ingesting certain medications, foods, and dietary supplements, especially those containing the B vitamin riboflavin, can alter urine's color.

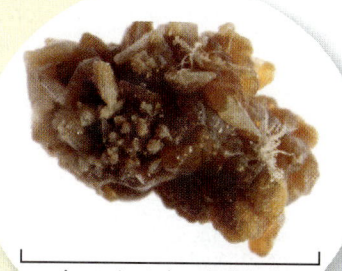

TASTY Tidbits

Sometimes, minerals settle out of urine and collect into crystals. If the crystals enlarge, they can form hard masses called "kidney stones." Such stones can be quite painful when they move from the kidneys and are eliminated in urine. Dehydration increases the chances that stones will form in people who are likely to develop them.

Approximate length: ⅕ inch
Jonathan Kim: Stockbyte/Getty Images

dehydration condition characterized by inadequate body water

diuretic substance that increases urine production

water intoxication condition that occurs when too much water is consumed in a short time period or the kidneys have difficulty filtering water from blood

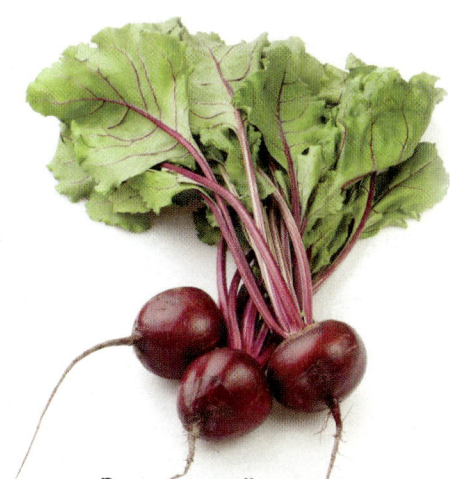

Beets naturally contain a reddish pigment. Thus, eating beets may cause your urine to turn pink or red, temporarily.

Getty Images/iStockphoto

9.3d From the Tap or Bottle?

The Environmental Protection Agency (EPA) regulates the sanitation of public water supplies in the United States. Safety standards for bottled water are similar to those established by the EPA for tap water. Therefore, most Americans can trust the safety of their tap water because the vast majority of municipal water systems in the United States are regulated by the Safe Drinking Water Act. As a result of this law, most tap water undergoes a purification process and is constantly tested for safety. If such testing indicates the local water supply poses a threat to consumers, a "boil order"—a requirement to boil water for 10 minutes to kill harmful microorganisms—may be issued for the public to follow.

The tap water in your community may be a source of minerals that can add to your daily intake. "Hard" water naturally contains a variety of minerals, including calcium, magnesium, sulfur, iron, and zinc. Fluoride is often added to public water supplies. Although fluoride isn't an essential nutrient, the mineral strengthens bones and teeth (see Section 9.2a).

Many people drink bottled water as a substitute for tap water because they think bottled water tastes better and it's safer. In fact, the water in some bottled water products actually comes from a municipal water supply. For most Americans, drinking bottled water is usually unnecessary and expensive. However, when public water supplies are disrupted by water main breaks, natural disasters, or environmental contaminants, drinking bottled water may be your only safe option.

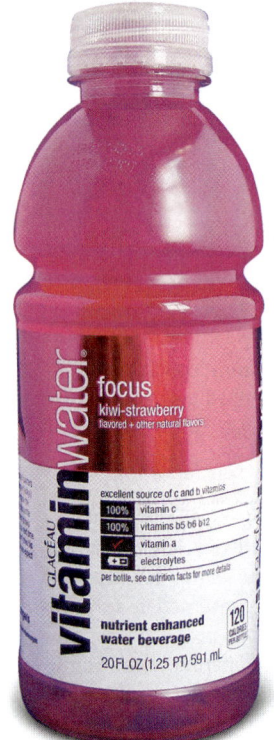
Wendy Schiff

The Food and Drug Administration (FDA) regulates bottled water products that are marketed for interstate commerce. According to FDA regulations, bottled water manufacturers are responsible for producing safe products. Bottled water must be sealed in containers and have no added ingredients other than a substance that prevents the growth of microbes, such as bacteria. Bottled water may have the tooth- and bone-strengthening mineral fluoride added, but amounts must meet FDA guidelines. If bottled water manufacturers add flavorings or other ingredients to their products, the name of the product must indicate the added ingredients—"Bottled Water with Cherry Flavor," for example. These drinks are often called "flavored water beverages." A growing number of flavored waters also have added nutrients, such as vitamins, sodium, potassium, and amino acids. The beverage's label must identify the additives in the list of ingredients.

Although bottled water is safe to drink, the plastic used to contain it may contain harmful substances. Bisphenol A (*biss'-feen-ol*) (BPA) is a chemical used to make polycarbonate plastics and epoxy resins. Polycarbonate plastics are in many consumer products that come in contact with foods and beverages, including some water bottles. The epoxy resin that contains BPA is used to coat the inside of certain food cans. The coating prevents the can's metal from coming in contact with and being damaged by the food (**Fig. 9.18**). However, BPA can leach from polycarbonate plastic containers or epoxy resin–coated cans and enter the food or beverage stored within them.

In 2012, the FDA banned the use of BPA in plastic baby bottles and sipping cups that babies use to prepare for drinking out of cups. Concern over the safety of BPA has encouraged many plastic bottle manufacturers to discontinue using the chemical in their products.

To reduce exposure to BPA, consider taking the following actions:

- Avoid buying used plastic baby bottles and "sippy" cups because they may have been made before the FDA baned the use of BPA in such plastic products;
- Use water bottles and plastic containers that are not made with BPA, as indicated on the label;
- Don't wash polycarbonate containers in the dishwasher or with harsh detergents;
- Reduce your intake of canned foods that are in epoxy resin–coated containers;
- Cook or store foods and beverages in glass, porcelain, or stainless steel containers; and
- Avoid using polycarbonate dishware, cups, or eating utensils for serving foods (especially hot foods or liquids).

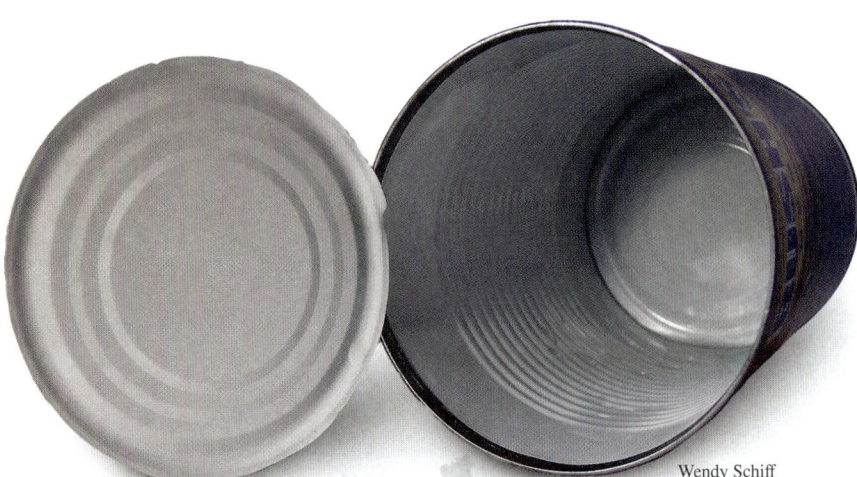
Wendy Schiff

Figure 9.18 BPA and epoxy resins.

■ *Why do some cans have an epoxy coating on their insides?*

Module 9.4

Drink to Your Health?

9.4 - Learning Outcomes

After reading Module 9.4, you should be able to

1. Define all of the **key terms** in this module.
2. Describe the amounts of beer, malt liquor, liquor, and wine that represent a standard drink.
3. Discuss how alcohol affects your body.
4. Identify factors that influence the blood alcohol concentration.
5. Discuss how your alcohol use can affect others.

Alcohol (ethanol) is a mind-altering depressant drug that's often classified as a food. When consumed in moderation, alcoholic beverages can make social situations more enjoyable. Many people, however, experience serious social and physical problems as a result of their drinking habits. This module focuses on alcohol, including its effects on the body.

9.4a What's Alcohol?

Alcohol is a simple nonnutrient that supplies energy but is poisonous (toxic) to cells. Alcohol dissolves in water (it's water soluble), and alcoholic beverages generally contain a lot of water.

- Beers are typically 3 to 6% alcohol.
- Wines are 8 to 14% alcohol.
- Malt liquors are about 7% alcohol by volume.
- Hard liquors (for example, whiskey, bourbon, and vodka) are generally 40 to 50% alcohol.

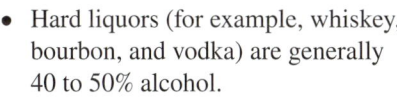

TASTY Tidbits

You can determine the percentage of alcohol in hard liquor by dividing the "proof" declaration on the label by two. Gin, for example, is "80 proof," or 40% alcohol.

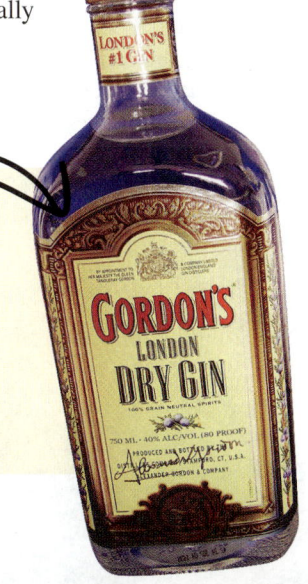

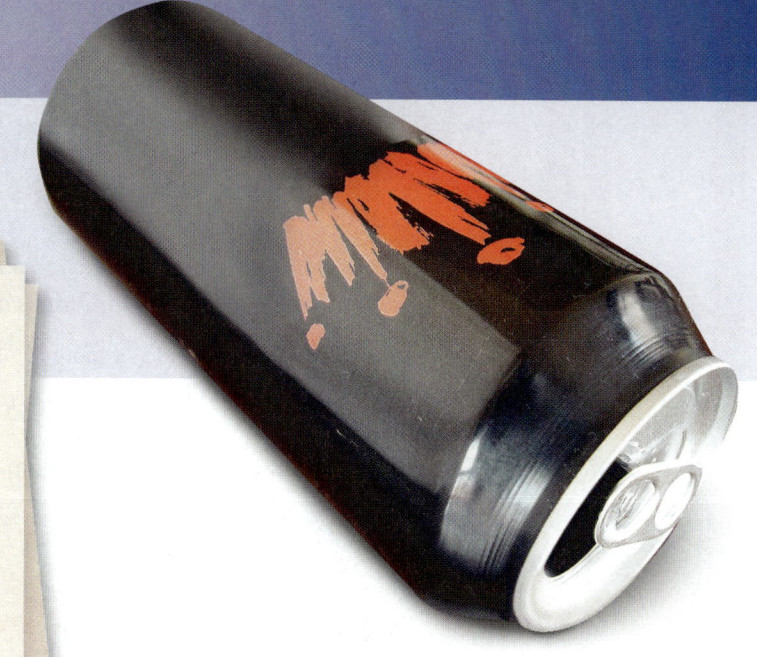

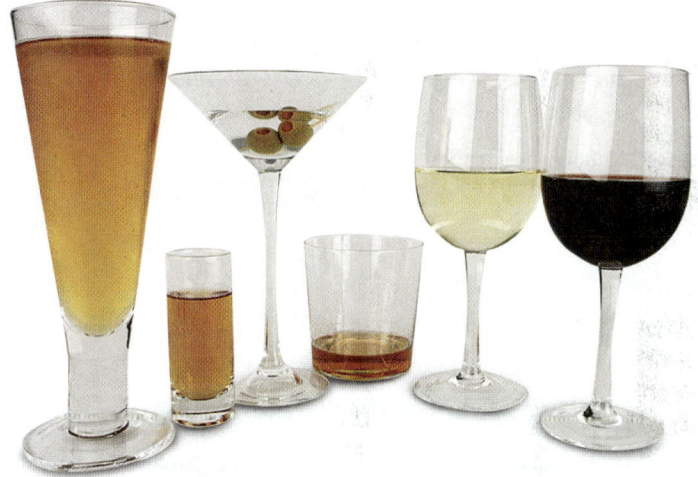

Figure 9.19 What's a standard drink?

Although alcohol is a nonnutrient, each gram of the substance provides 7 kcal. Beer and wine contain simple carbohydrates and small amounts of certain minerals and B vitamins. Distilled spirits have essentially no nutritional value other than water; preparing "cocktails" by adding mixers to spirits provides small amounts of nutrients to the drinks. A *standard drink* is approximately 12 ounces of beer, 8 to 9 ounces of malt liquor, 5 ounces of wine, or 1½ ounces of liquor. Each standard drink contains 13 to 14 grams of alcohol **(Fig. 9.19)**.

9.4b Classifying Drinkers

People who drink alcohol can be classified according to their usual intake patterns. **Table 9.20** indicates this classification scheme, which includes binge drinkers. Binge drinking is a serious public health concern. In the United States, one in six adults binge drinks about four times a month. Males are twice as likely to binge drink than females.[34]

Binge drinking is often associated with driving while drunk. Furthermore, the practice may increase a person's later risk of alcoholism and can result in death. If you drink alcohol, which type of drinker are you?

Empty can, Bottle of gin, Wendy Schiff; Alcoholic beverages: Jill Braaten/McGraw-Hill Education

263

Unit 9 Key Minerals, Water, and the Nonnutrient Alcohol

Table 9.20 Classifying Drinkers

Level	Amount of Standard Alcoholic Drinks Consumed	
	Males	Females
Moderate	Up to 2 drinks/day	Up to 1 drink/day
Heavy	15 or more drinks/week	8 drinks or more/week
Binge drinker	5 or more drinks/occasion (2-hour period)	4 or more drinks/occasion (2-hour period)

Source: Centers for Disease Control and Prevention: *Fact sheets—alcohol use and your health.* 2018. https://www.cdc.gov/alcohol/fact-sheets/alcohol-use.htm Accessed: July 6, 2019

Ingram Publishing/AGE Fotostock

9.4c How Your Body Processes Alcohol

Alcohol requires no digestion and readily passes into the bloodstream through the tissues lining the inside of your stomach and small intestine. When alcohol is consumed with meals, food delays its absorption from the stomach and slows the rate at which the drug enters the bloodstream.

Detoxification is the process of converting alcohol to less-damaging compounds. Detoxification begins in the stomach, where a specific enzyme metabolizes up to 20% of the alcohol. In the small intestine, the absorptive cells remove nearly all of the remaining alcohol. After entering the bloodstream, the alcohol circulates to the liver. The liver is the primary site for metabolizing the substance. In the liver, alcohol can be metabolized completely to form carbon dioxide (CO_2) and water (H_2O), or the alcohol can be used to make fatty acids.

alcohol (ethanol) a mind-altering depressant drug that's often classified as a food

blood alcohol concentration (BAC) estimated percentage of alcohol in blood

What's Blood Alcohol Concentration?

Until the liver can detoxify all the alcohol that has been consumed, the toxic chemical circulates in the bloodstream and passes into the watery fluids within and surrounding cells. The lungs eliminate some of the alcohol; that's why you can smell alcohol on the breath of someone who's been drinking. Law enforcement officials use special devices to analyze the alcohol in blood, urine, or expired air to estimate a person's **blood alcohol concentration (BAC).** BAC is the estimated percentage of alcohol in the bloodstream and indicates the drinker's level of intoxication.

Table 9.21 describes typical nervous system effects when BAC reaches various levels. At present, a BAC of 0.08% is the legal limit for intoxication for motor vehicle operators. Some officials want to reduce the limit to 0.05%. To estimate your BAC after consuming one or more standard drinks, use the "0.08 BAC law in Wisconsin" estimator at Wisconsin's Department of Transportation's website http://wisconsindot.gov/Documents/safety/education/drunk-drv/08law.pdf.

Table 9.21 Typical Nervous System Effects of Alcohol at Various BAC Levels (Adults)

BAC	Typical Effects*
up to 0.05	Mild speech, memory, coordination, and balance impairments; relaxation
0.06 to 0.15	Increased aggression, in some people
	Major impairments in ability to drive or operate other machinery
	Increased risk of injury to self or others
0.16 to 0.30	Speech, memory, coordination, balance, reaction time seriously impaired
	Judgment and decision making seriously impaired
	Blackouts, vomiting (sign of alcohol poisoning), and loss of consciousness
0.31 to 0.45	Life-threatening alcohol poisoning
	Coma
	Major risk of death

*Effects may vary among adults. Moderate to heavy drinkers may not display these effects until higher BACs are reached.

Source: Adapted from: National Institutes of Health, U.S. National Library of Medicine: Rethinking drinking. *MedlinePlus Magazine* 9(1):18, 2014. https://medlineplus.gov/magazine/issues/spring14/articles/spring14pg23.html Accessed: July 6, 2019

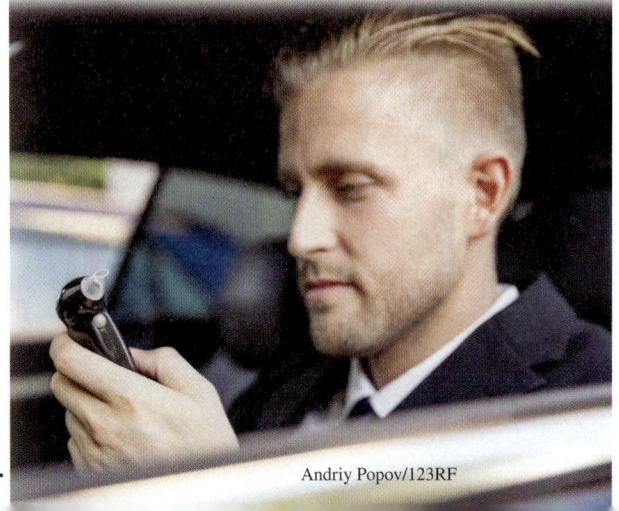

You can buy a device that checks your BAC before you drive.

Andriy Popov/123RF

Nutrition Fact or Fiction?

Drinking strong coffee, running around the block, or taking cold showers can help you sober up quickly.

Drinking caffeinated beverages, exercising, taking cold showers, and following other popular recommendations for sobering up aren't useful. Why? These actions don't increase your body's rate of alcohol detoxification. To sober up, you must stop consuming alcohol and give your liver time to metabolize the chemical.

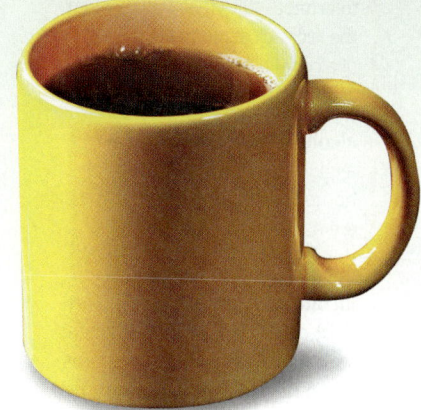

Don Farrall/Photodisc/Getty Images

Factors That Influence BAC You may have noticed that a few of your friends who drink can "hold their liquor" better than others. Why? Many factors influence the rate at which a person becomes noticeably affected by his or her alcohol consumption.

- *Amount and timing of alcohol consumption*

  A person who drinks six beers in an hour will become more intoxicated than if he or she drinks one beer in an hour.

- *Sex, body size, and body composition*

  Compared to women, men generally make higher amounts of the enzyme that's needed to metabolize alcohol.

The average man is larger than the average woman. Larger people have bigger livers that detoxify more alcohol at a time. As a result, men generally can drink more alcohol and not become intoxicated as quickly as women.

Women tend to have more body fat than men. Alcohol doesn't move easily into fatty tissues, so the chemical circulates in the bloodstream longer in women (**Fig. 9.20**).

- *Eating food along with the alcohol*

  As mentioned earlier, having food in the stomach delays alcohol's absorption.

- *Prior drinking history*

  People who drink alcohol regularly develop tolerance to the substance.

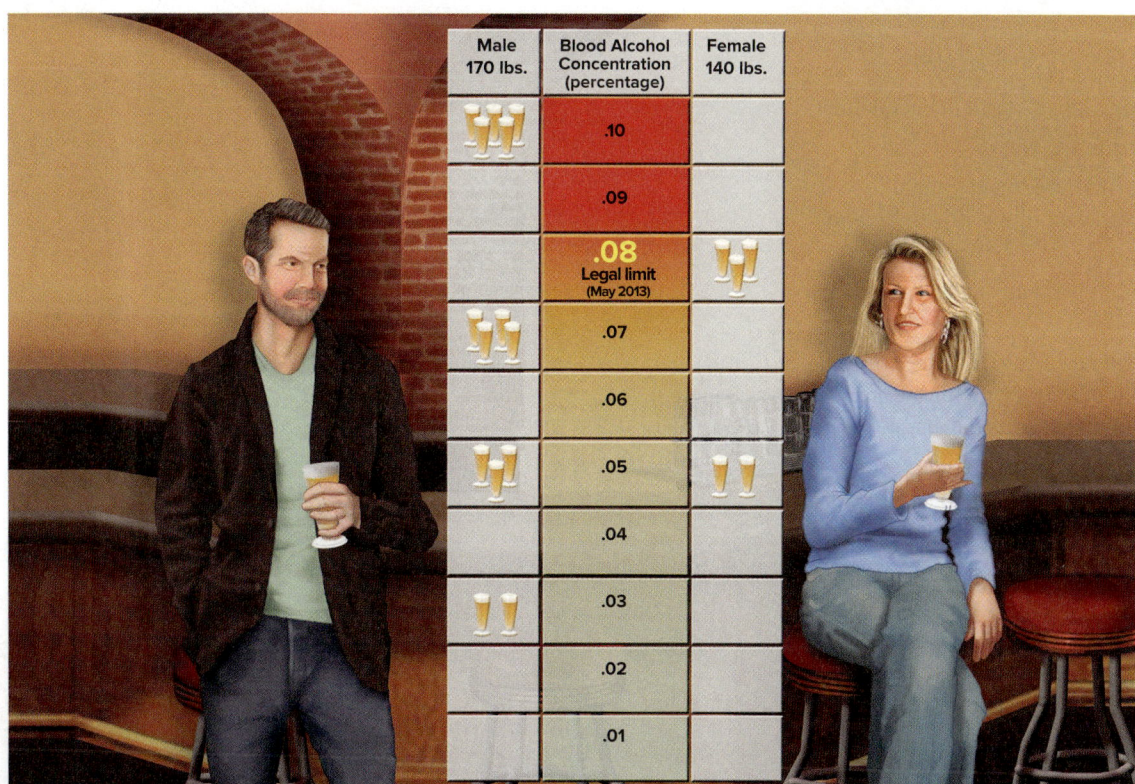

Figure 9.20 Alcohol consumption and approximate BAC.

■ *How does a person's sex influence his or her ability to metabolize alcohol?*

tolerance state that occurs when the liver adjusts to the usual amount of alcohol that's been consumed and metabolizes it more quickly

alcohol abuser person who experiences problems at home, work, and school that are associated with his or her drinking habits

alcoholic person who is dependent on alcohol and experiences withdrawal signs and symptoms when he or she hasn't consumed the drug

Tolerance occurs when the liver adjusts to the usual amount of alcohol that's been consumed and metabolizes it more quickly. As a result of tolerance, a regular drinker eventually needs to consume more alcohol to achieve the same mind-altering effects as in the past. Tolerance can lead to alcohol dependence (alcoholism).

What's Alcohol Poisoning?
On March 15, 2004, Jason Reinhardt was living in a fraternity house at Minnesota State University, Moorhead. While celebrating his twenty-first birthday with friends in a bar, Jason rapidly drank 16 shots of alcohol. Although he managed to return to the fraternity house and go to bed, his lifeless body was discovered a few hours later. The young man's BAC was 0.361, close to the deadly range. What makes binge drinking so dangerous?

Binge drinking increases a person's BAC rapidly and to a point at which signs of alcohol poisoning occur. An individual suffering from alcohol poisoning

- is confused,
- "passes out" and cannot be aroused,
- breathes slowly and irregularly, and
- has pale or bluish skin.

The heart rate of a person with alcohol poisoning slows and becomes irregular. If a "passed out" person vomits, his or her stomach contents can enter the lungs, causing the person to choke to death. Additionally, the lungs of the person who has alcohol poisoning can stop functioning, resulting in death. Jason died in his sleep from the effects of alcohol poisoning. It's important to recognize that alcohol poisoning is a life-threatening condition. If you suspect someone has consumed a deadly amount of alcohol, call 911 immediately.

Alcohol Use Disorders
When a person's drinking behavior creates serious problems for him- or herself, the condition may be classified as an *alcohol use disorder*. Alcohol abuse and alcoholism are two forms of alcohol abuse disorder. An **alcohol abuser** experiences problems at home, work, and school that are associated with his or her drinking habits.

An **alcoholic** is a person who is dependent on alcohol (addicted) and experiences *withdrawal* signs and symptoms, such as shakiness, when he or she hasn't consumed the substance. Both abusers and alcoholics engage in behaviors that place themselves and others in danger, such as drinking and driving. **Table 9.22** lists possible signs of alcohol use disorder. For more information about alcoholism visit the National Institute on Alcohol Abuse and Alcoholism: www.niaaa.nih.gov/alcohol-health.

TABLE 9.22 POSSIBLE SIGNS OF ALCOHOL USE DISORDER

Not everyone who drinks alcohol regularly abuses the drug, but you might be abusing alcohol. Have you

- Had times when you drank more than you intended?
- Wanted to reduce or stop drinking, or you tried to but couldn't?
- Had a strong need or urge to drink?
- Felt that drinking or its effects interfered with your ability to take care of your personal responsibilities, do your job, or keep up with school work?
- Continued to drink even though it was causing trouble with your family or friends?
- Gotten into situations while or after drinking that increased your chances of being harmed, such as driving, swimming, using machinery, walking in a dangerous area, or having unsafe sex?
- Continued to drink even though it was making you feel depressed or anxious, or was causing other health problems?
- Continued to drink even after having a memory blackout?
- Found that when the effects of alcohol were wearing off, you had withdrawal symptoms, such as trouble sleeping, shakiness, irritability, anxiety, depression, restlessness, nausea, or sweating?

If you've had one or more of these signs, your alcohol use may already be a concern for you and others. Seek professional help.

Source: Adapted from: National Institutes of Health, National Institute of Alcohol Abuse and Alcoholism: *Alcohol use disorder*. ND. www.niaaa.nih.gov/alcohol-health/overview-alcohol-consumption/alcohol-use-disorders Accessed: July 6, 2019

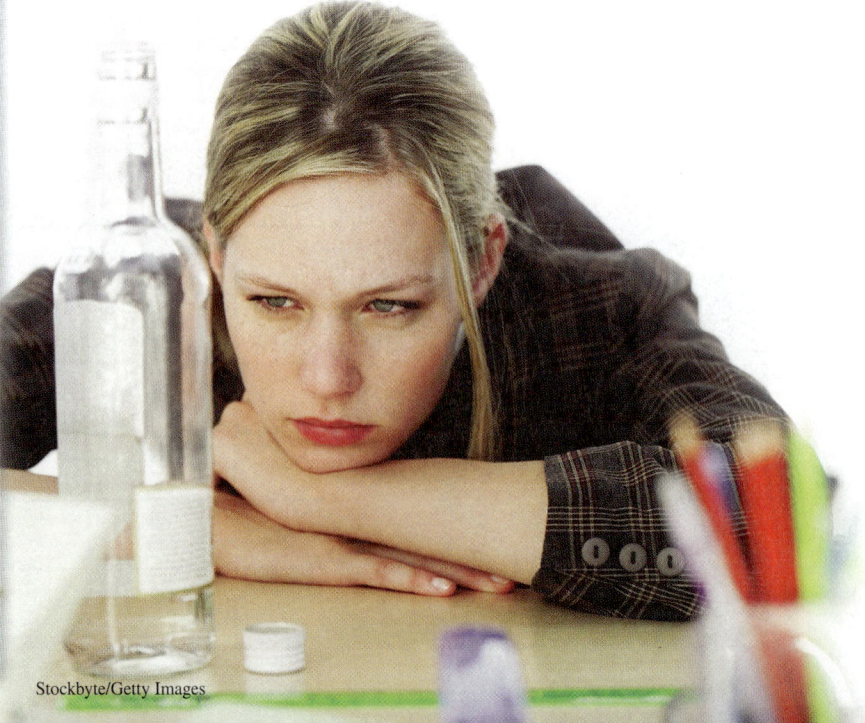

Stockbyte/Getty Images

9.4d Alcohol and Health

Alcohol is a central nervous system depressant. Thus, mild alcohol intoxication often produces pleasant sensations and relaxed inhibitions. Consuming large amounts, however, depresses the ability to control thought processes and muscular movements, including those needed for safe driving. Excessive alcohol use is responsible for 1 in 10 deaths of Americans who are of working age (20 to 64 years of age).[35] Alcohol is often involved in motor vehicle accidents, falls, and drownings, as well as acts of violence and abuse. An estimated 88,000 Americans die each year as a result of excessive alcohol use.[35] Additionally, many people suffer physical injuries and have damaged interpersonal relationships related to excess alcohol consumption.

Alcohol affects every cell in the body, and when consumed in excess, the drug damages every system in the body, particularly the digestive, nervous, and cardiovascular systems.

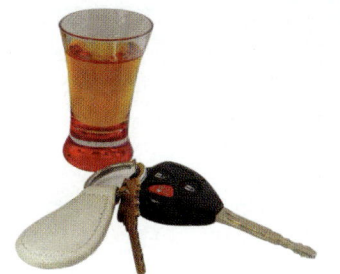

According to the U.S. Department of Transportation, approximately one-third of all deadly traffic accidents involve drunk drivers.

Some Serious Effects of Alcohol on the Body

If you have consumed distilled spirits without adding mixers, you probably felt a burning sensation as the alcohol entered your throat and stomach. This sensation is an indication of alcohol's irritating effects on the lining of your gastrointestinal tract. Not surprisingly, chronic drinking contributes to ulcer formation, particularly in the esophagus and stomach.

Alcohol's effects on the brain appear within a few minutes of having a drink. Alcohol slows the transmission of messages between nerve cells (neurons). Long-term consumption of excessive amounts of alcohol can cause the brain's neurons to shrink, and the organ develops other structural abnormalities. Confusion and memory loss are common signs of the extensive brain damage that occurs in a chronic heavy drinker.

In addition to harming the brain, alcohol can damage the liver. After a heavy-drinking episode, the liver makes an excess of fatty acids that accumulate in liver cells, causing a condition called "fatty liver." Fatty liver is reversible; if the affected person is healthy and avoids alcohol for an extended period, the liver metabolizes the fat, and the organ eventually heals itself. If the person continues to drink, the buildup of fat destroys his or her liver cells, and tough scar tissue replaces them. This irreversible condition is called liver **cirrhosis** ("hardening of the liver"). Liver cirrhosis can cause the organ to fail. Alcoholics are also prone to develop a form of **hepatitis,** inflammation of the liver. Hepatitis can cause cirrhosis and increases the risk of liver cancer. People who consume alcohol have an increased risk of other cancers, including mouth, throat, esophagus, breast (women), and colon cancers.[35]

When consumed in moderate intakes (1 to 2 drinks/day), alcohol may reduce the risk of heart disease. Excess consumption, however, can damage heart muscle and elevate blood pressure to dangerous levels. As a result, chronic alcoholics often have enlarged but weakened hearts and suffer strokes. **Figure 9.21** summarizes the major damaging effects of alcohol on the body.

Alcohol and Body Water

Billboard and media advertisements for alcoholic beverages often show sweaty, physically active young adults gulping down beer or liquor to relieve their thirst. These ads are misleading. Alcohol is not a good thirst quencher because it's a diuretic that causes the kidneys to produce more urine, and the body loses water and certain vitamins and minerals along with it. If a dehydrated drinker consumes even more alcohol to relieve thirst, this response only increases his or her water losses. Drinking water and other nonalcoholic drinks is the best way to keep the body well hydrated.

Alcohol's Effects on Your Nutritional Status

When consumed in moderation, alcohol stimulates the appetite. Alcohol, however, lowers blood glucose levels and raises blood triglycerides. Alcohol also interferes with the absorption, metabolism, and storage of fat, proteins, and various vitamins and minerals. Furthermore, alcohol increases the excretion of water-soluble micronutrients, particularly magnesium and calcium.

Many alcoholics consume a considerable portion of their energy intake as alcohol. As a result, alcoholic beverages often displace nutrient-dense foods from alcoholics' diets. Chronic excessive alcohol intake contributes to malnutrition. Deficiencies of magnesium, vitamin A, vitamin C, and the B vitamins thiamin and folate are common among alcoholics.

cirrhosis hardening of tissues, such as the liver

hepatitis inflammation of the liver

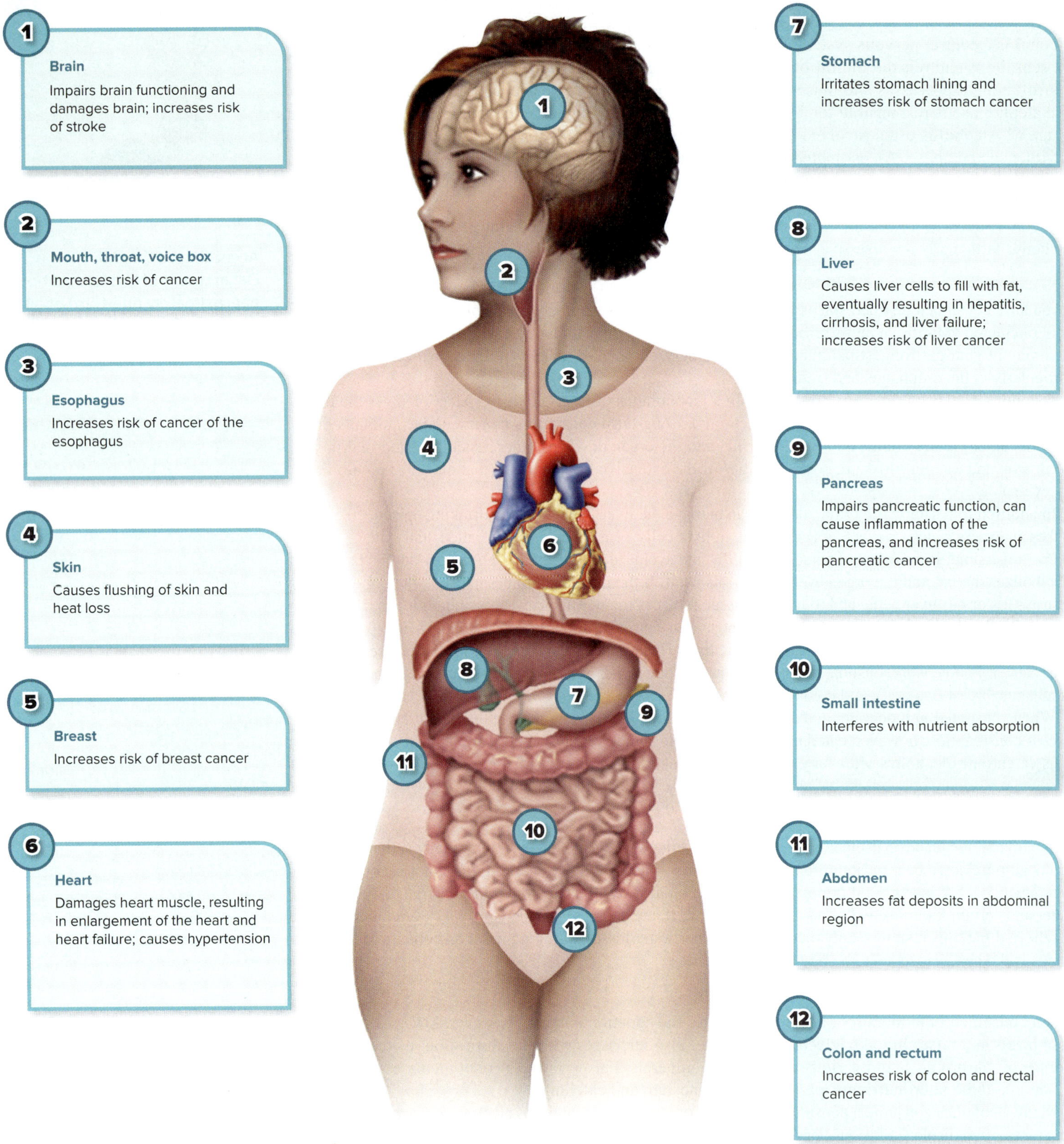

1 Brain
Impairs brain functioning and damages brain; increases risk of stroke

2 Mouth, throat, voice box
Increases risk of cancer

3 Esophagus
Increases risk of cancer of the esophagus

4 Skin
Causes flushing of skin and heat loss

5 Breast
Increases risk of breast cancer

6 Heart
Damages heart muscle, resulting in enlargement of the heart and heart failure; causes hypertension

7 Stomach
Irritates stomach lining and increases risk of stomach cancer

8 Liver
Causes liver cells to fill with fat, eventually resulting in hepatitis, cirrhosis, and liver failure; increases risk of liver cancer

9 Pancreas
Impairs pancreatic function, can cause inflammation of the pancreas, and increases risk of pancreatic cancer

10 Small intestine
Interferes with nutrient absorption

11 Abdomen
Increases fat deposits in abdominal region

12 Colon and rectum
Increases risk of colon and rectal cancer

Figure 9.21 Some effects that alcohol can have on your body.

TASTY Tidbits

People who abuse alcohol are prone to develop hepatitis. Hepatitis can cause cirrhosis of the liver and increases the risk of liver cancer. Chronic alcohol abuse is a major cause of liver failure among adult Americans.

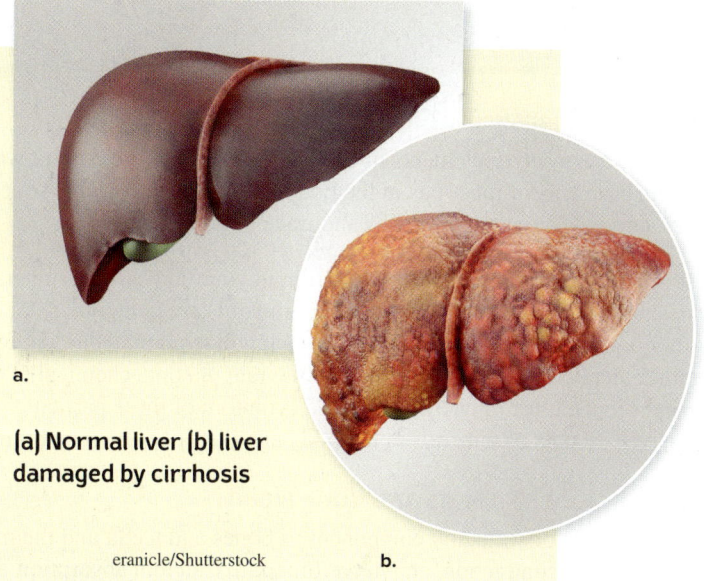

(a) Normal liver (b) liver damaged by cirrhosis

eranicle/Shutterstock

Fetal Alcohol Spectrum Disorder

When a pregnant woman drinks alcohol, her developing embryo/fetus is exposed to the alcohol as it circulates through its mother's bloodstream. Alcohol consumption during pregnancy can result in the birth of a baby with **fetal alcohol spectrum disorder (FASD)**. Babies with FASD experience delayed and abnormal physical and intellectual development. Fetal alcohol syndrome (FAS) is a severe form of FASD. A child with FAS is born with certain facial and heart defects as well as irreversible nervous system damage that causes intellectual disability (**Fig. 9.22**).

The amount of alcohol that can be safely consumed by a pregnant woman has not been determined. Therefore, if you or someone you know is trying to conceive or is pregnant, you or that person should "play it safe" and avoid alcohol completely.

Health Benefits of Alcohol

Consuming light to moderate amounts of alcohol raises HDL cholesterol levels, reduces blood levels of an important blood-clotting factor, and decreases platelet stickiness.[36] *Platelets* are cell fragments involved in the blood-clotting process. Reducing the likelihood of blood clot formation lowers the risk of heart attack and certain types of strokes.

Results of studies suggest that all alcoholic beverages may provide the same heart-healthy benefits, as long as they are consumed in moderation.[36] (See Table 9.20 for the definition of "moderate" drinkers.) Although drinking small amounts of alcohol seems to reduce the risk of heart disease, consuming moderate to excessive amounts of alcohol is associated with increased risks of addiction, hypertension, heart failure, certain cancers, liver damage, and motor vehicle accidents. More research is needed to determine if alcohol alone or other compounds present in certain alcoholic beverages provide beneficial effects on health when consumed in moderation.

9.4e Where to Get Help for Alcohol Abuse or Dependence

If you think you are abusing alcohol or are dependent on the substance, seek help from your personal physician. For information about alcohol abuse, you can contact the Substance Abuse and Mental Health Services Administration's National Helpline at 1-800-662-HELP. You can also visit the websites of Alcoholics Anonymous (www.aa.org/) or Al-Anon /Alateen (www.al-anon.alateen.org/).

fetal alcohol spectrum disorder (FASD) condition characterized by abnormal physical and intellectual development that affects newborns of women who consumed alcohol during pregnancy

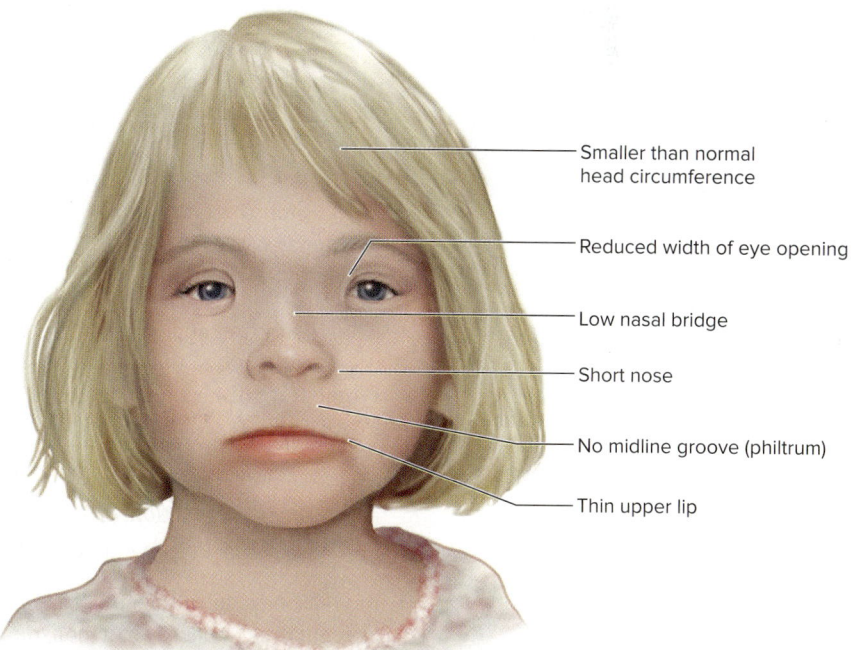

Figure 9.22 Some physical signs of fetal alcohol syndrome.

■ *How much alcohol can a pregnant woman drink safely?*

In a Nutshell

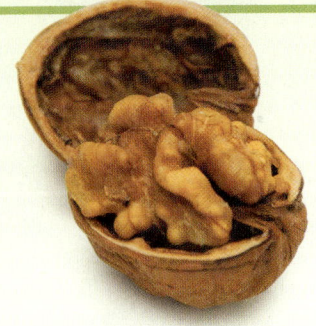

Module 9.1 Minerals for Life

- Minerals are a group of elements in Earth's rocks, soils, and natural water sources. About 15 mineral elements have known functions in the body and are necessary for your health. The two primary groups of dietary minerals are major minerals and trace minerals.

- Most minerals have more than one function in your body. Some minerals function as inorganic ions or structural components of tissues; other minerals are components of various enzymes, hormones, or other organic molecules. Cells cannot metabolize minerals for energy. The body, however, needs certain minerals as cofactors to speed up the rate of some chemical reactions that release energy from macronutrients. Lack of energy is often a symptom of these particular mineral deficiency disorders. Excessive amounts of minerals in the body can disrupt normal cell functioning, causing toxicity.

Module 9.2 Key Minerals and Your Health

- Calcium is a major structural component of bones and teeth, and the mineral is necessary for blood clotting, muscle contraction, and nerve function. Calcium absorption depends on vitamin D. Most dairy foods are rich calcium sources. Although people, especially women, are at risk of developing osteoporosis as they age, various lifestyle modifications help reduce this risk. Fluoride works with calcium to strengthen bones and teeth.

- Potassium, the major positively charged ion found inside cells, is vital for maintaining normal fluid balance and nerve functioning. The typical American diet doesn't supply enough potassium. Plant foods, meat, and milk are good sources of potassium.

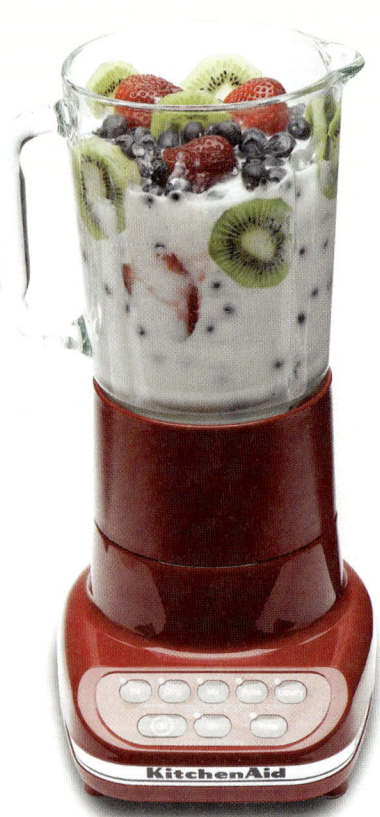

A smoothie made with reduced-fat yogurt and a variety of fresh fruit is a good source of calcium and potassium.

Ken Karp/McGraw-Hill Education

- Sodium, the major positively charged ion found outside cells, has some functions that are similar to those of potassium. The typical American diet provides high amounts of sodium, primarily from processed foods. Diets high in sodium are associated with increased risk of hypertension.

- Hypertensive individuals have greater risk of CVD, kidney failure, and damage to other organs than people with normal blood pressures. Advanced age, African-American ancestry, obesity, physical inactivity, cigarette smoking, and excess alcohol and sodium intakes are major risk factors for hypertension. Treatment for hypertension usually includes following dietary modifications and making some other lifestyle changes.

- Iron is a critical component of hemoglobin, myoglobin, and a group of proteins that help release energy from macronutrients. Hemoglobin in RBCs transports oxygen from the lungs to the tissues.

- Iron deficiency can result in iron deficiency anemia, a condition characterized by low hemoglobin levels. People suffering from anemia become fatigued easily and lack interest in activities. Iron deficiency during pregnancy can result in giving birth to a premature baby or low-birth-weight baby. In children, anemia interferes with normal growth and development.

- Iron absorption depends on the body's need for the mineral and the form of iron in food. Heme iron is better absorbed than nonheme iron. Meat and liver are among the best sources of dietary iron. Women of childbearing age often have higher needs for iron than men because of menstrual blood loss. Iron deficiency is the leading cause of anemia.

- Magnesium is a cofactor for numerous chemical reactions and is needed for energy metabolism, and nerve and heart function. Cases of magnesium deficiency rarely occur among healthy members of the population. Plant foods are good sources of magnesium.

- In your body, selenium and copper help reduce free radical damage. Iodine, zinc, and chromium function as regulators of energy metabolism. Iodine deficiency can cause goiter and cretinism.

Module 9.3 Water: Liquid of Life

- In the body, water is a major component of body fluids. Water is a solvent that often participates directly in chemical reactions. Water's other physiological roles include transporting substances, removing waste products, lubricating tissues, and regulating body temperature and acid-base balance. Water doesn't provide energy for the body. Depending on a person's age, sex, and body composition, about 45 to 75% of his or her body is water.

- The body maintains a balance between intracellular and extracellular fluids primarily by controlling concentrations of electrolytes (ions) in each fluid compartment. If the normal concentrations of these ions change too much, water shifts out of a compartment, and cells shrink or swell as a result.

- Total water intake includes water from beverages and foods. About 80% of a person's total water intake is from beverages. Metabolic water is another source of water for the body.

- A healthy body loses water in urine, sweat, exhaled air, and feces. A healthy person's average daily total water input equals his or her average output. Environmental factors, physical condition, and lifestyle practices can alter your body's fluid balance.

- The kidneys are the major regulator of the body's water content and ion concentrations. In a healthy person, the kidneys maintain proper hydration by filtering excess ions from blood. When the kidneys remove ions such as sodium, water follows and becomes the main component of urine.

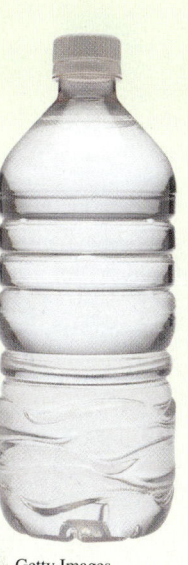
Getty Images

- To avoid overheating, your body must release the excess heat into the environment, primarily by perspiration. When water evaporates from your skin, it takes some heat along with it, cooling your body.

- Thirst is the primary regulator of fluid intake. The majority of healthy people meet their AI for water by letting thirst be their guide. Under certain conditions, however, older adults, sick persons, and people who work or exercise outdoors, especially in hot conditions, are at risk of dehydration.

- In the United States, bottled water is often derived from a municipal water supply. When public water supplies are disrupted, drinking bottled water may be the only option. The EPA regulates the sanitation of public water supplies in the United States. The FDA regulates bottled water products that are marketed for interstate commerce. Bottled water may have fluoride added, but amounts must meet FDA guidelines. If bottled water manufacturers add flavorings or other ingredients to a product, the name of the product must indicate the added ingredients, and the beverage's label must identify the additives in the list of ingredients.

Module 9.4 Drink to Your Health?

- Alcohol is a simple nonnutrient substance that supplies energy but is toxic to cells. Beers are typically 3 to 6% alcohol, wines contain about 8 to 14% alcohol, and malt liquors are about 7% alcohol by volume. Each gram of alcohol provides 7 kcal, but alcohol isn't a nutrient; it's a mind-altering drug.

- A standard drink (approximately 12 ounces of beer, 5 ounces of wine, 8 to 9 ounces of malt liquor, or 1½ ounces of liquor) contains 13 to 14 grams of alcohol.

- Alcohol requires no digestion and readily passes through the tissues lining the inside of the mouth, esophagus, stomach, and small intestine. The body detoxifies alcohol by converting the chemical into less-damaging compounds. Until the liver has had enough time to metabolize all the alcohol that has been consumed, the amount of the substance that remains circulates in the bloodstream.

- Binge drinking is a major public health problem in the United States.

- Although drinking small amounts of alcohol raises HDL cholesterol, excessive amounts of the substance damage every system in the body, particularly the gastrointestinal, nervous, and cardiovascular systems. Alcohol has especially devastating effects on an embryo. Infants born with fetal alcohol syndrome have certain facial and heart defects as well as extensive, irreversible nervous system damage that causes intellectual disability. Therefore, pregnant women should not drink alcohol.

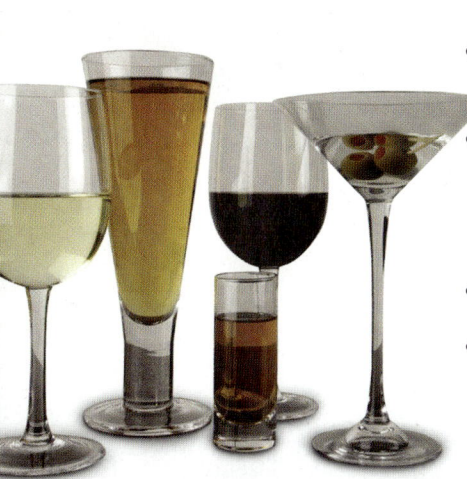
McGraw-Hill Education/Jill Braaten

What's in Your Diet?!

Using the DRIs: Minerals

1. Refer to your 3-day food log from the "What's in Your Diet?!" feature in Unit 3.

   a. Find the DRI (RDA/AI) for minerals under your life stage/sex group category in the DRI tables (see **Appendix E**). Write those values under the "My RDA/AI" column in the table below.

   b. Review your personal dietary assessment. Find your 3-day average intakes of potassium, sodium, calcium, magnesium, iron, and zinc. Write those values under the "My Average Intake" column of the table.

   c. Calculate the percentage of the DRI you consumed for each mineral by dividing your intake by the DRI amount and multiplying the figure you obtain by 100. For example, if your average intake of iron was 9 mg/day, and your RDA for the mineral is 18 mg/day, you would divide 18 mg by 9 mg to obtain 0.50. To multiply this figure by 100, simply move the decimal point two places to the right, and replace the decimal point with a percentage sign (50%). Thus, your average daily intake of iron was 50% of the RDA. Place the percentages for each mineral under the "% of My RDA/AI" column.

   d. Under the ">, <, or =" column, indicate whether your average daily intake was greater than (>), less than (<), or equal to (=) the RDA/AI (DRI value).

2. Use the information you calculated in the first part of this activity to answer the following questions:

   a. Which of your average mineral intakes equaled or exceeded the DRI value?

   b. Which of your average mineral intakes was below the DRI value?

   c. What foods would you eat to increase your intake of the minerals that were less than the DRI levels? (Review food sources of the minerals in Unit 9, including those listed in tables.)

Mineral	My RDA/AI	My Average Intake	% of My RDA/AI	>, <, or =
Iron				
Calcium				
Zinc				
Sodium				
Potassium				

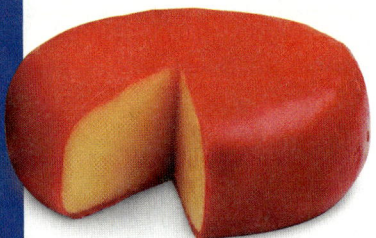
D. Hurst/Alamy

Sodium Intake Assessment

For each question, place a check in the column that best describes your sodium intake habits.

How Often Do You...	Rarely	Often	Daily
1. Eat processed meat, such as bacon, sausage, hot dogs, ham, and other luncheon meats?			
2. Eat canned vegetables?			
3. Eat commercially prepared meals or soups?			
4. Eat processed cheeses, such as cheese spreads?			
5. Eat salted nuts, popcorn, pretzels, corn chips, or potato chips?			
6. Add salt to cooking water for vegetables, rice, or pasta?			
7. Add salt, seasoning mixes, or condiments—such as soy sauce, steak sauce, pickles, and catsup—to foods during preparation?			
8. Salt your food before tasting it?			
9. Ignore the Nutrition Facts panel for sodium content when buying foods?			
10. Choose salty menu items when dining out?			

Scoring: The more checks you put in the "often" or "daily" columns, the higher your sodium intake is. Adapted from: USDA: *Home and Garden Bulletin*, No. 232–6, April 1986.

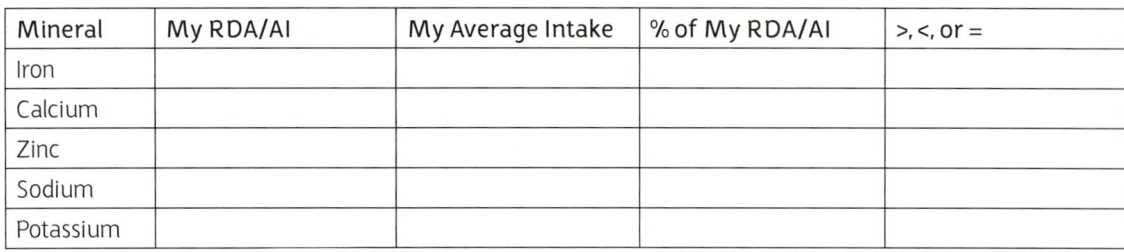
Wendy Schiff

Consider This...

1. A friend of yours refuses to drink her community's tap water because it has been fluoridated. She's heard that fluoride is toxic. She drinks only bottled water. What advice about fluoride and bottled water would you give your friend?

2. Paul is a total vegetarian (vegan), and he doesn't like soy-based foods. Based on this information, identify at least three minerals that are likely to be lacking in his diet.

3. Consider your family history and lifestyle to determine whether you're at risk of osteoporosis. If you're at risk, what steps can you take at this point in your life to reduce your chances of developing this disease?

4. Consider your family history and lifestyle to determine whether you're at risk of hypertension. If you're at risk, what steps can you take at this point in your life to reduce your chances of developing this disease?

5. In a televised interview, a person claiming to be a doctor recommends taking megadoses of chromium and selenium supplements to enhance muscular strength and endurance. Discuss why you would or wouldn't follow this person's advice.

6. If you drink alcohol, consider assessing your alcohol use habits by answering the questions listed in Table 9.22. According to your responses, are you at risk for alcoholism? If your answer is "yes," what can you do to obtain help?

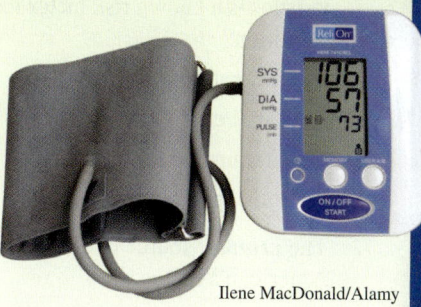

Ilene MacDonald/Alamy

Test Yourself

Select the best answer.

1. Which of the following statements is false?
   a. Lean tissue contains more water than fat tissue.
   b. Water is a major solvent.
   c. Generally, young women have more body water than do young men.
   d. Water doesn't provide energy.

2. If the extracellular fluid has an excess of sodium ions,
   a. sodium ions move into cells.
   b. intracellular fluid moves to the outside of cells.
   c. phosphate and calcium ions are eliminated in feces.
   d. blood levels of arsenic and oxalate increase.

3. Which of the following foods has the lowest percentage of water?
   a. Tomatoes
   b. Oranges
   c. Whole-grain bread
   d. Vegetable oil

4. In the United States, table salt is often fortified with
   a. iron.
   b. selenium.
   c. potassium.
   d. iodine.

5. Which of the following foods isn't a good source of calcium?
   a. Butter
   b. Cheddar cheese
   c. Canned sardines
   d. Kale

6. Henry is concerned about his risk of osteoporosis. Which of the following characteristics is a known risk factor for this chronic condition?
   a. Occupation
   b. Racial/ethnic background
   c. Vitamin B-12 intake
   d. Iron exposure

7. The primary source of sodium in the typical American's diet is
   a. bottled water.
   b. milk.
   c. fruit.
   d. processed food.

8. Bioavailable sources of heme iron include
   a. fortified grain products.
   b. beef.
   c. spinach.
   d. cast-iron cookware.

9. Which of the following populations has the highest risk of hypertension?
   a. People with African-American ancestry
   b. Young, physically active Asian men
   c. Hispanic women who don't drink alcohol
   d. Young adults who consume high amounts of fruit

10. In the United States, the most common cause of anemia is _____ deficiency.
    a. iodine
    b. cobalt
    c. iron
    d. calcium

11. Cretinism is caused by a deficiency of ____ during pregnancy.
    a. iron
    b. sodium
    c. copper
    d. iodine

12. Which of the following statements is true?
    a. Safety standards for bottled water are similar to those for tap water.
    b. Most brands of water bottled in the United States contain unsafe amounts of arsenic and lead.
    c. The EPA inspects and certifies water bottling facilities at least three times a year.
    d. The majority of Americans should drink bottled water because water from municipal systems is unsafe.

13. Many Americans have low intakes of
    a. potassium.
    b. chloride.
    c. phosphorus.
    d. manganese.

Answers: 1. c 2. b 3. d 4. d 5. a 6. b 7. d 8. b 9. a 10. c 11. d 12. a 13. a

A Answer This (Module 9.2e)
Iodine

References → See Appendix D.

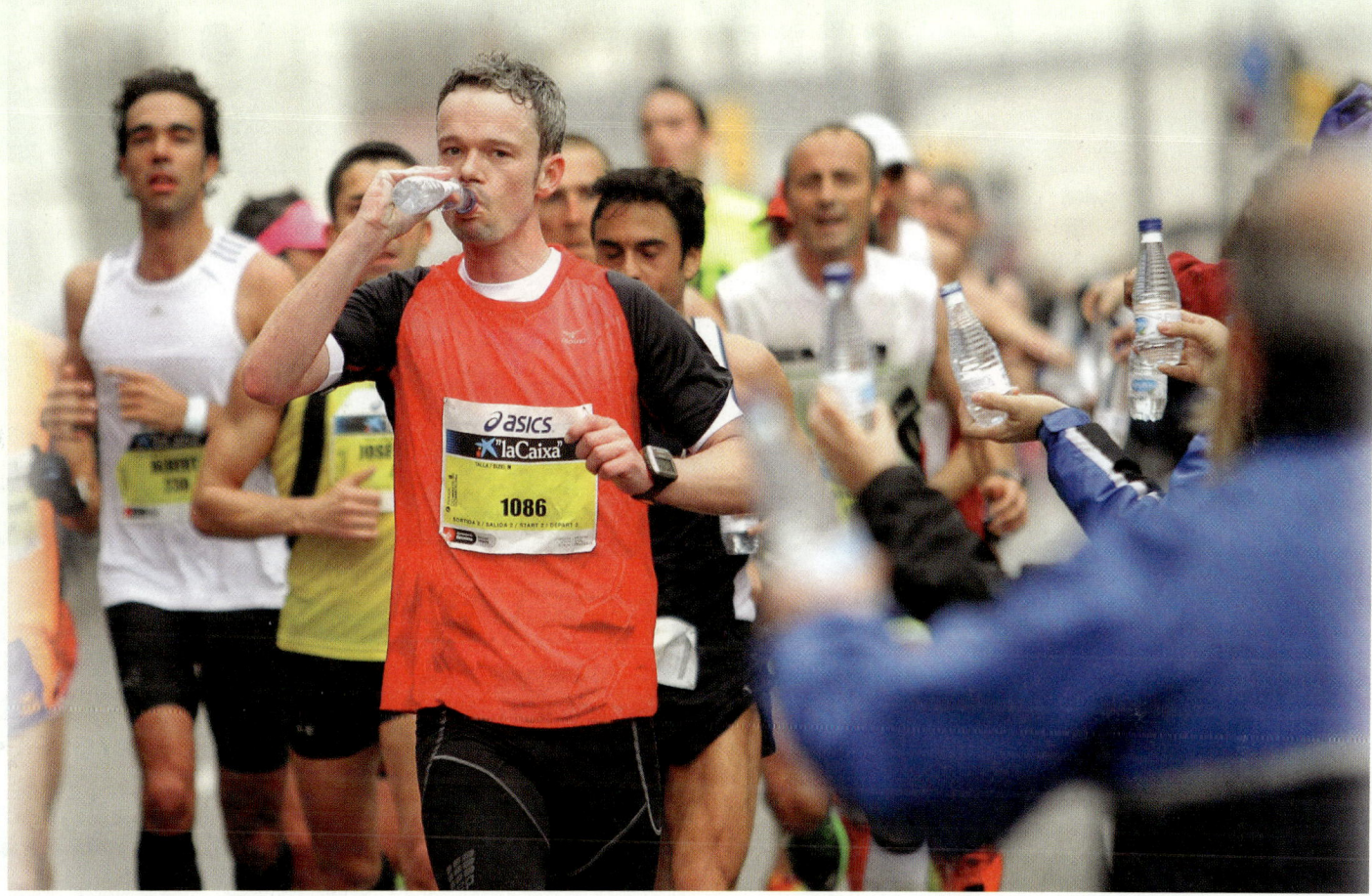

sportgraphic/123RF

Design elements: Spiral notebook paper background, Stacked paper with clip background, Marginal note clip, and Culture & Cuisine globe icon: ©McGraw-Hill Education; In a Nutshell walnut: ©McGraw-Hill Education/Mark A. Dierker, photographer; Test Yourself red pepper: Iconotec/Glow Images

Unit 10

Nutrition for a Healthy Weight and Fit Body

What's on the Menu?

Module 10.1
Overweight or Obese?

Module 10.2
Factors That Influence Your Body Weight

Module 10.3
Managing Your Weight Safely

Module 10.4
Disordered Eating and Eating Disorders

Module 10.5
Get Moving; Get Healthy!

Pixtal/AGE Fotostock

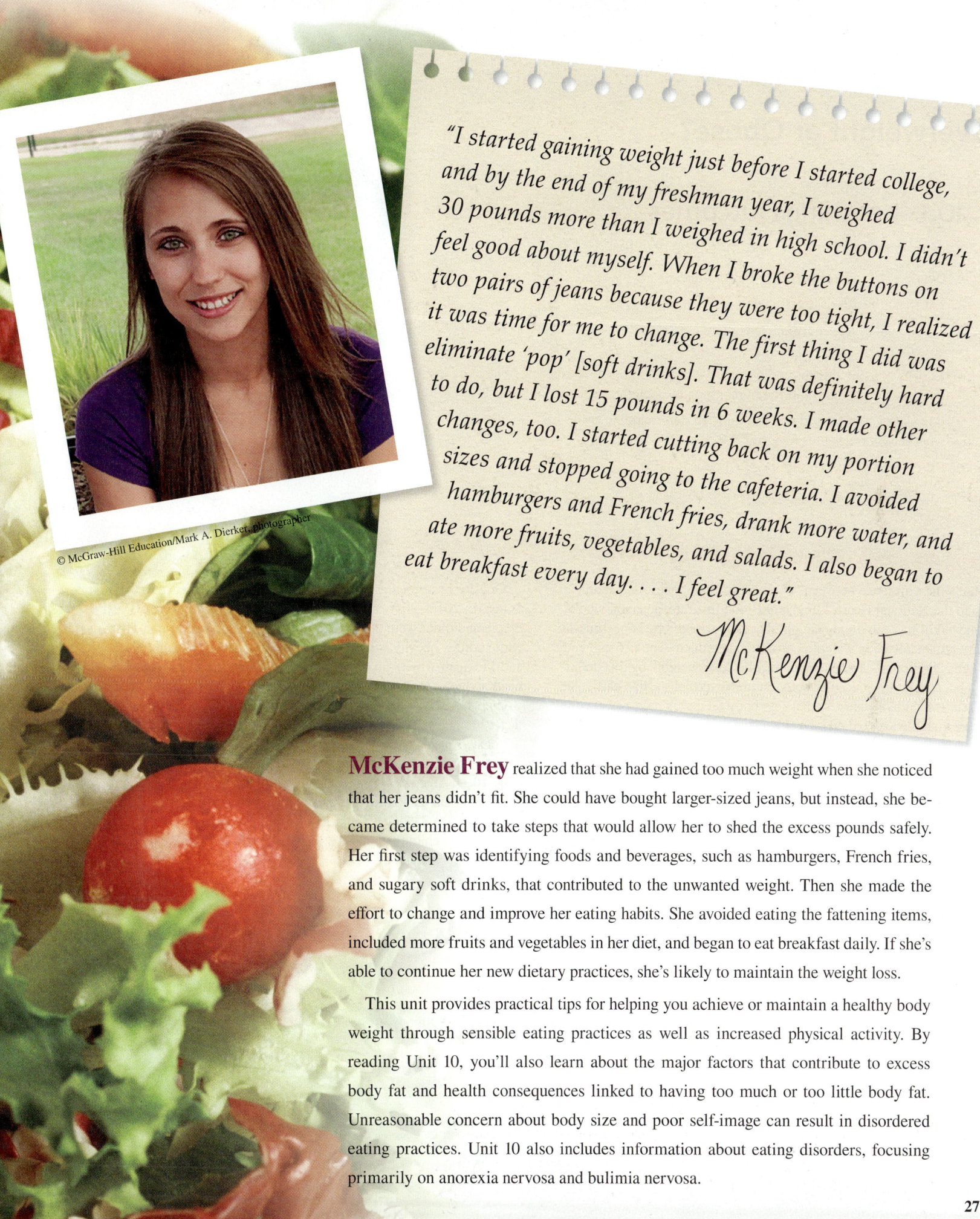

"I started gaining weight just before I started college, and by the end of my freshman year, I weighed 30 pounds more than I weighed in high school. I didn't feel good about myself. When I broke the buttons on two pairs of jeans because they were too tight, I realized it was time for me to change. The first thing I did was eliminate 'pop' [soft drinks]. That was definitely hard to do, but I lost 15 pounds in 6 weeks. I made other changes, too. I started cutting back on my portion sizes and stopped going to the cafeteria. I avoided hamburgers and French fries, drank more water, and ate more fruits, vegetables, and salads. I also began to eat breakfast every day. . . . I feel great."

McKenzie Frey

McKenzie Frey realized that she had gained too much weight when she noticed that her jeans didn't fit. She could have bought larger-sized jeans, but instead, she became determined to take steps that would allow her to shed the excess pounds safely. Her first step was identifying foods and beverages, such as hamburgers, French fries, and sugary soft drinks, that contributed to the unwanted weight. Then she made the effort to change and improve her eating habits. She avoided eating the fattening items, included more fruits and vegetables in her diet, and began to eat breakfast daily. If she's able to continue her new dietary practices, she's likely to maintain the weight loss.

This unit provides practical tips for helping you achieve or maintain a healthy body weight through sensible eating practices as well as increased physical activity. By reading Unit 10, you'll also learn about the major factors that contribute to excess body fat and health consequences linked to having too much or too little body fat. Unreasonable concern about body size and poor self-image can result in disordered eating practices. Unit 10 also includes information about eating disorders, focusing primarily on anorexia nervosa and bulimia nervosa.

Module 10.1
Overweight or Obese?

10.1 - Learning Outcomes

After reading Module 10.1, you should be able to

1. Define all of the **key terms** in this module.
2. List major health risks associated with excess body fat.
3. Explain differences between subcutaneous fat and visceral fat.
4. Explain why the distribution of body fat may be more important to health than the percentage of body fat.
5. Calculate your BMI and use the value to determine whether your weight is healthy.
6. Describe ways to measure body composition.

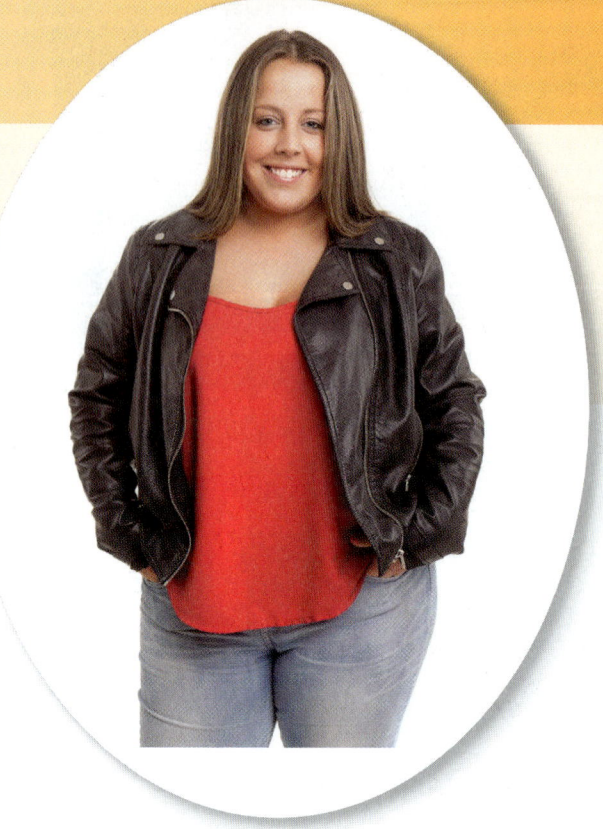

Hugo Felix/Alamy Stock Photo

10.1a The Modern Epidemic

What's the difference between "overweight" and "obese"? According to the National Heart, Lung, and Blood Institute, a person who's **overweight** has extra body weight that's contributed by bone, muscle, body fat, and/or body water.[1] A professional athlete who is 6' tall and weighs 200 pounds, for example, may be "overweight" by this definition because of his muscular body build. Nevertheless, this particular athlete is healthy because he has less body fat and is more physically active than the average man who's his height, weight, and age. Many people, however, have too much body fat (**"overfat"**). **Obesity** is a condition characterized by excessive and unhealthy amounts of body fat. Unless otherwise noted, we'll generally use the term *overweight* when referring to people who are overfat but not obese. Overweight and obese people have greater risk of developing serious chronic diseases, including type 2 diabetes, hypertension, and cardiovascular disease (CVD) than people who aren't overweight or obese.[1]

Obesity is a *prevalent* (common) nutritional disorder in the United States. In 2015–2016, almost 40% of Americans who were 20 years of age and older were obese (**Table 10.1**).[2] Compared to non-Hispanic white adults, obesity is more common among non-Hispanic black and Mexican-American adults, particularly among non-Hispanic black women. In 2015–2016, almost 55% of non-Hispanic black women were obese.[2] Cultural, behavioral, and environmental factors may be largely responsible for racial/ethnic differences in obesity rates.

In the United States, obesity has reached epidemic proportions (**Fig. 10.1**). An epidemic is a widespread health problem. Between 1988–1994 and 2015–2016, the percentage of obese adult Americans rose by almost 73% (see Table 10.1). Public health experts are also concerned about childhood obesity. In 2015–2016, 18.5% of children who were 2 to 19 years of age were obese.[3]

overweight having extra weight from bone, muscle, body fat, and/or body water

overfat having too much body fat

obesity condition characterized by an excessive and unhealthy amount of body fat

TABLE 10.1 AGE-ADJUSTED PREVALENCE OF OVERWEIGHT AND OBESITY AMONG U.S. ADULTS AGED 20 AND OVER

Weight Status	1988–1994	2015–2016
Overweight	33.1%	31.6%
Obese	22.9%	39.6%

Source: Data from: Fryar CD and others: Prevalence of overweight, obesity, and severe obesity among adults aged 20 and over: United States, 1960–1962 through 2015–2016. *National Center for Health Statistics, E-Stats.* September 2018. www.cdc.gov/nchs/data/hestat/obesity_adult_15_16/obesity_adult_15_16.pdf Accessed: July 21, 2019

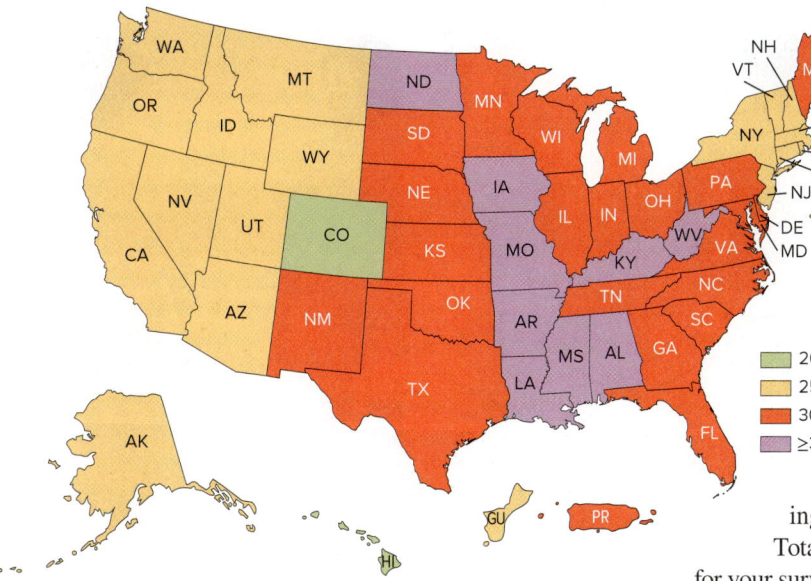

Figure 10.1 Adult obesity map of the United States (2018).
Source: Centers for Disease Control and Prevention.

Legend:
- 20%–<25%
- 25%–<30%
- 30%–<35%
- ≥35%

Rates of overweight and obesity are also increasing rapidly throughout the world ("globesity"). The World Health Organization (WHO) estimated that worldwide, more than 1.9 *billon* people, 18 years of age or older, were overweight and 650 million of these persons were obese in 2016.[4] In most countries, overweight and obesity are responsible for more deaths than the number caused by being underweight.

10.1b Body Composition and Adipose Tissue

Your body is composed of two major compartments: **fat-free mass** (lean tissues) and **total body fat.** Fat-free mass is comprised of body water, mineral-rich tissues such as bones and teeth, and protein-rich tissues, including muscles and organs.

Total body fat includes "essential fat" and fat tissue. Essential fat is vital for your survival—every cell in your body contains some essential fat in its cell membrane. Furthermore, essential fat is also in certain bones and nervous tissue.

Adipose Cells

Fat tissue is actually a very large organ that's in the endocrine system (see Table 4.1). Unlike other organs that have distinct structures, such as the brain, heart, and kidneys, fat tissue is located under the skin and throughout the body.

Body fat contains two main types of adipose ("fat") cells. White adipose cells, which are shown in **Figure 10.2,** remove fatty acids from the bloodstream and store the lipid as a large droplet of triglycerides (see Figure 6.12).[5] White adipose cells can also remove excess glucose from the bloodstream and convert the simple sugar into fatty acids. These cells also make and secrete numerous proteins, some of which have roles in regulating food intake, glucose metabolism, and immune responses. Thus, having some white adipose cell tissue is necessary for good health, but overweight and obese people have excessive amounts of this type of fat tissue.

Compared to white adipose cells, brown adipose cells aren't designed to store and release fat. Brown fat cells' primary function is to burn triglycerides, which releases heat. This action helps maintain normal body temperature. Adults have far more white fat cells than brown fat cells. Therefore, this unit focuses primarily on white fat tissue.

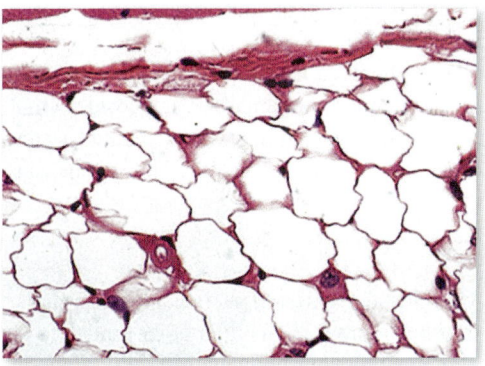

Figure 10.2 White fat (adipose) cells.
© McGraw-Hill Education. Dennis Strete, photographer

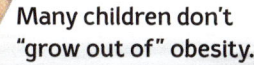

Many children don't "grow out of" obesity.

fat-free mass lean tissues

total body fat essential fat and storage fat tissue

Ingram Publishing/SuperStock

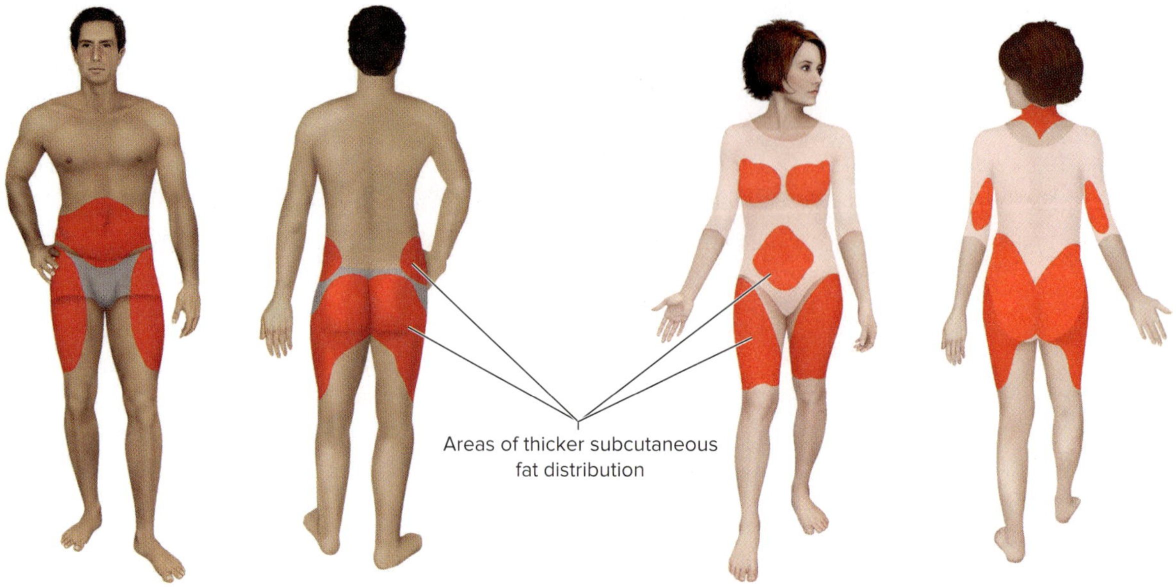

Areas of thicker subcutaneous fat distribution

Figure 10.3 **Uneven subcutaneous fat distribution in men and women.** Subcutaneous fat is the layer of fat that's directly under the skin. This type of fat is thicker in certain regions of the body.

Too Many White Adipose Cells The body forms new white fat cells during periods of rapid growth, such as before birth and during the teenage years. However, the body can also form new adipose cells throughout a person's lifetime, and especially in response to eating a high-calorie diet that supplies too much fat.[6]

As the amount of fat stored in white adipose cells increases, the size of each cell expands, and the body gains weight. When the body needs energy, its white adipose cells release fat into the bloodstream for other cells to use as fuel. As each adipose cell loses some fat, it shrinks. The body eventually loses weight and appears slimmer, as a result. The fat cell, however, remains alive and is capable of storing fat again. Once adipose cells form, they can live for about 10 years, under normal conditions.[6]

Although white fat cells can enlarge by allowing fat to enter them, there's a limit to their ability to expand. Once they reach that point, the adipose cells cannot take in any more fat, and the triglycerides circulate in the bloodstream as a result.[6] The excess fat is taken up by other organs that aren't designed to accumulate large amounts of triglycerides, particularly the liver and pancreas. When this occurs, the organs can become inflamed, and conditions such as nonalcoholic fatty liver disease develop (see Unit 4).

Subcutaneous Fat and Visceral Fat

Subcutaneous (*sub-qu-tay'-nee-us*) tissue holds skin in place over underlying tissues such as muscles. Subcutaneous tissue also contains fat cells. When subcutaneous tissue has more fat cells than other kinds of cells, it's referred to as **subcutaneous fat.**[6] Subcutaneous fat helps insulate your body against cold temperatures and protects muscles and bones from bumps and bruises. This layer of fat is thicker in certain regions of men's and women's bodies, especially in the abdominal area, thighs, and buttocks **(Fig. 10.3).**

Your body also has **visceral** (*viss'-eh-rol*) **fat.** Visceral fat is adipose tissue that's under your abdominal muscles and hangs over your stomach and intestines like a protective apron **(Fig. 10.4).** Women generally have more subcutaneous fat than men, whereas men tend to have more visceral fat than women.[5] Excessive visceral fat and/or subcutaneous abdominal fat result in what's commonly called a "beer belly" or the "middle-age spread." The following section of this module explains why having too much visceral fat can be unhealthy.

subcutaneous fat layer of tissue that's under the skin and has more fat cells than other kinds of cells

visceral fat adipose tissue that's under the abdominal muscles, which forms a protective apron over the stomach and intestines

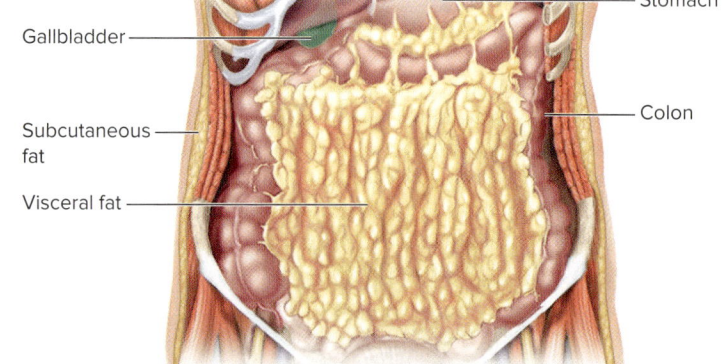

Figure 10.4 Visceral and subcutaneous fat.

■ *Why is it unhealthy to have too much visceral fat?*

Nutrition Fact or Fiction?
Cellulite is toxic wastes trapped under the skin.

This statement is false because the body doesn't store toxic wastes under the skin. Whenever possible, your body detoxifies poisonous substances or eliminates them. Nearly all women have dimpled-appearing skin ("cellulite") on their buttocks and thighs.[7] Cellulite is simply subcutaneous fat that's held in place by irregular bands of connective tissue. Despite claims by cosmetic manufacturers that their products eliminate cellulite, there are no nonmedical treatments that can smooth the skin's dimpled appearance.

Anetlanda/Shutterstock

10.1c Health Effects of Excess Fat

Several chronic health problems that affect millions of Americans are associated with excessive body fat. Obese people have increased risks of

- heart disease,
- type 2 diabetes,
- certain cancers (uterine, breast, liver, kidney, gallbladder, and colon),
- hypertension (high blood pressure),
- high total cholesterol or high triglyceride levels,
- stroke,
- gallbladder disease,
- sleep apnea and other breathing problems,
- osteoarthritis (breakdown of joint tissues), and
- all causes of death (mortality).[8]

A person's mental health and self-esteem can be negatively affected by his or her "weight problem." Many Americans admire people with slim and muscular body builds. Thus, overweight and obese people often suffer from poor self-images because they think their bodies are unattractive. The general public tends to view obesity as a condition that results from lack of willpower and the inability to "push oneself away from the table." People who aren't overfat or obese often characterize obese persons as lazy, lacking in willpower, and not intelligent.[9] Thus, many obese people must deal with the negative attitude that slimmer people have toward them.

Body Fat Distribution: Effects on Health

The distribution of a person's excess body fat is closely associated with the risk of obesity-related diseases. Central-body obesity is characterized by a large amount of visceral fat ("spare tire") that causes the waistline to spread beyond the buttocks and thighs. A person with **central-body obesity** is sometimes described as having an "apple" body shape (see **Fig. 10.5a**). People with central-body obesity have higher risks of CVD and type 2 diabetes than people who have waists that don't extend beyond their hips.[5] Fat cells, particularly visceral fat, make substances that cause inflammation in the body. These inflammatory factors may increase risks of type 2 diabetes and CVD.

Some people, especially women, tend to store extra subcutaneous fat below the waist, primarily in the buttocks and thighs (see **Fig. 10.5b**). Having a "pear shape" pattern of fat distribution adds stress to hip and knee joints that must carry the extra weight, which can lead to osteoarthritis (breakdown of joint tissues). This particular type of body fat distribution, however, isn't associated with increased risk of more serious chronic diseases such as type 2 diabetes.[5]

central-body obesity condition characterized by having a large amount of visceral fat and an "apple" shape

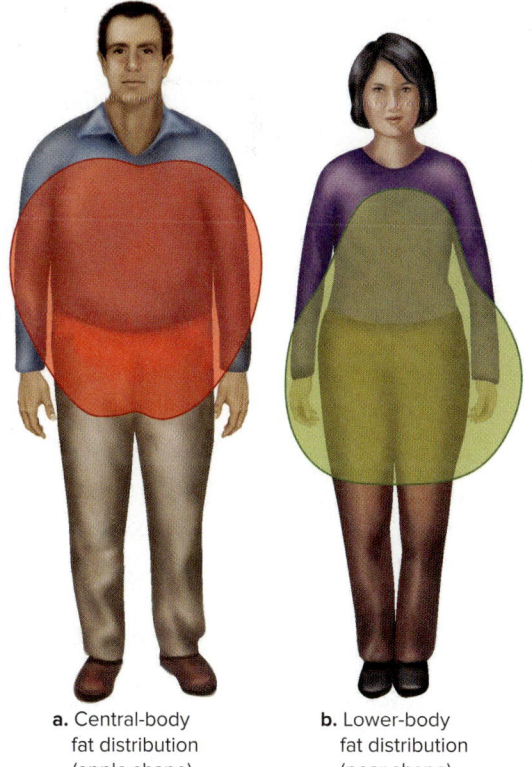

a. Central-body fat distribution (apple shape)

b. Lower-body fat distribution (pear shape)

Figure 10.5 Body fat distribution: Typical sex differences.

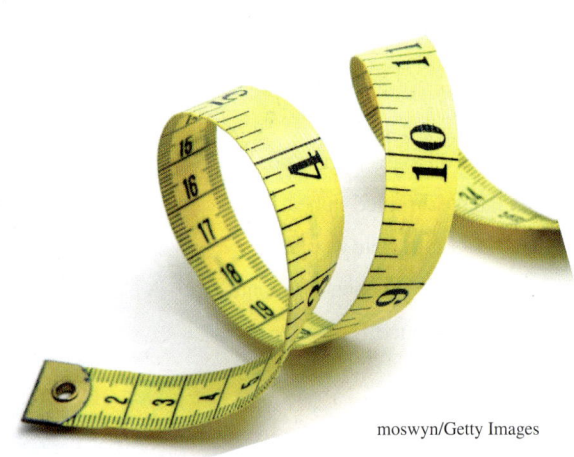
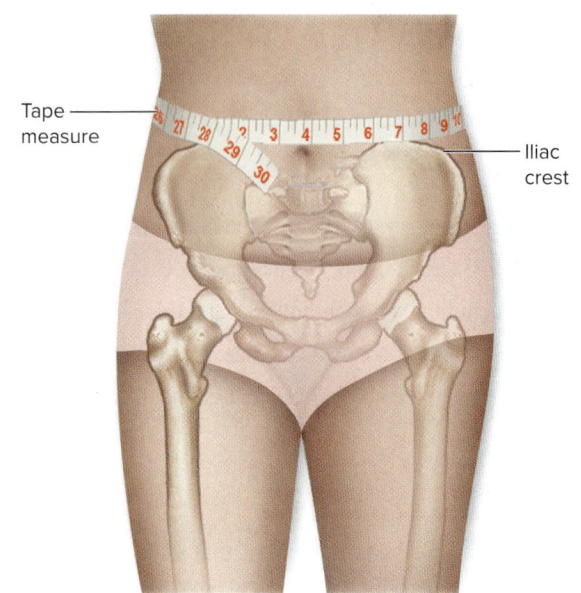

moswyn/Getty Images

Figure 10.6 Measuring waist circumference.

■ *What is the waist circumference of a man who has central-body obesity? What is the waist circumference of a woman with central-body obesity?*

body mass index (BMI) numerical value that's used to relate body weight and risk of chronic health problems associated with excess body fat

A quick and easy method to determine whether you have an unhealthy amount of visceral fat is to measure your waist circumference. **Figure 10.6** shows the recommended placement of the tape measure. Note the positioning of a measuring tape at the top of the hip bones and not necessarily at the narrowest point.[10] A person with central-body obesity has a waist circumference that's greater than 40 inches (men) and greater than 35 inches (women).[10]

How can you determine whether your weight is within the healthy range for your height? How much body fat is unhealthy? The following sections of this module answer these questions.

10.1d What's Body Mass Index?

At one time, people referred to height/weight tables to determine whether their body weights were "ideal" or "desirable." Although it's easy to step on a scale and weigh yourself, knowing that number doesn't always provide good information about your health status. Today, medical experts use the **body mass index (BMI)** to judge whether an adult's weight is healthy. BMI is a numerical value that's used to relate body weight and risk of chronic health problems associated with excess body fat.

How to Calculate Your BMI

To calculate your BMI, you can use the following formula:

$$\text{weight (lb)} \div [\text{height (in)}]^2 \times 703$$

For example, let's calculate the BMI of a person who weighs 140 pounds and is 5'3" (63"). Fill these numbers into the formula: $[140 \div (63)^2] \times 703$

Do the math:

Step 1: 63^2 is 63×63, which $= 3969$

Step 2: $[140 \div 3969] = 0.03527$

Step 3: $0.03527 \times 703 = 24.8$

This person's BMI is 24.8. To determine your BMI, replace the numbers in the formula with your height and weight values. You can also use the BMI calculator at www.nhlbi.nih.gov/health/educational/lose_wt/BMI/bmicalc.htm. What's your BMI?

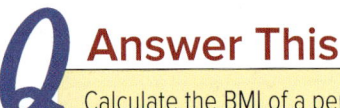

Answer This

Calculate the BMI of a person who weighs 157 pounds and is 5'6". You can find the answer on the last page of this unit.

BMI Categories

Table 10.2 presents adult weight status classifications based on standard BMI ranges. Such classifications apply to people with white, African, and Mexican-American ancestry. According to the standards, healthy BMIs range from 18.5 to 24.9.

As BMI increases, the risks of heart disease, hypertension, type 2 diabetes, gallstones, certain cancers, and breathing problems increase. Thus, obese and *extremely* obese people are far more likely to develop the serious chronic diseases associated with excess body fat and to die prematurely than are people who have BMIs that range from 18.5 to 30.0. Extremely obese adults have BMIs that are 40.0 and higher. In 2015–2016, 7.7% of adult Americans were extremely obese.[2] This percentage is 175% higher than the percentage of adults who were extremely obese in 1988 to 1994.

Limitations of the BMI

Muscle is denser than fat. Therefore, a muscular person whose BMI is in the overweight range may actually have a healthy percentage of body fat. For example, a college athlete with a BMI of 27.5 is more likely to be healthy than a nonathletic college student who also has a BMI of 27.5. The BMI may underestimate body fat in people who have lost muscle tissue as a result of aging or illness.[11] Therefore, BMIs should be used with caution when assessing the health of highly muscular individuals, people who are elderly, or chronically ill persons. However, people with BMIs of 30 or higher generally have excess body fat.

Your BMI doesn't provide the entire picture regarding your chances of developing diseases, especially CVD and type 2 diabetes, that are associated with having excess body fat. You should also consider whether you have major risk factors for such diseases, including family history of CVD, high blood pressure, a large waistline, and an inactive lifestyle.

Table 10.2 Adult Weight Status Categories (Standard BMI)

BMI	Weight Status
Below 18.5	Underweight
18.5 to 24.9	Healthy
25.0 to 29.9	Overweight
30.0 to 39.9	Obese
40 and above	Extremely obese

Source: National Institutes of Health, National Heart, Lung, and Blood Institute: Classification of overweight and obesity by BMI, waist circumference, and associated disease risks. ND. www.nhlbi.nih.gov/health/educational/lose_wt/BMI/bmi_dis.htm Accessed: July 21, 2019

Culture & Cuisine

A healthy diet for people with Asian ancestry supplies a variety of vegetables, rice, noodles, seeds, nuts, fruit, and products made from soybeans. Such foods may be prepared with small amounts of fish and shellfish, eggs, chicken, and healthy oils (see Figure 3.7). When Asian people immigrate to Western nations, they often discard many of their healthy food-related practices and adopt some of the unhealthy dietary patterns that are popular in their new homelands. As a result, Asian immigrants' obesity rates as well as their risks of CVD, hypertension, and type 2 diabetes increase. Other factors, however, may contribute to the likelihood that a person with Asian ancestry develops serious, and often deadly, chronic diseases.

Compared to non-Hispanic white Americans, people with Asian ancestry have more abdominal subcutaneous fat and visceral fat, which can result in central-body obesity.[12] High waist circumference is a sign of central-body obesity and a risk factor for CVD. Furthermore, Chinese-American adults have a greater risk of developing CVD at lower BMIs when compared to the BMIs of non-Hispanic white Americans.[13] For Chinese-American adults, having a BMI of less than (<) 23.0 is within the healthy/underweight range; Americans with Chinese ancestry who have BMIs of 27.5 or more are obese.[13] Compare those values with the general BMI classifications shown in Table 10.2.

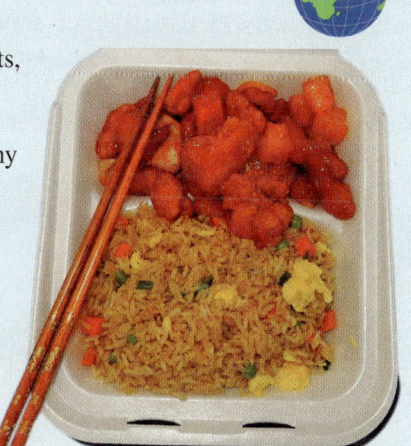

Chinese food—American style
Wendy Schiff

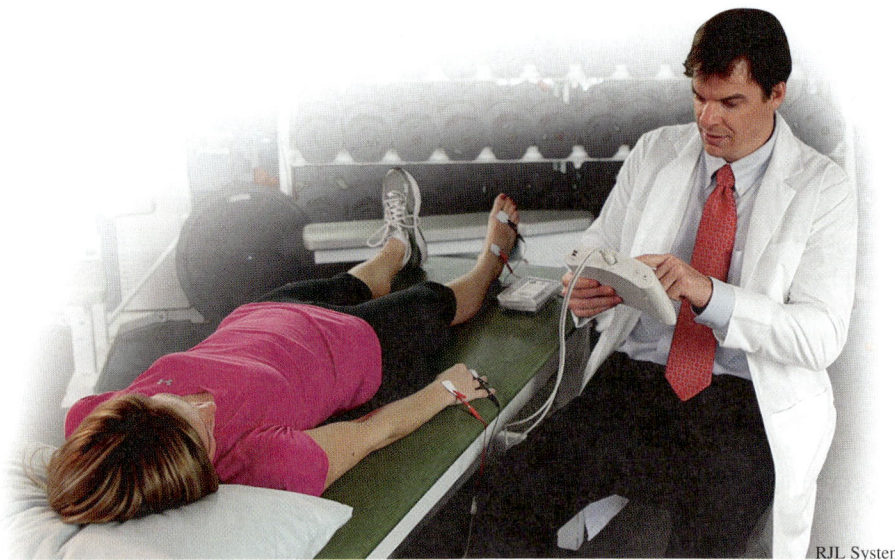

Figure 10.7 Measuring bioelectrical impedance.

10.1e Estimating Body Fat

There are some scientific methods of measuring body fat, but most involve large and expensive equipment. Let's take a closer look at a couple of less costly and more practical ways to estimate your level of body fat.

Bioelectrical Impedance

Bioelectrical impedance is a method that's based on the principle that water and electrolytes, such as sodium ions, conduct electricity. Fat tissue contains less water and electrolytes than does lean tissue. Therefore, body fat resists the flow of electricity more than lean tissue does.

The bioelectrical impedance device sends a painless, low-energy electrical current through a person's body via wires connected to electrodes placed on the subject's skin (**Fig. 10.7**). The device converts information about the body's resistance to the electrical current into an estimate of total body water. This information is used to predict the percentage of fat tissue in the body. The method is fairly accurate, as long as the subject's hydration status is normal. For home use, you can purchase a hand-to-hand bioelectrical impedance device that resembles a bathroom scale. Such devices are easy to use and can provide reliable results.[14]

bioelectrical impedance technique of estimating body composition in which a device measures the conduction of a weak electrical current through the body

skinfold thickness measurements technique of estimating body composition in which calipers are used to measure the width of skinfolds at multiple body sites

Skinfold Thickness

A commonly used technique for estimating total body fat involves taking **skinfold thickness measurements** at multiple body sites, including the triceps muscle of the arm (**Fig. 10.8**). The width of a skinfold indicates the depth of the subcutaneous fat at that site. To perform the measurements, a trained person pinches a section of the subject's skin, gently pulls it away from underlying muscle tissue, and uses special calipers to measure the thickness of the fat. After taking the measurements, the values are incorporated into a mathematical formula that provides a fairly accurate estimate of the subject's amount of body fat.

Skinfold thickness measurements are relatively easy and inexpensive to perform, but the method's accuracy largely depends on the number of sites that are measured and skill of the person performing the measurements. Also, the technique may underestimate total body fat when used on obese subjects. However, by combining the information collected from skinfold, waist and hip circumference, and body frame measurements, researchers can obtain more reliable estimates of an individual's total body fat.[15]

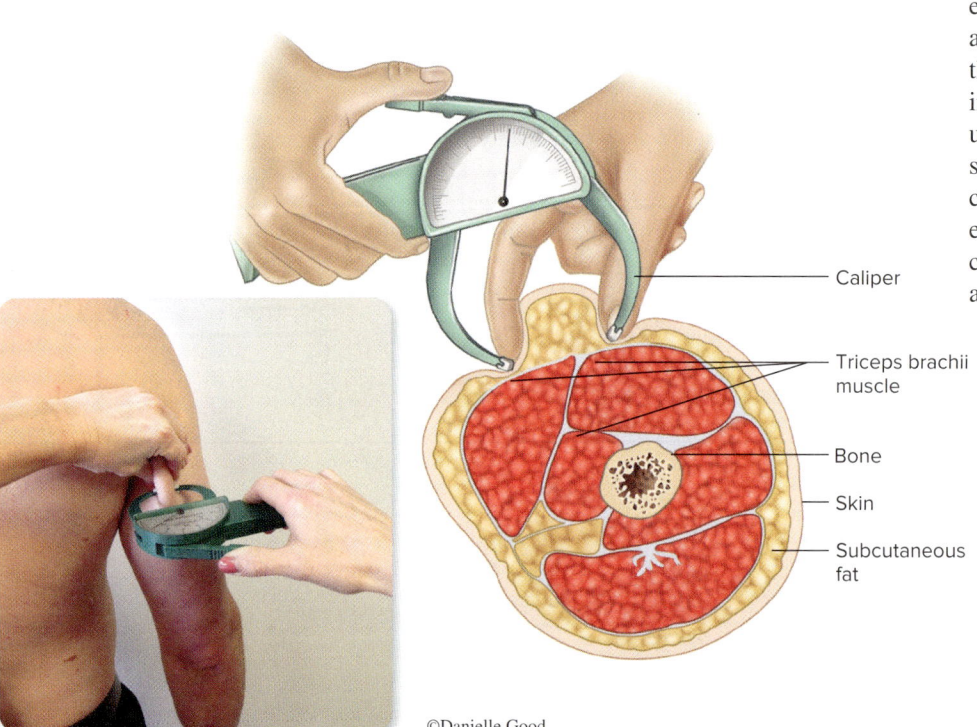

Figure 10.8 Measuring skinfold thickness.

10.1f How Much Body Fat Is Healthy?

Some body fat is essential for good health, but too much fat tissue can interfere with your body's ability to function normally. What percentage of body fat is too much for good health? **Table 10.3** classifies people into weight categories according to their percentage of body fat. A man is overweight when his body is 22 to 25% fat; a woman is overweight when her body is 32 to 37% fat.[16] A man is obese when fat comprises 26% or more of his body; a woman is obese when fat makes up 38% or more of her body. The average healthy young woman has more body fat than the average healthy young man because she needs the extra fat for reproductive purposes.

Adults tend to gain fat tissue as they age, but for older adults, some additional fat doesn't necessarily contribute to serious health problems. The extra fat may actually provide some health benefits, such as providing an energy reserve for a very ill person who cannot eat. Furthermore, the extra padding of fat may protect a person from being injured by falling.

TABLE 10.3 ADULT BODY WEIGHT CLASSIFICATION BY PERCENTAGE OF BODY FAT

Classification	Body Fat (%) Men	Body Fat (%) Women
Healthy	13 to 21%	23 to 31%
Overweight	22 to 25%	32 to 37%
Obese	26 to 31%	38 to 42%
Extremely obese	32% or more	43% or more

Source: Adapted from: Food and Nutrition Board: *Dietary Reference Intakes for energy, carbohydrate, fiber, fat, fatty acids, cholesterol, protein, and amino acids.* Table 5.5, page 126, 2005. www.nap.edu/catalog/10490/dietary-reference-intakes-for-energy-carbohydrate-fiber-fat-fatty-acids-cholesterol-protein-and-amino-acids Accessed: September 15, 2019.

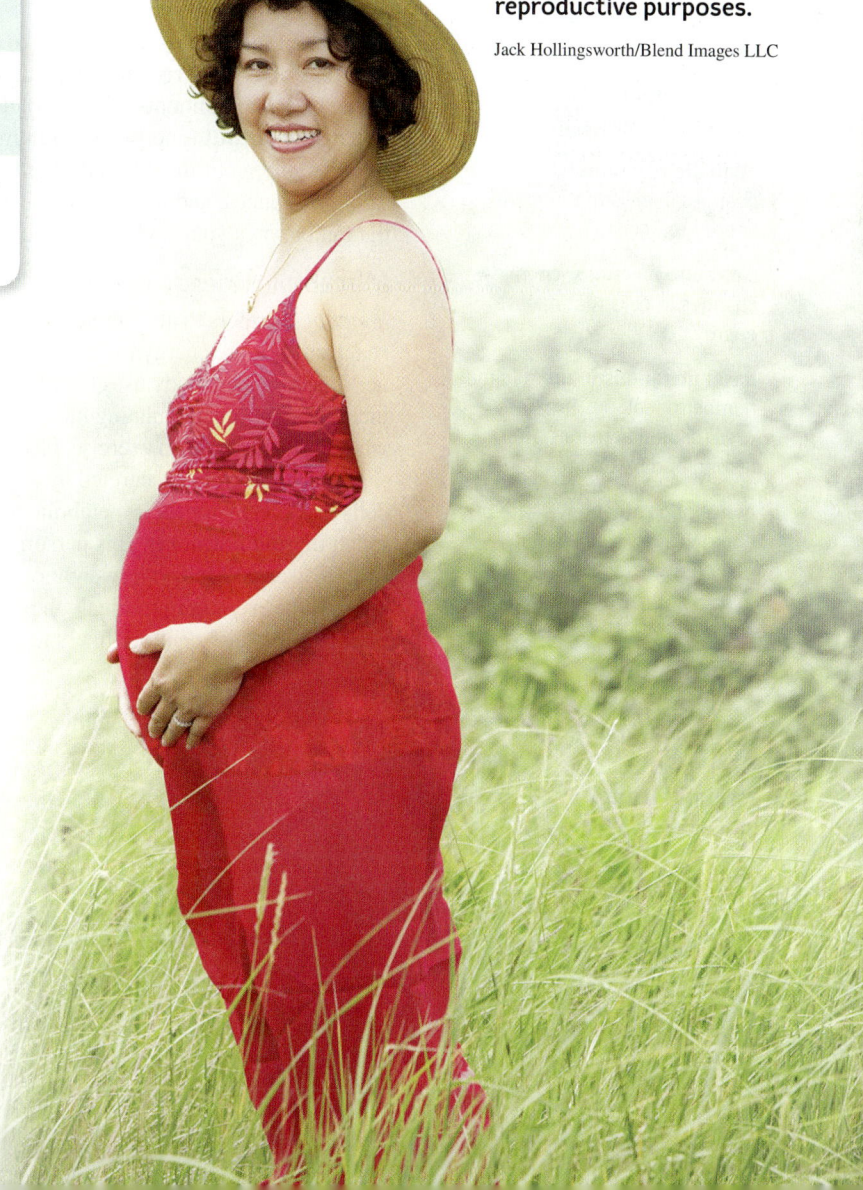

Women need more body fat than men for reproductive purposes.

Jack Hollingsworth/Blend Images LLC

Module 10.2
Factors That Influence Your Body Weight

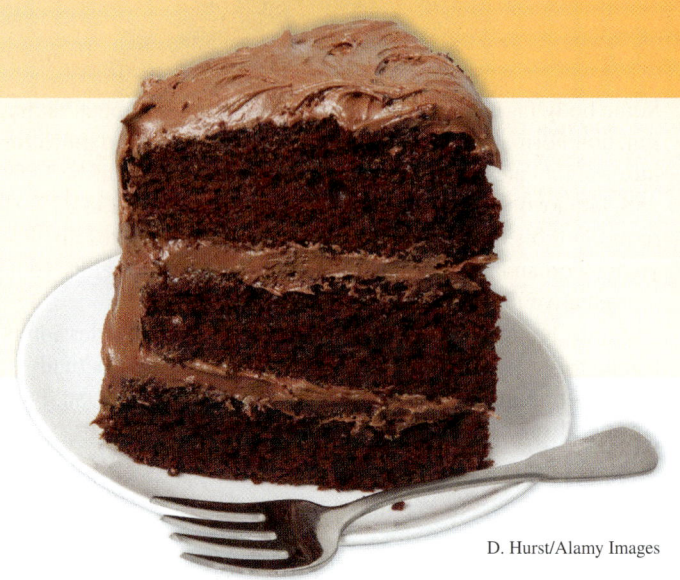

10.2 – Learning Outcomes
After reading Module 10.2, you should be able to
1. Define all of the **key terms** in this module.
2. Describe the uses of energy by the body, and explain the concept of energy balance.
3. Identify factors that influence the development of excess body weight.

energy intake calories from foods and beverages that contain macronutrients and alcohol

energy output calories cells use to carry out their activities

anabolic reactions chemical changes in cells that require energy to occur

catabolic reactions chemical changes in cells that release energy

basal metabolism the minimal number of calories the body uses for vital activities after fasting and resting for 12 hours

metabolic rate body's rate of energy use a few hours after resting and eating

10.2a Calories In; Calories Out

Just as a car engine uses a mixture of gasoline, ethanol, and oxygen to run properly, your body uses a mixture of biological fuels and oxygen to do its work. Biological fuels are foods and beverages that contain macronutrients (**energy intake**). Under normal conditions, our cells metabolize primarily glucose and fatty acids, but small amounts of amino acids are also used for energy.

Energy output (energy expenditure) refers to the energy (calories) cells use to carry out their activities. For example, your muscle cells need energy to contract, liver cells use energy to convert toxic compounds to safer substances, and intestinal cells need energy to absorb certain nutrients. The following sections discuss the major ways your body uses food energy.

Metabolic Energy Needs

Metabolism refers to all chemical changes, or reactions, that constantly occur in living cells. **Anabolic reactions** require energy to occur; **catabolic reactions** release energy. **Basal metabolism** is the minimal number of calories the body uses for vital activities after fasting and resting for 12 hours. Vital metabolic processes include breathing, circulating blood, and maintaining constant liver, brain, and kidney functions. For people who don't obtain much exercise, basal metabolism accounts for most of their bodies' total energy use.[16]

Thyroid hormone, secreted by the thyroid gland, regulates the **metabolic rate,** that is, the rate at which cells use energy for their metabolic activities. A person who has an overactive thyroid gland produces too much thyroid hormone. This person has a higher-than-normal metabolic rate and loses weight as a result of this disease. Many overweight or obese people have thyroid hormone levels that are within the normal range. However, an individual who secretes slightly less thyroid hormone than other persons may have lower caloric needs and be more likely to become obese as a result.[17]

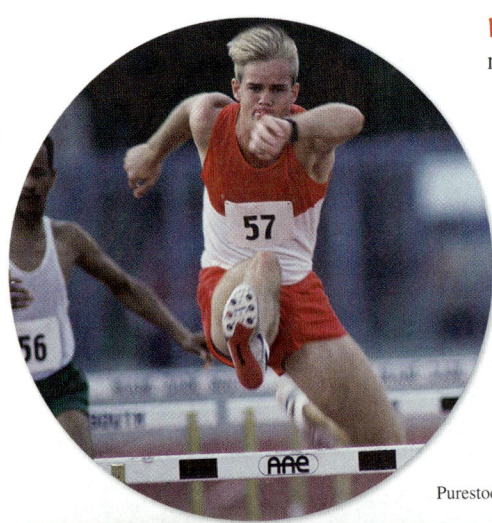

Males generally have higher metabolic rates than women.

What Influences the Metabolic Rate? In addition to thyroid hormone, numerous factors can increase or decrease basal metabolic rates:

- *Body composition:* Lean body mass is the major factor that influences the metabolic rate.[16] Muscle tissue, a component of lean body mass, is more metabolically active than fat tissue. In general, a person who has more muscle mass will have a higher metabolic rate than someone with less muscle tissue.
- *Sex:* Males generally have higher metabolic rates than women because they tend to have more lean body mass.
- *Age:* Basal metabolism declines as one grows older, primarily due to the loss of fat-free tissues such as muscle. As many adults grow older, they think their muscles have "turned into" fat. A muscle cell, however, cannot transform itself into a fat cell. During the aging process, lean tissue mass shrinks, as cells from muscle, bone, and organs die and aren't replaced.

Fat cells, however, can continue to develop throughout life, especially when a person overeats consistently. When fat tissue expands in size, it can fill in the spaces formerly occupied by muscle and organ tissues. Regular exercise helps build and preserve lean body mass, so to some extent, you can reduce the decline in the metabolic rate by being physically active as you grow older.

- *Calorie intake:* Calorie intake also affects the metabolic rate. The body conserves energy when calorie intakes are very low or lacking altogether. Because following a very-low-calorie diet (fewer than 800 kcal/day) can reduce the metabolic rate, such diets aren't generally recommended for weight loss.

Calculating Metabolic Energy Needs Your basal metabolic rate is fairly constant from day to day.[18] Thus, you can estimate your daily metabolic rate by following a "rule of thumb" formula:

$$\text{Formula for men} = 1.0 \text{ kcal/kg/hr}$$

$$\text{Formula for women} = 0.9 \text{ kcal/kg/hr}$$

To estimate the number of kcal you need for your basal metabolism, first convert your weight in pounds to kilograms by dividing your weight by 2.2. (A kilogram is approximately 2.2 pounds.)

$$\_\_\_\_\_ \text{ lb} \div 2.2 \text{ lb/kg} = \_\_\_\_\_ \text{ kg}$$

Then, depending on your sex, use one of the following formulas:

$$\_\_\_\_\_ \text{ kg} \times 0.9 \text{ (women)} = \_\_\_\_\_ \text{ kcal/hr}$$

$$\_\_\_\_\_ \text{ kg} \times 1.0 \text{ (men)} = \_\_\_\_\_ \text{ kcal/hr}$$

Finally, use this hourly basal metabolic rate to estimate your basal metabolic rate for an entire day by multiplying the hourly value by 24.

$$\_\_\_\_\_ \text{ kcal/hr} \times 24 \text{ hr} = \_\_\_\_\_ \text{ kcal/day}$$

These calculations provide only an estimate of your daily metabolic rate. To estimate your Estimated Energy Requirement (EER) for a 24-hour period, you need to add kilocalories used for physical and other activities to your BMR figure.

Energy for Physical Activity

Physical activity increases energy output above basal metabolic needs. The number of kilocalories expended for a particular physical activity depends largely on the type of activity, how long it's performed (duration), the degree of effort used while performing the activity, and the weight of the person. A heavy person expends more kilocalories when performing the same activity, for the same duration, and at the same intensity than a lighter person. Why? The muscles of the heavier person must work harder to move the larger body.

Table 10.4 lists various physical activities and the approximate number of kilocalories an individual who weighs 150 pounds expends while performing each activity for 30 minutes. For example, a 150-pound person who walks for 30 minutes (3.5 mph) burns approximately 130 kcal during the walk. The number of kilocalories you need for physical activity can vary widely, depending on how active you are each day. Because you can control the type, intensity, and duration of your physical activities, you can manipulate your energy output to increase, decrease, or maintain your weight. When you are sedentary (physically inactive), you don't burn as many calories as when you are moderately or vigorously active.

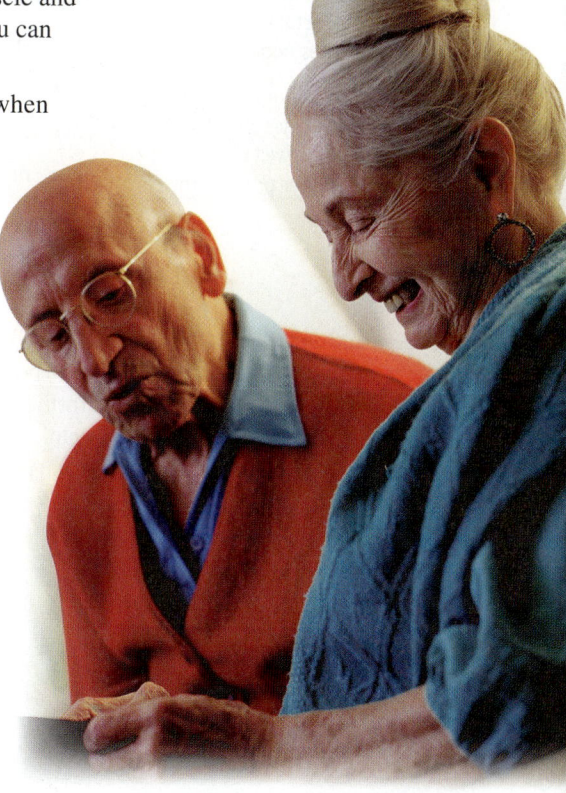

The metabolic rate declines as people grow older.

Steve Mason/Getty Images

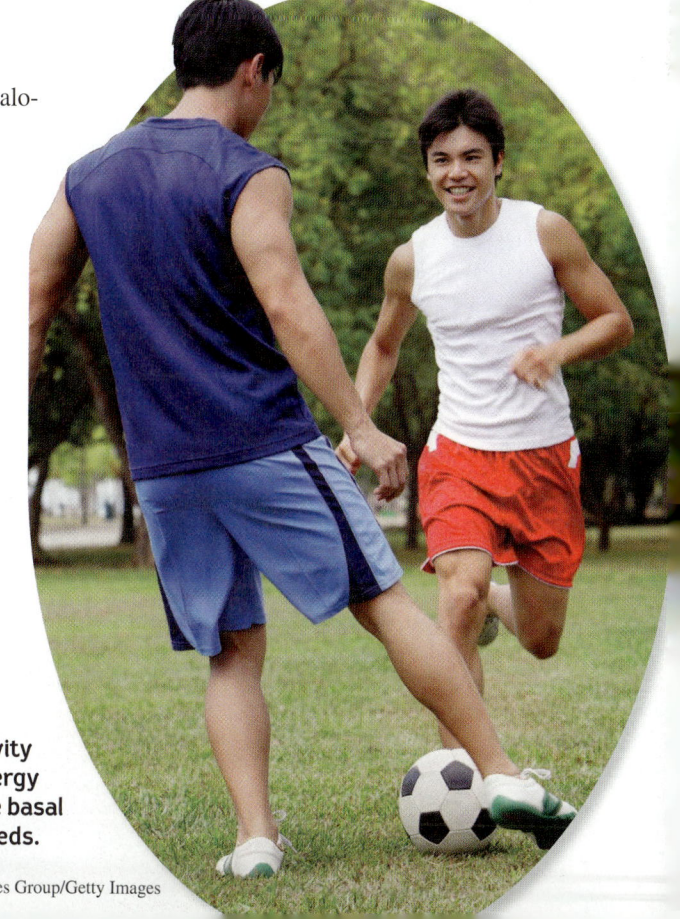

Physical activity increases energy output above basal metabolic needs.

Asia Images Group/Getty Images

nonexercise activity thermogenesis (NEAT) involuntary skeletal muscular activities such as fidgeting

thermic effect of food (TEF) energy used to digest foods and beverages as well as absorb and further process the macronutrients

Nonexercise Activity Thermogenesis (NEAT) **Nonexercise activity thermogenesis (NEAT)** refers to physical activity that a person doesn't consciously control. NEAT activities include

- shivering,
- fidgeting,
- maintaining muscle tone, and
- maintaining body posture when not lying down.

Some individuals may resist weight gain from overeating because they have higher-than-average energy expenditures for NEAT. Nevertheless, NEAT's contribution to overall calorie needs is minor for most people.

Thermic Effect of Food (TEF)

The body needs a relatively small amount of energy to digest foods and beverages as well as to absorb and further process the macronutrients. The energy used for these tasks, generally 5 to 10% of total caloric intake, is referred to as the **thermic effect of food (TEF).** For example, if your energy intake was 3000 kcal/day, TEF would account for 150 to 300 kcal.

TABLE 10.4 APPROXIMATE CALORIC OUTPUT/30 MINUTES OF PHYSICAL ACTIVITY (150-POUND PERSON)

Physical Activity	Approximate kcal/30 min.
Cycling (15 mph)	408
Swimming (vigorous)	339
Running/jogging, steady pace (6 mph)	339
Martial arts	339
Cycling (12–13 mph)	270
Touch football	270
Tennis (singles)	270
Hiking	204
Walking (4 mph)	168
Walking (3.5 mph)	129
Dancing (casual)	102
Weight training	102
Housework	102
Sitting and sewing	33

Source: American Council on Exercise: *Tools & calculators: Physical activity calorie counter.* ND. www.acefitness.org/education-and-resources/lifestyle/tools-calculators/physical-activity-calorie-counter Accessed: July 21, 2019

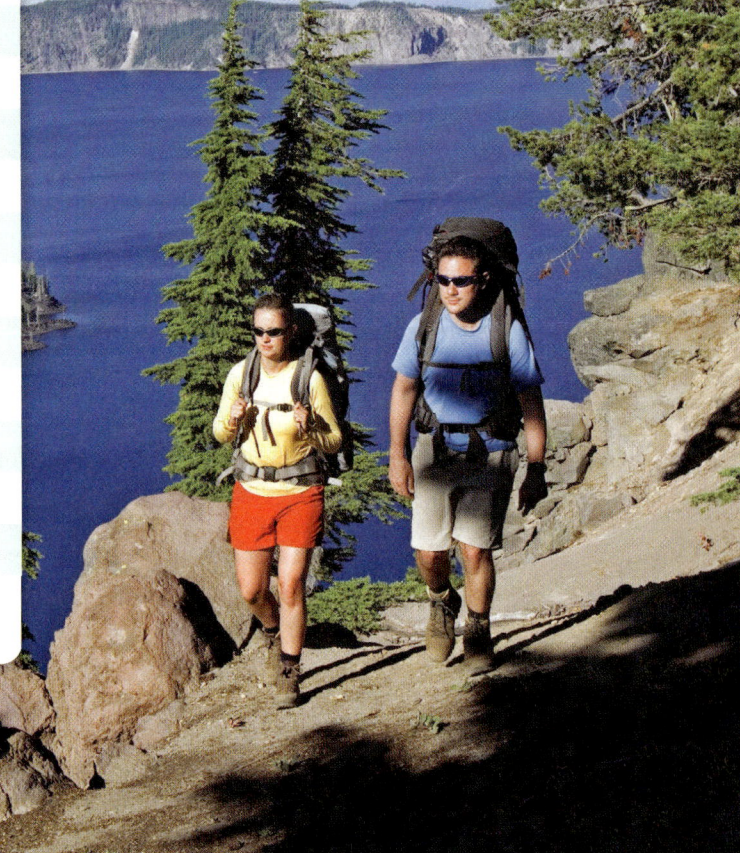

Aurora Open/SuperStock

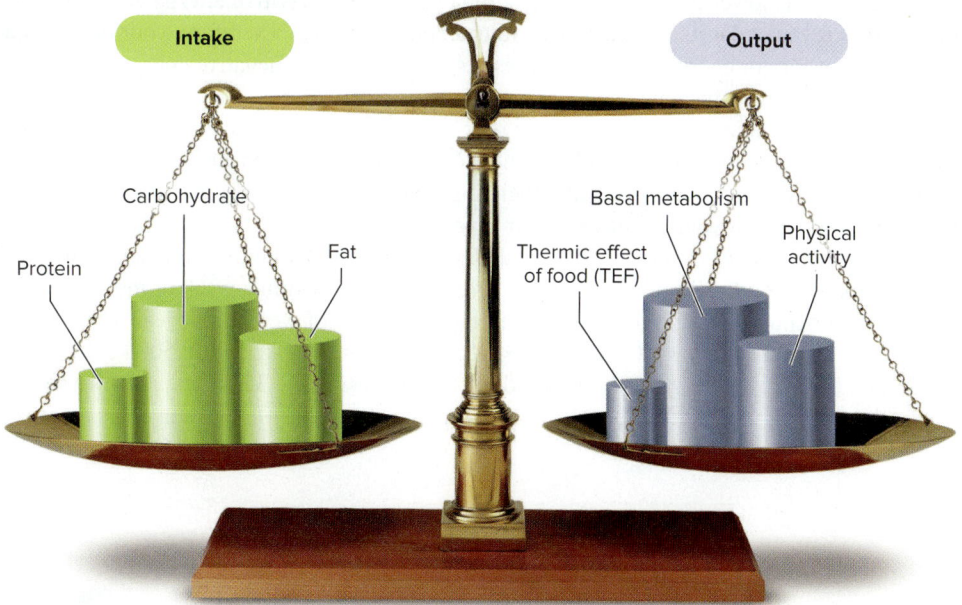

Figure 10.9 **Energy balance.** In addition to macronutrients, energy intake includes alcohol consumption.

■ *What will happen to your weight if your energy intake is consistently greater than your energy output?*

10.2b Energy Balance

Understanding the concept of energy balance is critical to understanding why people gain, lose, or maintain weight. Your body is in a state of **energy balance** when your calorie intake from food and beverages equals your calorie output for basal metabolism, physical activity, and TEF (**Fig. 10.9**). By maintaining a balanced energy state, your weight will remain relatively stable over time.

energy balance calorie intake equals calorie output

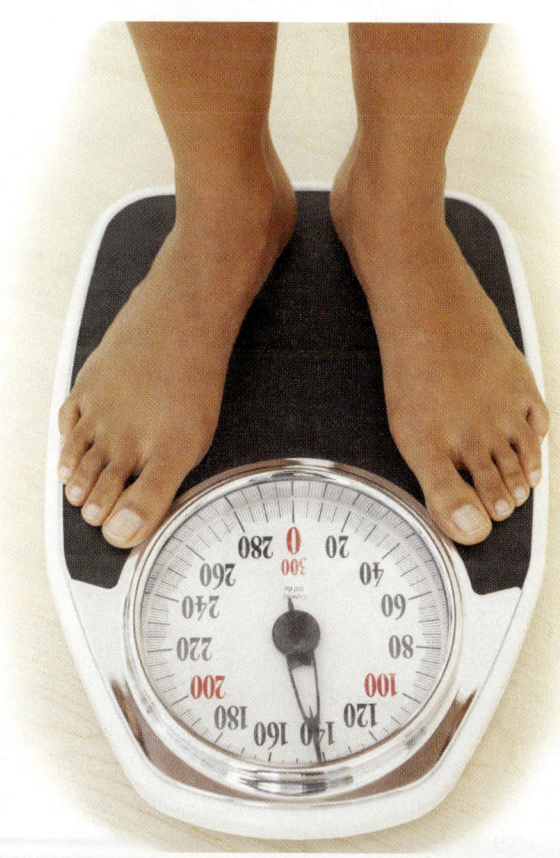

One pound of body fat represents about 3500 kcal.

Stockbyte/Getty Images

negative energy state calorie intake is less than calorie output

positive energy state calorie intake is greater than calorie output

If your calorie intake is lower than your calorie output, you're in a **negative energy state.** Your body needs more calories to carry out its activities than your diet is supplying. Therefore, your body metabolizes more stored fat than usual for energy. Weight loss results from being in a negative energy state. Over time, you'll notice your clothes have become baggy as your fat tissue shrinks.

If your calorie intake is greater than your calorie output, you're in a **positive energy state.** Your body stores excess dietary fat in adipose cells. Additionally, your body converts surplus dietary carbohydrate and protein to fat and stores that fat in adipose cells. Weight gain results from being in a positive energy state, and eventually, you notice that your clothes seem to have shrunk.

One pound of body fat represents about 3500 kcal. This fact is often used to estimate how much you should reduce or increase your calorie intake to lose or gain a pound within a week or month. According to the "3500-kcal rule-of-thumb," you'll lose approximately 52 pounds of weight in a year if you reduce your usual caloric intake by 500 kcal/day (500 kcal/day × 365 days = 182,500 kcal; 182,500 kcal ÷ 3500 kcal/pound = ~52 pounds). Scientific studies, however, don't support using the 3500-kcal rule-of-thumb for predicting weight change over the long term.[19] Losing or gaining weight over time involves more factors

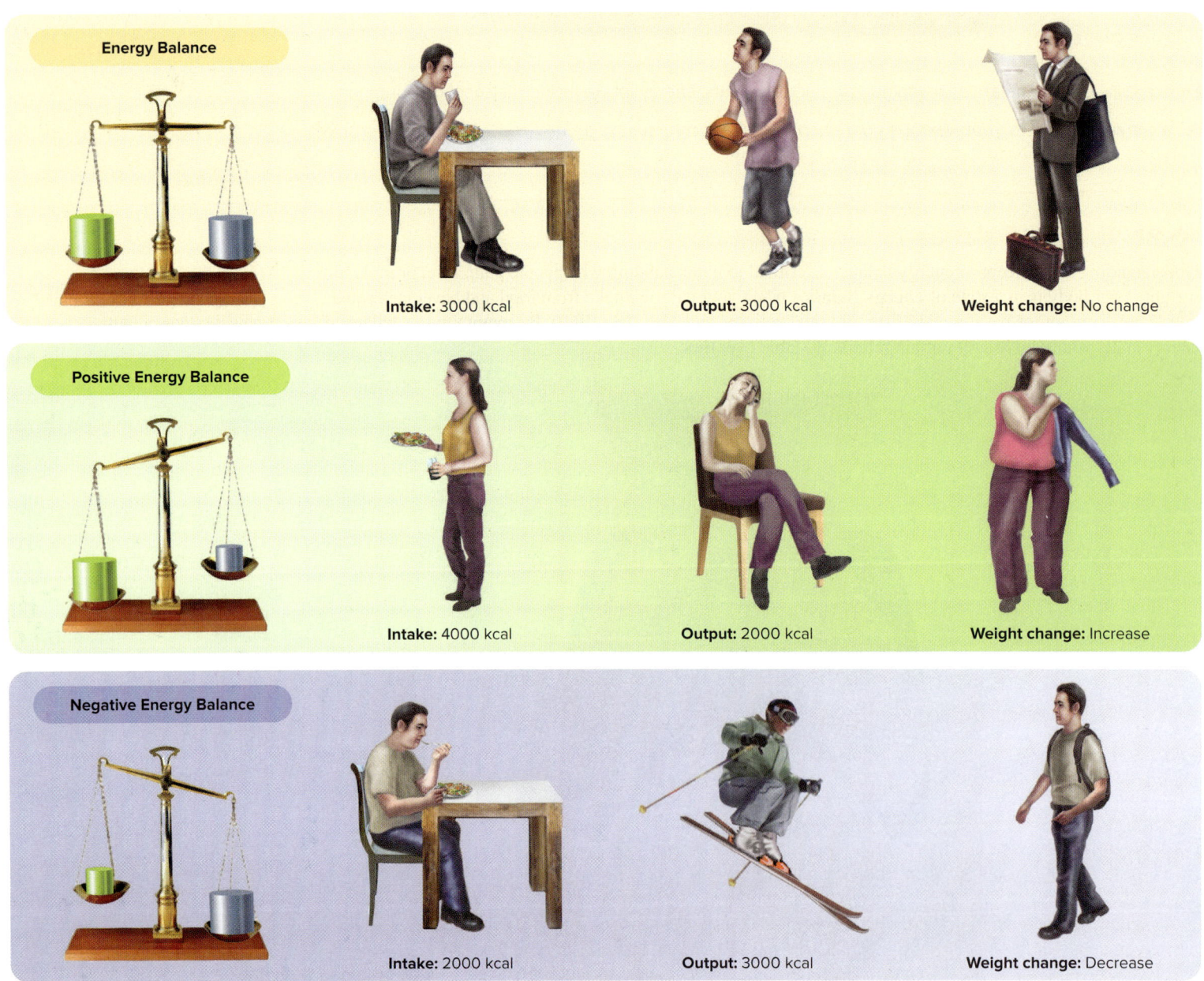

Figure 10.10 Your body's possible energy states.

(current weight, height, age, and physical activity level, for example) than simply cutting calories. Scientists developed a new formula that takes into account these factors. To estimate your caloric intake to achieve weight change by using this formula, visit www.nih.gov/ and type "body weight planner" in the search box.

Maintenance of energy balance—matching calorie intake to calorie output over the long term—is critical for controlling body weight **(Fig. 10.10)**. To lose weight, you need to create a negative energy state by eating significantly fewer calories, expending more calories than the amount consumed, or taking both actions. If you're like many people, however, it isn't easy to make major changes to your calorie input and output and maintain the new lifestyle.

Putting It All Together

To estimate your daily energy expenditure, add the kilocalories you burned for basal metabolism, physical activity, and TEF in a day. An easy way to calculate your "calories in" is to keep track of your daily food and beverage intakes. Then, enter the information into a computerized dietary analysis program such as NutritionCalc Plus.

10.2c Factors That Influence Weight Gain

Does your mood influence your eating behavior? Many people eat not because they are hungry but because they are bored, anxious, angry, or depressed. Other factors, including biological and environmental forces, also influence your calorie intake and output.

Biological Factors

Hunger and satiety are key sensations that regulate eating behavior. **Hunger** is an uncomfortable feeling that drives a person to consume food. **Satiety** is the sense that enough food or beverages have been consumed to satisfy hunger. A small area of the brain helps control hunger and satiety.

The size of your stomach also influences satiety. During meals, your stomach stretches as it fills. The sensation that the stomach has reached its capacity can make you stop eating. Nevertheless, many overfat persons don't recognize the sensation of stomach fullness, and as a result, they may eat even when they shouldn't be hungry.

The stomach, intestines, and fat tissue produce certain proteins that stimulate nerve cells involved in the regulation of hunger and satiety. **Ghrelin** (*greh'-lin*), a hormone secreted mainly by the stomach, stimulates eating behavior. Some scientists think that reducing ghrelin production or activity is the key to helping people lose or maintain their weight. Fat cells secrete **leptin,** a hormone that reduces hunger and inhibits fat storage in the body. Studies involving humans generally find that obese people produce high amounts of leptin, but their bodies resist the hormone's hunger-suppressing action.[20]

Genetic Factors Several genes contribute to human fatness. Researchers are interested in developing medications that regulate these genes. If such medications are safe and effective, they could help people manage their weight over the long term.

If you gain weight easily, you may have inherited a *thrifty metabolism*. A person with a thrifty metabolism has a body that's more efficient at storing excess energy as fat than a person who doesn't have such a metabolism. An energy "thrifty" person is more likely to survive periods of starvation than other persons. In the United States, however, high-calorie "convenience" foods are available 24 hours a day and starvation is unlikely. Therefore, having a thrifty metabolism is not beneficial for most Americans because depositing excess body fat often results in serious health problems.

According to the **set-point theory,** the body's fat content is genetically predetermined. The set point acts like a home thermostat, except that it regulates body weight instead of temperature. For example, a person infected with an intestinal virus may lose a pound or two because he or she has no interest in eating for a few days. During and after recovery, the person generally regains the lost weight. This may explain why the majority of people who intentionally lose weight regain the weight over time.

Environmental Influences

Appetite is the desire to eat appealing food. If you often eat when you're not hungry, then you're probably aware of the effect your environment can have on your appetite. For example, do you get the urge to eat when you see an open bag of candy or a clock that indicates it's "lunch time"?

Food advertising is an aspect of the environment that has a powerful influence on your food choices. To entice you to buy their products, food manufacturers usually appeal to your senses, emphasizing the appearance and taste of food, in particular. How do you respond when you see food advertisements on television? Do the ads make you hungry or eager to try a new food product?

---

hunger uncomfortable feeling that drives a person to consume food

satiety sense that enough food or beverages have been consumed to satisfy hunger

ghrelin protein that stimulates eating behavior

leptin hormone that reduces hunger and inhibits fat storage in the body

set-point theory scientific notion that body fat content is genetically predetermined

appetite desire to eat appealing food

Food advertisers also try to appeal to your emotions. You may choose to purchase "supersized" portions of foods because you like the idea of getting more for your money. In many instances, however, "more" means more fat and calories per serving. Not surprisingly, people tend to eat more when they're offered more food.[21]

Your environment also affects whether you choose to be sedentary or physically active. At home, you may rely on a variety of "energy-saving" devices such as floor-hugging automatic vacuum sweepers, TV remote controls, and garage door openers to work for you. Outside your home, you may use cars, elevators, escalators, and other motorized devices, instead of your feet, to move from place to place. With the help of machines, your life is considerably easier, but you may not be burning enough calories every day as a result.

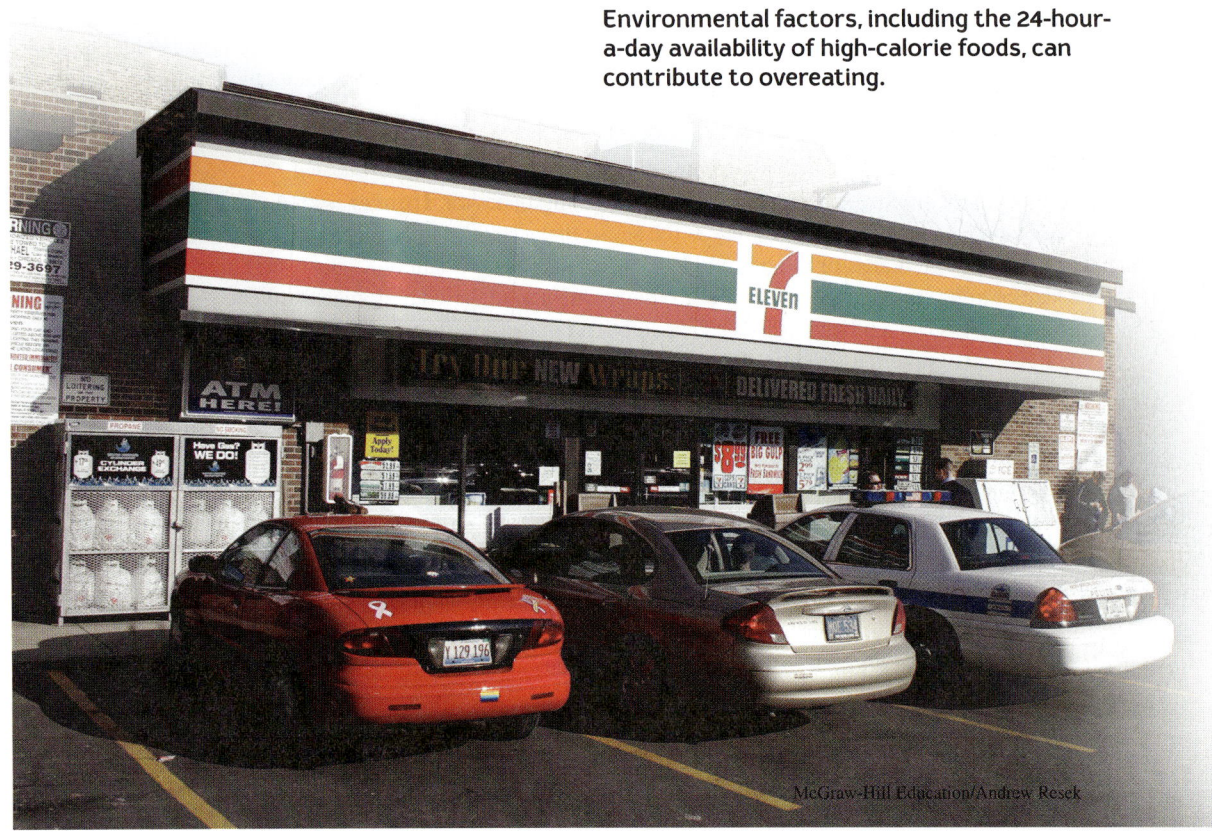

Environmental factors, including the 24-hour-a-day availability of high-calorie foods, can contribute to overeating.

Module 10.3

Managing Your Weight Safely

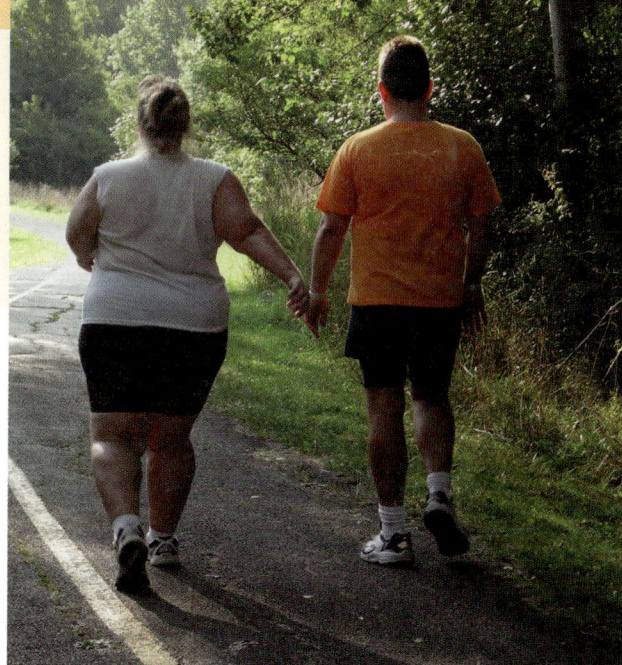
Frances L Fruit/Shutterstock

10.3 - Learning Outcomes

After reading Module 10.3, you should be able to

1. Define all of the **key terms** in this module.
2. Evaluate weight-reduction diets for safety and long-term effectiveness.
3. Identify medical options for overweight and obesity.
4. Identify key factors for successful weight loss and maintenance.
5. Plan a long-term weight-loss regimen that's safe and effective.
6. Discuss ways to gain weight safely and sensibly.

10.3a Features of Medically Sound Weight-Loss Plans

An overweight or obese person doesn't have to shed a lot of weight to reduce risk factors associated with CVD, stroke, and type 2 diabetes. Just losing 5 to 10% of excess body fat can increase beneficial high-density lipoprotein levels (HDL cholesterol), reduce elevated blood pressure, and lower blood glucose and triglyceride levels.[11]

Despite claims made in Internet advertisements and TV infomercials, there are no quick cures for overweight and obesity. No particular diet or food has a "metabolic advantage" by promoting greater calorie burning by the body. A dieter's goal should be reducing total calorie intake while obtaining all essential nutrients.

A sound weight-loss plan

- is safe and effective;
- meets nutritional, psychological, and social needs;
- incorporates a variety of common foods from all food groups;
- doesn't require costly devices or diet books;
- accommodates family and restaurant meals, parties and special occasions, ethnic foods, and food likes;
- doesn't make you feel deprived;
- emphasizes readily available nutritious foods;
- promotes changing habits that encourage overeating;
- encourages regular physical activity;
- provides suggestions for obtaining social support; and
- can be followed for a lifetime.

McKenzie, the young woman featured in the unit opener, lowered her intake of total calories by reducing her consumption of added sugars and fats.

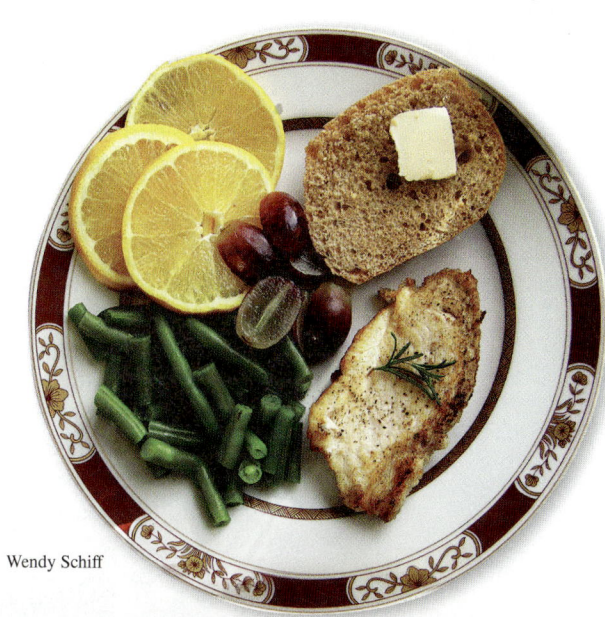
Wendy Schiff

TASTY Tidbits

In 2013–2016, almost 50% of adult Americans reported trying to lose weight during the past year.[22] According to the survey's results, women were more likely to try to lose weight than men. The most common methods used for losing excess body fat were exercising, cutting calories, and eating more fruits, vegetables, and salads.

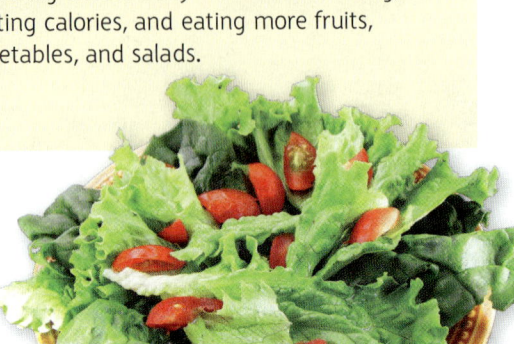
Wendy Schiff

10.3b Weight Loss: Key Factors for Success

The motivation to lose weight and keep it off requires an overfat person to recognize that there's a need to change his or her behaviors. Furthermore, the person is committed to making those changes permanent. For some people, this recognition occurs when they are diagnosed with a serious health disorder that's associated with excess body fat. The commitment to lose weight, maintain the lost weight, and enjoy better health must become far more important than the desire to overeat.

Successful weight-loss treatments and long-term weight maintenance often include making lifestyle changes and changing behaviors. The following sections provide some basic information and practical tips for achieving and maintaining a healthy weight.

Setting Goals

For many overfat people, the first step to losing excess body fat is to set a realistic weight-loss goal. Overfat adults should strive to lose at least 5 to 10% of their current weight over a 6-month period.

Making Lifestyle Changes

Lifestyle includes diet and physical activity. To make your lifestyle healthier, you need to identify what needs to change. What or how much do you eat? How do your food choices contribute to your excess body fat? During a typical day, how physically active are you? For example, are your portion sizes too generous, do you eat fast foods and/or drink sugary soft drinks too often, or do you sit too much?

Calorie Reduction A reasonable rate of weight loss for an obese person is 1 to 2 pounds per week.[23] People who have excess body fat can usually accomplish this rate of loss by reducing their calorie intake or increasing their physical activity (energy output). Although many overweight and obese people would like to shed more than 2 pounds per week, registered dietitians recommend a slow and steady rate.

In general, the more weight a person needs to lose, the faster he or she will lose weight when following a calorie-restricted diet. However, an obese dieter's rate of weight loss tends to slow down as his or her weight reaches a healthier level.

Certain diets severely limit food intake and provide fewer than 800 kcal/day. Such very-low-calorie diets generally require a physician's supervision.[24] Patients (especially women) who follow a very-low-calorie diet and lose weight rapidly often develop gallstones. Obese people often lose a lot of weight during the first few months of following a very-low-calorie diet. However, they are likely to regain the weight quickly after they "go off" the diet and return to their former eating and physical activity habits.

Physical Activity When combined with reduced calorie intake, regular physical activity is critical for weight loss and maintenance. The more physically active you are, the more calories you'll burn. Module 10.5 focuses on physical activity, including the health benefits of a physically active lifestyle.

TASTY Tidbits

Regular exercise, such as walking, can shrink abdominal fat, but it isn't possible to "spot-reduce" by exercising a fatty body part intensely.[25] The energy needed to fuel muscle activity comes from fatty deposits within muscle tissue and the rest of the body. Exercise, however, can improve muscle tone, so that fat tissue appears less flabby.

Fancy Collection/SuperStock

Changing Your Food- and Exercise-Related Practices

Consider the following suggestions, which may help you lose excess weight as well as maintain a lower, healthier body weight.

- *Planning Menus*
  1. Plan meals and snacks to cover three or more days, then use the plan to prepare grocery lists.
  2. When menu planning, include sources of protein, unsaturated fat, and complex carbohydrates in meals and snacks.
  3. Avoid labeling certain foods as "off limits." Depriving yourself of such items can result in bingeing on the "forbidden" food. Analyze why you have difficulty controlling your intake of these foods. Then develop strategies to learn how to reduce your intake of them.

- *Shopping Carefully*
  1. To reduce the likelihood of making impulsive food choices, shop for food after eating.
  2. Shop from a grocery list.
  3. Read food labels to compare calorie and saturated fat contents per serving.

- *Preparing and Serving Your Food*
  1. Reduce the use of solid fat in cooking; bake, broil, or roast meats instead of frying them.
  2. Add less solid fat to foods such as cooked vegetables before serving or eating them.
  3. Prepare only enough food to provide one limited-size portion for yourself. Using measuring cups and a small scale for weighing food can be helpful.
  4. Remove serving dishes from the table. Keeping foods or their containers in sight can encourage overeating.

- *Eating Smart*
  1. Keep nutrient-dense, low-calorie snack foods, such as fresh fruits and vegetables, on hand.
  2. Eat meals and snacks at scheduled times; don't skip meals, especially breakfast.
  3. Eat all food in a "dining" area; avoid eating while engaged in other activities, such as when reading a book, texting, or watching television.
  4. Slow down the pace of meals by eating more slowly.
  5. Leave some food on your plate.

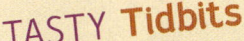
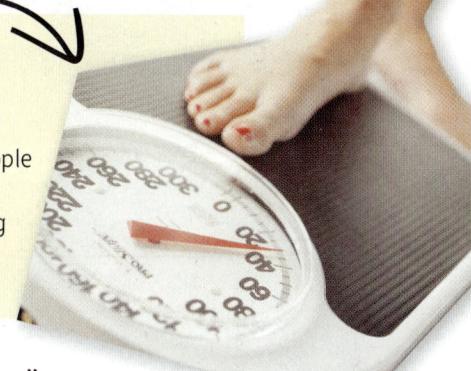
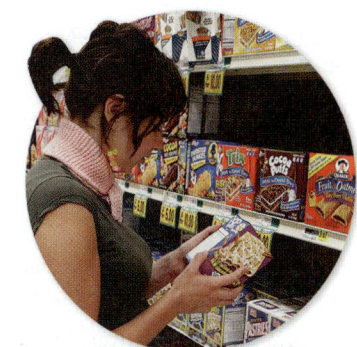

TASTY Tidbits

According to limited data, approximately 20% of overweight and obese people who intentionally lose weight can avoid regaining most of the weight for at least 5 years.[26]

  6. Become a "defensive eater." Practice ways to refuse food graciously or request smaller portions. Be aware of people, especially relatives and friends, who sabotage your weight-loss efforts. Examples of such sabotage include a person who repeatedly offers calorie-dense foods to you, even though you have turned down the food and this person knows you're trying to lose weight.

- *Preparing for Holidays and Parties*
  1. Consider limiting your food intake earlier in the day of the special occasion to avoid consuming too many calories at the event.
  2. Eat a low-calorie snack about an hour before the occasion.
  3. Drink fewer alcoholic and sugar-sweetened beverages. Replace such beverages with ice water.

- *Using Caution at Restaurants*
  1. Avoid eating regularly at fast-food outlets.
  2. Choose pasta with red sauce instead of white sauce.
  3. Request salad dressing "on the side" so you can control the amount.
  4. Don't be a member of the "clean plate club." Ask your server for a carryout box when he or she brings your order to the table. Be sure to refrigerate the leftovers within 2 hours after the meal, and eat them for a meal the following day.
  5. If you choose a dessert item, share it with others.
  6. Avoid fried menu items or those made with butter, gravy, or cream sauce.
  7. When at fast-food outlets, make substitutions:
     - regular hamburger instead of a specialty burger,
     - roasted chicken sandwich instead of a breaded and fried chicken sandwich,
     - plain water instead of a regular soft drink, and
     - baked potato instead of fries, if possible.

- *Exercising Regularly*
  - Walk or bicycle as much as possible to your destinations.
  - If your college or community has a gym, use it often.
  - Reduce the amount of time you spend sitting.

Woman on bathroom scale: Photodisc/Getty Images; Woman grocery shopping: Andrew Resek/McGraw-Hill Education; Food scale: Wendy Schiff

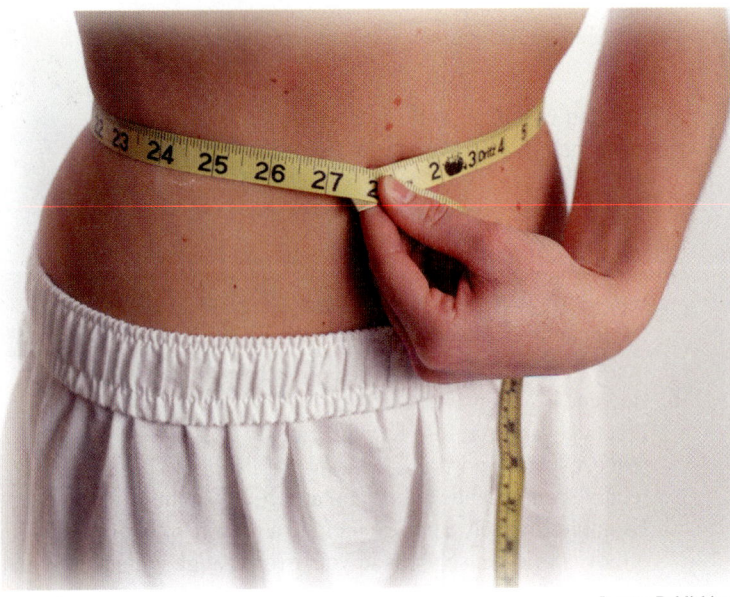

Ingram Publishing

- *Self-Monitoring*
  1. Set reasonable weight-loss goals, for example, losing 1 to 4 pounds in 1 month. When you achieve that goal, set another reasonable goal, and continue with this process until the goal weight is achieved.
  2. Keep a special notebook to use as a food and exercise diary where you can see it—near the kitchen table or refrigerator, for example.
  3. In the diary, note the time and place of eating as well as the type and amount of food eaten. Also record your mood when you ate meals and snacks. Use the diary to identify your food-related problem areas, such as eating when bored or depressed.
  4. In the exercise section of the diary, record the form of moderate-intensity exercise you performed and the number of minutes you spent engaging in that activity each day.
  5. Measure your waistline weekly and record the measurements in the diary.
  6. Weigh yourself several times a week, preferably at the same time of day and without clothing. However, don't rely only on your weight as an indication of your progress. Regular exercise often increases muscle mass that can result in weight gain or failure to lose weight. Still, adding muscle mass is healthier than maintaining too much body fat.

- *Obtaining Social Support*
  1. Consider joining a group weight-loss program. You may make new friends and benefit from others' experiences and support as a result.
  2. Encourage family and friends to provide praise and encouragement for your efforts to manage your weight. Let family, friends, and associates know that you're trying to lose weight and you would appreciate their help and support.

- *Changing Negative Thought Patterns*
  1. Don't get discouraged by occasional setbacks—relapses can be expected when changing behaviors. For example, instead of thinking, "I can't lose weight. I'm a failure," say to yourself, "OK, so I lost control and had too much to eat at the wedding. I just need to get back on track. I'll pull in the reins on my eating for the next day and exercise more."
  2. Think positively about progress. "I didn't lose any weight this week, but I didn't gain any either. I must be losing fat and getting trimmer—those jeans fit better than they did 2 months ago."
  3. Counter negative thoughts with positive statements. "This afternoon, I'll just have to walk a little longer and harder to burn off those extra calories."

Successful Dieters—How Do They Manage Their Weight?

The National Weight Control Registry tracks a group of over 10,000 adult Americans, mostly women, who have lost an average of 66 pounds and maintained the weight loss for at least 5.5 years.[27] Registry members tend to

- eat a low-calorie, low-fat diet;
- exercise, on average, for about an hour daily;
- eat breakfast daily;
- watch less than 10 hours of television per week; and
- weigh themselves at least once a week.

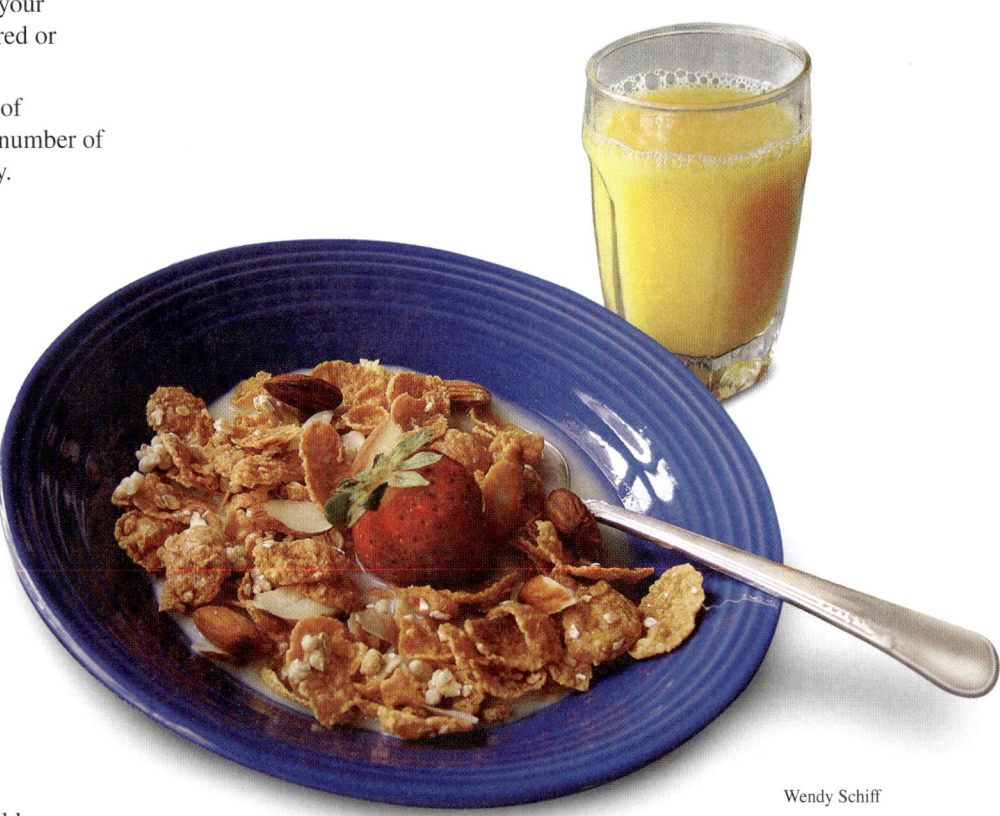

Wendy Schiff

Overfat people may find it easier to lose weight by eating regular meals, including breakfast.

10.3c Medical Treatments for Obesity

Obese patients are often unsatisfied with the amount of weight they lose while following fad as well as conventional diets. The frustration of repeated dieting leads some obese persons to turn to physicians for medications and even surgical procedures to help lose weight.

Weight-Loss Medications

As of July 2019, the only medications approved by the U.S. Food and Drug Administration (FDA) for long-term use for weight loss were orlistat ("Alli"), Contrave, Saxenda, Belviq, and Qsymia.[28] Orlistat reduces some fat absorption by the small intestine; Belviq and Qsymia suppress hunger. These medicines can aid weight-loss efforts, but they don't replace the need to reduce calorie intake and increase physical activity.

Popular Surgical Procedures

Bariatric (*bar-ee-a'-tric*) **medicine** is the medical specialty that focuses on the treatment of obesity. Such surgical procedures drastically reduce the size of an obese person's stomach, markedly limiting food intake. Bariatric surgeries result in weight loss partly because the stomach pouch fills quickly with food; patients experience satiety sooner than they did prior to surgery. Moreover, overeating causes discomfort or vomiting. Thus, people who undergo such surgical procedures must make major lifestyle changes, such as learning to plan and consume frequent, small meals.

Patients often achieve normal blood pressure, glucose levels, and triglyceride levels after bariatric surgery.[29] Furthermore, such surgeries are relatively safe; fewer than 1% of patients die as a result of a bariatric surgical procedure.[30]

In the United States, bariatric surgery is commonly used to treat extreme obesity. **Figure 10.11a** illustrates the appearance of the stomach and intestine after the *Roux-en-Y* operation. This procedure involves using surgical staples to reduce the obese patient's stomach capacity to about 1.5 oz, which is approximately the volume of one egg. Additionally, the surgeon cuts the small intestine and attaches the lower end of it to the newly formed stomach pouch (see Figure 10.11a). The "bypassed" section of the intestine doesn't receive food, so digestion and absorption are reduced as a result of the surgery.

Sleeve gastrectomy also reduces the stomach's size (**Fig. 10.11b**). During this procedure, the surgeon staples the stomach to form a banana-shaped pouch that holds about 2 to 5 ounces of food. The surgery doesn't involve bypassing a section of the small intestine, so nutrient absorption isn't reduced. These patients lose weight because they aren't as hungry as they were before having the surgery. Why? The portion of the stomach that secretes ghrelin is removed during surgery, and as a result, hunger sensations are reduced (see Figure 10.11b). Sleeve gastrectomy surgery is irreversible because the unused portion of the stomach is removed.

Complications often associated with gastric bypass surgery include intestinal blockage and bleeding, leaks along the staple site, blood clot formation, and wound infections. After surgery, gastric bypass patients can develop micronutrient deficiencies and some bone loss. However, patients can reduce their risk of nutrient deficiencies by taking vitamin and mineral supplements.

The adjustable gastric banding procedure creates a small stomach pouch with an adjustable band instead of fixed surgical staples

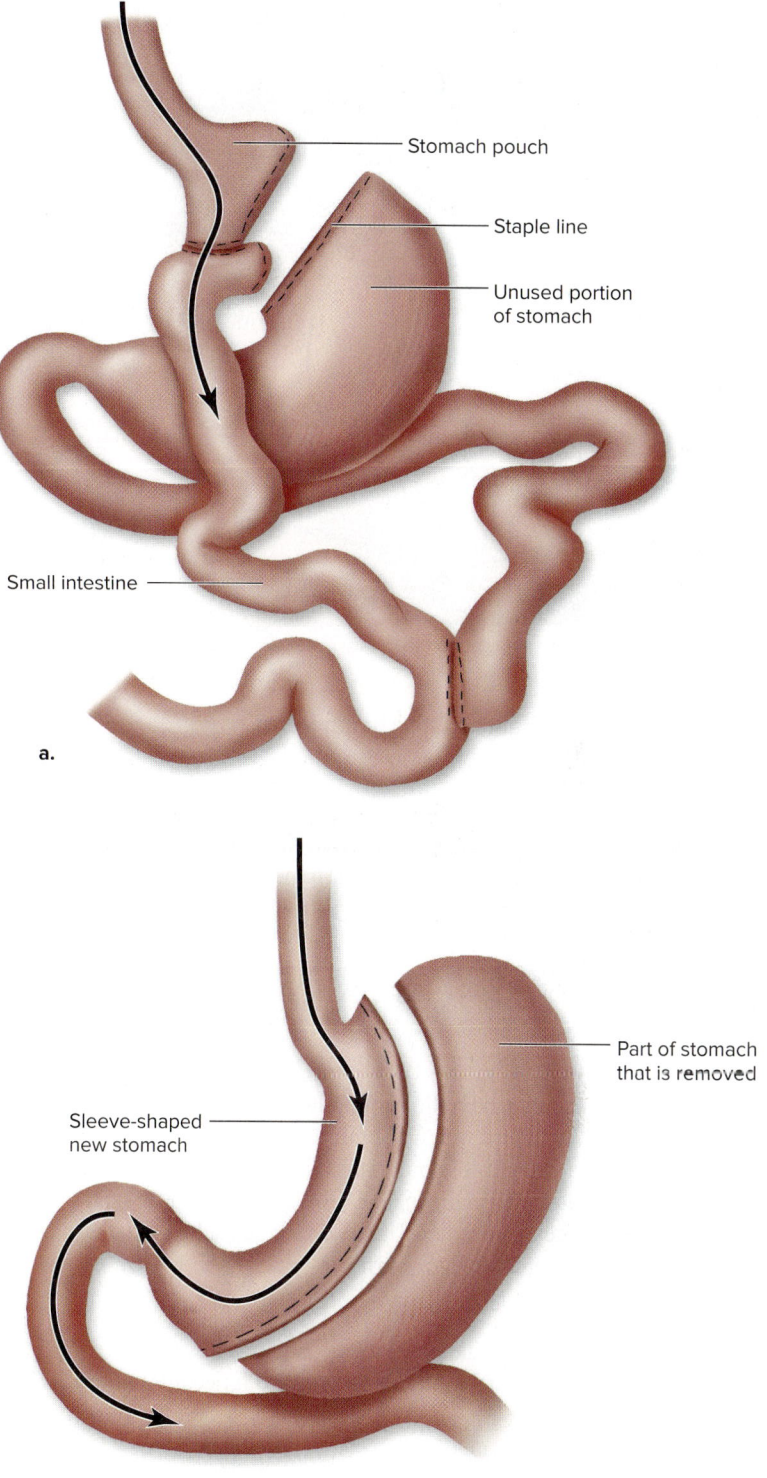

Figure 10.11 Common bariatric surgical procedures. (a) Gastric bypass (Roux-en-Y procedure); (b) sleeve gastrectomy.

■ *How do bariatric surgeries aid in weight loss?*

bariatric medicine medical specialty that focuses on the treatment of obesity

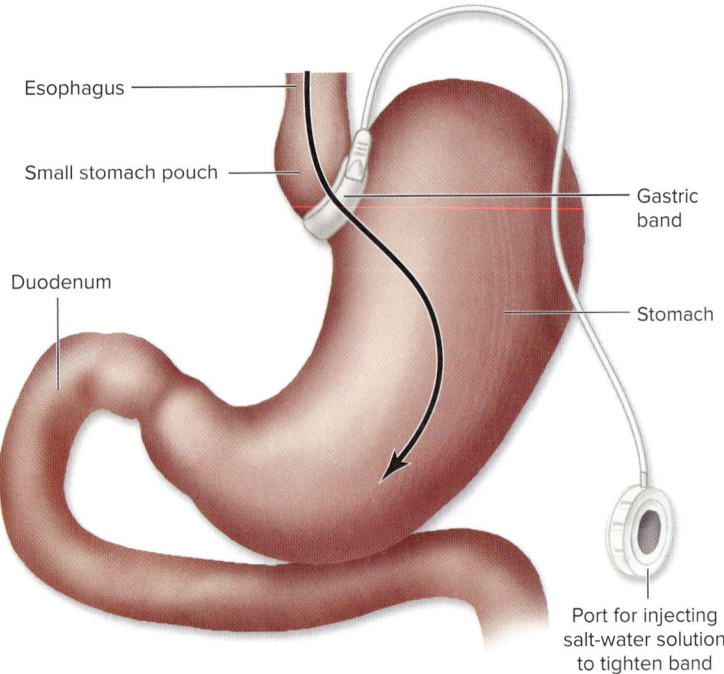

Figure 10.12 Adjustable gastric banding.

(Fig. 10.12). By adjusting the tightness of the band, the surgeon determines the size of the stomach. Compared to the other surgical procedures, adjustable gastric banding is easier to perform and reversible. However, patients who have adjustable gastric banding experience more complications after the procedure than people who undergo gastric bypass or sleeve gastrectomy procedures.[31] As a result, adjustable gastric banding has lost much of its popularity.

10.3d Unreliable Weight-Loss Methods

Each year, Americans spend billions of dollars on products and services promoted to help them lose weight. Some people who have excess body fat join commercial weight-loss programs that can be useful for encouraging safe weight loss and maintenance. However, many overweight and obese people seek "quick fixes" to lose weight, such as fad diets and dietary supplements promoted to "burn" or "melt" fat fast.

Fad Diets

A **fad** is a trendy practice that has widespread appeal. After a period, however, people lose interest in the practice, and it becomes no longer fashionable. Fad diets often rely on *gimmicks*. A gimmick is an unusual feature or food, such as "raspberry ketones" and "green tea extract," that makes the diet seem to be unique and more likely to work than other diets. Some fad diets use the gimmick of emphasizing one food or food group while excluding almost all others. The grapefruit diet, for example, promotes eating this single food.

Dieters may lose some weight while following eating plans that restrict food variety, but the weight loss occurs because the diet is low in calories, not because grapefruit, açai berries, or other "diet food" contains compounds that cause rapid weight loss. Eventually, dieters abandon such restrictive menu plans because they crave a slice of bread and cannot face another bowl of grapefruit. If they return to their prior eating and other lifestyle habits, fad dieters usually regain much of the weight that they lost while on the diet.

If you examine any diet plan carefully, you can determine whether it's probably a fad. A typical fad diet

- promotes rapid weight loss without calorie restriction and increased physical activity;
- limits food selections from a few food groups and requires specific rituals, such as eating only fruit for breakfast or eating only certain food combinations;
- requires buying a book or various gimmicks, such as expensive dietary supplements, weight-loss patches, or beverages that contain "secret" weight-loss ingredients; or
- relies on testimonials from famous people or connects the diet to trendy places such as Hollywood, California and South Beach, Florida.

Low-Carbohydrate Approaches Fad weight-loss diets that limit carbohydrate intakes and are high in protein and saturated fat include the Atkins' Diet, the "Keto" Diet, the Low-Carb Paleo Diet, and the early phases of the South Beach and the Dukan Diets. A weight-reduction diet is low carbohydrate if it eliminates or severely restricts the intake of carbohydrate-rich foods such as breads, cereals, fruits, starchy vegetables, and sweets.

Low-carbohydrate diets usually produce rapid weight loss initially, primarily because the body loses water. Why? The body produces less glycogen when carbohydrate intake is low and uses much of its stored glycogen to supply glucose for energy. Tissues maintain about 3 grams of water with each gram of glycogen, so a reduction in body glycogen content results in the need for less water to store with it. The kidneys eliminate the excess water in urine.

Carbohydrate-restricted diets often improve high-density lipoprotein ("good cholesterol") and serum triglyceride levels. Such diets can be helpful for losing weight, controlling blood glucose levels, and reducing the risk of CVD.[32] More studies, however, are needed to determine whether low-carbohydrate diets are safe and reduce the risk of CVD when followed for long periods.

Very-Low-Fat Approaches Very-low-fat diets, such as the Pritikin Diet and the "Eat More, Weigh Less" diet plan, supply approximately 5 to 10% of calories from fat. Such diets generally result in rapid weight loss. Although very-low-fat diets aren't harmful for healthy adults, they are difficult to follow for the long term. Fat contributes to the flavor and texture of foods. Therefore, very-low-fat diets aren't tasty, and they eliminate many foods that are usually high on people's favorite foods lists, such as ice cream and meat.

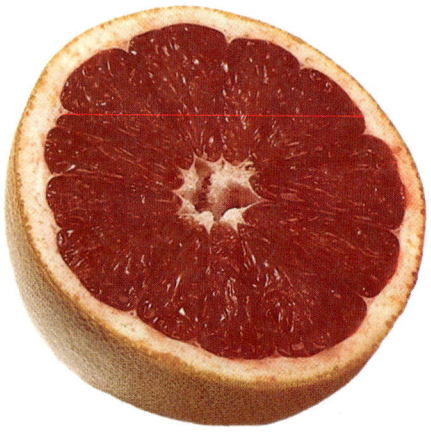

fad trendy practice that has widespread appeal for a period, then becomes no longer fashionable

Burke Triolo Productions/Getty Images

Intermittent Fasting Fasting is the practice of not eating or severely limiting food and calorie-containing beverage intakes for a period of time. Fasting is an ancient practice; followers of many religions, including Islam, Judaism, and Catholicism, may practice fasting during certain holidays. Intermittent fasting is a dietary pattern that includes a day of fasting that's followed by a day of usual (unrestricted) food intake. People who are overfat may use intermittent fasting to lose weight or improve their blood cholesterol, glucose, and/or blood pressure levels. Although more long-term research is needed, currently there's no scientific evidence that indicates intermittent fasting is better for losing weight than following a daily diet that's calorie-reduced.[33] Women who are pregnant or breastfeeding, or people who have diabetes or eating disorders, shouldn't fast. Fasting increases the production of ketone bodies, which can upset the body's normal blood chemistry (see section 5.2b).

What About Dietary Supplements for Weight Loss?

Many overweight and obese people are attracted to dietary supplements for weight loss because they believe promoters' claims that their products are "magic bullets" for shedding unwanted weight quickly and effortlessly. In general, there's a lack of scientific evidence that supports claims of their effectiveness or long-term safety. At this point, medical experts don't recommend any dietary supplement for weight loss, including products containing green tea extracts, chitosan, or other substances presented in **Table 10.5**.

TABLE 10.5 SELECTED WEIGHT-LOSS SUPPLEMENTS: EFFECTIVE OR NOT EFFECTIVE?

Supplement	Usefulness	Side Effects/Safety Concerns (Usual Doses)
Bitter orange	May increase metabolic rate and suppress appetite. Mixed results concerning weight loss	Some negative effects reported, including chest pain and increased blood pressure and heart rate
Chitosan	Little effect on weight loss	May cause allergic response and gastrointestinal discomfort including nausea, constipation, and intestinal gas
Chromium	May enhance weight loss to a small extent	Headache, diarrhea, dizziness
Conjugated linoleic acid	Has minimal effect on reducing body weight	Appears to be safe, but can cause gastrointestinal upset
Garcinia cambogia (hydroxycitric acid, HCA)	Overall evidence does not suggest usefulness	Safety concerns; may cause headache, nausea, gastrointestinal discomfort, mania, and liver damage
Glucomannan	Little or no effect on body weight	Tablet forms can block the esophagus. Diarrhea, intestinal gas, and abdominal discomfort
Green tea and green tea extracts	May enhance weight loss to a small extent	Contains caffeine. Concentrated extracts linked to severe liver damage
Guar gum	Not effective	May cause diarrhea and intestinal gas
Hoodia	Few studies involving humans have been conducted; not effective, according to one study	Increases blood pressure and heart rate; may cause headaches, dizziness, nausea, and vomiting
Pyruvate	Possible minimal effect of weight loss	Abdominal discomfort; may reduce "good" cholesterol levels
Raspberry ketone	More research is needed	Unknown
Yohimbe	Not effective, according to a few studies	Serious negative effects, including hypertension and rapid heart rate

Source: National Institutes of Health, Office of Dietary Supplements: *Dietary supplements for weight loss.* Updated June 2019. https://ods.od.nih.gov/factsheets/WeightLoss-HealthProfessional/ Accessed: July 21, 2019

What IS That?

Promoters of products that contain açai, such as açai juice, claim the tropical fruit has numerous healthful benefits, including stimulating weight loss. Although açai is a source of antioxidants that may reduce inflammation, there is little scientific evidence to support any claims for weight loss.[34]

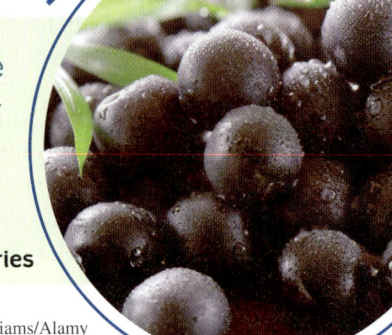

Açai berries

funkyfood London/Paul Williams/Alamy

Analyzing Advertising Hype

Be wary of weight-loss claims that the product or service

- *Causes rapid and extreme weight loss.* Ads commonly use outrageous claims such as "Lose up to 18 pounds in one week!" to attract consumers. The use of the modifier "up to" means that the person using the product could lose considerably less than 18 pounds a week.

- *Requires no need to change dietary patterns or physical activity.* Principles of energy balance don't support claims such as "Lose weight without dieting or strenuous exercise" and "Eat as much as you want—the more you eat, the more you'll lose."

- *Results in permanent weight loss.* Claims such as "Discover the secret to permanent weight loss" and "Lose weight and keep it off" often appear in ads. These claims target consumers who have lost weight but gained it back and are wary of weight-loss products. Long-term weight loss is difficult to achieve without calorie reduction and regular exercise, and claims that permanent weight loss can result simply from using a product are questionable.

- *Is scientifically proven or doctor endorsed.* Some ads claim their product or service has been "clinically tested," "scientifically proven," or "physician recommended." Scientific testing of the product or service supposedly occurred at "leading" medical centers or universities. However, most ads don't provide information about testing sites or journals where the results were published. Endorsements by medical professionals can be misleading.

- *Displays before-and-after photos.* If you read carefully, you may find disclaimers in small print, such as "results not typical," at the bottom of the "after" photo.

- *Includes a money-back guarantee.* Consumers should recognize that a product doesn't necessarily work just because it's guaranteed. The FTC frequently sues companies that fail to return money to dissatisfied consumers as their ads guarantee.

- *Is safe or natural.* Ads may include safety-related claims, such as "proven 100% safe" or "safe, immediate weight loss." Despite such assurances, weight-loss supplement manufacturers usually have little scientific evidence to support safety claims, particularly concerning long-term use of their products. Furthermore, "natural" doesn't indicate safety. Mushrooms are natural, but many kinds of mushrooms are highly toxic and even deadly.

- *Is supported by satisfied customers.* Testimonials generally provide little reliable information about what consumers can expect from using the product.

10.3e Gaining Weight

In 2015–2016, 2.5% of Americans who were 20 to 39 years of age were underweight.[35] An underweight individual has a BMI that's less than 18.5. Many underweight individuals want to gain weight, especially muscle mass.

For an underweight person, gaining weight can be just as challenging as losing weight is for an overfat person. To gain weight, underweight adults can gradually increase their consumption of calorie-dense foods, especially those high in healthy fats. Fatty fish (such as salmon), olives, avocados, seeds, low-fat cheeses, nuts and nut butters, bananas, and granola made with dried fruit, seeds, and nuts are high-calorie nutritious food choices with low saturated-fat content. Additionally, underweight people can replace beverages such as soft drinks with more nutritious calorie sources, such as 100% fruit juices, smoothies, and milkshakes made with peanut butter and fat-reduced ice cream. Encouraging a regular meal and snack schedule also aids in weight gain and maintenance.

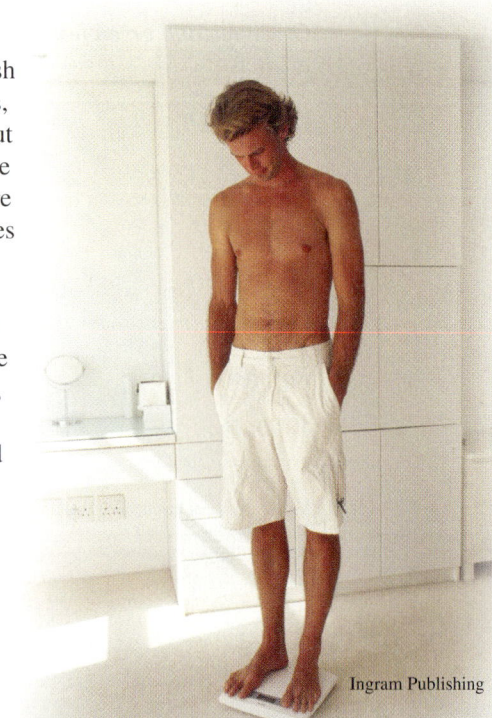

Ingram Publishing

Module 10.4

Disordered Eating and Eating Disorders

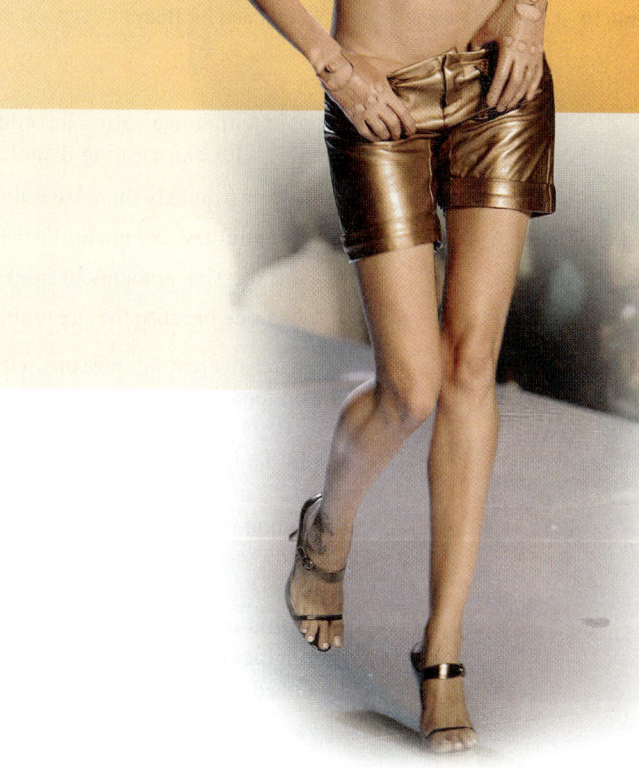

Lars A. Niki/McGraw-Hill Education.

10.4 - Learning Outcomes

After reading Module 10.4, you should be able to

1. Define all of the **key terms** in this module.
2. Explain why disordered eating practices and eating disorders are common among young Americans.
3. Identify major kinds of eating disorders, and discuss signs and symptoms, risk factors, and treatments for these conditions.

With the prevalence of obesity rising rapidly in the United States, it isn't surprising that many American adolescents and young adults are concerned about their body shape and weight. Furthermore, the media constantly bombard us with images of the "ideal" body. Television shows and movies often portray thin women or muscular men as happy, confident, and successful. Excessive concern about body size and social pressure to avoid weight gain can lead to abnormal food-related practices such as skipping meals, limiting food choices, following fad diets, and bingeing on food. Such *disordered eating* behaviors are temporary and often occur when a person is under a lot of stress or wants to lose weight to improve his or her appearance. When a person adopts disordered eating behaviors as a lifestyle, the practices can become harmful and difficult-to-treat eating disorders.

Eating disorders are psychological disturbances that lead to serious health problems. In the United States, physicians can diagnose three major types of eating disorders: anorexia nervosa, bulimia nervosa, and binge-eating (overeating) disorder.[36] The causes of eating disorders are unknown, but genetic, social, and psychological factors contribute to their development.

Anorexia nervosa and bulimia nervosa are more likely to develop during adolescence. Binge-eating disorder tends to occur during the adult years. However, these conditions can begin at any age.

Known risk factors for eating disorders include

- being a female (females are more likely to develop eating disorders),
- having a history of frequent dieting to control weight,
- being overly concerned or dissatisfied with body shape and weight,
- having low self-esteem and a poor self-image,
- being in a sport or occupation that emphasizes a lean body,
- having a history of being a victim of bullying or sexual abuse, and
- having a close relative (mother or sister, for example) who has an eating disorder or certain forms of mental illness (especially a depressive or anxiety disorder).[37]

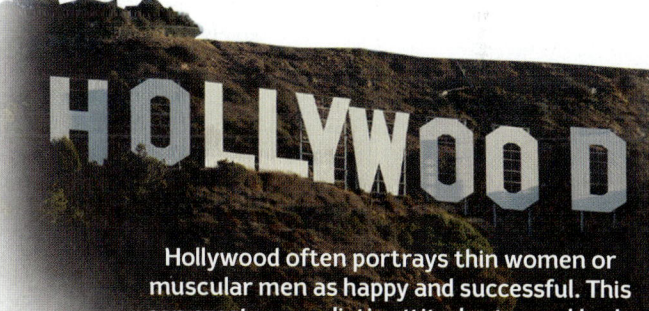

Hollywood often portrays thin women or muscular men as happy and successful. This can create unrealistic attitudes toward body image, especially in young people.

Ingram Publishing/SuperStock

eating disorders psychological disturbances that lead to certain physiological changes and serious health complications

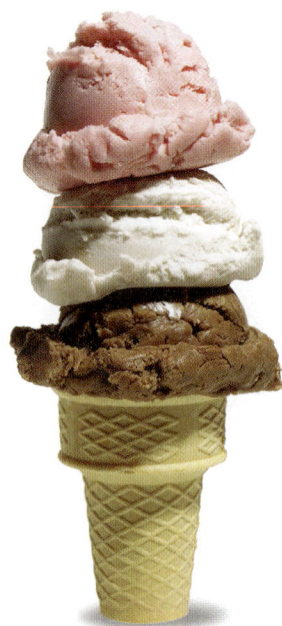

Alex Cao/Getty Images

10.4a Binge-Eating Disorder

People with binge-eating disorder (BED) often eat an unusually large amount of food at one time (bingeing). People with binge-eating disorder also may eat

- more quickly than usual during binge episodes,
- until they feel uncomfortably full,
- excessive amounts of food even when they're not hungry, and
- alone because they're embarrassed about their overeating behavior.

After overeating, persons with BED feel disgusted, depressed, or guilty. Individuals with the disorder often feel they cannot control their eating behavior. Unlike someone with bulimia nervosa, a person who has BED doesn't purge (try to eliminate the excess calories) following an episode of binge eating.

In the United States, BED is the most common eating disorder.[38] An estimated 3.5% of American women and 2% of American men have binge-eating disorder. Although anyone can have BED, the disorder is more common in people who are extremely obese.

10.4b Bulimia Nervosa

Bulimia nervosa (BN) is characterized by reoccurring episodes of bingeing. Food binges often consist of high-calorie foods and are followed by attempts to purge the calories consumed during binges by self-induced vomiting, as well as abusing laxatives, diuretics, or enemas. Repeated vomiting can cause

- blood chemistry abnormalities; blood potassium can drop dramatically, altering heartbeat and increasing risk of sudden death;
- swelling of the throat;
- tears and bleeding of the esophagus;
- sores or scars on the knuckles (from self-induced vomiting); and
- tooth decay (from self-induced vomiting).

About 1.5% of women in the United States develop BN during their lifetimes.[39] People with BN are often disgusted with their binge-purge practices. As a result, they often try to hide these behaviors from others. Individuals who have bulimia may be difficult to identify by their appearance because they tend to have BMIs in the healthy range.[40] However, they may view themselves as being overweight and rely excessively on body shape and weight to judge themselves. It is important to recognize that people with bulimia may have a history of anorexia nervosa.

10.4c Anorexia Nervosa

Anorexia nervosa (AN) is a severe psychological disturbance characterized by self-imposed starvation that results in malnutrition and extreme underweight. A person with AN maintains a body weight that's 15% or more below the normal weight for his or her height.[41] In the United States, 0.9% of women develop AN during their lifetimes.[39]

People with AN

- limit calorie intake, which leads to very low body weight;
- are emotionally disturbed about their body weight and shape;
- have an intense fear of gaining weight or becoming fat, despite their very low weight; and
- deny that they have a serious illness.

bulimia nervosa (BN) eating disorder characterized by cyclic episodes of bingeing and calorie-restrictive dieting

anorexia nervosa (AN) severe psychological disturbance characterized by self-imposed starvation

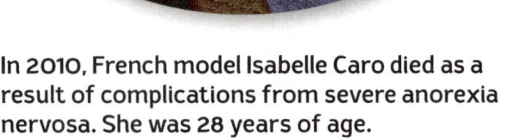

In 2010, French model Isabelle Caro died as a result of complications from severe anorexia nervosa. She was 28 years of age.

Mercier Serge/ZUMAPRESS/Newscom

In addition to extreme thinness, signs and symptoms of AN generally include

- confusion or slowed thinking;
- widespread delicate, dense, white hairs on the skin;
- shrunken breasts and buttocks;
- emotional depression;
- low blood potassium levels; and
- tooth decay (from self-induced vomiting).

To lose weight or prevent weight gain, people with AN often avoid eating, especially in front of others, and they may engage in one or more of the following practices:

- self-induced vomiting,
- abuse of laxatives or diuretics,
- excessive exercise regimens, and
- use of appetite suppressants.

With treatment, patients may recover and achieve a healthy weight, but it's not unusual for them to return to their unhealthy eating and physical activity practices. At least 5 to 6% of people with AN eventually die as a result of the disorder.[42]

Other Related Conditions: The Female Athlete Triad

Athletes participating in appearance-based competitive sports that require low body mass, such as gymnastics, swimming, and figure skating, are at risk of developing health problems because they often limit their energy intake.[43] The **female athlete triad** is characterized by low energy intakes (with or without disordered eating), abnormal menstrual cycles, and bone mineral irregularities. Severe food restriction can result in lower blood estrogen levels that, in turn, can cause the absence of menstrual cycles. Young women with low estrogen levels have bones that are less dense and weaker than normal. As a result, these women have an increased risk of bone fractures such as "stress" fractures. Male athletes who limit their energy intake also experience reproductive and bone health problems. For more information, visit The Female and Male Athlete Triad Coalition at www.femaleandmaleathletetriad.org.

10.4d Treating Eating Disorders

A team of health professionals, including registered dietitians, physicians, nurses, and mental health counselors, are usually involved in the treatment of eating disorders. A key goal of therapy is for patients to achieve and maintain healthy BMIs without using unhealthy food-related behaviors.

Treatment for eating disorders generally includes *cognitive behavioral therapy,* which teaches people ways to monitor their eating behavior and change their unhealthy eating habits. Such therapy also helps patients develop more positive feelings about their body shape and weight. Medication, particularly antidepressants, may also be included as part of treatment.

If you or someone you know has an eating disorder, it's important to seek help for the condition as early as possible—before the affected person's life is at risk. Professional help is often available at student health centers and student guidance/counseling facilities on college campuses.

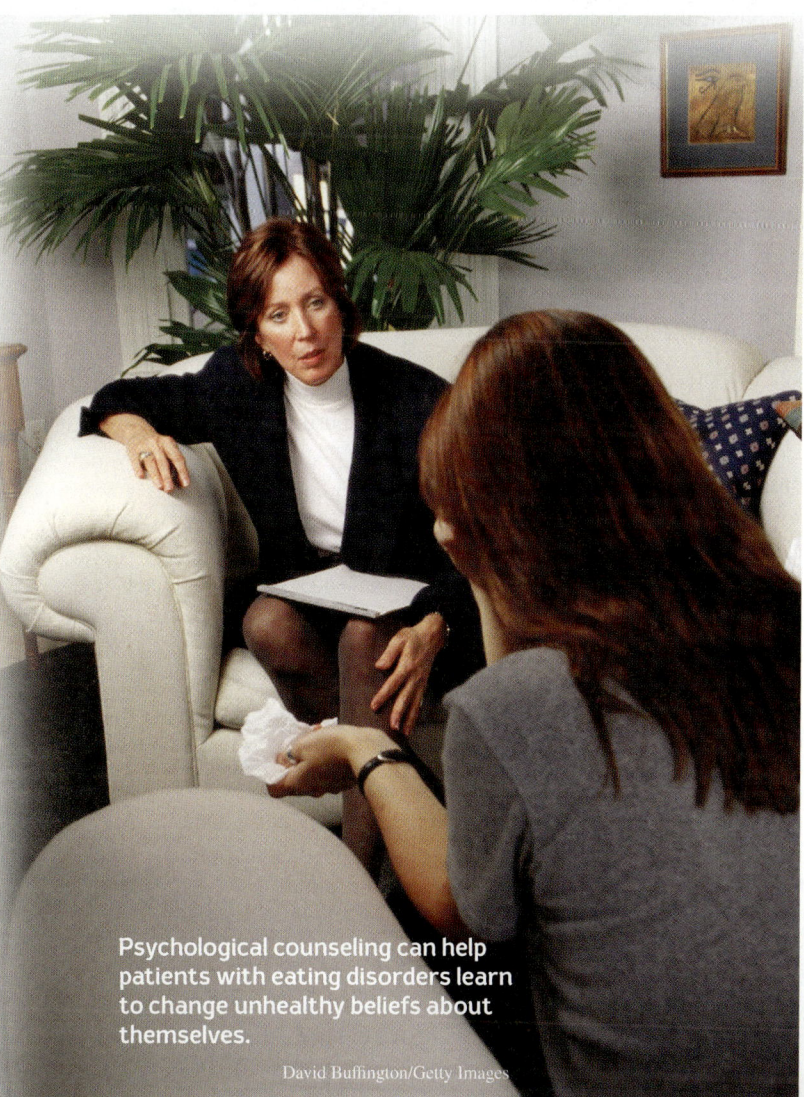

Psychological counseling can help patients with eating disorders learn to change unhealthy beliefs about themselves.

David Buffington/Getty Images

female athlete triad condition characterized by low energy intakes, abnormal menstrual cycles, and bone mineral irregularities

Module 10.5

Get Moving; Get Healthy!

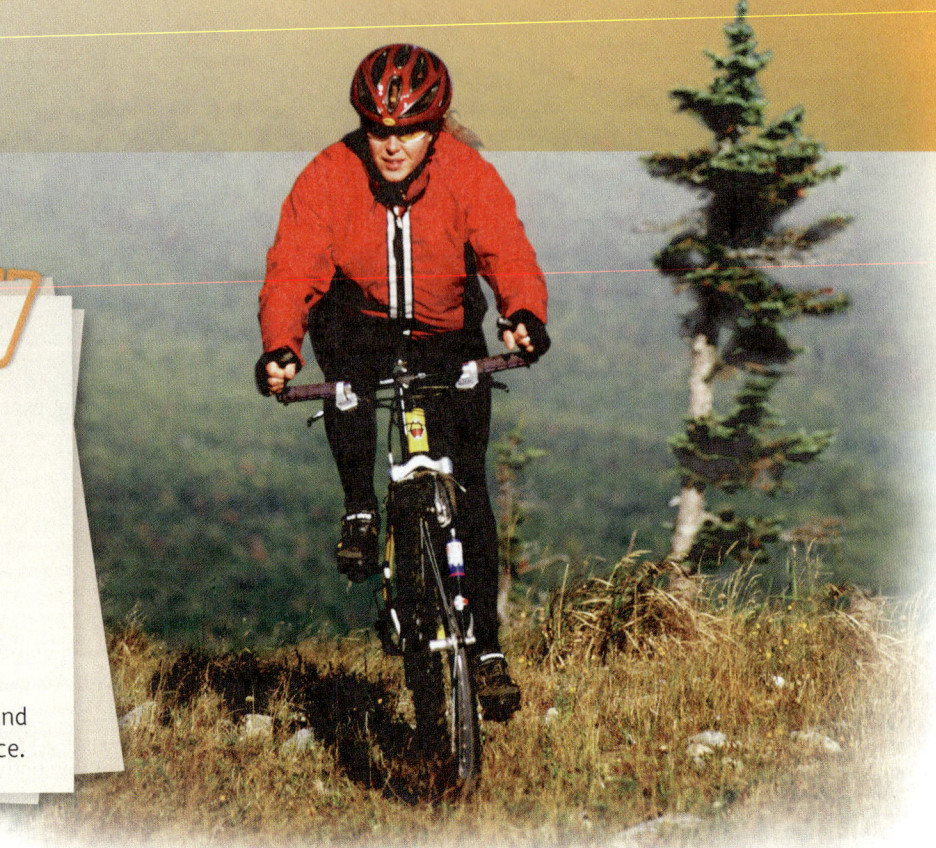

10.5 - Learning Outcomes

After reading Module 10.5, you should be able to

1. Define all of the **key terms** in this module.
2. List five health benefits of a physically active lifestyle.
3. Distinguish moderate-intensity activities from vigorous-intensity activities.
4. Plan nutritionally adequate, high-carbohydrate menus.
5. Estimate an athlete's energy and protein needs.
6. List at least five ergogenic aids that athletes often use, and describe their effects on health and physical performance.

Pixtal/AGE Fotostock

The human body is designed for **physical activity**—movement that results from skeletal muscle contraction. Most of the physical activities you perform each day are unstructured, for example, shopping for groceries or doing household tasks. **Exercise** refers to physical activities that are usually planned and structured for a particular purpose, such as having fun, losing weight, or increasing muscle mass. Both forms of physical activity can benefit your health.

10.5a Health Benefits of Regular Exercise

Millions of Americans suffer from chronic illnesses that can be prevented or improved by exercising more often. Exercising regularly can help

- control your weight;
- reduce your risk of CVD;
- reduce your risk for type 2 diabetes;
- reduce your risk of dementia (loss of memory and other thought processes) and colon, bladder, uterine lining (female), kidney, lung, stomach, esophagus, and breast cancer;
- strengthen your bones and muscles;
- improve your psychological well-being; and
- increase your chances of enjoying a longer, healthy life.[44]

Simply put, Americans should move more and sit less.[44]

physical activity movement resulting from contraction of skeletal muscles

exercise physical activities that are usually planned and structured for a purpose

physical fitness ability to perform moderate- to vigorous-intensity activities without becoming excessively fatigued

intensity degree of effort used to perform a physical activity

Darlene Schueller

Performing household chores often involves low-intensity physical activity.

10.5b What's Physical Fitness?

Physical fitness is the ability to perform moderate- to vigorous-intensity activities without becoming excessively tired. If you're physically fit, you have the strength, endurance, flexibility, and balance to meet the physical demands of daily living, exercise, and sports. Proper nutrition is essential for optimal physical fitness and sports performance.

Determining the Intensity of Physical Activity

Intensity refers to the level of exertion (physical effort) used to perform an activity. Duration and type of physical activity, as well as body weight, influence the intensity of skeletal muscle movement. Thus, activities such as walking and swimming can be classified as either moderate- or vigorous-intensity physical activity, depending on the rate at which the activities are performed as well as the weight of the person performing them.

Low-intensity, unstructured physical activities include your usual daily living activities, such as routine household chores. Moderate-intensity activities make your muscles work harder than usual and cause your breathing and heart rates to increase above their usual rates. When doing a moderate-intensity activity, you can talk but you can't sing.[45] When performing a vigorous-intensity activity, you're breathing much faster than usual, and you can't say more than a few words without trying to catch your breath. For examples of activities that can be classified as moderate or vigorous intensity, visit www.heart.org/HEARTORG/HealthyLiving/PhysicalActivity/FitnessBasics/Moderate-to-Vigorous-What-isyour-level-of-intensity_UCM_463775_Article.jsp.

The Physical Activity Pyramid

The physical activity pyramid shown in **Figure 10.13** serves as a visual model to help people add more physical activity into their daily routines. This pyramid presents various activities that need to be performed regularly and discourages physical inactivity.

Performing *aerobic exercise* at least three times a week raises your heart rate, giving your heart a more effective workout. **Aerobic exercise** involves sustained, rhythmic contractions of large muscle groups in the legs and arms. Running, jogging, rapid walking, and swimming are aerobic activities. Performing resistance exercises, such as weight lifting, increases muscle mass and strength, and can also increase bone mass. Stretching activities improve flexibility. You may achieve even greater health benefits by increasing the duration, frequency, and intensity of your exercise routine. For example, you'll exert more physical effort and expend more energy if you "jog" instead of "walk" the dog.

Recommendations for Physical Activity

According to recommendations issued by the U.S. Department of Health and Human Services in 2018, healthy adults should perform

- moderate-intensity physical activity for at least 150 to 300 minutes a week,

or

- vigorous-intensity physical activity for about 75 to 150 minutes a week,

and

- muscle-strengthening exercises (moderate to vigorous) focusing on all major muscle groups on at least 2 days a week.[46] Strengthening activities should give your major muscle groups a workout.

Performing a minute of vigorous-intensity physical activity equals 2 minutes of moderate-intensity physical activity.[47] It's also a good idea to spread the activities out over a week.

> **aerobic exercise** physical activities that involve sustained, rhythmic contractions of large muscle groups

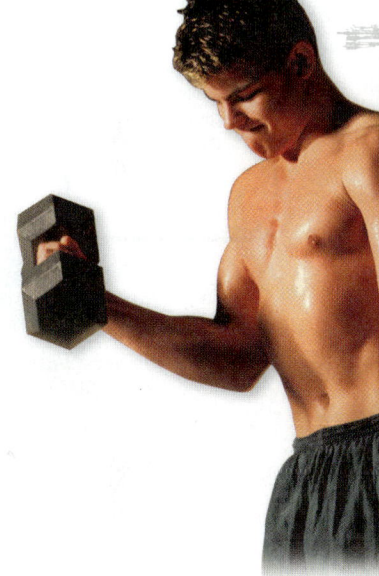

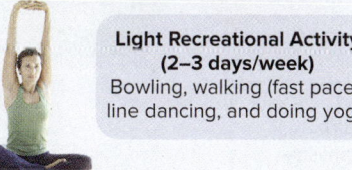
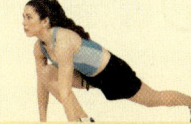
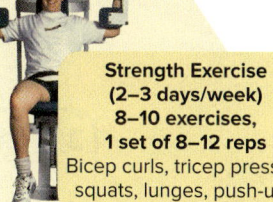
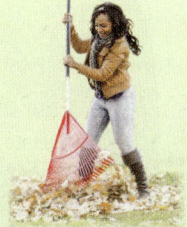
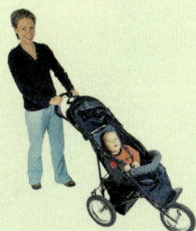

Sedentary Activity (occasionally)
Sitting, driving, watching TV, using a computer, texting, or talking on a phone

Light Recreational Activity (2–3 days/week)
Bowling, walking (fast pace), line dancing, and doing yoga

Moderate-Intensity Aerobic Exercise (3–5 days/week)
Running, cycling, in-line skating, stair stepping

Flexibility Exercise (2–3 days/week)
Static stretching of major muscle groups. Holding each stretch for 10–30 seconds.

Strength Exercise (2–3 days/week) 8–10 exercises, 1 set of 8–12 reps
Bicep curls, tricep presses, squats, lunges, push-ups

Activities of Daily Living (Most days of the week, accumulate 30+ minutes)
Gardening, raking leaves, mowing the lawn, walking the dog, cleaning the house, playing with your children

Figure 10.13 A physical activity pyramid.

Man using laptop: BJI/Blue Jean Images/Getty Images; Woman doing yoga: Fancy Collection/SuperStock RF; Bicyclist: Ljupco Smokovski/123RF; Woman doing forward lunge: Ingram Publishing/Alamy; Man at the gym: Ingram Publishing/Alamy RF; Woman raking leaves: Amble Design/Shutterstock; Woman with stroller: Ingram Publishing/Fotosearch RF; Man exercising with weights: Ingram Publishing

10.5c Fueling Exercise

As mentioned in Unit 4, cells obtain energy by means of a series of chemical reactions ("metabolic pathways") that break down macronutrients to release the energy that's stored within them. Cells capture some of the energy in special compounds such as adenosine triphosphate (ATP). ATP is the primary source of direct energy for all cells.

Aerobic Versus Anaerobic Conditions

In **aerobic** conditions, muscle cells have plenty of oxygen. As a result, the cells can metabolize glucose completely to CO_2 and H_2O. Aerobic conditions enable cells to produce far more ATP-energy than the amount cells can produce when oxygen isn't available. The ability to obtain this amount of energy is useful for endurance athletes because it allows their muscle cells to contract repeatedly for hours.

Gram for gram, fat supplies more ATP-energy than carbohydrate. Fatty acids, however, aren't a very useful fuel for intense, brief exercise, such as a 100-meter sprint. Why? A fatty acid molecule has fewer oxygen atoms in relation to carbon atoms than there are in a glucose molecule. Thus, cells need more oxygen to metabolize a fatty acid molecule than to burn a glucose molecule. During a brief bout of intense exercise, the heart and lungs don't have enough time to deliver much oxygen to muscles. When cells don't have much oxygen (**anaerobic** conditions), glucose is a major source of energy. Under these conditions, muscle cells, however, lack enough oxygen to metabolize glucose completely. **Essential Concept 10.1** illustrates what happens under anaerobic conditions and how your body forms glucose from another substance.

> **aerobic** conditions that include oxygen
>
> **anaerobic** conditions that lack oxygen
>
> **pyruvate** compound that results from anaerobic breakdown of glucose
>
> **lactic acid** compound formed from pyruvate during anaerobic metabolism

Essential Concept

10.1 Glucose Recycling

1 Cells convert glucose to **pyruvate** and then convert pyruvate to **lactic acid**.

2 The breakdown of glucose to lactic acid produces a small amount of ATP—only enough to sustain maximum physical exertion for 10 seconds to approximately 2 minutes.[48] Lactic acid accumulates in muscles and converts to a related substance, lactate.

3 Although certain muscle cells can use lactate as a fuel, some of the compound enters the bloodstream.

4 The liver can convert lactate into glucose. The liver can then release the glucose into the bloodstream to help meet muscles' demand for fuel or use the simple sugar to make glycogen.

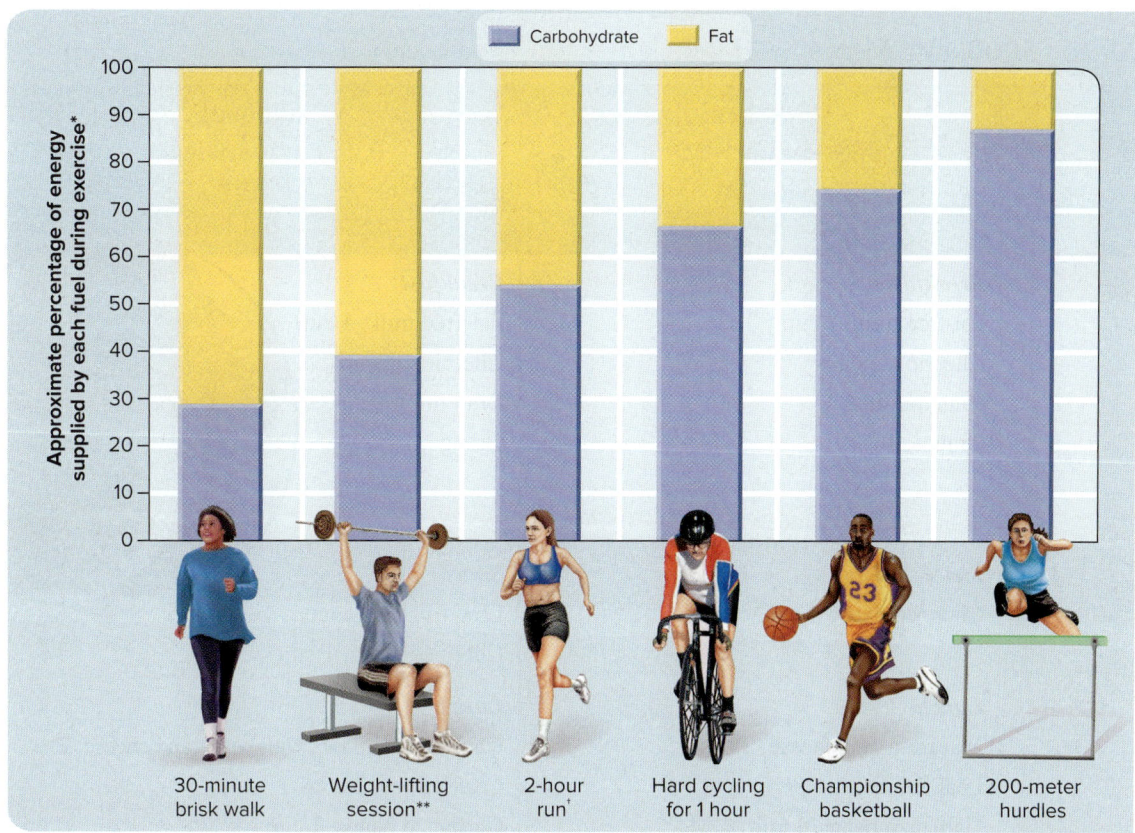

*Protein supplies a minor percentage of energy.
**Fat use generally is higher because much of the time spent weight lifting is for rest periods.
†The values shown are for a runner consuming carbohydrate during the run; more fat and less carbohydrate would be used if carbohydrates were not consumed.

Figure 10.14 Carbohydrate or fat?

Fat or Carbohydrate for Fuel?

The intensity and duration of a physical activity largely influence the relative amounts of fatty acids and glucose that muscles metabolize for energy. Fat is the primary fuel that muscles use while resting or engaged in low- to moderate-intensity physical activities. During prolonged high-intensity exercise, muscles use more glucose than fat for energy. To supply glucose, muscles and the liver break down glycogen. The chart in **Figure 10.14** illustrates rough estimates of carbohydrate and fat metabolism during six forms of exercise.

10.5d General Dietary Advice for Athletes

Compared to nonathletes, athletes generally need more energy to support their physically active lifestyles. Athletes who don't consume enough food energy can lose muscle mass and bone density, experience fatigue and menstrual problems (females), and be at risk of injury.[48]

Male athletes who train or compete aerobically for more than 90 minutes daily need at least 50 kcal/kg/day; their female counterparts need 45 to 50 kcal/kg/day.[49] Thus, athletes may require 3000 kcal/day or more to support their energy needs and maintain their weight. **Table 10.6** presents three sample daily menus that are nutritionally adequate, are high in carbohydrates, and supply approximately 3000, 4000, and 5000 kcal/day. Unit 3 provides general information to help you plan nutritious menus using MyPlate.

TASTY Tidbits

A pedometer is a small device that records the number of steps a person takes while engaging in physical activities. A reasonable goal is to take at least 10,000 steps per day. Even if you take 7,000 steps per day, this level of activity is better for your health than spending most of your time engaging in sedentary activities. You can purchase an inexpensive pedometer online or at a sporting goods store.

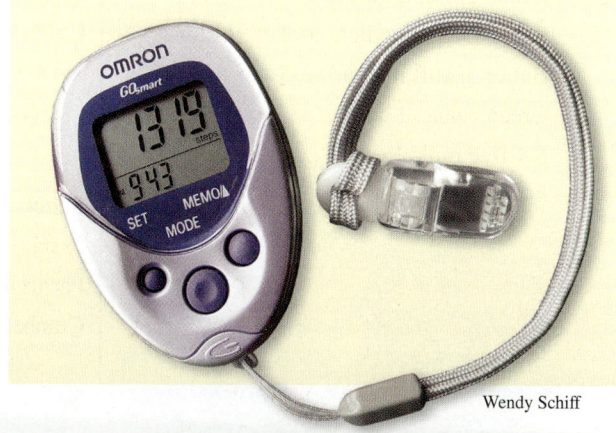

Wendy Schiff

Table 10.6 Sample Daily 3000, 4000, and 5000 kcal Menus

3000 kcal 62% carbohydrate 20% fat 18% protein	4000 kcal 66% carbohydrate 19% fat 15% protein	5000 kcal 62% carbohydrate 21% fat 17% protein
Breakfast Fat-free milk, 1 cup Cheerios, 2 cups Bagel, 1 Cherry preserves, ½ Tbsp Oat bran muffin, 1 Low-fat cream cheese, 1 Tbsp	**Breakfast** Fat-free milk, 1 cup Cheerios, 2 cups Bran muffins, 2 Orange, 1	**Breakfast** Fat-free milk, 1 cup Cheerios, 2 cups Bran muffins, 2 Orange, 1
Snack Oatmeal-raisin cookie, 1	**Snack** Chopped dates, 1 cup	**Snack** Low-fat plain yogurt, 1 cup Chopped dates, 1 cup
Lunch Chicken breast, skinless roasted, 2 oz Whole-wheat bread, 2 slices Provolone cheese, 1 oz Mayonnaise, 1 tsp Raisins, ½ cup Cranberry juice, 1½ cups Low-fat vanilla yogurt, 1 cup	**Lunch** Macaroni and cheese, 2 cups Leaf lettuce, 2 cups Garbanzo beans, 1 cup Grated carrots, ½ cup French dressing, 2 Tbsp Apple juice, 1 cup	**Lunch** Chicken enchilada, with beans and cheese, 2 Leaf lettuce, 2 cups Garbanzo beans, 1 cup Shredded carrots, ¾ cup Chopped celery, ½ cup Seasoned croutons, ½ cup French dressing, 2 Tbsp Whole-wheat bread, 2 slices Butter or soft margarine, 1 Tbsp
Snack Banana, 1 Oatmeal-raisin cookie, 1	**Snack** Whole-wheat bread, 2 slices Peanut butter, 1 Tbsp Grape jelly, 2 Tbsp Fat-free milk, 1 cup	**Snack** Banana, 1 Bagel, 1 Cream cheese, 1 Tbsp Fat-free milk, 1 cup
Dinner Lean broiled beef, 3 oz Leaf lettuce, 2 cups Garbanzo beans, ½ cup Italian dressing, 2 Tbsp Spinach egg noodles, cooked, 1 cup Butter or soft margarine, 1 tsp Green beans, 1 cup Fat-free milk, ½ cup	**Dinner** Skinless, roasted turkey breast, 2 oz Mashed potatoes, 1 cup Peas, 1 cup Butter or soft margarine, 2 tsp Fat-free milk, 1 cup	**Dinner** Lean broiled beef or pot roast, 6 oz Mashed potatoes, 2 cups Butter or soft margarine, 2 tsp Spinach egg noodles, cooked, 1½ cups Grated parmesan cheese, ¼ cup Green beans, 1 cup Oatmeal-raisin cookies, large, 3 Fat-free milk, 1 cup
	Snack Pasta, 1 cup cooked Parmesan cheese, 2 Tbsp Cranberry juice, 1 cup	**Snack** Whole-wheat bagel, 1 Peanut butter, 1 Tbsp Raisins, ½ cup Cranberry juice, 1½ cups

Wendy Schiff

Focusing on Carbohydrate Intake

Recall from Unit 5 that carbohydrate "spares" protein from being used for energy. If your diet doesn't supply enough carbohydrate to burn for energy, your cells may break down protein into amino acids to use for fuel. Thus, having an adequate carbohydrate intake enables you to conserve the protein in your muscles.

Recommended diets for athletes should supply adequate amounts of energy from carbohydrates. To maintain adequate muscle glycogen, endurance athletes should consume 3 to 10 grams of carbohydrate per kilogram of body weight daily.[48] Athletes who obtain more than 4 hours of moderate- to high-intensity exercise daily may need as much as 12 grams of carbohydrate per kilogram of body weight. **Table 10.7** lists energy and macronutrient information for several carbohydrate-rich foods. By consuming several servings of grains, starchy vegetables, and fruits daily, an athlete can obtain enough carbohydrate to maintain adequate liver and muscle glycogen stores.

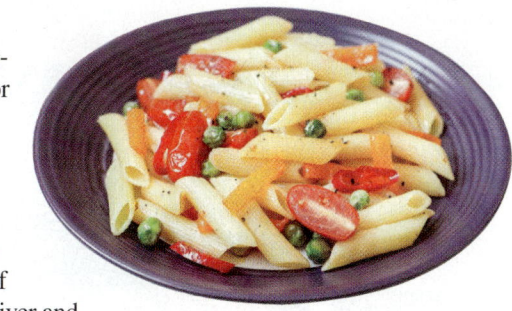

What's Carbohydrate (Glycogen) Loading?
Endurance athletes who have more glycogen in their muscles at the start of an event may be able to exercise longer than those who don't have as much muscle glycogen. Carbohydrate, or glycogen, loading involves altering dietary and physical activity patterns a few days before an event to increase muscle glycogen stores well above the normal range. The practice may help delay fatigue in athletes participating in events lasting more than 90 minutes.[48]

Table 10.7 Examples of Carbohydrate-Rich Foods

Food and Amount	kcal	Carbohydrate (g)	Protein (g)	Fat (g)
Spaghetti, cooked, 1 cup	239	46.60	8.76	1.49
Rice, instant, white, cooked, long-grain, 1 cup	205	44.15	3.60	0.82
Corn, canned, drained, 1 cup	166	40.82	5.06	1.05
Macaroni, plain, cooked, 1 cup	209	40.47	7.66	1.23
Egg noodles, cooked, 1 cup	221	40.26	7.26	3.31
Baked potato, ½ large, flesh	139	31.62	3.74	0.19
Oatmeal, regular, cooked with water, plain, 1 cup	166	28.08	5.94	3.56
Bagel, ½, 4" diam.	144	28.04	5.51	0.84
Cornflakes, 1 cup	130	28.00	2.00	0.00
Grapes, green, 1 cup	104	27.33	1.09	0.24
Banana, 1 med. (approx. 7" long)	105	26.95	1.29	0.39
Baked beans, canned, plain, ½ cup	119	26.85	6.03	0.47
English muffin, plain, 1	134	26.22	4.39	1.03
Pretzels, hard, 1 oz	109	22.79	2.85	0.83
Orange juice, unsweetened, from frozen concentrate, 1 cup	92	21.91	1.49	0.15
Soy milk, plain, 1 cup	131	15.26	7.95	4.25
Tortilla, flour, refrigerated, ready-to-cook, 6" diam. (1)	92	14.81	2.46	2.40
Crackers, 6 squares, saltines	75	13.33	1.70	1.56
Bread, white, 1 slice	67	12.29	2.98	0.60
Fat-free milk, 1 cup	86	11.98	8.40	0.44
Yogurt, low-fat, plain, 6-oz. container	107	11.97	8.93	2.63

USDA: *National Nutrient Database for Standard Reference Legacy Release,* April 2018. https://ndb.nal.usda.gov/ndb/search/list?home=true Accessed: January 9, 2019
Bowl of pasta: nesavinov/Shutterstock; Fruit: Wendy Schiff; Placemat: McGraw-Hill Education/Mark A. Dierker, photographer

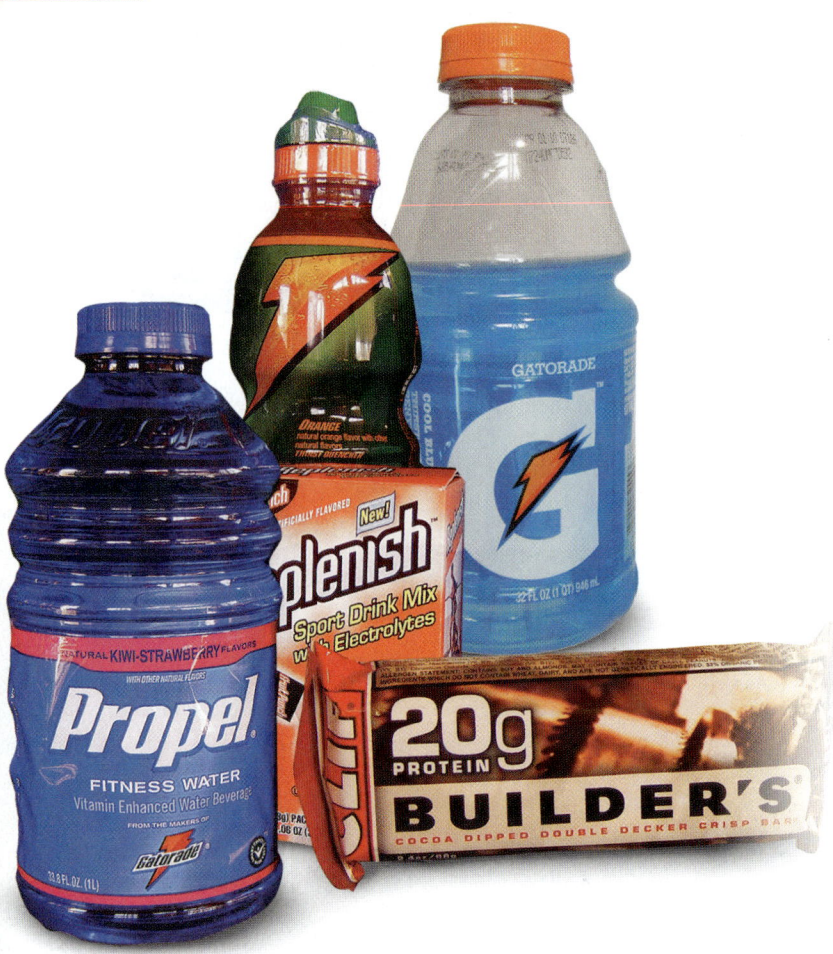

together. Proteins aren't "quick energy" sources because the liver must process amino acids before they can be used for energy. Granola bars, oatmeal cookies, and fresh or dried fruits are less expensive and more natural sources of energy and nutrients than are energy or sports bars.

Protein Intake

Under normal conditions, carbohydrate and fat are the primary fuels for cellular activity. Protein provides no more than 15% of the body's energy needs. During prolonged physical activity, muscles lose some protein because they metabolize certain amino acids for energy. Therefore, the RDA for protein may not apply to athletes involved in training or competition. Such athletes should consume more protein than the RDA of 0.8 gram per kilogram of body weight. When in training or competition, athletes should consume the RDA for protein and an additional 0.3 gram of high-quality protein per kilogram of body weight.[48] Ideal sources of high-quality protein include foods such as milk, lean meats, and dietary supplements that contain whey, casein, soy, and egg proteins.

Replenishing Fluids

Athletes should avoid losing more than 2% of their body weight during exercise.[48] Athletes can weigh themselves prior to exercising and then calculate 2% of their body weight. After working out, athletes should weigh themselves again. If the difference between preexercise and postexercise body weights is more than 2%, fluid replacement is needed during such activities. In general, you can replace each pound of water lost during exercise by drinking about 2 to 2.5 cups of a suitable replacement fluid.[50]

Sports drinks provide some nutritional benefits beyond those of plain water. These beverages usually contain simple carbohydrates and electrolytes, such as sodium, that can enhance performance during endurance activities. Recommended products contain about 21 g of carbohydrate per 12-ounce serving, or about 6% carbohydrate by weight. Drinks with a sugar content above 10%, such as soft drinks or fruit juices, aren't recommended because they may cause intestinal discomfort. Sodium and other electrolytes in sports beverages help maintain blood volume, enhance the absorption of water and carbohydrate from the intestinal tract, and stimulate thirst.

Consuming Carbohydrate During Events While performing prolonged physical activity (active for 1 to 2.5 hours), athletes can delay fatigue by consuming 30 to 60 g of carbohydrate per hour of activity.[48] Athletes who engage in ultra-endurance exercise (active for more than 2.5 hours) should aim to consume as much as 90 grams of carbohydrates per hour of activity. Commercially available sports drinks are often used as a source of carbohydrates during physical activity. These beverages are usually sweetened with nutritive sweeteners such as sucrose, glucose, fructose, or maltodextrin. Sports drinks typically provide 15 to 27 g of carbohydrate per 12-ounce serving. Sports gels are also good sources of simple carbohydrate, but they generally supply very little fluid. Therefore, it's important for athletes who consume these products to drink enough water to maintain proper hydration during endurance events.

Carbohydrates for Exercise Recovery After completing exhaustive physical activity, trained athletes can replenish their glycogen stores by consuming approximately 1.0 to 1.2 grams of carbohydrate per kilogram of body weight per hour during the first 4 to 6 hours after the activity.[48] To restore their supply of muscle glycogen quickly after an event, athletes can consume sports drinks, fruit, or fruit juices. During a post-event meal, starchy foods such as whole-grain bread, mashed potatoes, rice, and pasta can be served to boost athletes' carbohydrate consumption.

What About Energy Bars? Energy, or sports, bars are essentially cookies made from soy and milk proteins that are fortified with vitamins, minerals, and fiber. Sugary syrups hold these ingredients

TASTY Tidbits

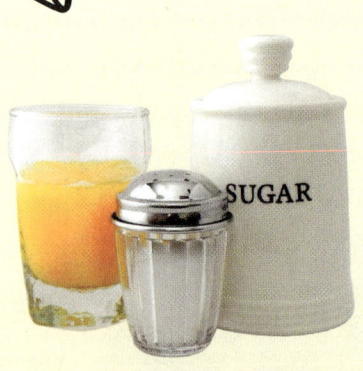

Compared to commercially available sports drinks, diluted fruit juices with added sugar and salt are less expensive sources of water, sodium, and simple sugars. You can prepare your own "sports" drink by adding ¼ cup of orange juice, ¼ cup of sugar, and ⅛ tsp of table salt to 30 oz of water or club soda. Pour the beverage into a quart pitcher, cover, and refrigerate until needed.

Protein bar, Sports drinks, Salt, sugar, and juice: Wendy Schiff

Should you drink water or a sports drink during competition? Sports drinks can improve physical performance when vigorous-intensity activities last more than an hour.[50] Although electrolytes are lost in sweat, the quantities lost in shorter periods can be easily replaced by consuming foods and beverages, such as water or fruit juice, after the event.

Water Intoxication

Water intoxication can occur when people drink too much water, which dilutes the level of sodium in their blood. Although sports drinks generally contain sodium, these beverages are mostly water; therefore, consuming excessive amounts of sports drinks can contribute to overload. Signs and symptoms of water intoxication include confusion, nausea or vomiting, weight gain, and muscle cramps. If not treated promptly, death can result. To avoid water intoxication, athletes should drink water according to their thirst.

Heat-Related Illness

Even a small degree of dehydration can lead to declines in an athlete's endurance, strength, and overall performance. Moreover, body temperature rises when dehydration occurs, increasing the risk of heat-related illness, including heat exhaustion and heat stroke. **Table 10.8** presents warning signs and symptoms of heat-related illnesses.

Heatstroke is a medical emergency that needs to be treated by trained medical staff. If you suspect that a person has heatstroke, summon emergency medical assistance immediately (call 911) and move the victim to a cool environment. Cool the person by soaking him or her in cold water.[51] If the person is alert and not vomiting, give him or her small amounts of cool water or a sports drink to swallow. According to recommendations, provide ½ cup of cool water every 15 minutes.[51] To reduce the risk of heat illnesses, you should avoid exercising under extremely hot, humid conditions. Furthermore, you should replace fluid losses that occur during prolonged exertion.

> **heatstroke** most dangerous form of heat-related illness
>
> **ergogenic aids** foods, devices, dietary supplements, or drugs used to improve physical performance

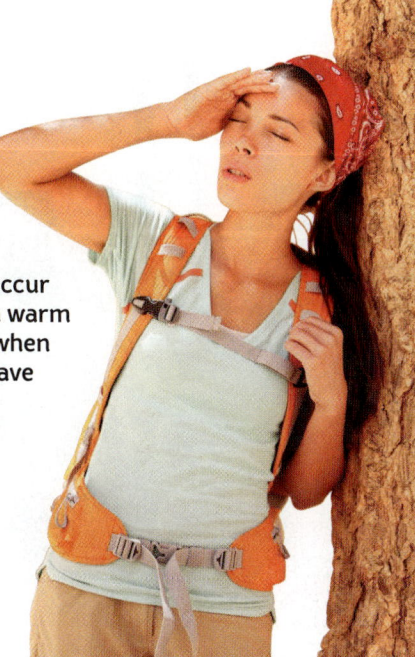

Heat exhaustion can occur after heavy exercise in warm conditions, especially when fluid and salt intakes have been inadequate.

maridav/123rf

TABLE 10.8 HEAT-RELATED ILLNESSES: WARNING SIGNS AND SYMPTOMS

Heat Cramps	Heat Exhaustion	Heatstroke
Painful muscle spasms ("heat cramps")	Dark urine	High fever (over 104°F)
Very heavy sweating	Cool, moist skin	Red, hot, dry skin
Tiredness	Weakness	Rapid, shallow breathing
Thirst	Nausea, dizziness, vomiting	Confusion
	Headache	Seizures
		Loss of consciousness

Source: National Library of Medicine, MedlinePlus: *Heat emergencies*. Reviewed October 2017. https://medlineplus.gov/ency/article/000056.htm Accessed: July 21, 2019

10.5e Ergogenic Aids: Separating Fact from Fiction

Athletes often use **ergogenic aids**—foods, devices, dietary supplements, and even drugs ("doping")—to improve their physical performance. Bee pollen, dried adrenal glands from cattle, seaweed, freeze-dried liver food, and ginseng are among the dietary supplements that athletes consume as they hope to gain the competitive edge over their rivals. However, no reliable scientific evidence supports the effectiveness of most dietary supplements purported to have ergogenic effects. Nevertheless, many athletes firmly believe in

caffeine naturally occurring stimulant drug

the value of the performance-enhancing aids that they use. **Table 10.9** summarizes science-based findings regarding some dietary supplements and ergogenic aids that are popular among athletes.

A few dietary practices can enhance physical performance. These ergogenic aids include consuming sufficient water, electrolytes, and carbohydrates, and eating a balanced, varied diet consistent with MyPlate recommendations. For athletes, meeting carbohydrate and fluid needs—along with overall nutrient needs—is the most important ergogenic aid.

"Energy" Drinks

Caffeine is a naturally occurring stimulant drug in coffee and tea. When consumed in moderate amounts, caffeine can increase alertness and decrease fatigue. Sugar-sweetened energy drinks provide calories, but their quick "energy" boost is a result of caffeine or other stimulants that are in the products. **Table 10.10** compares the caffeine and calorie contents of popular beverages, including some energy drinks.

Some energy drinks also contain the amino acid *taurine* and herbal substances such as ginseng. Although your body uses taurine, humans don't require the compound. Ginseng may enhance the stimulating effects of caffeine.

Caffeine Toxicity Excess caffeine is toxic. Toxicity signs and symptoms include heartbeat irregularities, increased blood pressure, dehydration, and sleep disturbances. As the popularity of energy drinks has increased in the United States, so has the number of people seeking emergency room treatment after consuming the beverages. In 2011, 1 in 10 Americans 12 years of age or older who visited emergency rooms for energy drink–related health problems required hospitalization.[52] In 2011, a 14-year-old girl with a heart condition died after consuming two 24-ounce energy drinks.

The practice of combining energy drinks with alcohol is very dangerous. The caffeine in the energy drink masks the central nervous system depressant effects of the alcohol. As a result, the drinker doesn't realize his or her level of intoxication and consumes too much alcohol.

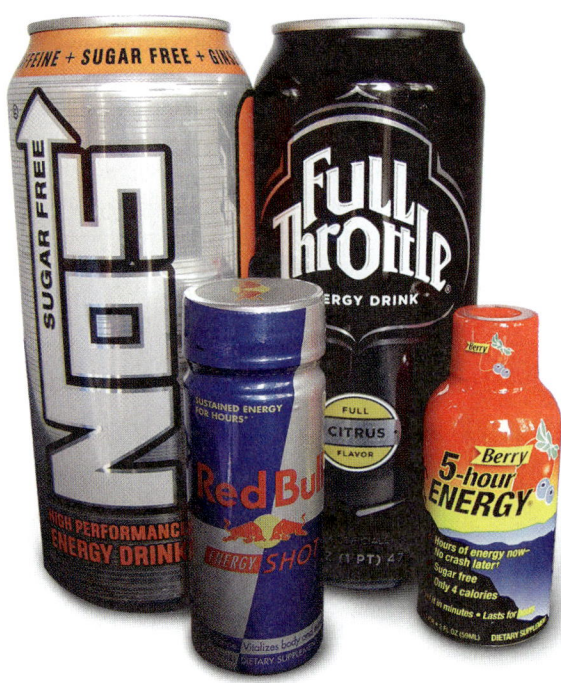

TASTY Tidbits

The seeds of the Brazilian shrub *guarana* (*Paullinia cupana*) are a concentrated source of caffeine. At present, the FDA doesn't require manufacturers to include information on food or beverage labels concerning amounts of caffeine provided by guarana or other herbal ingredients.

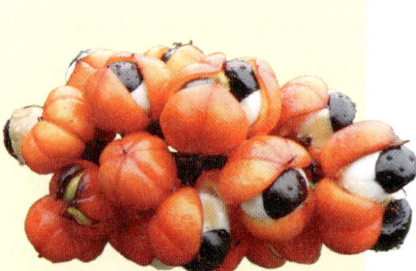

Guarana seeds

Football player: Purestock/SuperStock; Energy drinks: Wendy Schiff; Guarana: guentermanaus/Shutterstock

TABLE 10.9 **EVALUATION OF SOME POPULAR ERGOGENIC SUPPLEMENTS/AIDS**

Substance	Claim	Current Science-Based Findings Concerning Claims	Side Effects
Beta-alanine	May enhance training capacity and improve performance during brief bouts of intense exercise	Seems to be effective	May cause tingling sensation in skin of the face, neck, and hands
Beta-hydroxy-beta-methylbutyrate (HMB)	Decreases protein metabolism, increasing muscle mass	May increase muscle mass, but evidence is weak	None reported, but results of long-term use are unknown
Branched chain amino acids (BCAA)	Provide energy for muscles	May enhance muscle recovery after intense physical activity	None reported
Caffeine	Enhances fat metabolism; Increases alertness	Increases alertness and decreases fatigue but doesn't increase fat metabolism during exercise	High doses can cause increased heart rate, nervousness, shakiness; may contribute to death when consumed in high amounts
Calcium pyruvate	Increases endurance and promotes weight loss	Not effective	Gastrointestinal upset; May be harmful
Chromium	Increases lean mass	No benefit	Toxic level: intakes above 400 mcg daily
Coenzyme Q_{10}	Enhances cardiac function, delays fatigue	No benefit	Long-term safety unknown
Creatine	Enhances muscular endurance and strength; Increases lean muscle mass	Increases lean and total body mass, improves performance for intense activities that aren't endurance activities, increases strength; Such positive effects are not consistent among athletes	May cause weight gain and gastrointestinal upset
Ginseng	Combats fatigue and improves stamina	Doesn't improve performance but may decrease muscle damage during exercise	May cause gastrointestinal upset, itching, sleeplessness, and, in rare cases, allergic reactions and liver damage
Nitrate	Improves exercise tolerance and performance	Benefits aren't as evident in highly trained athletes	Concentrates, such as beetroot juice, may cause intestinal upset and red urine
Sodium bicarbonate (baking soda)	Reduces lactic acid accumulation	May enhance performance	May cause nausea and vomiting

Sources: Position of the Academy of Nutrition and Dietetics, Dietitians of Canada, and the American College of Sports Medicine: Nutrition and athletic performance. *Journal of the Academy of Nutrition and Dietetics* 116(3):501, 2016; Trexler ET and others: International society of sports nutrition position stand: Beta-alanine. *Journal of the International Society of Sports Nutrition* 12(1), 2015; Kreider RB and others: ISSN exercise and sport nutrition review: Research and recommendations. *Journal of the International Society of Sports Nutrition* 7(7):1, 2010; NIH, *MedlinePlus: American ginseng* 2017. https://medlineplus.gov/druginfo/natural/967.html Accessed: July 21, 2019

Terry Wild Studio/McGraw-Hill Education

TABLE 10.10 **CAFFEINE CONTENT OF SELECTED BEVERAGES (APPROXIMATE)**

Beverage (8 fl oz)	Kcal	Caffeine (mg)
Coffee, brewed from grounds, unsweetened*	5	92
Mtn Dew® AMP® Energy Strawberry Limeade**	110	78
Caffé Latte, short, 2% milk Starbucks†	100	75
Red Bull*	103	76
Coffee, instant, plain, prepared*	5	62
Tea, black, brewed, unsweetened*	2	47
Mtn Dew® **	113	36
Cola, sugar-sweetened, with caffeine*	103	22
Tea, AriZona®, ready-to-drink, extra sweet††	100	15
Chocolate-flavored drink, whey- and milk-based, 8 oz*	120	2

*U.S. Department of Agriculture, Agricultural Research Service, *USDA National Nutrient Database for Standard Reference Legacy Release, April 2018.* https://ndb.nal.usda.gov/ndb/search/list?home=true Accessed: July 5, 2019
**Nutrition information: www.pepsicobeveragefacts.com/.
†Nutrition information: www.starbucks.com/.
††https://www.drinkarizona.com/product/extra-sweet-tea

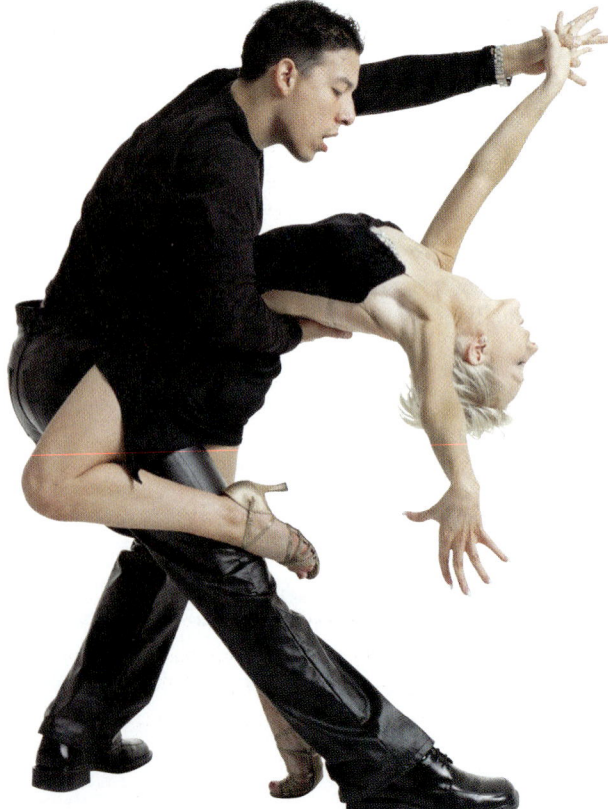

10.5f Physically Active for a Lifetime

When developing your personal physical fitness plan, first consider your fitness goals. For example, if you want to lose weight, how much do you want to lose and how many weeks will it take to lose that amount? Do you want to focus more on strengthening your muscles or on improving your aerobic capacity? Then determine when you can work out and whether you'll need to join a fitness facility such as a gym or purchase special equipment, such as handheld weights. For a comprehensive fitness program, make sure to include aerobic, resistance, and stretching activities in your weekly exercise regimen. Consider the following tips:

1. *Choose* physical activities that you enjoy and can do without the need for expensive equipment.
2. *Increase* the time you spend walking each day. Keep walking shoes where you can see them.
3. *Reduce* the amount of time you spend sitting. For example, do more household chores yourself.
4. *Take* stairs instead of elevators or escalators whenever possible.
5. *Park* your car farther from your destination and walk, if you feel it's safe to do so.
6. *Lift* handheld weights while watching television.
7. *Adopt* moderate-intensity activities for your leisure time. For example, join a co-ed volleyball club or take a ballroom dancing class.

Placemat: McGraw-Hill Education/Mark A. Dierker, photographer; Cup of coffee: McGraw-Hill Education; Tango couple: Mark Andersen/Getty Images

In a Nutshell

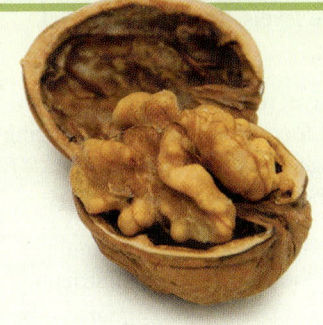

Module 10.1 Overweight or Obese?

- A person who's overweight has extra body weight that's contributed by bone, muscle, body fat, and/or body water. Obesity is a condition characterized by excessive and unhealthy amounts of body fat. Obese people have a greater risk of developing type 2 diabetes, hypertension, certain cancers, and cardiovascular disease than people who aren't obese.

- Obesity is the most prevalent nutritional disorder in the United States. In 2015–2016, almost 40% of American adults 20 years of age and older were obese. The prevalence of obesity among American children is a public health concern. Obese children have higher risk of maturing into obese adults than children who aren't obese. Rates of overweight and obesity are also increasing rapidly throughout the world ("globesity").

- Your body has fat-free mass and total body fat, which includes "essential fat" and fat (adipose) tissue. In addition to storing and releasing energy as fat, adipose cells secrete numerous proteins, some of which have roles in regulating food intake, glucose metabolism, and immune responses.

- Subcutaneous fat helps insulate your body against cold temperatures and protects muscles and bones from bumps and bruises. Visceral fat protects abdominal organs.

- Excess body fat distribution influences the risk of obesity-related diseases. People with "apple" body fat distribution have higher risks of CVD and type 2 diabetes than people with "pear" body shapes. Fat cells, particularly visceral fat, make substances that cause inflammation in the body.

- The BMI is a numerical value based on the relationship between body weight and risk of chronic health problems associated with excess body fat. Healthy BMIs range from 18.5 to 24.9. As BMI increases, the risks of serious chronic health problems increase. BMIs shouldn't be applied to highly muscular individuals, people who are elderly, or chronically ill persons.

- Bioelectrical impedance and skinfold thickness measurements are practical ways to estimate your percentage of body fat. A man is overweight when his body is 22 to 25% fat; a woman is overweight when her body is 32 to 37% fat. A man is obese when fat comprises 26% or more of his body; a woman is obese when fat makes up 38% or more of her body. Adults tend to gain fat tissue as they age, but for older adults, some additional fat doesn't necessarily contribute to serious health problems.

Module 10.2 Factors That Influence Your Body Weight

- Your cells generally metabolize primarily glucose and fatty acids, but small amounts of amino acids are also used for energy. Metabolism refers to all chemical changes, or reactions, that constantly occur in living cells. Anabolic reactions require energy to occur; catabolic reactions release energy. Basal metabolism generally accounts for most of the body's total energy use. Numerous factors can influence your metabolic rate, including thyroid hormone production, body composition, sex, age, and calorie intake.

- The amount of energy expended for a particular physical activity depends largely on the weight of the person, type of activity, and its duration and intensity.

- Total daily energy expenditure equals the sum of kilocalories burned for basal metabolism, physical activity, and TEF in a day. Energy balance occurs when calorie intake from food and beverages equals calorie output for basal metabolism, physical activity, and TEF. A negative energy state occurs when calorie intake is lower than calorie output. A state of positive energy state occurs when calorie intake is greater than calorie output.

- One pound of body fat represents about 3500 kcal. Losing weight requires a negative energy state.

- Hunger and satiety regulate eating behavior. Ghrelin stimulates eating behavior; leptin reduces hunger and inhibits body fat storage. Having a thrifty metabolism enables the body to store more excess energy as fat. According to the set-point theory, the body's fat content is genetically predetermined. Oversized portions of many restaurant foods may contribute to the widespread obesity problem in the United States.

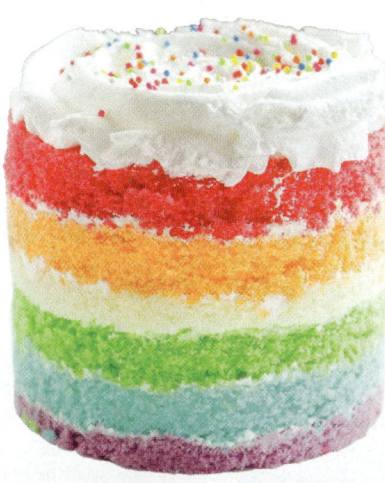

siraphol/123RF.com

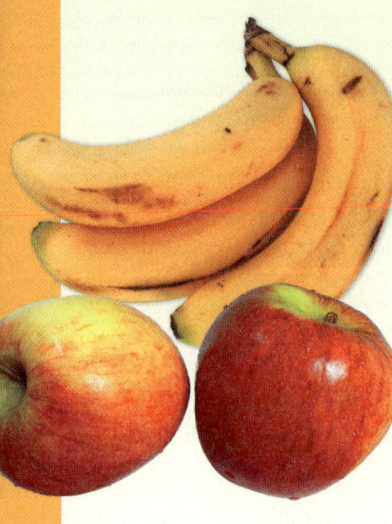

Module 10.3 Managing Your Weight Safely

- By losing 5 to 10% of excess body fat, an overfat person can increase beneficial high-density lipoprotein levels, reduce elevated blood pressure, and lower blood glucose and triglyceride levels. There are no quick cures for overweight and obesity.

- A reliable weight-loss plan has several features, including being safe and effective; meeting the dieter's nutritional, psychological, and social needs; including nutritious foods from all food groups; and encouraging regular physical activity. Successful weight loss and long-term weight maintenance involve motivation, calorie reduction, regular physical activity, and change in food-related behaviors.

- Actions that can help you lose excess weight and maintain a lower, healthier body weight include planning menus, monitoring food intake, shopping carefully, preparing and serving your food, and keeping nutrient-dense, low-calorie snacks on hand.

- At present, the FDA has approved few medications for long-term weight loss. Medications don't replace the need to reduce calorie intake and increase physical activity. The most common surgical procedures for weight loss drastically reduce the size of an obese person's stomach, markedly limiting food intake.

- Many overfat people use fad diets to lose weight. A typical fad diet promotes rapid, dramatic weight loss without calorie restriction and increased physical activity. Low-carbohydrate diets usually produce rapid weight loss initially, primarily because the body loses water. At this point, medical experts don't recommend any dietary supplement for weight loss.

- An underweight individual has a BMI that's less than 18.5. Many underweight individuals want to gain weight, especially muscle mass. To gain weight, underweight adults can gradually increase their consumption of calorie-dense foods, especially those high in healthy fats.

Module 10.4 Disordered Eating and Eating Disorders

- Disordered eating involves temporary chaotic and abnormal food-related practices. The practices can become harmful and difficult-to-treat eating disorders.

- Eating disorders are psychological disturbances that often lead to serious health complications. Anorexia nervosa, bulimia nervosa, and binge-eating disorder are major types of eating disorders. The causes of eating disorders are unknown, but genetic, social, and psychological factors contribute to their development.

- Treatment of eating disorders is complex, involving more than just dietary counseling. It's important to seek professional help for an eating disorder as early as possible—before the behavior becomes highly ingrained or the affected person's life is at risk.

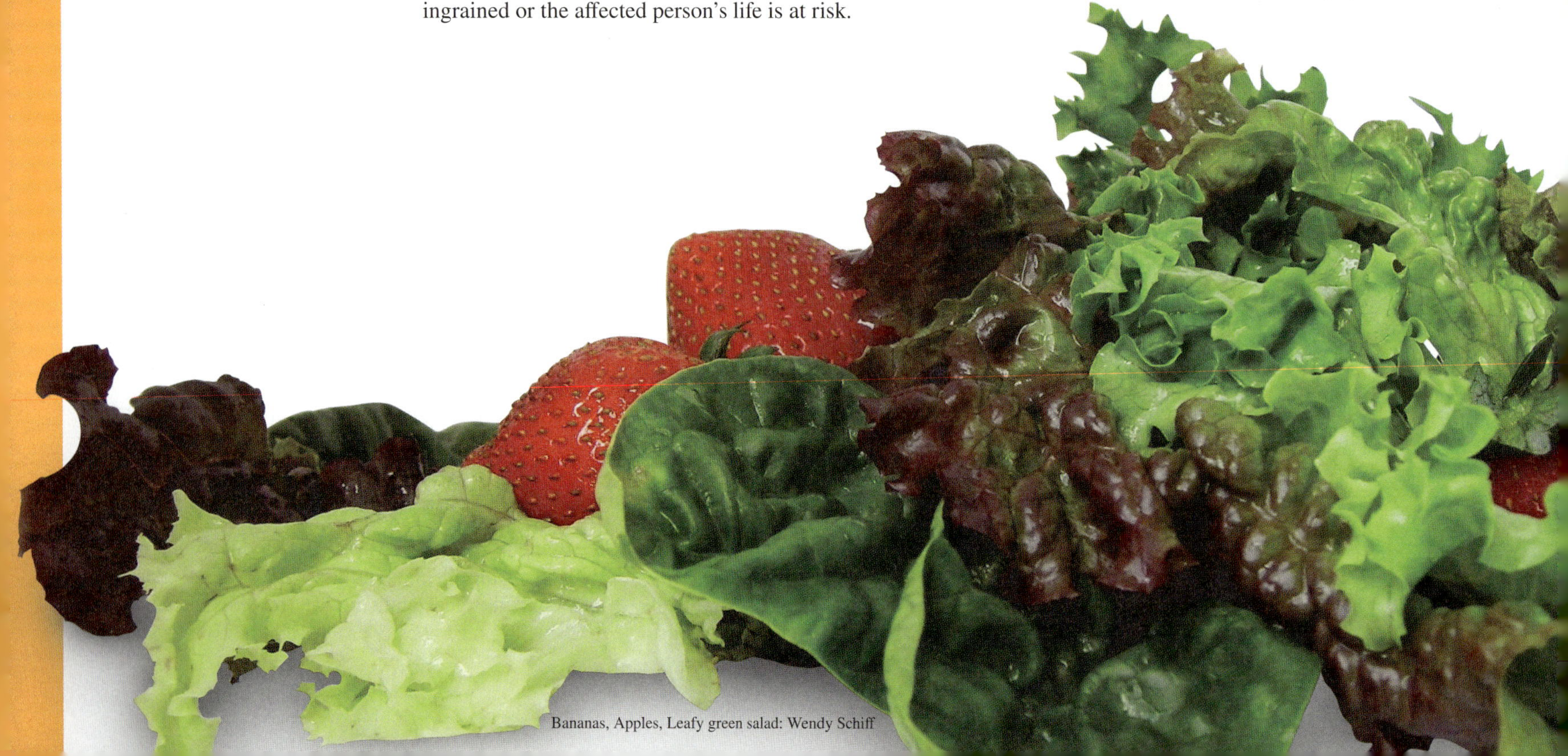

Bananas, Apples, Leafy green salad: Wendy Schiff

Module 10.5 Get Moving; Get Healthy!

- You can manage your weight more effectively and reduce your risk of developing the major causes of death and disability by becoming physically active. Healthy adults should perform moderate-intensity aerobic activity for at least 150 to 300 minutes a week or vigorous-intensity activities for about 75 to 150 minutes a week. In addition to aerobic activities, adults should perform strength training and flexibility exercises. Most people can achieve even greater health benefits by increasing the duration, frequency, and intensity of their physical activities.

- Regular exercise provides many benefits, such as reducing the risk of heart disease, diabetes, and certain cancers; aiding weight-control efforts; and promoting psychological well-being.

- ATP is the major form of direct energy used by cells. To generate ATP, muscle cells can metabolize carbohydrate, fat, and protein. In muscle cells, glucose molecules are broken down through a series of steps to yield lactic acid (in anaerobic conditions) or CO_2 and H_2O (in aerobic conditions).

- Fat is a key aerobic fuel for muscle cells, especially at rest and during low-intensity exercise. Little protein generally is used to fuel muscles. Under anaerobic conditions, muscle cells metabolize glucose rather than fat for energy, but their ability to sustain the release of energy for intense activity is limited. Muscle cells can obtain far more energy when in aerobic conditions.

- High-carbohydrate diets can be beneficial for athletes, and carbohydrate-rich foods should form the foundation of pre-event meals. Many athletes need more protein, including high-quality protein, than the RDA.

- Physically active people need to be concerned about their fluid intakes. Fluid replacement should be based on thirst and loss of body weight while exercising. Consuming a source of electrolytes, such as a sports drink, can be helpful, especially when the duration of intense exercise exceeds 60 minutes. It's important to avoid overconsumption of water because of the risk of water intoxication.

- Athletes often ingest certain substances, including caffeine and herbal products, because they believe these substances have ergogenic effects. Scientific evidence, however, doesn't suggest that most of these substances are effective. Furthermore, long-term safety of many ergogenic aids has not been determined.

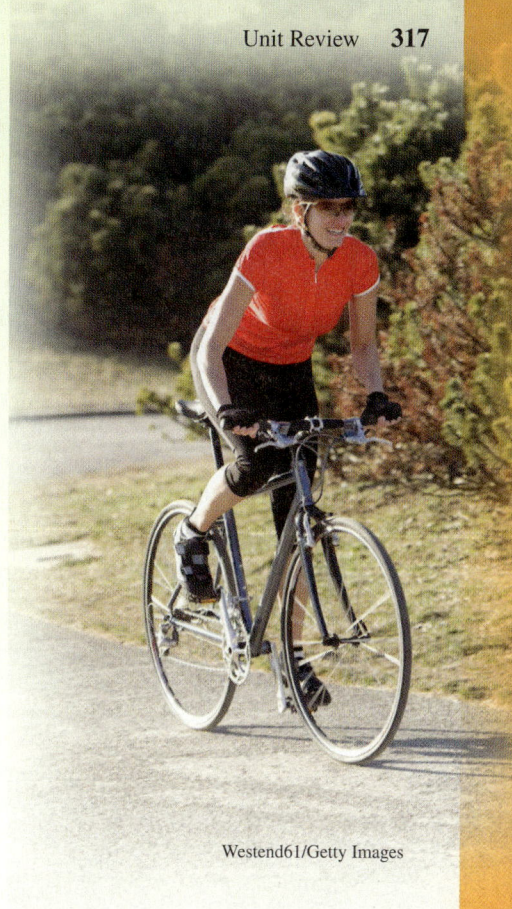
Westend61/Getty Images

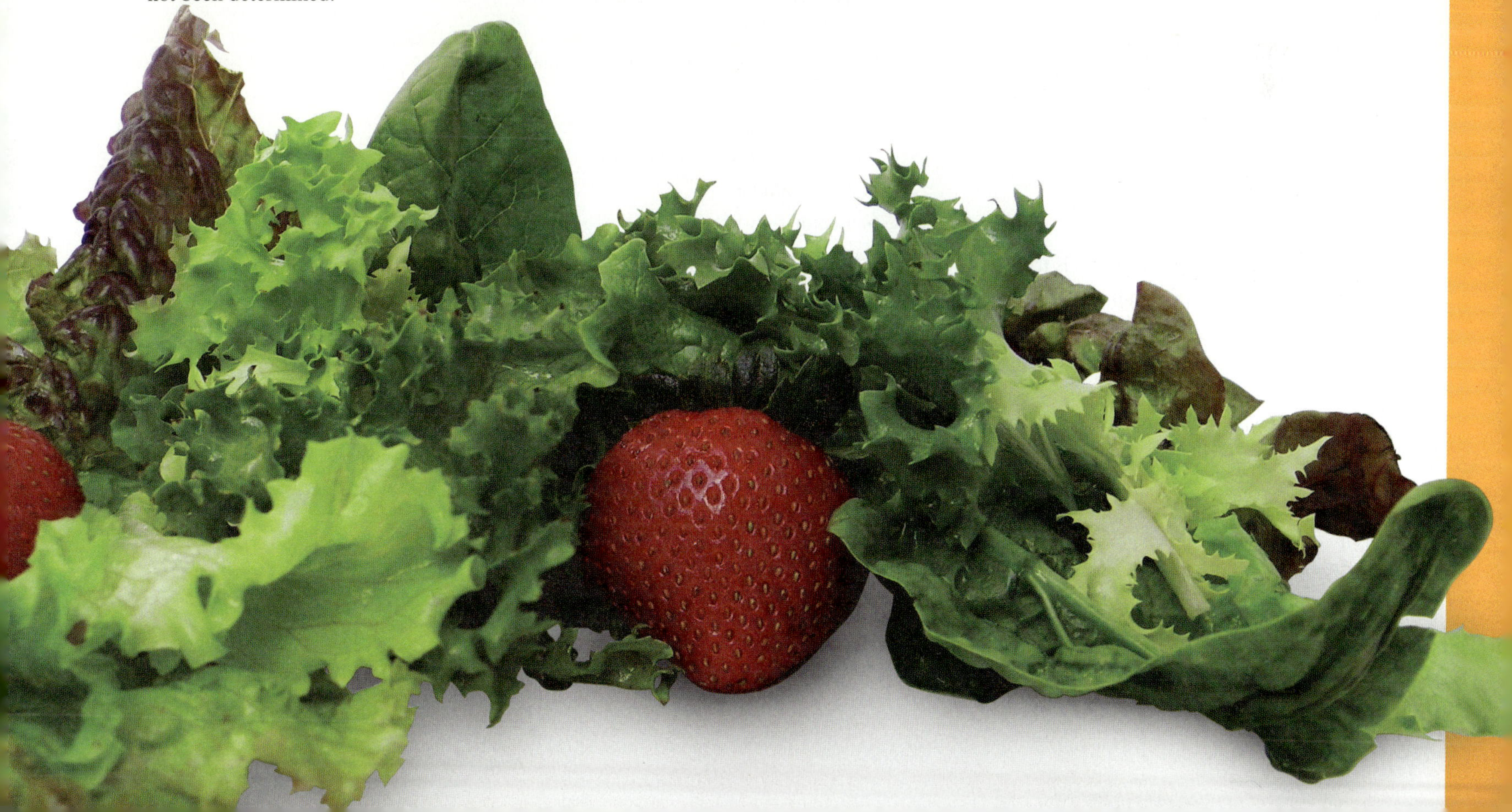

Consider This...

1. Why is it usually difficult to pinpoint a cause of obesity?
2. Why are most people who lose weight unable to maintain the lower body weight over time?
3. If your BMI is within the overweight or obese range, discuss your reasons for being interested or not interested in losing weight. If you want to lose weight, what lifestyle changes can you make to meet your weight-loss goal?
4. If your BMI is within the underweight range, discuss your reasons for being interested or not interested in gaining weight. If you want to gain weight, what lifestyle changes will you make?
5. If your BMI is in the healthy range, discuss steps you can take to maintain a healthy body weight as you grow older.
6. Analyze your weekly physical activity habits. Does your participation in various physical activities meet the minimum recommendations? If not, which physical activities are you willing to include in your weekly routine to improve your fitness level?

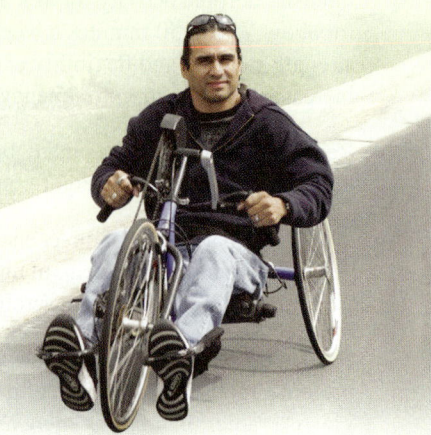
Realistic Reflections

Test Yourself

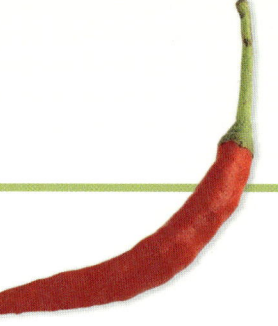

Select the best answer.

1. _____ fat is in a layer under the skin.
   a. Cellulite
   b. Visceral
   c. Subcutaneous
   d. Metabolic

2. Basal metabolism includes energy needs for
   a. breathing and circulating blood.
   b. performing physical activity.
   c. digesting food.
   d. absorbing nutrients.

3. Which of the following statements is true?
   a. Women generally have higher metabolic rates than men.
   b. Thyroid hormone levels influence the metabolic rate.
   c. A person who has more muscle mass will have a lower metabolic rate than someone with less muscle tissue.
   d. When your thyroid gland produces too much thyroid hormone, your metabolic rate drops below normal.

4. A negative energy state occurs when
   a. your body needs more calories than the diet supplies.
   b. fat storage in your body increases.
   c. your energy intake is higher than your energy output.
   d. the thermic effect of your food equals NEAT.

5. _____ is a hormone that reduces hunger and inhibits fat storage in your body.
   a. Glucosamine
   b. Leptin
   c. Ghrelin
   d. Creatine

6. Members of the National Weight Control Registry tend to
   a. weigh themselves once a month.
   b. follow low-carbohydrate/high-protein diets.
   c. exercise 2 to 3 times per week.
   d. eat breakfast.

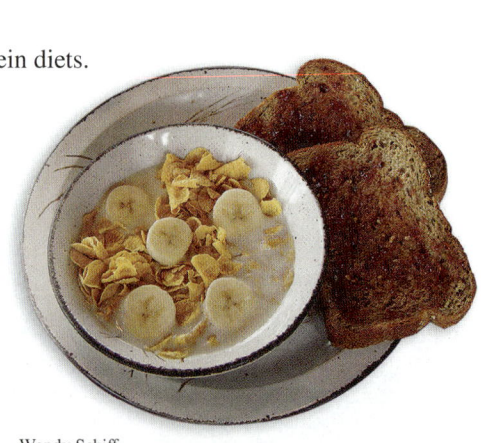
Wendy Schiff

7. Joseph's BMI is 23. When he's under a lot of stress, he eats a large amount of cookies and ice cream. Soon after eating these foods, he goes to a bathroom and makes himself vomit. Based on this information, Joseph probably has
   a. glycogen storage disease.
   b. anorexia nervosa.
   c. cystic fibrosis.
   d. bulimia nervosa.

8. Miranda is physically fit. Based on this information, she has
   a. an increased risk of osteoporosis.
   b. the strength, endurance, and flexibility to meet the demands of daily living.
   c. a greater need for vitamins and minerals than other women.
   d. more muscle and less bone tissue than other women who are her age.

9. Aerobic activities
   a. enable muscles to use less oxygen than normal.
   b. don't require voluntary muscular contractions.
   c. force muscle cells to use more vitamins and minerals for energy.
   d. involve sustained, rhythmic contractions of certain large skeletal muscles.

10. Which of the following statements is true?
    a. Resistance exercises don't help build bone mass.
    b. Sedentary activities don't require much energy to perform.
    c. Healthy adults should obtain at least 1 hour of vigorous-intensity activity daily.
    d. Older adults can reduce their metabolic rates by exercising regularly.

11. Amy is studying quietly. Under these conditions, her muscles are using primarily _____ for energy.
    a. fat
    b. glucose
    c. amino acids
    d. ketone bodies

12. Which of the following beverages is a common source of caffeine?
    a. Mineral water
    b. Iced tea
    c. Lite beer
    d. Orange drink

13. Under aerobic conditions, cells break down glucose to form
    a. carbon dioxide and water.
    b. nitrogen and DNA.
    c. beta-carotene and vitamin B-6.
    d. sodium and ATP.

14. _____ is an immediate and direct source of energy for cells.
    a. DNA
    b. Glycogen
    c. ATP
    d. Phospholipid

Answers: 1. c 2. a 3. b 4. a 5. b 6. d 7. d 8. b 9. d 10. b 11. a 12. b 13. a 14. c

Answer This (Module 10.1d)

25.3

References → See Appendix D.

Design elements: Spiral notebook paper background, Stacked paper with clip background, Marginal note clip, and Culture & Cuisine globe icon: ©McGraw-Hill Education; In a Nutshell walnut: ©McGraw-Hill Education/Mark A. Dierker, photographer; Test Yourself red pepper: Iconotec/Glow Images

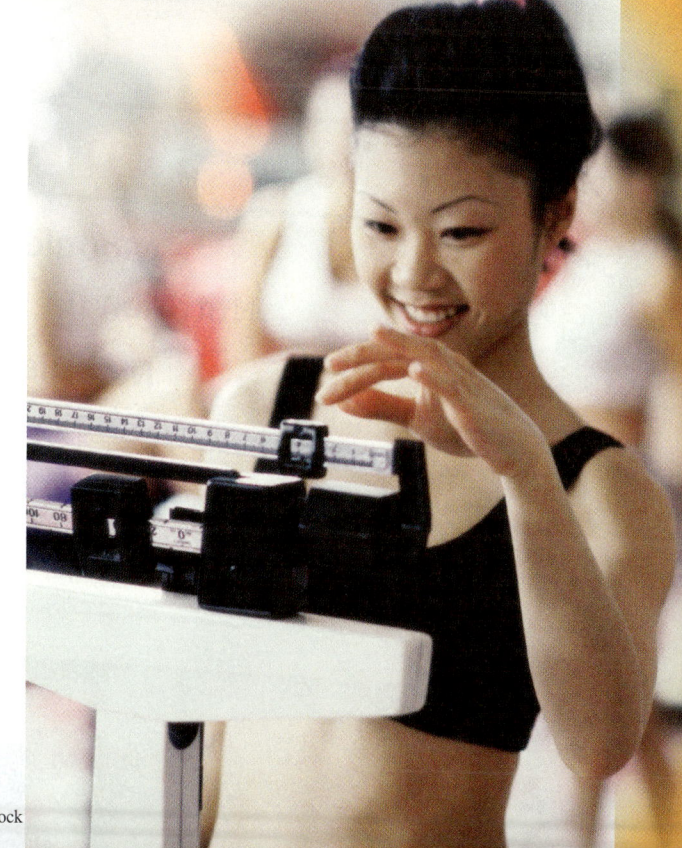

Purestock/SuperStock

Unit 11
Nutrition for Your Life, Environment, and World

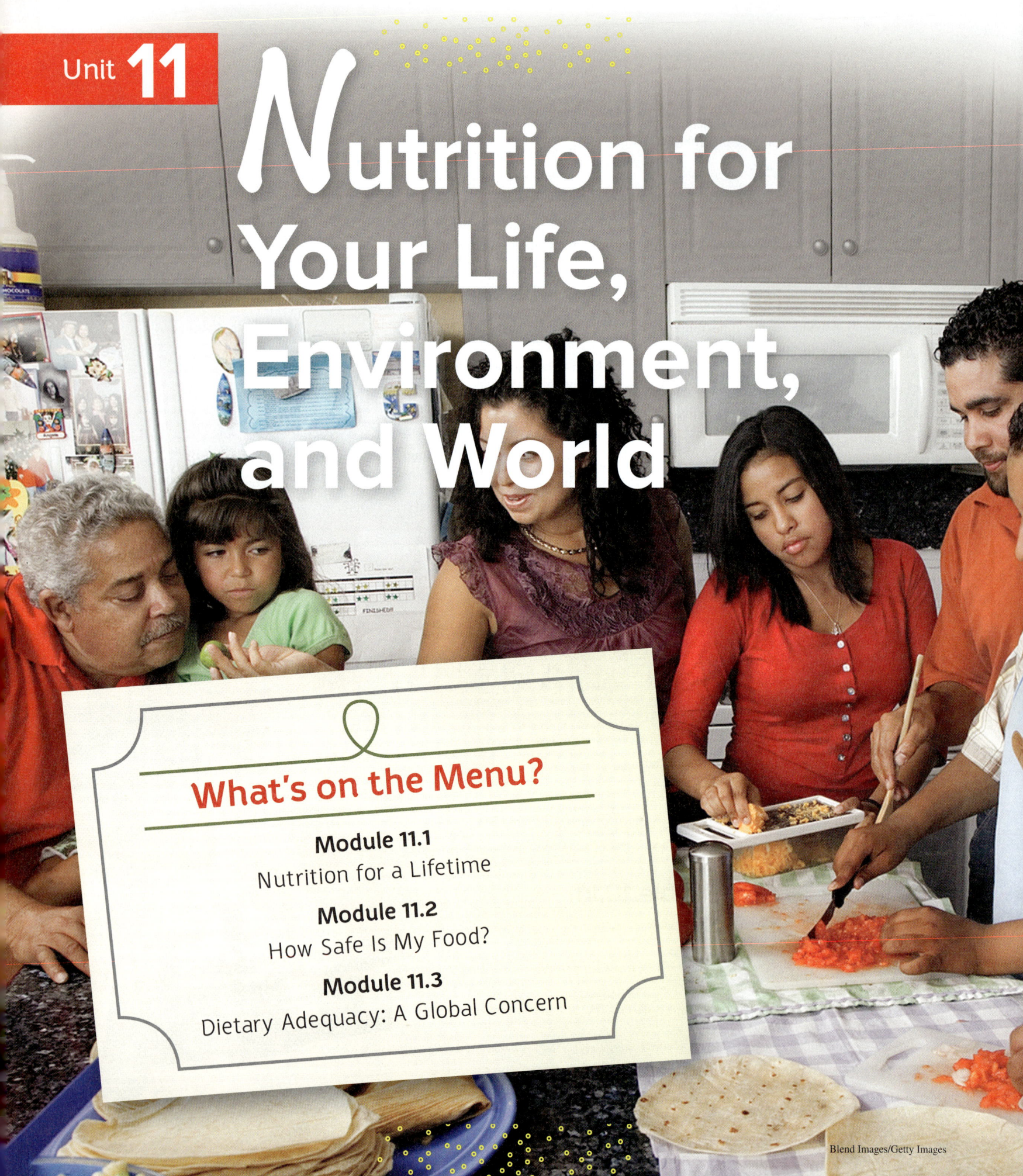

What's on the Menu?

Module 11.1
Nutrition for a Lifetime

Module 11.2
How Safe Is My Food?

Module 11.3
Dietary Adequacy: A Global Concern

Blend Images/Getty Images

"I can't seem to exercise and eat the way I did before Elijah was born. I find myself snacking with him regularly, plus I don't have the time to work out. When I structure my time and my diet, I feel energetic, but it doesn't last. Within a few weeks, I'm feeling heavy again. I can't keep off the extra pounds I've gained. . . . it's driving me crazy!

"We try to 'eat smart,' but planning meals and snacks is very much a challenge. Eating healthy foods has to become a habit with me, so my son will know what's good for him as he grows."

Theresa Washington

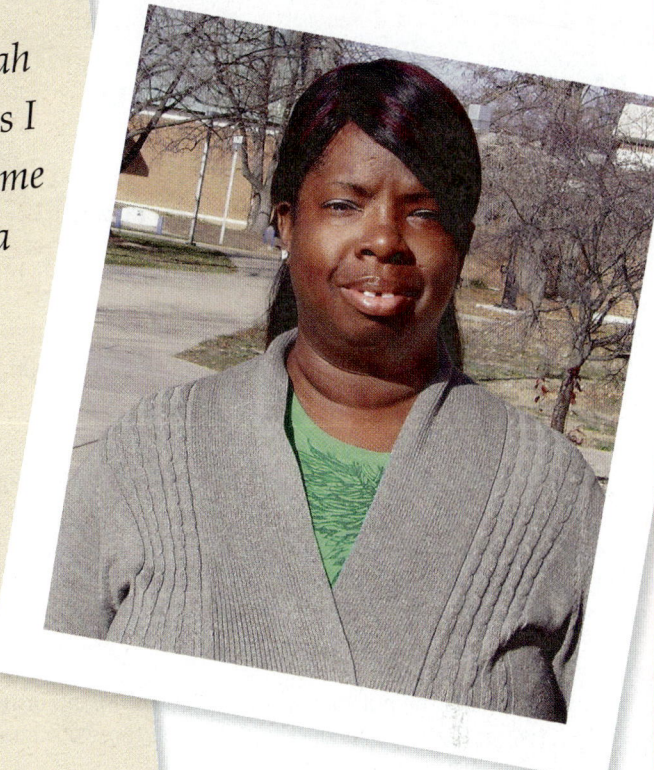

Wendy Schiff

Theresa Washington is a nontraditional college student, majoring in business administration at St. Louis Community College. Her busy lifestyle makes it difficult for her to "eat right," but she's determined to make the effort because she wants to lose weight and set a good example for her young son. Is snacking such a bad practice? What can parents and other caregivers do to improve their children's eating habits?

This unit covers three major topics that are important for you and your future. The first part of this unit focuses on nutrition during specific periods of the life cycle, including infancy and the older adult years. Then we'll discuss food-borne illness and the safety of our food supply—concerns of all Americans, regardless of their ages. Finally, we'll provide some basic information about global nutrition, including ways to produce enough nutritious food for the world's population without destroying the Earth's valuable natural resources.

Module 11.1

Nutrition for a Lifetime

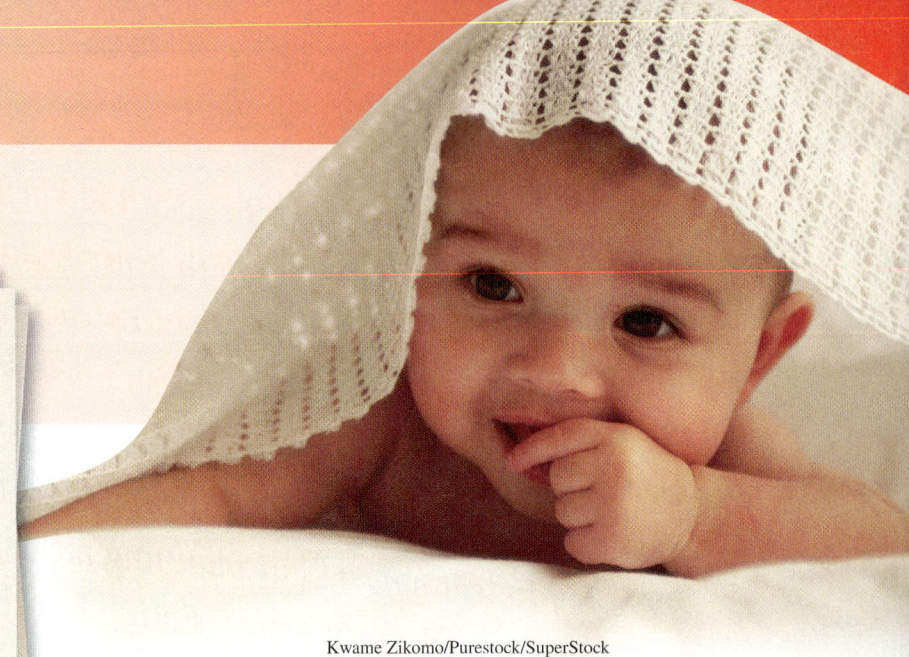

Kwame Zikomo/Purestock/SuperStock

11.1 - Learning Outcomes

After reading Module 11.1, you should be able to

1. Define all of the **key terms** in this module.
2. Discuss why proper nutrition is important for having a healthy pregnancy and baby.
3. Classify weight gained during pregnancy according to recommendations that are based on a woman's weight before pregnancy.
4. List nutrients that may need to be supplemented during pregnancy.
5. Describe major physical processes involved in lactation and breastfeeding.
6. Compare the nutritional composition of infant formula with breast milk, and identify at least three advantages of breastfeeding.
7. Explain the rationale for delaying the introduction of solid foods to infants until they're 4 to 6 months of age.
8. Summarize practical suggestions for encouraging healthy eating habits among children.
9. Identify some major nutrition-related health concerns facing American children and teenagers.
10. Identify at least three physical changes that occur during the normal aging process.
11. Explain how growing older affects your nutrient needs.

If you are a woman, are you pregnant or considering pregnancy? Do you already have children? If you have children, were they breastfed or fed a synthetic beverage that simulates human milk (**infant formula**)? Do you live with and help to care for an elderly parent or grandparent? These may seem to be very personal questions, but many undergraduate college students don't fit the stereotype of being 18 to 22 years of age, having no children, and residing away from home. Most of the nutrition recommendations presented in this textbook apply to people who are "adults"—loosely defined as the period when a person is 19 to 70 years of age.[1] A person's nutrient needs, however, vary according to life stage. This module focuses on the differing nutrition needs and health concerns of people who are in specific life stages—the **prenatal period** (from conception to birth), pregnancy, **lactation** (milk production for breastfeeding), infancy, childhood, and older adulthood.

Why is it important to learn some basic information about nutrition-related concerns during the life cycle? If you don't have children, you may become a parent in the future. If your parents and grandparents are relatively young and vigorous now, you can expect them to experience declining physical functioning as they grow older. Finally, you need to recognize that most of these changes are normal and will occur in you as well.

infant formula synthetic beverage that simulates human milk

prenatal period time between conception and birth

lactation milk production

embryo human organism during the first 8 weeks after conception

fetus human organism from 8 weeks after conception until birth

placenta organ of pregnancy that connects the uterus to the embryo/fetus via the umbilical cord

11.1a The Prenatal Period

The prenatal period begins with conception and ends with birth. This stage of life lasts about 40 weeks and is often divided into three, 13-week trimesters. During the first 8 weeks, the fertilized egg divides rapidly to form a mass of cells that increases in size and begins to form organs. At this stage, the developing human being is an **embryo**. From 8 weeks after conception until birth, the developing human being is referred to as a **fetus**. During the second and third trimesters, the fetus continues to develop and grow to the point that it's physically mature enough to be born. Birth ends the prenatal period.

The first trimester is a critical stage because nutrient deficiencies or excesses and exposure to toxic compounds, such as alcohol, are most likely to have devastating effects on the embryo/fetus. However, many women who are in their first trimester don't realize they're pregnant.

Throughout the prenatal period, the embryo/fetus develops in the uterus and depends entirely on its mother for survival. During most of the pregnancy, the expectant mother nourishes her embryo/fetus through the **placenta,** the organ of pregnancy that connects the mother's uterus to the embryo/fetus via the umbilical cord

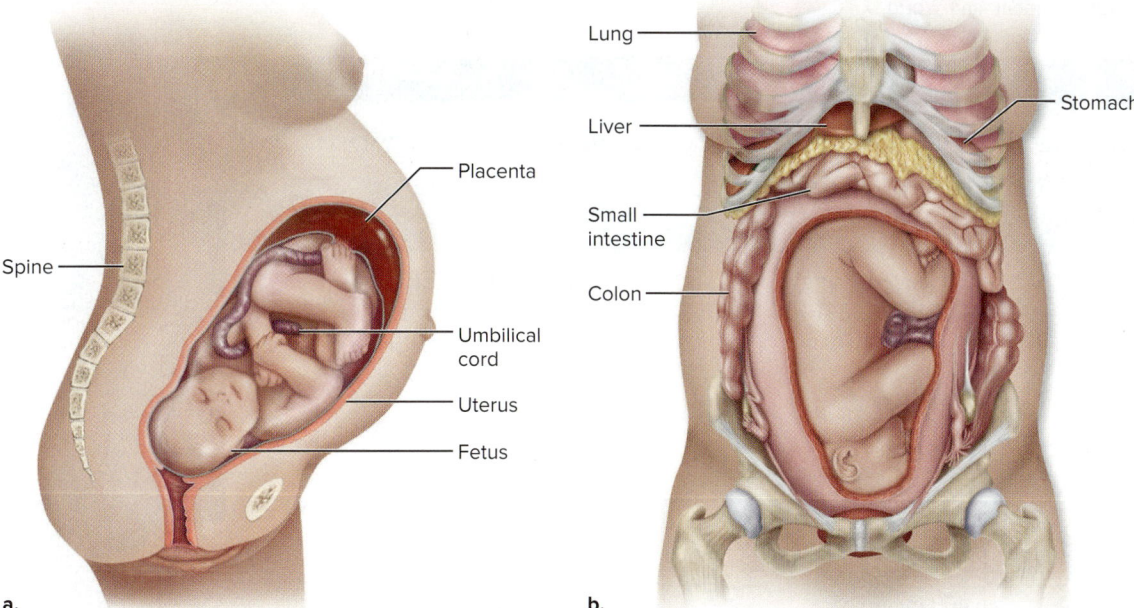

premature describes infant born before 37 weeks of pregnancy

low-birth-weight (LBW) infant generally weighing less than 5½ pounds at birth

Figure 11.1 Getting ready for birth. (a) The placenta transfers nutrients and oxygen from the mother's bloodstream to the fetus. This organ of pregnancy also conveys waste products from the fetus to the mother's bloodstream for elimination. (b) This illustration shows the position of a full-term fetus and the mother's abdominal organs.

■ *Why is having a healthy placenta critical for having a healthy baby?*

(Fig. 11.1). The role of the placenta is to transfer nutrients and oxygen from the mother's bloodstream to the embryo/fetus. Additionally, the placenta transfers wastes from the embryo/fetus to the mother's bloodstream, so her body can eliminate them. The placenta, however, doesn't allow the mother's blood to mix with the blood of her fetus.

Unfortunately, the placenta doesn't filter many infectious agents and toxic substances, such as alcohol and nicotine, from the mother's blood. Thus, the embryo/fetus can become harmed or killed by infectious diseases and poisonous chemicals that are in her bloodstream.

What's Prematurity?

A developing human being generally needs to spend at least 37 weeks within the uterus to survive after birth without the need for special care. A fetus that's born before the 37th week of the prenatal period is **premature.** In 2017, about 10% of American infants were born prematurely.[2] When compared to "full-term" infants (babies born between 39 and 41 weeks of pregnancy), premature infants are more likely to die before their first birthday.

The Importance of Birth Weight

Birth weight is another major factor that determines whether a baby is healthy and survives his or her first year of life. At birth, a healthy, mature fetus usually weighs about 6 to 8 pounds and is 19 to 21 inches long. **Low-birth-weight (LBW)** infants generally weigh less than 5½ pounds. In 2017, about 8% of infants born in the United States were low birth weight.[2] A fetus's weight depends on the supply of nutrients that it receives through the placenta. If the placenta fails to grow properly, the developing fetus may be premature and be lighter than average at birth. Low birth weight and prematurity are among the leading causes of death among American infants who are less than 1 year of age.[3]

11.1b Nutrition in Pregnancy

During pregnancy, a woman's body undergoes major physical changes, such as increased blood volume and breast size, increased absorption of many nutrients, and higher levels of several hormones. These adaptations enable her body to nourish and maintain the developing embryo/fetus, as well as produce milk for her infant after its birth. However, some of the changes are troublesome and even dangerous for the pregnant woman.

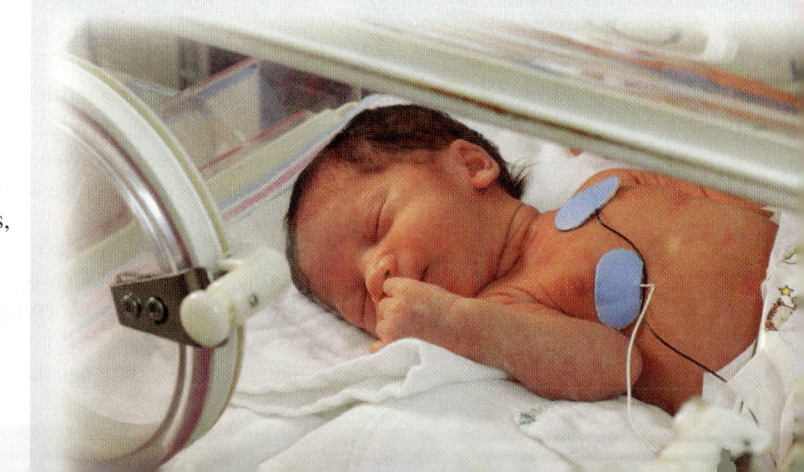

Premature baby being cared for in a special hospital nursery

Larry Mulvehill/Corbis

Table 11.1 Comparing Selected DRIs: 25-Year-Old Nonpregnant and Pregnant Women

Energy/Nutrient*	Nonpregnant	Pregnant
Kilocalories	Estimated Energy Requirement (EER)	First trimester = EER + 0 Second trimester = EER + 340 Third trimester = EER + 452
Protein	46 g/day	71 g/day
Vitamin C	75 mg/day	85 mg/day
Thiamin	1.1 mg/day	1.4 mg/day
Niacin	14 mg/day	18 mg/day
Folate	400 mcg/day	600 mcg/day
Vitamin D	15 mcg/day	15 mcg/day
Calcium	1000 mg/day	1000 mg/day
Iron	18 mg/day	27 mg/day
Iodine	150 mcg/day	220 mcg/day

*RDA.

Source of data: Institute of Medicine: *Dietary Reference Intakes.* Available from *Nutrient recommendations: Dietary Reference Intakes (DRIs)*. http://ods.od.nih.gov/Health_Information/Dietary_Reference_Intakes.aspx

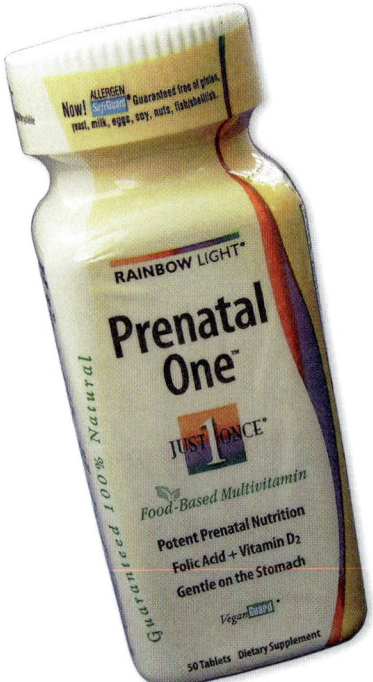

Eating for Two?

The mother-to-be should follow a diet that meets her own nutritional needs as well as those of her developing offspring. Otherwise, she's likely to become deficient in certain nutrients, especially iron and calcium, as her fetus removes them from her bloodstream to meet its needs. Depending on the trimester, an expectant woman's requirements for energy (calories), protein, and many other nutrients are greater than her needs were prior to pregnancy. Nevertheless, a pregnant woman doesn't need to double her usual food intake just because she is "eating for two." **Table 11.1** compares Recommended Dietary Allowances (RDAs) for energy and selected nutrients that apply to healthy 25-year-old nonpregnant and pregnant women.

Folate and Iron Needs

As Table 11.1 indicates, a pregnant woman's requirements for folate and iron are 50% higher than those of a nonpregnant woman. It's important for women to enter pregnancy with adequate folate status because embryos need the vitamin to support rapid cell division. Pregnant women who are folate deficient have high risk of giving birth to infants with neural tube defects, such as spina bifida (see Unit 8).

During pregnancy, a woman's blood volume expands. Thus, her need for iron increases because her body must use the iron to make more hemoglobin for the extra red blood cells. Additionally, the woman's body transfers iron to the fetus to build its stores of the mineral. If women fail to meet their iron needs during pregnancy, they can develop iron deficiency anemia. Pregnant women who are iron deficient have high risk of giving birth prematurely and having low-birth-weight infants.[4] According to the Dietary Guidelines for Americans, iron is a nutrient of public health concern for pregnant women.

To obtain adequate folate and iron, pregnant women should include food sources of the micronutrients in their diets. Units 8 and 9 provide information about foods that supply these micronutrients. Most physicians also recommend prenatal multiple vitamin/mineral supplements that contain folic acid and iron for their pregnant patients.

What's Morning Sickness?

During the first trimester, most women experience physical signs that they're pregnant, such as "morning sickness." The name **morning sickness** is misleading because the queasy stomach and vomiting can occur at any time of the day. Some women find that eating crackers and drinking some water helps to reduce the likelihood of feeling nauseated, especially before they get out of bed in the morning. Furthermore, eating

morning sickness nausea and vomiting associated with pregnancy

Placemat: McGraw-Hill Education/Mark A. Dierker, photographer; Orange juice, Prenatal supplement: Wendy Schiff

smaller but more frequent meals and nutritious snacks can be helpful. If the vomiting is severe, the pregnant woman should check with her physician. In most instances, morning sickness ends by the beginning of the second trimester.

What About Cravings?

The stereotype of a pregnant woman who craves pickles and ice cream isn't simply a myth. Food cravings are common during this stage of life and aren't limited to any particular food. Ask pregnant women to identify the foods they crave and you're likely to get a variety of responses. The causes of cravings are unknown, but they may be responses to the hormonal changes associated with pregnancy or to the emotional state of the mother-to-be. Unless food cravings supply too many empty calorie foods or contribute to excess weight gain, they're generally harmless.

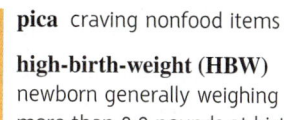

Some women develop **pica,** the craving of nonfood items such as laundry starch, chalk, cigarette ashes, and soil. Pica may be linked with iron and zinc deficiency, but it's not clear if pica is the result or the cause of such deficiencies. Pregnant women should avoid practicing pica, especially eating clay or soil. Soil may contain substances that interfere with the absorption of minerals in the intestinal tract. Furthermore, eating soil can be harmful because the dirt may be contaminated with toxic substances, such as lead and pesticides, and disease-causing microbes.

11.1c Weight Gain During Pregnancy

Nearly all pregnant women experience weight gain. In fact, gaining an appropriate amount of weight is crucial during pregnancy. Women who don't gain enough weight during pregnancy have a high risk of giving birth to a LBW baby. On the other hand, women who gain too much weight during pregnancy can develop serious health problems and may have difficulty losing the excess weight after delivery. **Table 11.2** indicates the typical distribution of weight that's gained during this life stage.

How much weight a woman should gain depends on her prepregnancy weight and the number of fetuses she is carrying. **Table 11.3** presents recommended ranges of weight that women should gain during pregnancy (single fetus). Weight gain recommendations are higher for women who are pregnant with more than one fetus. For example, a healthy woman who is carrying twins can expect to gain as much as 54 pounds during pregnancy.[5]

Women who are obese when they become pregnant are more likely to give birth to **high-birth-weight (HBW)** babies.[6] HBW newborns generally weigh more than 8.8 pounds. Pregnant women with poorly controlled diabetes have a higher risk of giving birth to an HBW infant than mothers who don't have this disorder.

When compared to newborns with healthy weights, HBW infants have higher risk of being injured during the birth process and of having birth defects.[6] Furthermore, HBW infants are more likely to develop obesity later in life.[7]

pica craving nonfood items

high-birth-weight (HBW) newborn generally weighing more than 8.8 pounds at birth

TABLE 11.2 DISTRIBUTION OF WEIGHT GAIN DURING A HEALTHY PREGNANCY

Tissue	Approximate Pounds
Maternal	
Blood	4
Breasts	2
Uterus	2
Fat, protein, and retained fluid	11
Fetus	7.5
Placenta	1.5
Amniotic fluid*	2.0

*Fluid that surrounds fetus.
Adapted from www.marchofdimes.org/pregnancy/weight-gain-during-pregnancy.aspx
Accessed: July 27, 2019

TABLE 11.3 RECOMMENDED RANGES OF WEIGHT GAIN DURING PREGNANCY

Prepregnancy BMI Category	Recommended Range of Weight Gain (lb)
Underweight	28–40
Healthy weight	25–35
Overweight	15–25
Obese	11–20

Source: www.marchofdimes.org/pregnancy/weight-gain-during-pregnancy.aspx
Accessed: July 27, 2019

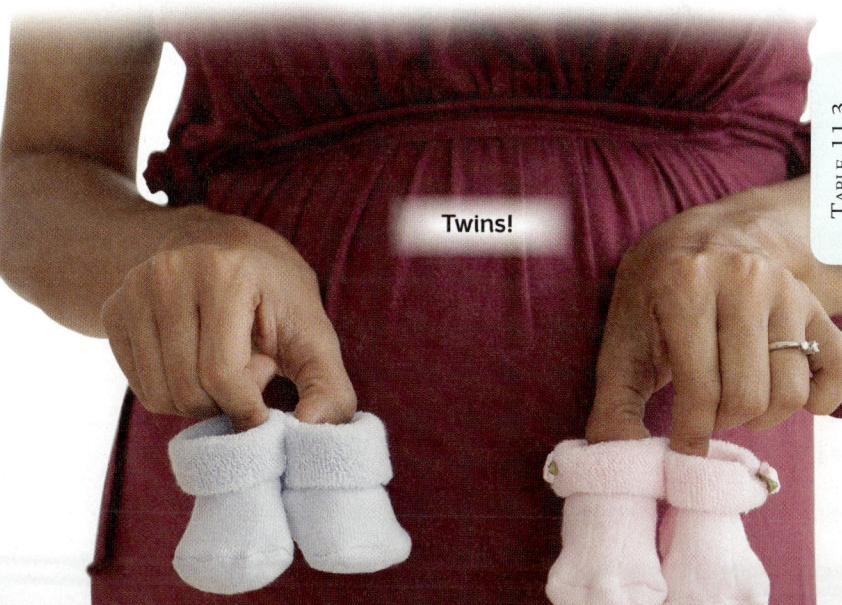

Jar of pickles: Photodisc/Alamy; Ice-cream cone: Photodisc/PunchStock; Pregnant woman: JGI/Blend Images LLC

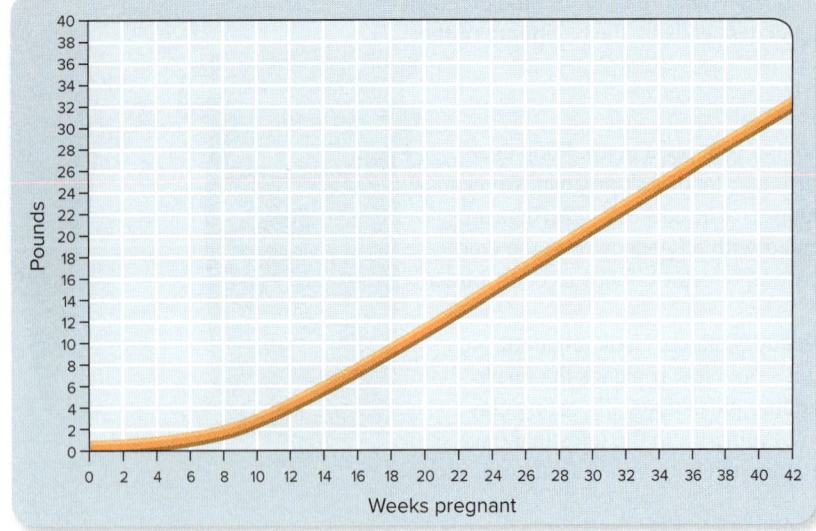

Figure 11.2 Rate of weight gain in a healthy pregnancy.

■ Why is it important to monitor a woman's weight gain during pregnancy?

Rate of Weight Gain

For an expectant mother, the rate of the weight gain is important, as well as the amount of weight gained. Pregnant women usually gain up to 4 pounds of weight during the first trimester. Throughout the rest of their pregnancies, women typically gain at a faster rate—about 1 pound per week. **Figure 11.2** charts the course of weight gain in a healthy pregnancy.

What's Gestational Hypertension?

High levels of certain hormones can cause various tissues to retain fluid during pregnancy. Although the extra fluid causes some minor swelling (mild edema), especially in the hands and feet, the condition is normal. Rapid weight gain, especially after the fifth month of pregnancy, could be a sign of a serious type of hypertension, **preeclampsia** (*pre-e-klamp'-see-a*). Preeclampsia is characterized by sudden, dramatic increase in weight that is due to edema, particularly of the hands or face; hypertension; and protein in urine **(Figure 11.3)**. Women with preeclampsia may also experience persistent headache, vision problems, and trouble breathing. An estimated 3 to 7% of pregnant women experience preeclampsia.[8] Treatment often includes medications to control high blood pressure. If a woman suffering from preeclampsia develops convulsions, her condition is called **eclampsia** (*e-klamp'-see-a*). In the United States and throughout the world, eclampsia is one of the leading causes of death among pregnant women.[9]

The only effective, emergency treatment for eclampsia is delivering the fetus, but infants born before the 24th week of pregnancy are unlikely to survive. If the fetus is older than 24 weeks, its mother may be hospitalized for treatment. This practice helps physicians monitor the mother's condition and enables the fetus to mature until it has a better chance of surviving after birth. Proper prenatal care is important to detect preeclampsia before it can damage the mother's kidneys and lead to eclampsia.

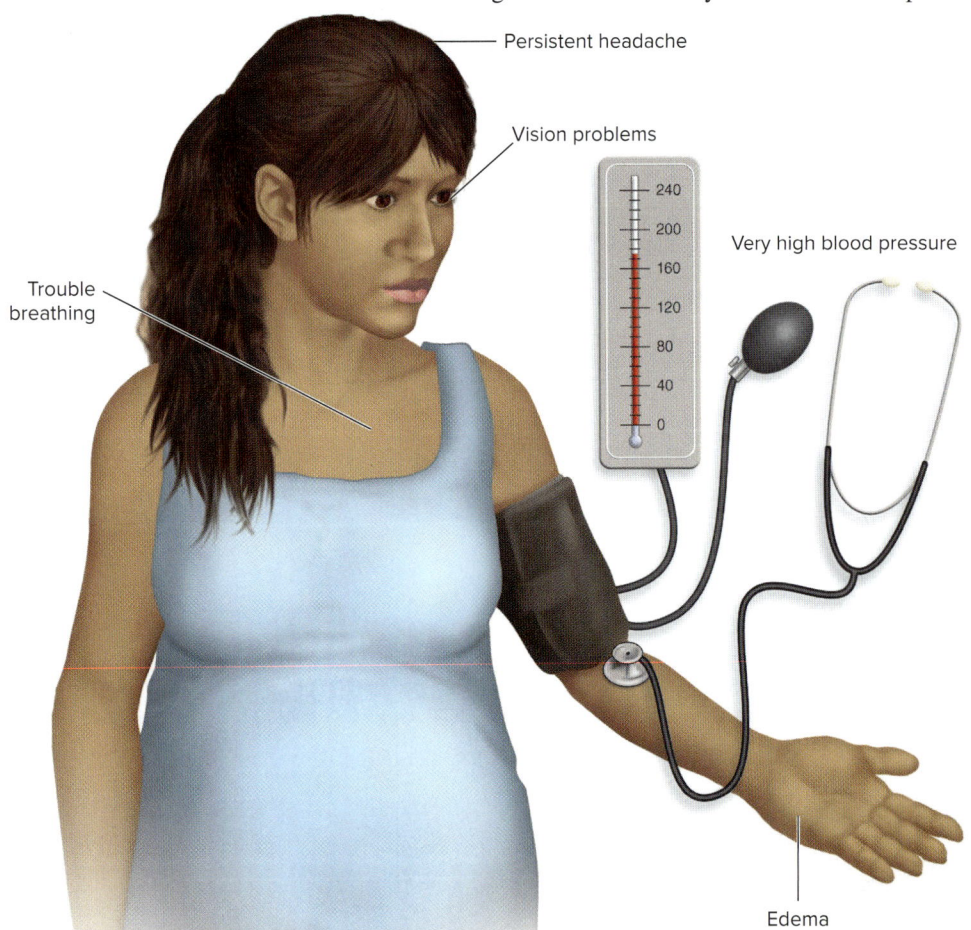

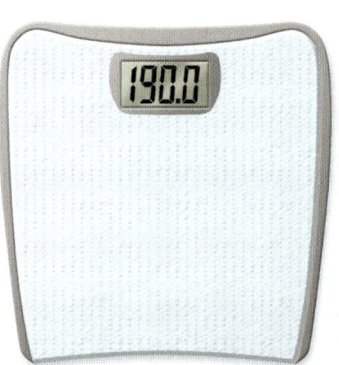

Sudden weight gain

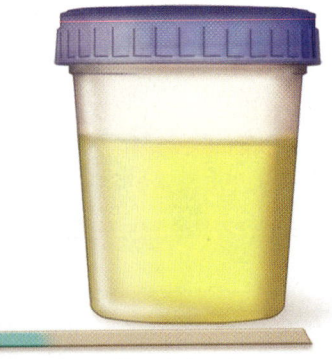

Protein in urine

Figure 11.3 Signs and symptoms of preeclampsia.

■ What is the only effective treatment for eclampsia?

preeclampsia common name for gestational hypertension

eclampsia condition that occurs when a woman with preeclampsia develops convulsions

colostrum initial form of breast milk that contains antibodies and immune system cells

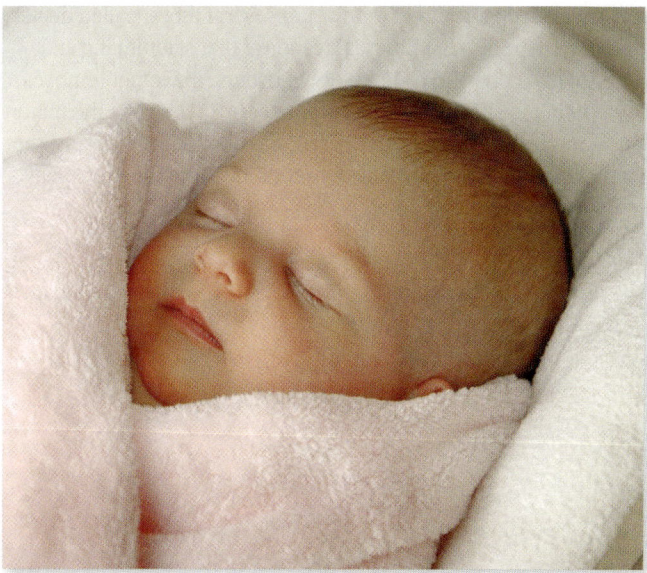
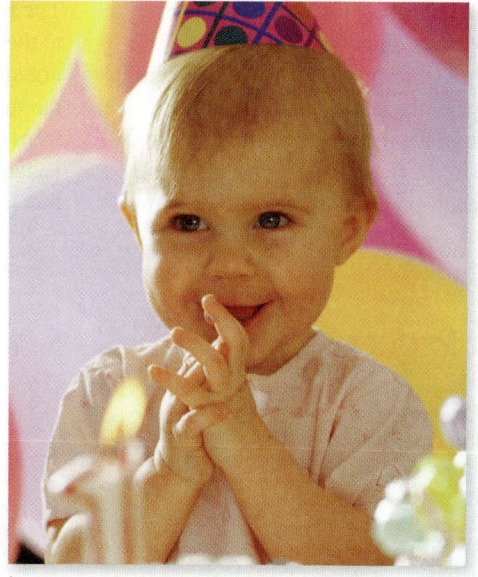

a.   b.

Figure 11.4 Babies' rapid growth rate. (a) Healthy newborn; (b) 1-year-old child.

■ *If this healthy baby weighs 6 pounds, 8 ounces at birth, how much would you expect her to weigh on her first birthday?*

11.1d Infant Nutrition

Rapid physical growth characterizes infancy, the life stage that extends from birth to about 1 year of age. During the first 4 to 6 months of life, a healthy baby doubles its birth weight, and by 1 year of age, an infant's birth weight has tripled. Additionally, an infant's length increases by 50% during its first year of life. Thus, if a baby girl weighs 7 pounds and is 20 inches long at birth, you would expect her to weigh 21 pounds and be 30 inches long by her first birthday **(Fig. 11.4)**.

Compared to older children, an infant needs more energy and nutrients per pound of body weight to support its rapid growth. If an infant's diet lacks adequate energy and nutrients, the baby's growth may slow or even stop. Furthermore, the child's brain development might be negatively affected. The following sections take a closer look at infant nutrition, including breastfeeding and other infant feeding practices.

Understanding Lactation

Lactation is a complex process that occurs after a woman gives birth. During the first couple of days after her baby is born, the new mother's breasts produce **colostrum** (*co-loss'-trum*), a yellowish fluid that doesn't look like milk.

Colostrum is a very important first food for babies because the fluid contains antibodies and immune system cells that can protect the infant's immature digestive tract from infections. Colostrum also contains a substance that encourages the growth of a type of bacteria, *Lactobacillus bifidus*, in the infant's GI tract. Such biologically active substances help an infant's body fight infections and hasten the maturation of the baby's immune system. Thus, breastfed infants, especially those who are exclusively breastfed for their first six months of life, have lower risks of allergies and gastrointestinal, respiratory, and ear infections than do formula-fed infants.[10]

By the end of the first week of lactation, colostrum has become mature milk. Breast milk is more watery than cow's milk and may have a slightly bluish color.

Human milk is a rich source of lipids, including cholesterol, and fatty acids such as linoleic acid, arachidonic acid (AA), and docosahexaenoic acid (DHA). An infant's nervous system, especially the brain and eyes, depends on AA and DHA for proper development. Furthermore, the fat in breast milk helps supply the energy needed to maintain the infant's overall growth.

Q Answer This

A healthy newborn's length is 18 inches. What should be the baby's approximate length when he or she is 12 months of age? You can find the answer on the last page of this unit.

Newborn: Travis VanDenBerg/Alamy; First birthday girl: Elyse Lewin/Getty Images; Woman breastfeeding her baby: Jiang Jin/Purestock/SuperStock

Breastfeeding may enhance a new mother's emotional bonding to her baby.

The Lactation Process When an infant suckles, nerves in the mother's nipple signal her brain to release **prolactin** and **oxytocin** (*ox-e-toe'-sin*) into her bloodstream. Prolactin stimulates specialized cells in breasts to form milk. These cells carry out the lactation process by making some nutrients and removing others from the mother's bloodstream and adding them to her milk. Oxytocin plays a different role in establishing successful lactation. This hormone signals breast tissue to "let down" milk.

The **let-down reflex** enables milk to travel in several tubes, called ducts, to the nipple area. A reflex is a physical response that's automatic and not under conscious control. When let-down occurs, the infant removes the milk by continued sucking. **Essential Concept 11.1** shows the major steps of the lactation process. Shortly before the flow of milk begins, the lactating woman often feels a tingling sensation in her nipples, a signal that let-down is occurring.

Essential Concept
11.1 The Lactation Process

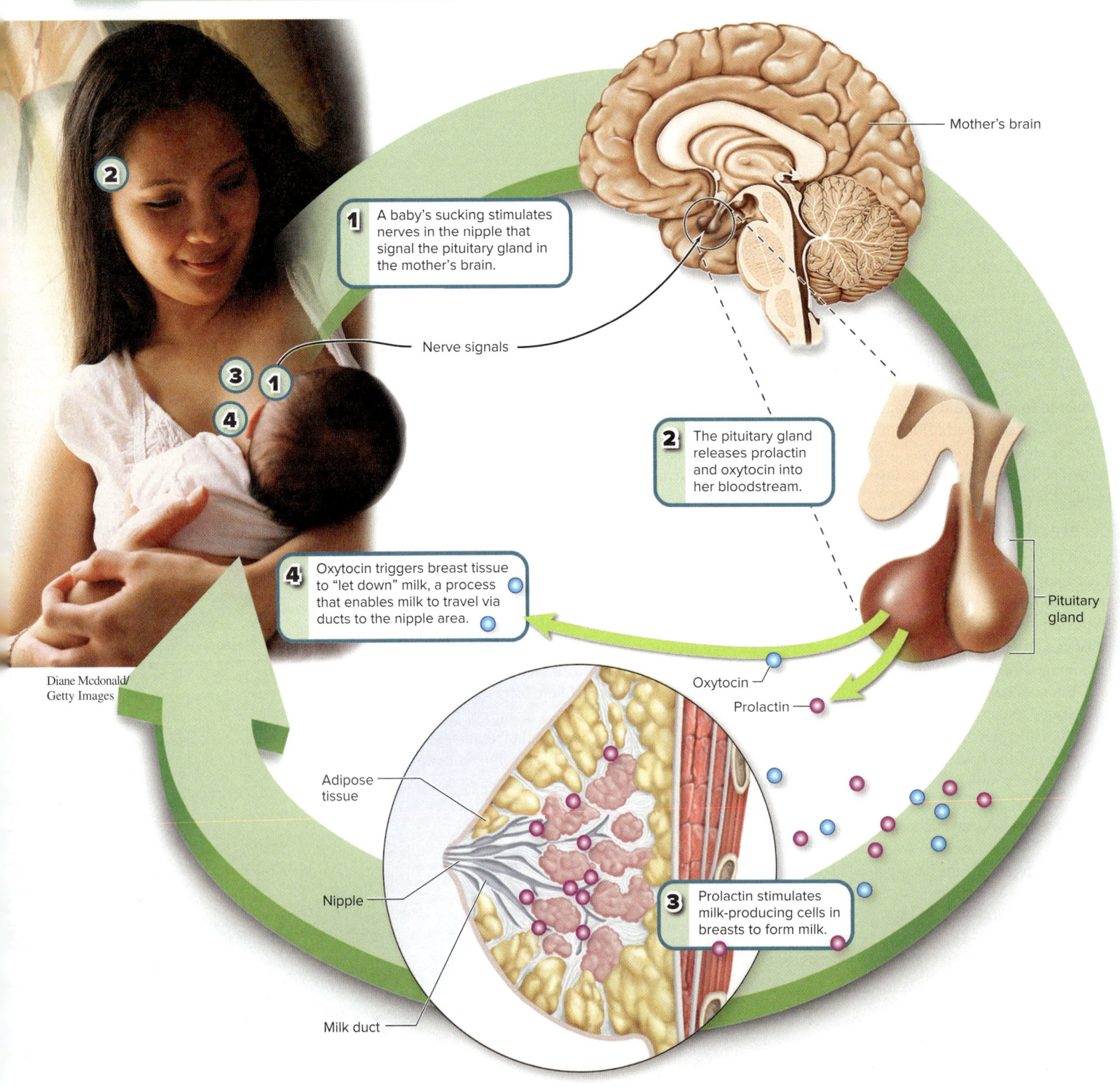

1. A baby's sucking stimulates nerves in the nipple that signal the pituitary gland in the mother's brain.
2. The pituitary gland releases prolactin and oxytocin into her bloodstream.
3. Prolactin stimulates milk-producing cells in breasts to form milk.
4. Oxytocin triggers breast tissue to "let down" milk, a process that enables milk to travel via ducts to the nipple area.

Diane Mcdonald/Getty Images

Embarrassment, emotional stress and tension, pain, and fatigue can easily block the let-down reflex. For example, if a lactating mother is tense or upset, let-down doesn't occur, and her infant will not be able to obtain milk when it suckles. When this happens, the hungry infant becomes frustrated and angry, and the mother may respond by becoming even more tense and upset, setting up a vicious cycle. At this point, new mothers often give up breastfeeding, reporting that they tried to suckle their babies but were unable to "produce" milk. It helps if new mothers are in a comfortable, relaxed environment when they breastfeed their babies.

It may take a few weeks for the new mother to feel confident as a member of a successful breastfeeding team with her baby. Milk production relies on "supply and demand." The more the infant suckles (demand), the more milk its mother's breasts produce (supply). However, if milk isn't fully removed from the breasts, milk production soon ceases. This is likely to occur when infants aren't hungry because they have been given baby food and formula to supplement breast milk feedings.

prolactin hormone that stimulates milk production after delivery

oxytocin hormone that causes the "let-down" response and the uterus to contract

let-down reflex automatic physical response to a breastfeeding infant that enables milk to reach the nipple area

Diet for a Lactating Woman No special foods are necessary to sustain milk production. However, a lactating woman should drink fluids to keep her body properly hydrated. For as long as she breastfeeds her baby, the lactating mother should limit her intake of alcohol-containing beverages because her body secretes the drug into her milk. A woman who breastfeeds her baby should also check with her physician before using any medications, even over-the-counter and herbal products, because such substances may also end up in her breast milk.

Breast Milk Is Best Milk

Breastfeeding offers several advantages for mother and child.[11]

For infants, human milk

- is free of bacteria as it leaves the breast;
- supplies antibodies and immune cells;
- is easily digested;
- reduces risk of food allergies, especially to proteins in infant formulas and cow's milk;
- changes in composition over time to meet the changing needs of a growing infant;
- contains zinc, iron, and other minerals in highly absorbable forms;
- decreases risks of ear, intestinal, and respiratory infections; and
- may reduce the risk of asthma, obesity, and type 1 diabetes in childhood.

For new mothers, breastfeeding

- reduces uterine bleeding after delivery,
- promotes shrinkage of the uterus to its prepregnancy size,
- decreases the risk of breast cancer (before menopause) and ovarian cancer,
- may promote maternal weight loss,
- may enhance emotional bonding with the infant, and
- is less expensive and more convenient than feeding infant formula.

For more information about breastfeeding, visit www.cdc.gov/ and search for "breastfeeding."

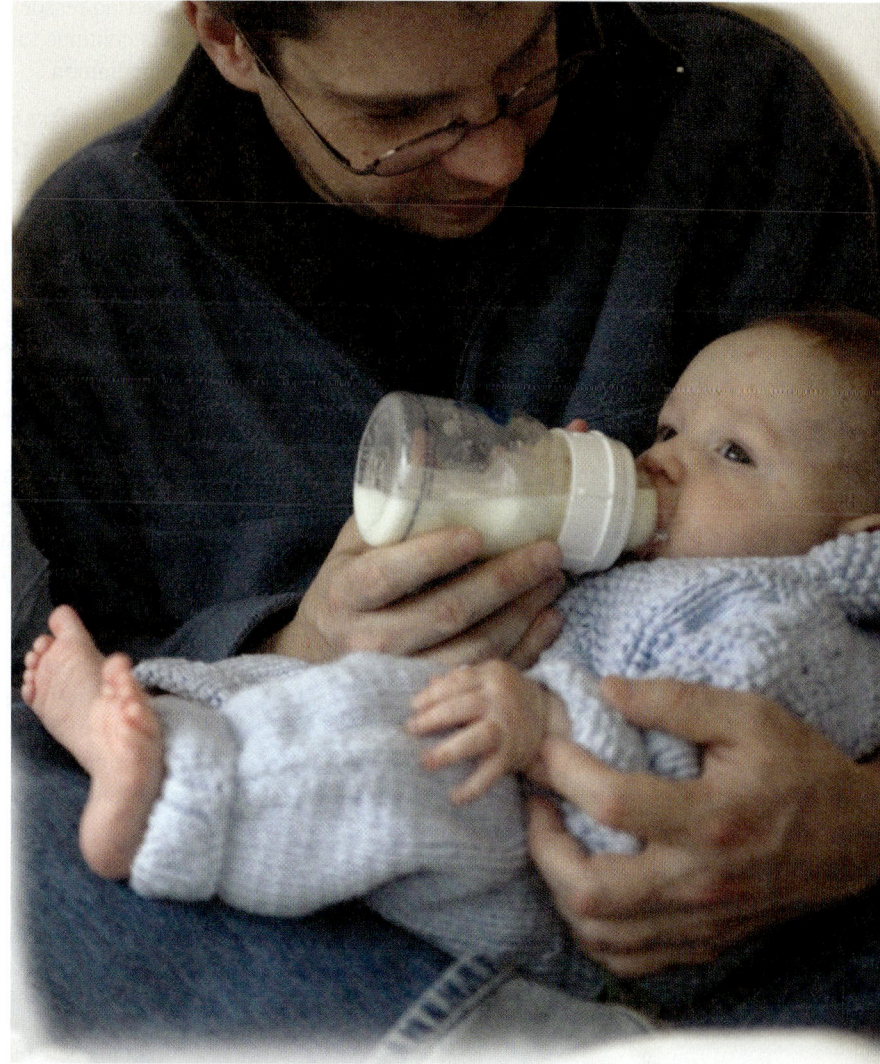

Aurora Photos/Alamy Stock Photo

A father can help meet his baby's nutritional needs by giving the infant breast milk that's been placed in a bottle.

Is Breast Milk a Complete Food? Registered dietitian nutritionists and pediatricians generally recommend that new mothers breastfeed their infants exclusively during their babies' first 6 months of life.[11] For most healthy infants, it's not necessary to supplement young infants' diets with other fluids, such as water, infant formula, and juices, or with solid foods, such as baby food. However, it is important to obtain prompt professional medical care to prevent a baby from becoming dehydrated, particularly if the infant is suffering from diarrhea, vomiting, or fever.

Although breast milk is highly nutritious, it's not a complete food for all infants. Human milk may contain inadequate amounts of vitamin D and the minerals iron and fluoride. The American Academy of Pediatrics (AAP) recommends all breastfed infants be given a supplement that supplies 400 IU of vitamin D per day.[11] Healthy breastfed newborns generally don't need an iron supplement until they're 4 months of age.[12] A fluoride supplement may be necessary for breastfed babies if the mother's water supply isn't fluoridated. Before giving any dietary supplements to their baby, parents or caregivers should discuss their infant's nutritional needs with the child's physician.

Kwame Zikomo/Purestock/SuperStock

After an infant reaches about 4 to 6 months of age, breastfeeding should continue, but the infant can also be offered some appropriate solid foods, especially foods that are sources of iron. Breastfeeding may be combined with infant foods until the child's first birthday. However, there's no reason why children cannot be breastfed for longer periods. Throughout the world, many mothers continue to nurse their babies well past the babies' first birthdays, but in the United States, this practice is uncommon.

Quitting Too Soon Nearly all healthy women are physically capable of breastfeeding their infants. In 2015, about 83% of American women started breastfeeding their babies soon after birth.[13] By their first birthday, only about 36% of the babies were still being nourished with their mother's milk.

Women who breastfeed their newborns often stop the practice within 6 months. There are many reasons why women discontinue nursing their infants too soon. New mothers often quit because they lack information about and support for breastfeeding their babies. Hospitals may employ lactation consultants who are trained to provide information and advice about breastfeeding to new mothers. An additional resource is La Leche League, an international organization dedicated to providing education and support for breastfeeding women (www.llli.org/).

Some women discontinue breastfeeding because of uncertainty over how much milk their babies are consuming. Baby bottles are marked to indicate ounces, so a mother who bottle-feeds her infant can easily measure the amount of formula consumed. A lactating mother, however, has to observe her baby for cues indicating the child's stomach is full. When a breastfeeding baby is no longer interested in nursing and stops, its mother has to assume the infant has had enough milk.

A well-nourished breastfed infant will gain weight normally and generally have six or more wet diapers as well as one or two bowel movements that consist of soft stools per day. Parents or caregivers who are concerned about their infants' food intake or nutritional status should consult their physician immediately.

Many new mothers discontinue breastfeeding too soon because they need to return to work and have caregivers feed their babies. Lactating women can learn to express milk from their breasts and chill it for later feedings (**Fig. 11.5**). However, many workplaces don't have comfortable, private facilities for women to express milk and then store it safely.

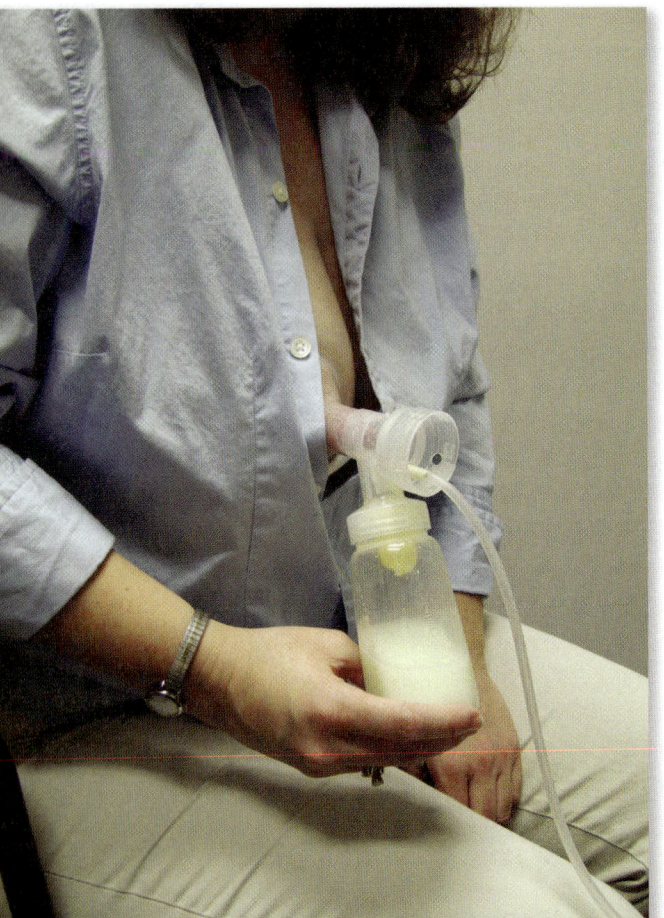

Wendy Schiff

Figure 11.5 Expressing milk. This new mother is expressing milk in a special room that was set up for this purpose at her workplace. She'll refrigerate the milk and take it home for later bottle feeding.

11.1e Infant Nutrition: Formula Feeding

Not every woman wants to breastfeed her baby and, in some instances, people other than the new mother must feed the infant when breast milk is not available. Infant formulas are nutritionally adequate and safe alternatives to mother's milk. Their nutrient compositions, however, aren't identical to human milk (**Table 11.4**). Furthermore, infant formulas do not supply human antibodies and other unique immune system factors that are in breast milk.

The fat content of human milk changes during each feeding, which usually lasts about 20 minutes. In the beginning of the session, the mother's milk is low in fat, but as her infant continues to suckle, the fat content of her milk gradually increases.[14] The higher fat content of the "hind milk" may make the baby feel satisfied and, as a result, discontinue feeding. Infant formulas, however, have uniform composition; that is, they don't change their fat content during a feeding session. Thus, the mother or infant caregiver is more likely to control the amount of formula the baby consumes, possibly leading to overfeeding.

Caregivers should provide an iron-fortified infant formula for babies who aren't breastfed. Not all infant formulas contain iron, so it's important to read the product's label before purchasing it. Formula-fed babies may also need a source of fluoride, but using municipal tap water that has been fluoridated to prepare concentrated infant formulas can ensure adequate fluoride intake.

Why Not Use Cow's Milk as a Formula?

Whole cow's milk shouldn't be fed to infants until they're 1 year of age.[12, 16] Cow's milk is too high in calcium, sodium, and protein, and it doesn't contain enough carbohydrate and essential fatty acids to meet an infant's needs. Essential fatty acids are critical for the development of an infant's nervous system, which includes the brain.

Infants have more difficulty digesting **casein** (*kay'-seen*), the major protein in cow's milk, than the major proteins in human milk. Cow's milk can also contribute to intestinal bleeding and iron deficiency.[12] Fat-reduced and fat-free cow's milk are too low in energy to be given to most children until they're 2 years of age. By then, the child should be eating a wide variety of foods in addition to milk, including sources of healthy fats and complex carbohydrates.

What About Allergies?
Compared to exclusively breastfed infants, formula-fed babies have a greater risk of developing allergic responses, especially *eczema* (patches of inflamed, itchy skin) and asthma.[17] Signs and symptoms of such allergies typically include the following:

- vomiting, intestinal pain, diarrhea, or constipation;
- eczema; and
- runny nose and breathing difficulties, such as asthma.

For babies who are allergic to infant formulas made from cow's milk proteins, similar products made with soy or other proteins are available.

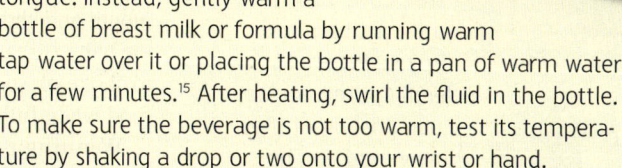

TASTY Tidbits

It's generally not recommended to heat bottles containing infant formula or human milk in a microwave oven. The heat can destroy immune factors in human milk and may create hot spots that can scald an infant's tongue. Instead, gently warm a bottle of breast milk or formula by running warm tap water over it or placing the bottle in a pan of warm water for a few minutes.[15] After heating, swirl the fluid in the bottle. To make sure the beverage is not too warm, test its temperature by shaking a drop or two onto your wrist or hand.

casein major protein in cow's milk

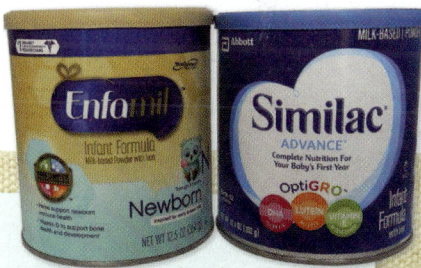

TABLE 11.4 COMPARING APPROXIMATE COMPOSITIONS OF HUMAN MILK AND IRON-FORTIFIED INFANT FORMULAS (PER OUNCE)

Milk or Iron-Fortified Formula	Energy (kcal/oz)	Protein (g/oz)	Carbohydrate (g/oz)	Fat (g/oz)	Cholesterol (mg/oz)	Iron (mg/oz)	Calcium (mg/oz)
Human milk	22.5	0.32	2.12	1.35	4.00	0.01	10.0
Cow's milk protein-based formulas							
Enfamil Premium Newborn®	20.0	0.42	2.25	1.06	0.00	0.36	16.0
Similac Advance®	20.0	0.41	2.10	1.06	1.12	0.36	16.0
Soy protein-based formulas							
ProSobee Lipil®	19.0	0.50	1.86	1.07	0.00	0.36	21.0
Similac Isomil Advance®	20.0	0.49	2.04	1.09	0.00	0.36	21.0

Microwave oven: Steve Wisbauer/Getty Images; Formula cans: Wendy Schiff; Placemat: McGraw-Hill Education/Mark A. Dierker, photographer

TASTY Tidbits

You can make your own baby food by taking plain, unseasoned cooked foods and pureeing them in a blender. If a large amount of the item is blended, the pureed food can be poured into an ice cube tray, covered with a plastic bag, and frozen. When it's feeding time, an ice cube portion of the baby food can be popped out of the tray and warmed.

extrusion reflex involuntary response in which a young infant thrusts its tongue forward when a solid or semisolid object is placed in its mouth

weaning gradual process of shifting from breastfeeding or bottle-feeding to drinking from a cup and eating solid foods

11.1f Infant Nutrition: Solid Foods

Many new parents are eager to start feeding their young infants solid food. Solid foods shouldn't be introduced to infants until they're about 6 months of age.[16] Why? Infants are born with the **extrusion reflex,** an involuntary response that occurs when a solid or semisolid object is placed in an infant's mouth. As a result of this reflex, a young baby thrusts its tongue forward, pushing the object out of its mouth. Thus, trying to feed the young infant solid foods is a messy, frustrating process because the child's tongue automatically pushes the food out of its mouth. Liquid foods, such as breast milk or infant formula, don't elicit the extrusion reflex, so the baby swallows fluids.

As the infant reaches about 4 to 6 months of age, the extrusion reflex disappears. Moreover, a 6-month-old infant can usually sit up with little or no back support and coordinate enough muscular control to open his or her mouth and show readiness to accept solid foods.[18] These signs indicate the baby is ready physically to swallow soft solid foods, is less likely to choke on such foods, and can turn his or her head away from food when full.

Weaning is the gradual process of shifting an infant from breastfeeding or bottle-feeding to drinking from a cup and eating solid foods. According to current recommendations, caregivers should begin introducing single-ingredient foods, along with breastmilk or formula, when the baby is between 4 and 6 months of age.[19] Typical first foods include rice cereal ("baby cereal"), ground meat or chicken mixed with breastmilk or formula, pureed green beans or squash ("baby vegetables"), and mashed bananas. If, after the child consumes the food for about 3 to 5 days, the new food appears to be tolerated by the baby, the caregiver should introduce another new food and watch the infant for any negative reactions, such as diarrhea, vomiting, skin rash, or runny nose.

In the past, highly allergenic foods, such as peanut butter, fish, and eggs, weren't introduced into a baby's diet until the child was at least 1 year of age. However, results of current studies indicate that *delaying* such foods may *increase* the child's risk of food allergies.[19] For example, feeding a small amount of peanut butter that has been diluted with water to a baby who is 4 to 6 months of age may prevent the infant from developing peanut allergy later in childhood. Foods that are often thought to be allergenic can be introduced to a baby in very small amounts after the typical first foods have been consumed without causing health problems.[20] If the infant doesn't show signs of an allergic reaction to the food, the child can be fed higher amounts of the item. Parents and other caregivers should always check with the infant's physician for advice on when to start feeding a new food to the child.

At about 6 to 8 months of age, the baby's first set of teeth, the "primary teeth," begin to appear. These teeth are important for proper nutrition because they help the child bite and chew food. By 8 to 12 months of age, most infants can use their fingers to pick up and chew "finger foods" such as crackers, toast, and cooked string beans. Babies can also hold a bottle and practice drinking from a special cup ("sippy cup") that has a lid with a spout **(Fig. 11.6).** By about 10 months of age, many infants are mastering self-feeding and making the transition from baby foods to menu items the rest of the family enjoys. Babies need to practice self-feeding skills, even if it means playing with food and creating messes.

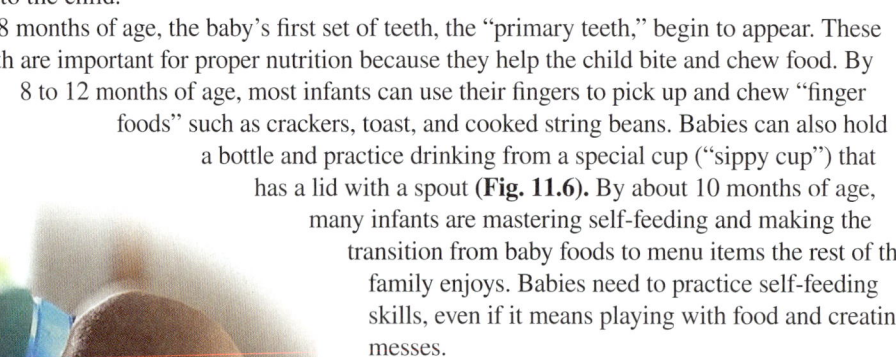

Figure 11.6 Drinking from a "sippy cup." Such cups as well as baby bottles can also provide food for molds and other microbes, so clean them thoroughly after each use.

Blender: PhotoSpin, Inc/Alamy; Baby food: Wendy Schiff; Toddler drinking from sippy cup: Amanda Ice

Nutrition Fact or Fiction?

Adding solid foods to infants' diets helps babies sleep through the night.

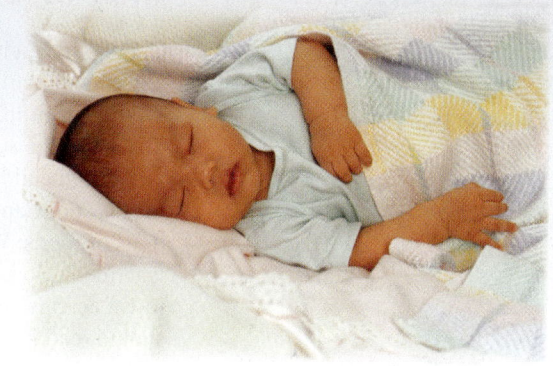

It's normal for young infants to fall asleep at night and wake up a few hours later. The developmental milestone of "sleeping through the night" generally occurs around 3 to 4 months of age, regardless of what infants are eating. Feeding solid foods to babies who are that age may actually help them sleep longer.[21]

What Not to Feed Infants

Certain foods and beverages are not appropriate for infants. Avoid feeding

- ***Honey.*** This product may contain spores of *Clostridium botulinum*, which can produce a potentially fatal toxin in children who are under 1 year old (see Unit 5).
- ***Semisolid baby food in a baby bottle that has the nipple opening enlarged.*** This practice may contribute to overfeeding and doesn't help the child learn self-feeding skills.
- ***Candy, flavored gelatin water, or soft drinks.*** These items provide few micronutrients and displace more nutritious fluids and foods from the infant's diet.
- ***Small pieces of hard or coarse foods.*** Foods such as hot dogs cut into "coin" shapes, whole nuts, grapes, chunks of cooked meat, raw carrots, popcorn, and spoonfuls of peanut butter can cause choking. Caregivers should supervise meals to keep young children from stuffing too much food in their mouths.
- ***Juice.*** The fructose contained in juice can lead to diarrhea. Also, if the infant drinks fruit juice or fruit drinks rather than breast milk or infant formula, the child may not be receiving adequate amounts of calcium and other essential minerals.
- ***Unpasteurized (raw) milk or juices.*** Unpasteurized milk and juice may be contaminated with bacteria or viruses.
- ***Goat's milk.*** Goat's milk is low in iron, folate, and vitamins C and D.

pasteurization process that kills the disease-causing microbes in foods and beverages as well as many microbes responsible for spoilage

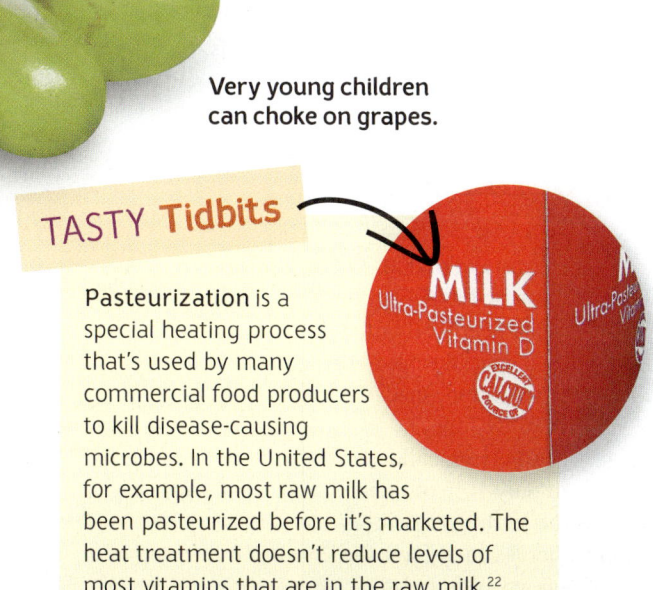

Very young children can choke on grapes.

TASTY Tidbits

Pasteurization is a special heating process that's used by many commercial food producers to kill disease-causing microbes. In the United States, for example, most raw milk has been pasteurized before it's marketed. The heat treatment doesn't reduce levels of most vitamins that are in the raw milk.[22]

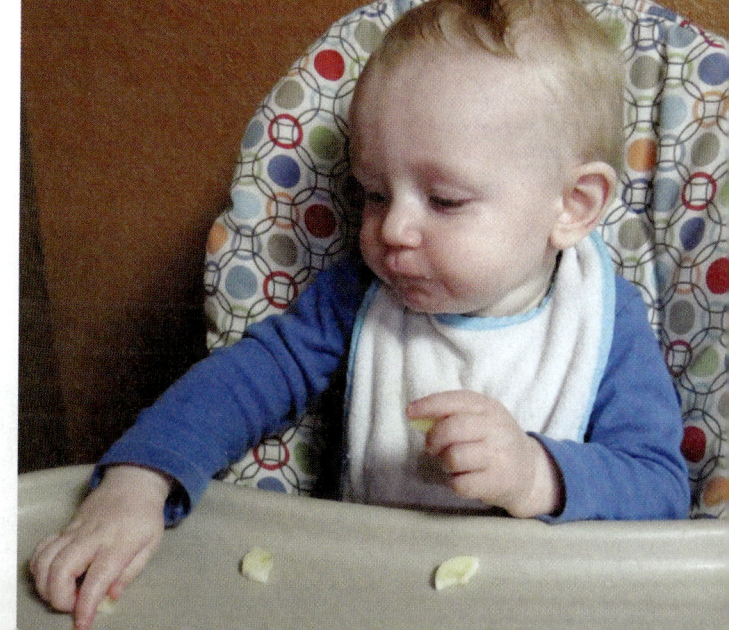

Sleeping baby: Elyse Lewin/Exactostock-1555/SuperStock; Grapes: Purestock/SuperStock; Milk carton: Wendy Schiff; Baby feeding himself: Stacy Schmitt

11.1g Nutrition for a Healthy Childhood

Childhood can be divided into the preschool period (2 to 5 years of age), the school-age period (6 to 11 years of age), and adolescence (12 to 19 years of age). The rapid growth rate that characterizes the first 12 months of life tapers off quickly during the preschool years and proceeds at a slow but steady rate until the end of the school-age period.

When a child's growth rate slows, the youngster's appetite decreases because he or she doesn't need as much food. Caregivers must recognize that children don't have the stomach capacity to eat adult-size portions of foods. When planning meals for children, caregivers should emphasize nutrient-dense foods, such as lean meats, low-fat dairy products, whole-grain cereals, fruits, nuts, and vegetables. Although many ready-to-eat cereals are sweetened with sugar, it's not necessary to eliminate such foods. Caregivers, however, should read product labels and choose varieties with less added sugar. Additionally, it's important to monitor children's intake of sweets because sugary items can crowd out more nutritious foods from their diets.

During adolescence, the child experiences **puberty,** the stage of life in which a person reaches physical maturity and is capable of reproduction. Adolescence also features a period of dramatic increases in height and weight that's referred to as the **adolescent growth spurt.** To provide the energy and nutrients needed to support such rapid growth rates, a youngster's food intake increases accordingly. If maturing boys and girls choose to eat nutritious foods and maintain a high level of physical activity, they can take advantage of their increased hunger and gain lean body mass without gaining excess body fat. The MyPlate food guide can provide the basis for healthy adolescents to plan nutritionally adequate meals and snacks.

Theresa, the mother featured in the unit opener, is concerned about the influence she has over her young child's snacking habits. She's his role model for food choices and physical activity habits. If she eats a variety of nutrient-dense foods and is more physically active, he's more likely to eat such foods and be active as well.

What About Snacks?

Snacking isn't necessarily a bad habit, especially if snacks are nutrient dense and fit into the child's overall diet and energy needs. Nutritious snacks can be offered at midmorning or midafternoon, when the child is likely to become hungry between meals. Some nutritious snacks include

- peanut butter spread on graham crackers;
- smoothies made with plain yogurt, orange juice, and fresh fruit;
- fruit salad, dried fruit, or cut-up fresh fruit;
- mini-pizzas (half an English muffin, topped with tomato sauce and Mozzarella cheese, and heated in toaster oven);
- ready-to-eat cereal;
- peanuts, cashews, or sunflower seeds;
- whole-wheat crackers with cheese cubes; and
- vegetable sticks dipped in hummus.

puberty stage of life in which a person matures physically and is capable of reproduction

adolescent growth spurt period associated with puberty when a child's height and weight rapidly increase

Culture & Cuisine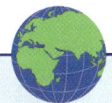

A recent study compared the snacking practices of over 3000 American and Chinese children who were between 4 and 13 years of age.[23] Results of the study indicated that nearly all of the American children consumed snacks, including fruit, flavored-water beverages, and candy. For the American children, snacks contributed about 25% of their daily calories. The Chinese youngsters were less likely to snack than the American children. Furthermore, the Chinese children consumed only 10% of their daily energy intake from snacks. Fruit was the leading calorie-containing snack of the Chinese children, whereas candy was the leading calorie-containing snack of the American youngsters. Regardless of one's age, consuming too many sugary snacks can contribute to an unhealthy amount of body fat.

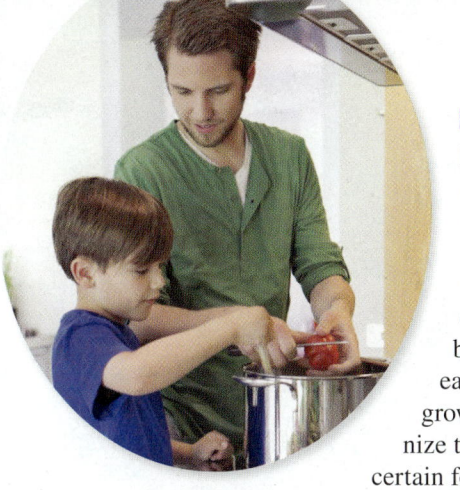

Fostering Positive Eating Behaviors

Parents often refer to their young children as "picky eaters" because the youngsters don't eat everything offered to them. Furthermore, it's not unusual for preschool children to have "food jags," periods in which they refuse to eat a food that they liked in the past or want to eat only a particular food, such as peanut butter and jelly sandwiches or cereal and milk. Picky eating and food jags may be expressions of a child's growing need for independence. It's important to recognize that everyone, including a child, is entitled to dislike certain foods. Caregivers should avoid nagging, forcing, and bribing children to eat. Instead, caregivers can offer the children a variety of healthy foods each day and allow the youngsters to choose which items and how much to eat.

Healthy children aren't in danger of starving if they skip a meal. A child who isn't hungry at mealtimes may have eaten a snack before the meal at a friend's home. If a child's lack of appetite persists, caretakers should consult the child's physician to rule out illness.

The following tips can help you improve your child's diet:

- Use the recommendations of MyPlate (see Unit 3) to guide your family's food choices and avoid dictating what they eat.
- Eat meals together as a family as often as possible.
- Encourage your child to help with food selection and preparation.
- Don't place your child on a restrictive diet unless the diet is recommended by the child's physician.
- Avoid using food as a reward or punishment.
- Encourage your child to drink water instead of sugar-sweetened beverages.
- Keep healthy snacks on hand.
- Serve at least five servings of fruits and vegetables each day.
- Discourage eating meals or snacks while watching TV.
- Encourage your child to eat a nutrient-dense breakfast daily.

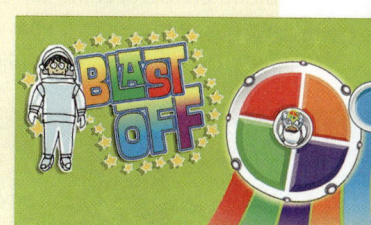

TASTY Tidbits

The MyPlate website has a special series of web pages for children over 5 years of age. Children can visit the website and play the interactive "Blast Off Game." To test this game and others, visit www.fns.usda.gov/tn/games-and-activities.

Source: USDA, https://www.fns.usda.gov/apps/BlastOff/BlastOff_Game.html Accessed: July 14, 2019

Common Nutrition-Related Concerns

Nutrition-related problems that often affect children are iron deficiency, poor calcium intake, and obesity.

Iron Deficiency Iron deficiency can lead to decreased physical stamina, learning ability, and resistance to infection. The best way to prevent iron deficiency in children is to provide foods that are good sources of iron, such as lean meat and enriched breads and cereals. Unit 9 provides more information about iron deficiency.

Poor Calcium Intakes Over the last 20 years, many adolescents have switched from drinking milk to drinking soft drinks, including energy drinks. Dietitians and other nutrition experts are concerned that many adolescents have inadequate calcium intakes because of this practice. Inadequate calcium intake during adolescence is associated with decreased bone mass and increased likelihood of bone fractures later in life. Adolescents should consume 3 cups/day of fat-free or low-fat milk or equivalent dairy products daily. Furthermore, teenagers need to be aware that physical activity can strengthen bones, whereas smoking cigarettes is a risk factor for osteoporosis (see Unit 9).

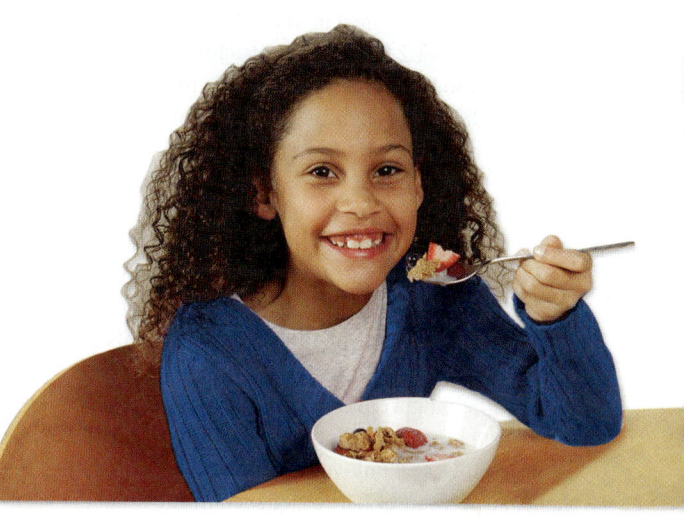

Caregivers should encourage older children to eat a nutrient-dense breakfast daily.

Cooks in the kitchen: Eric Audras/SuperStock; Blast Off game: United States Department of Agriculture (USDA); Girl eating cereal: McGraw-Hill Education/Eclipse Studios

Obesity The prevalence of obesity has increased for all American children over the past few decades. One in five children and adolescents is obese.[24] Obese children often have higher-than-normal blood pressure, cholesterol, and glucose levels.[25] Obese youngsters are also more likely to have low self-esteem, sleep apnea, heartburn, fatty liver disease, and musculoskeletal problems. Such children are at risk to develop hypertension, heart disease, and type 2 diabetes later in life. Furthermore, obese children are more likely to mature into obese adults than children who have healthy body weights.[25]

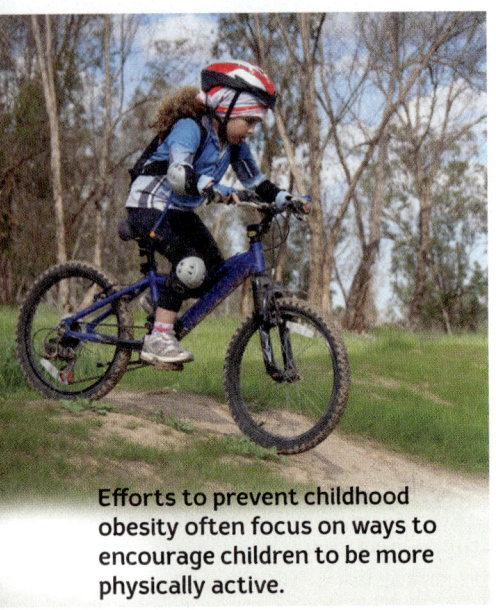

Efforts to prevent childhood obesity often focus on ways to encourage children to be more physically active.

There's no single cause of excess body fat in children, but researchers have identified factors that are associated with the development of the condition. These factors include having an obese mother who gained an excessive amount of weight during pregnancy and a high birth weight.[26] Furthermore, youngsters who consume too many energy-dense foods and beverages that are sources of empty calories are also at risk of gaining excess fat in childhood.[25]

A major challenge is preventing childhood obesity without negatively affecting normal growth and development. Caregivers may need to limit the obese child's intake of empty calories. These items often replace more nutrient-dense or lower-calorie foods in children's diets.

Aside from making poor dietary choices, physical inactivity also contributes to excessive weight gain in childhood.[25] For many children, media use, such as viewing television programs and playing computer games, replaces physical activities that burn more energy. Children who spend more than 2 hours a day watching TV or using a computer are more likely to be overweight or obese than children who spend less than 2 hours a day using such entertainment media.[27]

Public health efforts to prevent childhood obesity often focus on ways for children to be more physically active. Children need at least 60 minutes of aerobic physical activity most days of the week.[28] If children are not obtaining enough physical activity while at school, their caregivers can enroll them in after-school sports or community-based exercise programs. Being physically active will help children not only to attain healthy body weights but also to maintain healthy body weights later in life.

When helping a child lose weight, caregivers should avoid scolding or nagging the youngster because doing so can make the child rebel against adults, feel unloved and depressed, and dislike his or her body shape. As a result of harboring such negative feelings, an obese child may become vulnerable to developing disordered eating practices or eating disorders.

11.1h Nutrition for Older Adults

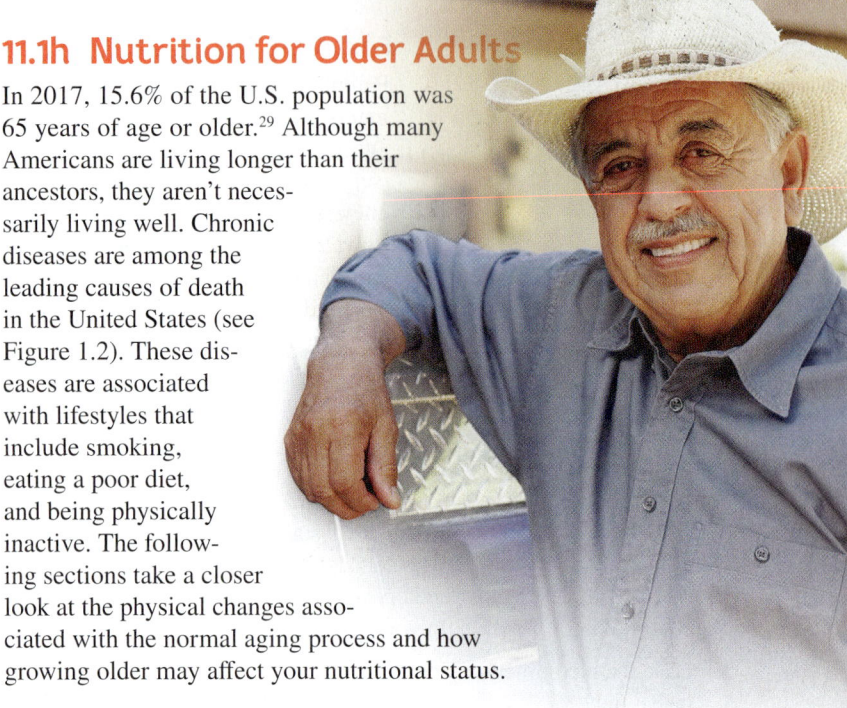

In 2017, 15.6% of the U.S. population was 65 years of age or older.[29] Although many Americans are living longer than their ancestors, they aren't necessarily living well. Chronic diseases are among the leading causes of death in the United States (see Figure 1.2). These diseases are associated with lifestyles that include smoking, eating a poor diet, and being physically inactive. The following sections take a closer look at the physical changes associated with the normal aging process and how growing older may affect your nutritional status.

The Aging Process

The aging process begins at conception and is characterized by numerous predictable physical changes. Your body ages, regardless of the dietary and other health-related practices you are following. By the time you're 70 years of age, you'll have reached the final life stage—older adulthood. Growing old is a normal and natural process. **Table 11.5** presents some of the physical changes you can expect to occur as your body ages.

As the human body ages, its need for energy decreases; muscle mass declines as some muscle cells shrink or die. The age-related loss of muscle mass (*sarcopenia*) leads to a decrease in muscular strength and basal metabolism. The aging body typically loses lean tissue and gains fat tissue. Increased body fat results from overeating and lack of physical activity, but even athletic men and lean women usually gain some central body fat after they're 50 years of age. Being overweight or obese may increase the bone density of older adults and result in stronger bones, but having too much body fat increases the risk of type 2 diabetes, hypertension, cardiovascular disease, and osteoarthritis.

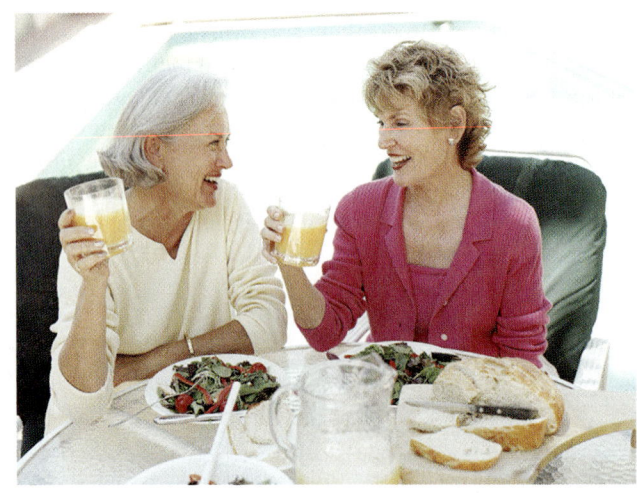

Child biking: Ilan Shacham/Getty Images; Man wearing hat: Dave and Les Jacobs/Blend Images LLC; Women having lunch: BananaStock/Alamy Stock Photo

Table 11.5 Aging: Normal Physical Changes

Body System	Changes
Digestive	Reduced saliva and stomach acid secretion; increased heartburn and constipation
Skin, hair, and nails (integument)	Graying hair; drier skin and hair; skin loses elasticity and forms wrinkles; skin bruises easily
Musculoskeletal	Bone-forming cells become less active, resulting in bone loss that can lead to tooth loss and bones that fracture easily; fractures heal more slowly; joints become stiff and painful; muscle mass declines, resulting in loss of strength and stamina
Nervous	Decreased brain weight, reduced production of chemicals that transmit information between nerves, delayed transmission of nervous impulses, loss of short-term memory, and reduced sensory abilities (e.g., vision, hearing, smell, and taste)
Lymphatic (immune)	Reduced functioning resulting in increased vulnerability to cancer and infections
Circulatory	Hardening of the arteries, reduced heart output, increased risk of blood clots
Endocrine	Decreased production of reproductive, growth, and thyroid hormones
Respiratory	Reduced lung capacity, increased vulnerability to respiratory infections
Urinary	Increased loss of functional kidney cells, resulting in decreased blood filtration rate; loss of bladder control

TASTY Tidbits

A few foods interfere with prescribed drugs. Grapefruit juice, for example, can alter the potency of certain medications that are used to lower blood pressure or cholesterol. Therefore, people who take such medications should avoid consuming grapefruits and grapefruit juice.

Wendy Schiff

Physical Inactivity Many of the undesirable physical changes we associate with growing old are the result of a lifetime of physical inactivity. A physically active lifestyle increases muscle strength and mobility, improves balance, slows bone loss, and boosts emotional well-being. Before embarking on a program to increase physical fitness, however, sedentary older adults should consult their physicians concerning appropriate activities.

Older Adults: Common Nutrition-Related Concerns

Compared to younger persons, older adults have greater risk of nutritional deficiencies because their food intake tends to decrease as their metabolic rates and physical activity levels decline. Nutrients that are very important for the health of older adults are protein, omega-3 fats, fiber, calcium, magnesium, potassium, and the vitamins folate, B-12, B-6, D, E, and K.[30] Despite having lower energy needs, however, older adults need the same or even higher amounts of vitamins and minerals.

Meeting micronutrient needs while eating less food can be difficult for older persons to accomplish. Older adults tend to consume more than recommended amounts of sodium, saturated fat, and added sugars. Their diets, however, generally don't provide enough fiber, calcium, magnesium, potassium, zinc, and vitamins A, B-6, C, D, E, and folate.[31]

MyPlate can provide the basis for planning nutritionally adequate meals and snacks for healthy older adults. However, amounts of foods recommended in these diet plans may not provide enough vitamin D and calcium for elderly persons. In many instances, older adults can also benefit from taking a daily multiple vitamin/mineral supplement. Older adults who live at home may need professional help planning nutritionally adequate diets.

Numerous factors can negatively influence an older person's nutritional status, including medications, lack of social support, and low income. Many older adults take one or more prescription drugs and/or herbal dietary supplements daily. Such medications and products may interfere with the body's absorption and/or use of certain nutrients. Older people who live alone and on fixed incomes are at risk of undernutrition. Social isolation and low incomes are associated with emotional depression and inability to afford adequate amounts of nutritious food.

Physical factors associated with the aging process also affect food intake. Older adults may eat less because they have lost the ability to taste, smell, and/or chew food. People who lack normal cognitive functioning (thought processes) may be unable to make decisions regarding planning nutritious meals, as well as to shop for and prepare food. Chronic health problems such as arthritis and osteoporosis can interfere with mobility and flexibility, and can also interfere with food shopping and preparation activities.

In many instances, very old people refuse to eat and, as a result, lose considerable amounts of weight—a situation that hastens their death. Monitoring the elderly individual's weight can indicate whether long-term food intake has been adequate. If weight loss becomes significant, a physician should be consulted to determine the cause.

Nutrition Resources for Older Adults

You can often obtain information regarding locally available nutrition services for older people from medical clinics, health departments, hospitals, and health maintenance organizations in your area. To learn more about nutrition and aging, as well as health conditions that often affect older adults, visit the National Institute on Aging, www.nia.nih.gov/. For information about nutrition support programs for older adults, visit Administration for Community Living, https://acl.gov/ and search for "nutrition services."

Module 11.2

How Safe Is My Food?

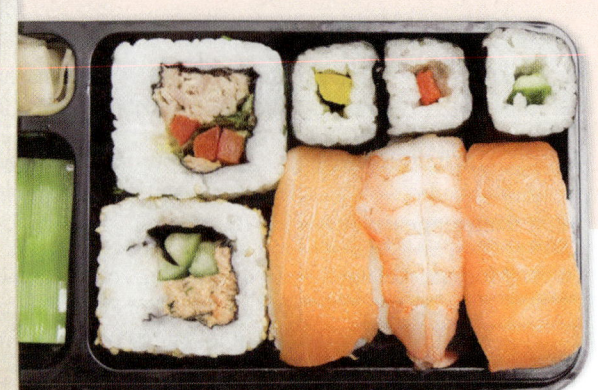

11.2 - Learning Outcomes

After reading Module 11.2, you should be able to

1. Define all of the **key terms** in this module.
2. Discuss the government's role in protecting the food supply.
3. List some common types and sources of pathogens that can cause food-borne illness.
4. Describe signs and symptoms of common food-borne illnesses.
5. Identify sources of contaminants in food.
6. Describe ways you can reduce the risk of food-borne illness.

Food-borne illness occurs when microscopic agents (microbes) or their toxic by-products enter food and they're consumed. Each year, about 1 in 6 Americans becomes sick from various food-borne illnesses.[32] Of those persons who contract such ailments, 128,000 require hospitalization and over 3000 die. In the United States, water-borne disease-causing agents aren't major health threats because municipal water supplies follow government guidelines for sanitation.

Which foods are most likely to be responsible for food-borne illness? How can you reduce the risk of contracting one of these illnesses? Which government agencies monitor the safety of the U.S. food supply? After reading Module 11.2, you'll know answers to these questions.

TASTY Tidbits

You cannot always rely on your senses to judge the wholesomeness of a food. A food can taste, smell, and appear safe to eat, but it may contain pathogens and/or their toxic by-products.

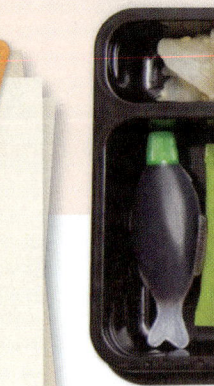

11.2a The Role of Government Agencies in Food Safety

The United States has one of the safest food supplies in the world, primarily the result of efforts conducted by cooperating governmental agencies that regulate and monitor the production and distribution of food. The Food and Drug Administration (FDA) of the U.S. Department of Health and Human Services and the U.S. Department of Agriculture (USDA) are the key federal agencies that protect consumers by regulating the country's food industry. Your local health department is responsible for inspecting grocery stores, dairy farms, food processing companies, and restaurants. In many communities, restaurants are required to post their sanitation rating where customers can easily see it.

After you obtain foods and bring them into your home, it becomes your responsibility to reduce the risk of food-borne illness by handling the items properly. However, if you suspect that something you consumed made you or a family member very sick, you should contact your physician for treatment. The physician may decide to report the case of food-borne illness to local public health officials so they can investigate and determine the source of your infection.

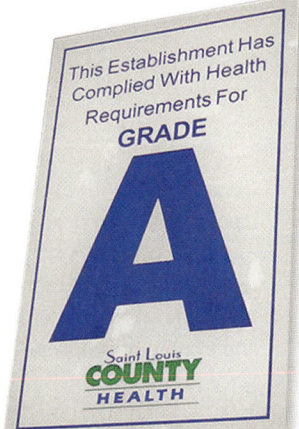

In many communities, local health departments inspect restaurants for food-related safety problems. The restaurants must display their rating for sanitation where customers can see it.

11.2b Potential Dangers in Your Food

For thousands of years, people have used certain microbes to produce a variety of foods, including hard cheeses, raised breads, pickled foods, and alcoholic beverages. Such microbes are desirable when they preserve foods and make foods more tasty. Other kinds of microbes grow and multiply in food, but their metabolic by-products spoil

food-borne illness infection caused by microscopic disease-causing agents in food

Sushi: Image Source/Glow Images; Nose: Ingram Publishing; FDA logo: U.S. Food and Drug Administration; Grade A sign: Wendy Schiff

What IS That?

Bioengineering involves scientific methods that alter an animal or plant's hereditary material (DNA). For example, genes that produce a desirable trait are transferred from one organism into the DNA of a second organism, altering its genes. According to a report published by the National Academy of Sciences in 2016, there's no scientific evidence that indicates bioengineered foods are unsafe for humans to consume or harmful to the environment.[33]

In 2016, the U.S. government passed the National Bioengineered Food Disclosure Law, which requires a national standard for identifying foods that are bioengineered or may be bioengineered. The U.S. Department of Agriculture (USDA) released the standard in 2018. A bioengineered food may be commonly referred to as a genetically modified organism (GMO) or having ingredients from genetically modified organisms.

By 2022, food manufacturers must use an approved method to identify a bioengineered food (BE food), such as the package logo shown in this feature. According to the Standard, **BE foods** contain detectable genetic material that's been modified by certain scientific methods. Furthermore, a BE food isn't found in nature or the result of conventional breeding techniques. For a list of BE foods, visit the USDA's Agricultural Marketing Service website (www.ams.usda.gov) and search for "list of bioengineered foods."

---

the food, making it unfit for human consumption. In some instances, disease-causing agents (**pathogens**) contaminate the food. When pathogens enter your food, they can cause vomiting, diarrhea, intestinal cramps, and other signs and symptoms of food-borne illness.

Food-borne pathogens include the following disease-causing agents:

- **Bacteria**—single-cell microorganisms, such as forms of *Clostridium* (*kloss-trid'-ee-um*), *Escherichia* (*esh'-er-ee'-ke-ah*), and *Salmonella* (*sall'-mo-nell'-ah*).
- **Viruses**—microscopic agents that can cause infections, such as norovirus and the virus that causes hepatitis A.
- **Molds**—simple microbes that live on dead or decaying organic matter. Scientists classify molds as *fungi*. Some fungi are beneficial and edible, such as baker's yeast, button mushrooms, and the mold in blue cheese. Other fungi contain toxins that can cause organ failure or liver cancer.
- **Protists**—generally tiny, single-cell organisms that can have the characteristics of animals, plants, or fungi. *Giardia* (*jee-ar'-dee-ah*) is a single-cell protist that often contaminates natural water sources such as ponds and lakes **(Fig. 11.7)**.
- **Parasitic worms**—worms that may be harmful to health because they live in the body. *Trichinella* (*trick'-in-el'-lah*) and *Anisakis* (*ah'-nah-say'-kis*) **(Fig. 11.8)** are parasitic worms that are food-borne pathogens.

Many kinds of food-borne pathogens can infect your digestive tract, inflaming the tissues and causing an "upset stomach" within a few hours after being ingested. A few types of food-borne pathogens multiply in your intestinal tract, enter your bloodstream, and cause general illness when they invade other tissues. When this happens, the sickness is called a food-borne infection. Other pathogens don't sicken you directly, but these microbes contaminate food and secrete poisons (toxins). When you eat the contaminated food, the toxins irritate your intestinal tract and cause a type of food-borne illness called **food intoxication** ("food poisoning"). Many of the foods you eat regularly, such as meats, eggs, milk, and products made from milk, are high-risk foods because they support the growth of food-borne pathogens.

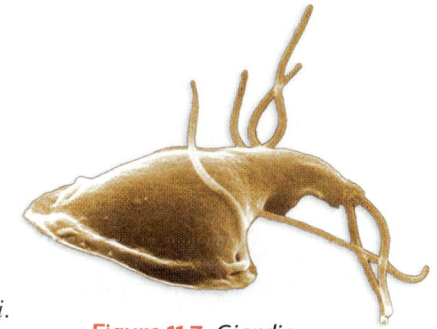

Figure 11.7 *Giardia*.

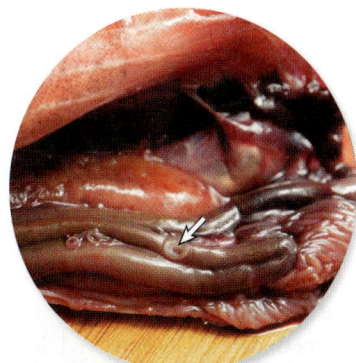

Figure 11.8 *Anisakis*.

BE foods foods that contain detectable genetic material that's been modified by certain scientific methods

pathogens disease-causing microbes

bacteria simple single-cell microorganisms

viruses microscopic agents that can cause infections

molds simple microbes that live on dead or decaying organic matter

protists tiny, single-cell organisms that can have the characteristics of animals, plants, or fungi

parasitic worms worms that are pathogens because they live in the body

food intoxication illness that results when poisons produced by certain microbes contaminate food and irritate the intestinal tract

Bioengineered logo: Source: U.S. Department of Agriculture (USDA); *Giardia*: Source: Dr. Stan Erlandsen and Dr. Dennis Feely/CDC; *Anisakis*: Purino/Shutterstock

incubation period a length of time in which pathogens need to multiply in food or the digestive tract before they can cause illness

11.2c Signs and Symptoms of Common Food-Borne Illnesses

In most cases, otherwise healthy individuals who suffer from common types of food-borne illness recover completely and without professional medical care within a few days. However, vomiting, diarrhea, and other signs of illness can be so severe that the patient requires hospitalization. You should consult a physician when an intestinal disorder is accompanied by one or more of the following signs:

- fever (oral temperature above 101.5°F),
- bloody bowel movements,
- prolonged vomiting that reduces fluid intake,
- diarrhea that lasts more than 3 days, and
- dehydration.[32]

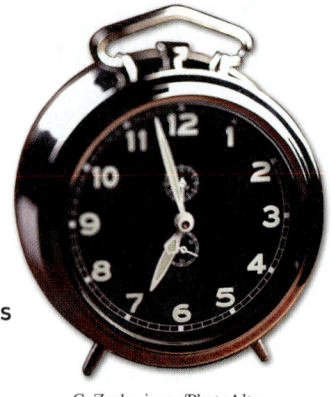

Some food-borne illnesses develop within 1 to 12 hours after eating the contaminated food.

C. Zachariasen/PhotoAlto

Most pathogens have an **incubation period,** a length of time in which they grow and multiply in food or the digestive tract before they can cause illness. Thus, if you develop signs and symptoms of a food-borne illness, you might have difficulty identifying the source of the infection or intoxication. Was the vomiting and diarrhea that you experienced at 7 A.M. the result of eating soft-cooked eggs 24 hours earlier or the sliced deli chicken you ate for lunch 2 days ago?

Many people mistakenly report that they have the "stomach flu," when they're actually suffering from a food- or water-borne illness. "Flu," or influenza, is an infectious disease caused by specific viruses that invade the respiratory tract. Influenza is characterized by coughing, fever, weakness, and body aches. On the other hand, food-borne illness primarily affects the digestive system and not the respiratory system. Intestinal cramps, diarrhea, and vomiting aren't typical signs and symptoms of influenza, and coughing isn't a usual sign of a food-borne illness. Thus, it's inaccurate to call a bout of diarrhea and intestinal cramps the "stomach flu."

Table 11.6 provides a summary of some common pathogens and signs and symptoms of the food-borne illnesses they cause.

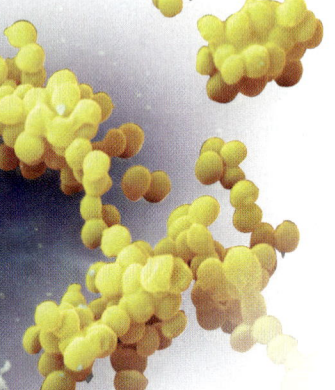

Staphylococcus aureus

Eye of Science/Science Source

Table 11.6 Common Sources of Food-Borne Illness

Pathogen	High-Risk Foods	Approx. Time of Onset	Typical Signs and Symptoms
Bacteria			
Campylobacter jejuni	Raw, undercooked poultry; raw milk; contaminated water	2–5 days	Diarrhea (often bloody), abdominal cramping, vomiting, fever
Clostridium botulinum (toxin)	Vacuum-packed foods, improperly canned foods, garlic-in-oil mixtures. Honey may contain spores.	18–36 hours	Vomiting, diarrhea, blurry or double vision, difficulty swallowing, muscular weakness. Can be fatal
Clostridium perfringens (toxin)	Cooked meat, poultry, casseroles, gravies	8–22 hours	Watery diarrhea, severe abdominal cramps
Escherichia coli O157:H7 (toxin)	Raw ground beef, raw seed sprouts, raw leafy greens, fresh fruit, raw milk, unpasteurized juices, foods contaminated with feces	2 hours to 6 days	Intestinal cramps, diarrhea (often bloody), kidney failure. Can be fatal
Listeria monocytogenes	Raw meat and poultry, raw milk, fresh soft cheese made from raw milk, liver paté, smoked seafood, deli meats and salads, hot dogs, produce	Unknown but probably more than 12 hours for GI tract signs and symptoms; probably a few days to 3 weeks for invasive disease	Fever, muscular aches, vomiting, diarrhea. In pregnant women, the infection can lead to stillbirth (birth of a dead fetus) or premature birth

TABLE 11.6 **COMMON SOURCES OF FOOD-BORNE ILLNESS** *(Concluded)*

Pathogen	High-Risk Foods	Approx. Time of Onset	Typical Signs and Symptoms
Bacteria (continued)			
Salmonella species	Raw or undercooked meat, poultry, seafood, and eggs; raw seed sprouts; raw vegetables; unpasteurized juice	6 hours–2 days	Nausea, vomiting, fever, chills, headache, abdominal cramps, diarrhea Infection can be fatal in infants, older adults, and people with serious chronic illness.
Staphylococcus aureus (toxin)	Meats, poultry, and eggs; foods made with eggs, such as potato, egg, macaroni, and egg salads; certain homemade ice creams, custards, and cream-filled pastries Cooked foods are often contaminated as a result of improper food handling practices.	1–6 hours	Diarrhea, nausea, vomiting, abdominal cramps, weakness
Viruses			
Hepatitis A (HAV)	Food or water that has been contaminated with HAV from feces	2–6 weeks	Fever, loss of appetite, nausea, vomiting, diarrhea, muscle aches, general weakness; may have yellow discoloration of skin and whites of eyes, liver enlargement, and dark-colored urine
Norovirus	Food or water that has been contaminated with infected feces, enabling the virus to be spread person-to-person	1–2 days	Vomiting; watery, nonbloody diarrhea; abdominal cramps; nausea; low-grade fever (occasionally)
Protists			
Cryptosporidium	Foods prepared with contaminated water or by people whose hands were contaminated with infected feces	2–10 days	Profuse, watery diarrhea; abdominal pain; fever; nausea; vomiting; weight loss
Giardia	Consumption of contaminated water, including water from lakes, streams, swimming pools High-risk groups include travelers to certain countries, hikers, and people who swim in or camp by lakes and streams.	1–2 weeks	Diarrhea, abdominal pain, loss of appetite
Toxoplasma	Raw or partially cooked infected meat, especially pork, lamb, or deer meat Accidentally ingesting infected cat feces	Difficult to determine because of uncertain timing of exposure	Fever, headache, muscle aches, rash Pregnant women should avoid contact with cat feces because the pathogen can infect their unborn offspring, causing eye or brain damage.
Parasitic worms			
Anisakis	Raw or undercooked infected seafood	1 hour to 2 weeks	Tickling sensation in throat during or after eating raw/undercooked seafood Severe abdominal pain that may be mistaken for appendicitis Vomiting or coughing up the worm may prevent infection.
Trichinella	Raw or undercooked infected meat, especially pork, bear, seal, and walrus meat	1–2 days	Initially: nausea, vomiting, diarrhea, fatigue, fever, abdominal discomfort Later: headaches, chills, cough, eye swelling, muscle and joint pain In severe cases, death can occur.

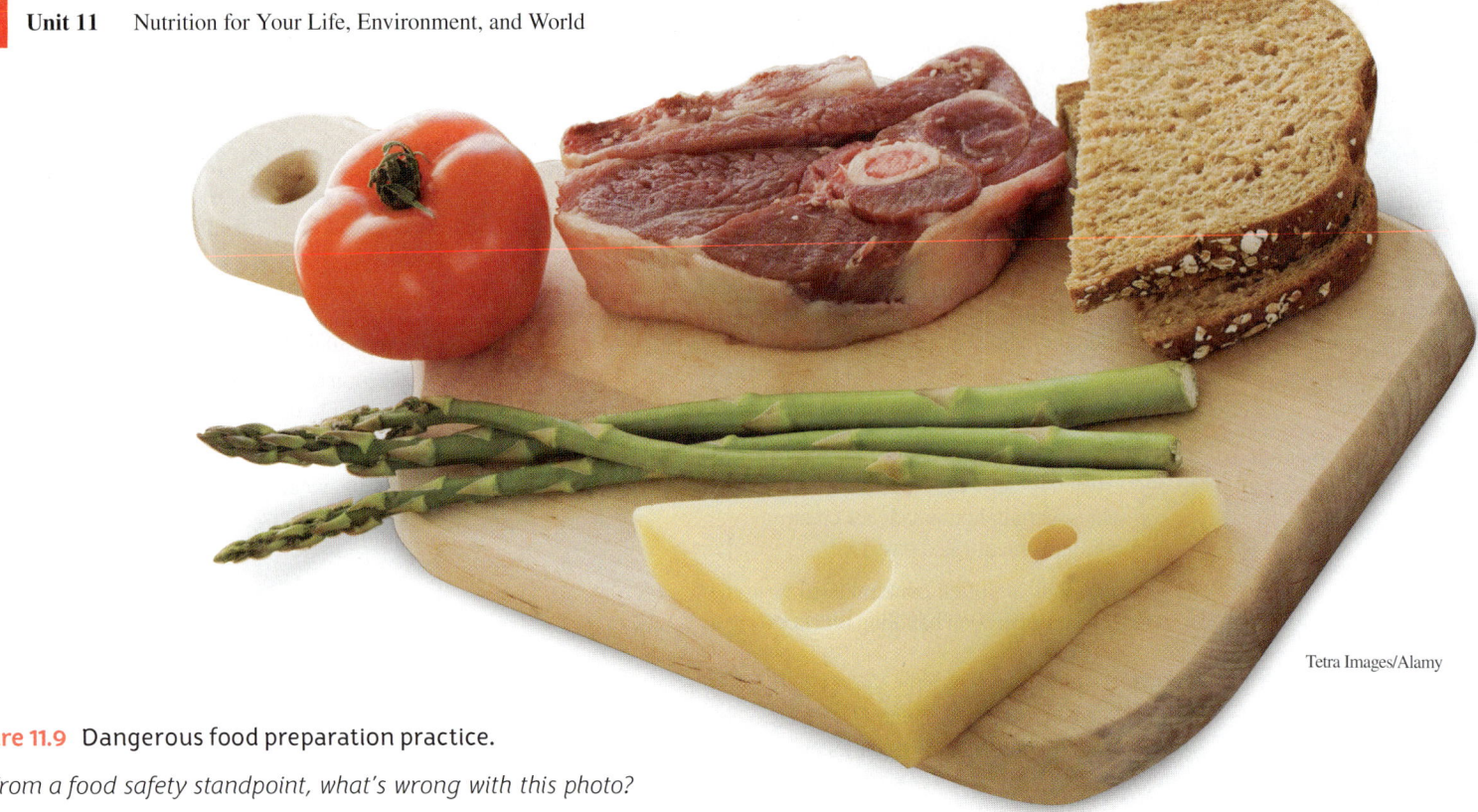

Figure 11.9 Dangerous food preparation practice.

■ *From a food safety standpoint, what's wrong with this photo?*

11.2d How Do Pathogens Get into Your Food?

Pathogens are found throughout your environment. Therefore, you need to be aware of how they can enter foods to prevent becoming sick as a result.

- Animals (*vermin*) that live around sewage or garbage, such as flies, cockroaches, mice, and rats, often carry pathogens on their bodies or in their urine and feces. When the vermin come in contact with food, they can transfer the pathogens to humans.
- Poor personal hygiene practices, especially failing to wash your hands frequently, can transmit pathogens to yourself and others.
- Improper food handling frequently results in food-borne illness. A common practice is failing to wash cutting boards and food preparation utensils after they come in contact with raw meat or poultry. The contaminated boards and utensils are then used to prepare other foods. As a result of this practice, **cross-contamination** is likely to occur because the pathogens in one food are transferred to another food, contaminating it. If that food is eaten raw, such as carrots in a salad, it carries a high risk of food-borne illness (**Fig. 11.9**).
- Failing to cook and store foods properly can also increase the likelihood of food-borne illness.

cross-contamination unintentional transfer of pathogenic microbes from one food to another

11.2e Preventing Food-Borne Illness

According to the USDA, pathogens usually grow well when the temperature of a high-risk food is between 40°F and 140°F—the "danger zone" (**Fig. 11.10**).[34] Cooking foods to the proper temperature destroys food-borne viruses and bacteria. To be safe, a product must be cooked to an internal temperature that's high enough to destroy harmful pathogens and certain bacterial toxins. Using a meat thermometer is a reliable way to ensure that meat, poultry, and thick

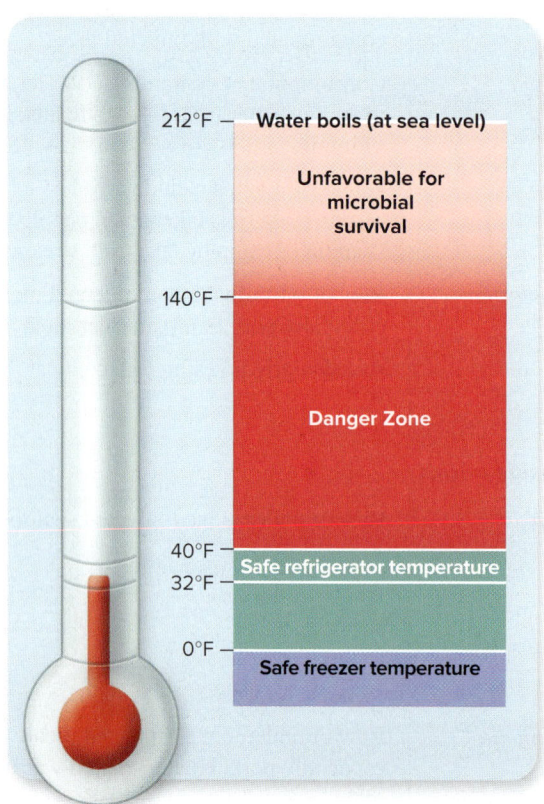

Figure 11.10 Temperature guide for food safety (USDA).

Table 11.7 USDA-Recommended Safe Minimum Internal Temperatures	
Food	**Safe Minimum Internal Temperature (°F)**
Beef steaks and roasts	145
Fish	145
Pork	145
Ground beef, pork, lamb, and veal	160
Egg dishes	160
Poultry products	165

Richard Griffin/Shutterstock

pieces of cooking foods have reached the proper internal temperature without overcooking. **Table 11.7** indicates recommended minimum internal temperatures for cooking these foods.

Chilling food slows the growth of microbes in the items, but some bacteria can grow even at proper refrigeration temperatures. Freezing doesn't kill bacteria or inactivate viruses in food; the process just halts the microbes' ability to multiply.[35] As frozen food thaws, the bacteria and viruses resume their activities and can cause illness.

To reduce your risk of food-borne illness when purchasing food, take the following steps.

- Select frozen foods and highly perishable foods, such as meat, poultry, or fish, last.
- Check "best by" dates on packaged perishable foods. Choose meats and other animal products with the latest dates.
- Don't buy food in damaged containers; for example, avoid containers that leak, bulge, or are severely dented, or jars that are cracked or have loose or bulging lids.
- Open egg cartons and examine eggs; don't buy cartons that have cracked eggs.
- Purchase only pasteurized milk, cheese, and fruit and vegetable juices (check the label).
- Purchase only the amount of produce needed for a week's menus. The longer you keep fresh fruits and vegetables, the more likely they're to spoil.
- Pack meat, fish, and poultry in separate plastic bags, so their drippings don't contaminate each other and your other groceries.
- Take groceries home immediately. Refrigerate or freeze meat, fish, egg, and dairy products promptly.
- Store whole eggs in their cartons, even if your refrigerator has a place for storing eggs. Egg cartons are designed to keep eggs fresh longer than a refrigerator's egg compartment.

Contaminated hands and food preparation surfaces spread pathogens.

The following tips can help reduce your risk of food-borne illness.

- Wash your hands before preparing food, especially after using the toilet, changing a baby's soiled diaper, or playing with pets.
  - Wash your hands in very warm, soapy water for at least 20 seconds before and after touching food. If clean water for hand washing isn't available, use sanitizing hand gels or wipes.
  - Use a fresh paper towel or clean hand towel to dry hands. Reserve dish towels for drying pots, pans, and cooking utensils that aren't washed and dried in a dishwasher.

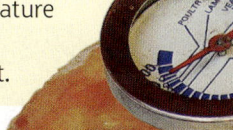

TASTY Tidbits

When using a meat thermometer, place the thermometer in the thickest part of the muscle tissue, away from bone, fat, or gristle. If the thermometer is inserted incorrectly or placed in the wrong area, the reading may not accurately reflect the internal temperature of the product.

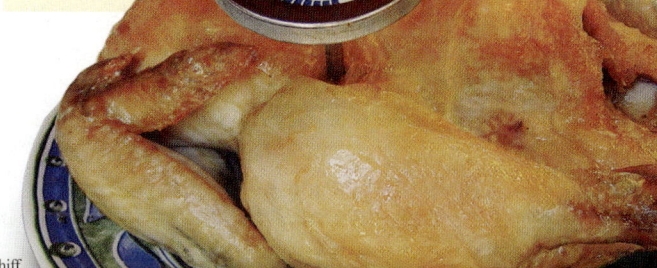

Wendy Schiff

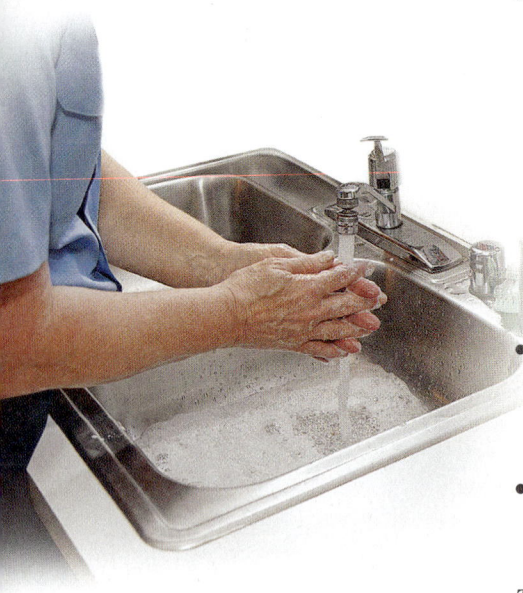

- Before preparing food, clean food preparation surfaces, including kitchen counters, cutting boards, dishes, knives, and other food preparation equipment, with hot, soapy water.
  - The FDA recommends cutting boards with unmarred surfaces made of easy-to-clean, nonporous materials, such as plastic, marble, or glass. If you prefer to use wooden cutting boards, make sure they're made of a nonabsorbent hardwood, such as oak or maple, and have no obvious seams or cracks.
  - You can kill most pathogens when you clean and sanitize food preparation surfaces and utensils with a solution made by adding a tablespoon of bleach to 1 gallon of water. You can also sanitize kitchen sponges with the dilute bleach solution.
  - Replace cutting boards when they become streaked with cuts because these grooves can be difficult to clean thoroughly and may harbor bacteria.
- Use a solution of 1 tablespoon of bleach mixed in 1 gallon of water to sanitize food preparation surfaces and equipment that have come in contact with raw meat, fish, poultry, and eggs. You can sanitize moist kitchen sponges by heating them in a microwave oven for 1 minute or by washing them in a dishwasher that has a heated dry cycle.[36] In addition, wash kitchen towels frequently.
- Before preparing fresh produce, carefully wash the foods under running water to remove dirt and bacteria clinging to the surface. Bacteria can be sticky, so scrub the peel with a vegetable brush. Even if you plan to remove the skin or peel, wash the produce before you cut it.

To reduce your risk of food-borne illness when preparing and serving food, take the following steps.

- Don't use foods from damaged containers and safety seals or expired "use by" dates.
- Don't taste or use food that spurts liquid or has a bad odor when the can is opened.
- Read product labels to determine whether foods need to be refrigerated after their packages are opened.
- Always thaw high-risk foods in the refrigerator, under cold running water, or in a microwave oven.
- Cook foods immediately after thawing.
- Marinate food in the refrigerator, and if marinating meat, fish, or poultry, discard the marinade.
- Chilled foods should be kept covered and served from a shallow container filled with ice. Hot foods should be kept covered and served from shallow, heated pans. The best simple advice to follow: "*Keep hot foods hot and cold foods cold.*"
- Avoid eating moldy foods.
- Don't allow hot foods to cool on the counter—place in refrigerator directly.
- When in doubt, throw the food out.

To reduce your risk of food-borne illness when cooking foods, take the following steps.

- Cook beef, poultry, pork, thick pieces of fish, and egg-containing dishes thoroughly, using a meat thermometer to check for doneness.
- Bake stuffing separately from poultry or wash the poultry cavity thoroughly and stuff the bird immediately before cooking. Make sure the temperature of the stuffing reaches 165°F. After cooking, transfer the stuffing to a clean bowl for serving or storage.

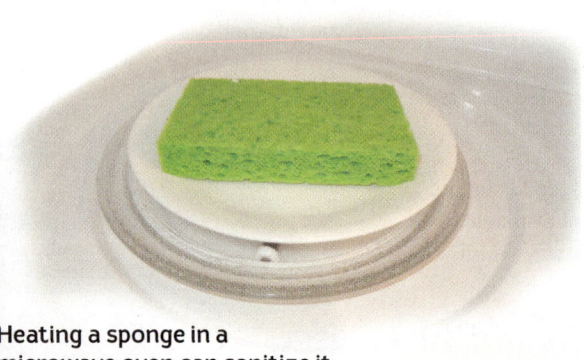

Heating a sponge in a microwave oven can sanitize it.

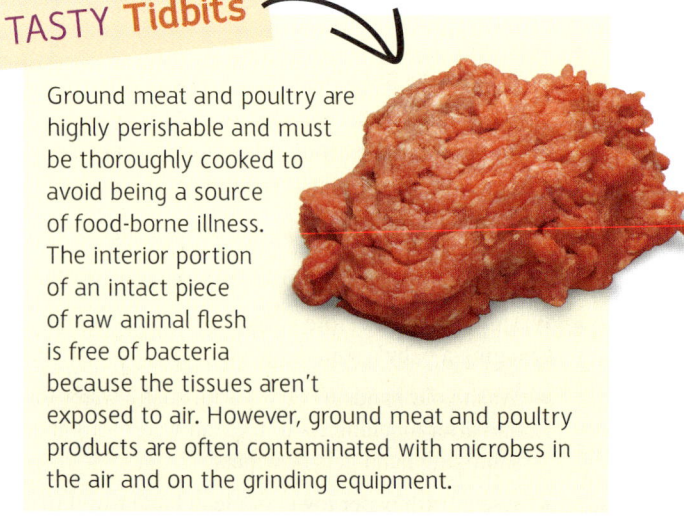

TASTY Tidbits

Ground meat and poultry are highly perishable and must be thoroughly cooked to avoid being a source of food-borne illness. The interior portion of an intact piece of raw animal flesh is free of bacteria because the tissues aren't exposed to air. However, ground meat and poultry products are often contaminated with microbes in the air and on the grinding equipment.

Handwashing: McGraw-Hill Education/Rick Brady; Bleach, sponge: Wendy Schiff; Ground beef: John A. Rizzo/Getty Images

Nutrition Fact or Fiction?

Food that drops on the floor will not pick up microbes if it's picked up within 5 seconds.

Studies have determined that this is a food-related myth. As soon as food touches a contaminated surface such as a floor, some microbes adhere to it.[37]

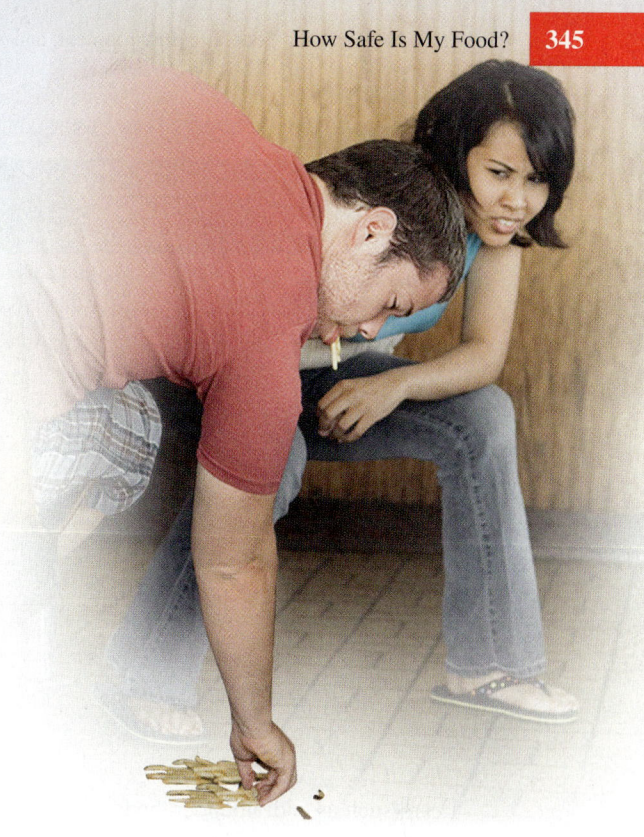

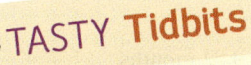
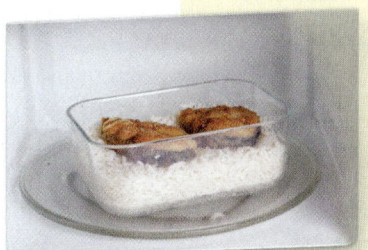

Microwave cooking often heats food unevenly, so microbes can survive in the cool spots. While cooking food in a microwave oven, stop the oven occasionally and stir the food to reduce uneven heating. Microwave cooking isn't recommended for stuffed foods because during cooking, the temperature of the stuffing may not be high enough to kill pathogens.[38]

- Serve meat, poultry, and fish on a clean plate. Never use the same plate that held the raw product. When grilling hamburgers, for example, don't put cooked items on the same plate that was used to carry the raw meat to the grill.
- Give picnic foods special attention because outdoor temperatures may favor rapid bacterial growth. Keep cold salads and desserts on ice. Meats should be cooked completely at a picnic site. Don't partially cook foods in advance and plan to finish cooking them at the picnic.

To reduce your risk of food-borne illness when storing and reheating food, take the following steps.

- Cover leftovers and refrigerate or freeze them as soon as you have finished eating, or within 2 hours. If environmental temperatures are above 90°F, refrigerate the leftovers within 1 hour.[39] It's dangerous to let hot foods cool before chilling or freezing them.
- Keep all foods, including leftovers, covered while they're in the refrigerator. Store raw meats, fish, poultry, and shellfish on lower shelves of the refrigerator, so they're separated from foods that are to be eaten raw.
- Check your refrigerator's temperature regularly to make sure it stays below 40°F. Keep the refrigerator as cold as possible without freezing milk and lettuce.
- Cook ground meats and poultry soon after purchasing. If this isn't possible, freeze the ground items.
- Note that raw fish, shellfish, and poultry are highly perishable. It's best to cook these foods or freeze them the day they're purchased.
- Use refrigerated ground meat and patties within 1 to 2 days, and use frozen meat and patties within 3 to 4 months after purchasing them. **Table 11.8** presents recommended time limits for refrigeration and freezer storage of foods. Foods that are stored in the freezer for longer than recommended periods often develop unappealing flavors.
- Use refrigerated leftovers within 4 days.
- Reheat leftovers to 165°F; reheat gravy to a rolling boil to kill pathogenic bacteria that may be present.

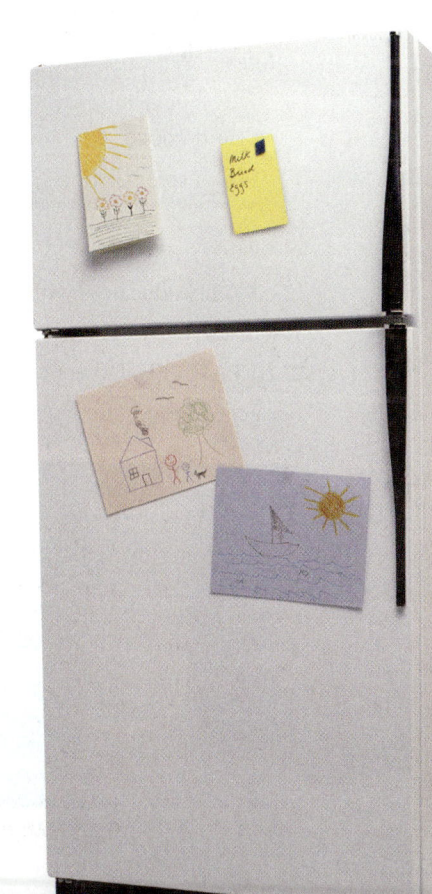

Man: McGraw-Hill Education/Susie Ross; Food in microwave oven: Михаил Аханов/123RF; Refrigerator: C Squared Studios/Getty Images

TABLE 11.8 COLD STORAGE TIME LIMITS FOR PERISHABLE FOODS

Product	Storage Period in Refrigerator (40°F)	Storage Period in Freezer (0°F)
Fresh meat		
Ground meat	1–2 days	3–4 months
Steaks and roasts	3–5 days	4–12 months
Fresh pork		
Chops	3–5 days	4–6 months
Ground	1–2 days	3–4 months
Roasts	3–5 days	4–6 months
Processed meat		
Luncheon meat (deli sliced or open package)	3–5 days	1–2 months
Luncheon meat (unopened package)	2 weeks	1–2 months
Sausage, raw	1–2 days	1–2 months
Gravy	3–4 days	2–3 months
Fresh fish		
Lean (such as cod, flounder, haddock)	1–2 days	—
Fatty (such as perch, salmon)	1–2 days	—
Fresh chicken or turkey		
Whole	1–2 days	12 months
Parts	1–2 days	9 months
Prestuffed, uncooked chicken breasts	1 day	Not recommended
Leftovers		
Cooked meat	3–4 days	2–3 months
Casseroles that contain meat	3–4 days	2–3 months
Eggs		
Fresh, in shell	3–5 weeks	—
Hard-cooked	1 week	—

Source: USDA, Food Safety and Inspection Service: *Basics of handling foods safely: Cold storage chart.* Updated 2015. www.fsis.usda.gov/wps/portal/fsis/topics/food-safety-education/get-answers/food-safety-fact-sheets/safe-food-handling/basics-for-handling-food-safely/ct_index Accessed: July 27, 2019

Food safety educators with the federal government have condensed food safety rules into four simple actions:

1. **CLEAN.** Wash hands and surfaces often.
2. **SEPARATE.** Do not cross-contaminate.
3. **COOK.** Cook to proper temperatures.
4. **CHILL.** Refrigerate promptly

For general food safety questions, you can call FDA's food information hotline at 1-888-723-3366.

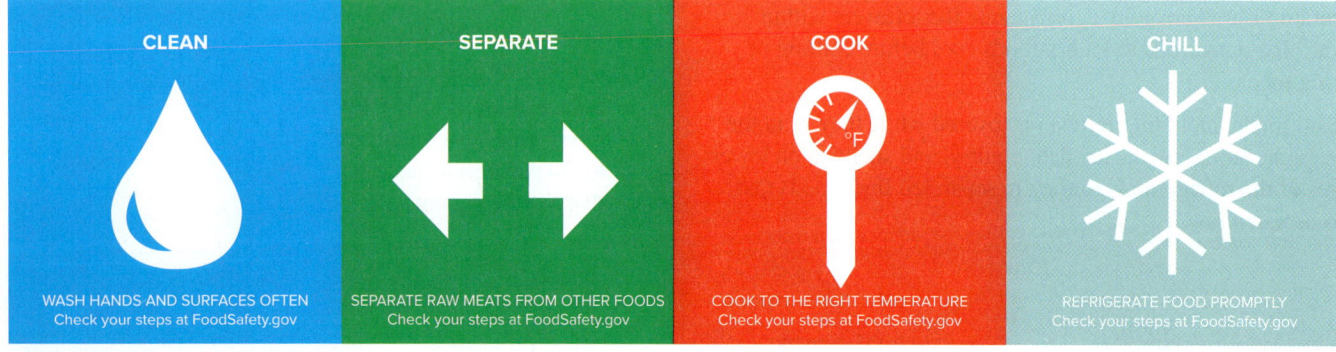

Centers for Disease Control and Prevention

What About Restaurant Foods?

In many instances, you cannot control the safety of foods that are prepared in restaurants or other places outside your home. However, you can greatly reduce your risk of food-borne illness by following some important rules, most of which require changing risky food selection, preparation, and storage practices. Be alert for signs of unsafe food handling practices when you eat out. The following tips also apply to foods prepared for dormitory residents:

- Make sure tabletops, dishes, and eating utensils are clean.
- Make sure servers who handle food directly are wearing gloves.
- Check custard, pudding, pies, and salad bar foods to make sure they're chilled and kept on ice.
- Make sure hot foods are served hot or served from a heated food bar.
- If your serving of meat, poultry, or fish doesn't appear to be thoroughly cooked, ask the server to return the item to the kitchen to be heated again.
- Be wary of perishable foods in vending machines, especially those that sell sandwiches.

> **TASTY Tidbits**
>
> The process of food irradiation preserves food by using a high amount of energy to kill pathogens. The energy passes through the food, as in microwave cooking, and no radioactive material is left behind. It's important to recognize that even when foods, especially meats, have been irradiated, once their packaging has been opened, the foods can still become contaminated.
>
> Radura symbol

If you or someone you know develops signs and symptoms of food-borne illness that probably resulted from products eaten at a restaurant or sold in a vending machine, call your physician or 911 for emergency care. For nonemergency cases involving food-borne illnesses, contact the staff of your local health department or FDA office https://www.accessdata.fda.gov/scripts/medwatch/index.cfm to report your experience.

11.2f Emergency Food Supply

Hurricanes, tornadoes, earthquakes, "superstorms"—enduring a natural disaster can easily disrupt your access to safe food. Therefore, you should store at least a three-day supply of food for emergency use. Choose foods that have a long storage life, require no refrigeration, and can be eaten without cooking, such as canned meats, fruits, and vegetables. If you have infants, you should also keep a supply of baby foods. **Table 11.9** lists foods that can be included in your emergency food supply. Also store a manual can opener, paper plates, and eating utensils. For more information about emergency preparedness, visit the Centers for Disease Control and Prevention's website: www.cdc.gov/disasters/foodwater/index.html.

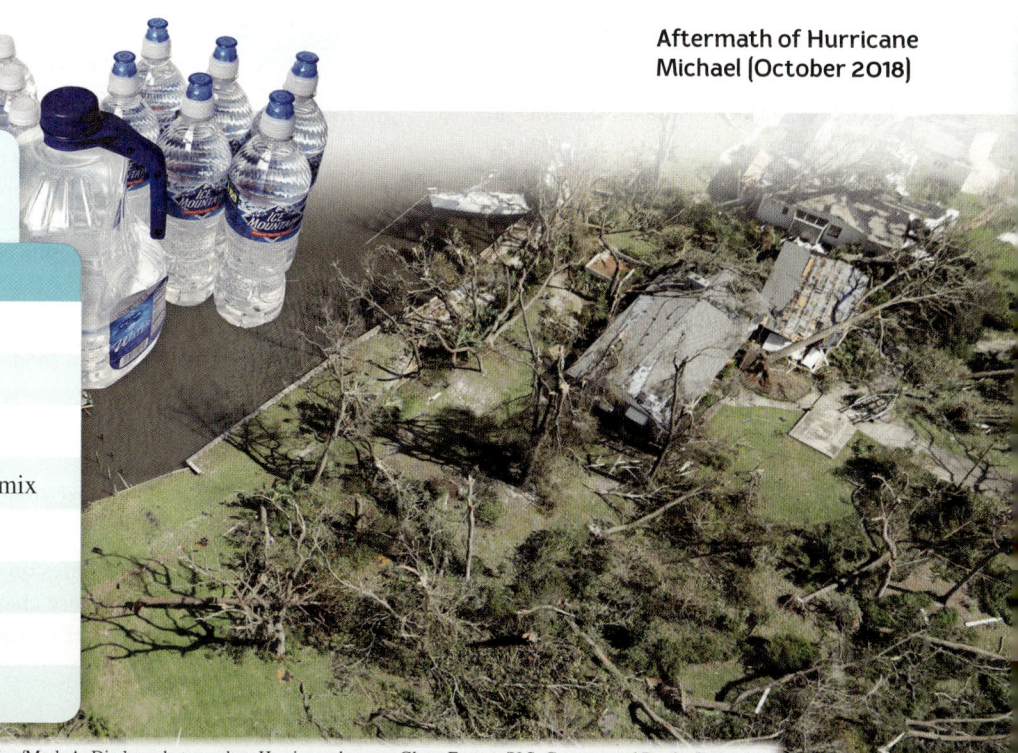

Aftermath of Hurricane Michael (October 2018)

Table 11.9 Foods to Store for Emergency Situations
Bottled water
Canned meats, fish, fruits, and vegetables
Canned fruit juices
Unopened boxes of cereal, low-salt crackers, and trail mix
Prewrapped fruit-filled granola bars
Peanut or other nut butters
Raisins and other dried fruit
Dry milk powder

Radura: U.S. Food and Drug Administration; Water bottles: McGraw-Hill Education/Mark A. Dierker, photographer; Hurricane damage: Glenn Fawcett/U.S. Customs and Border Protection

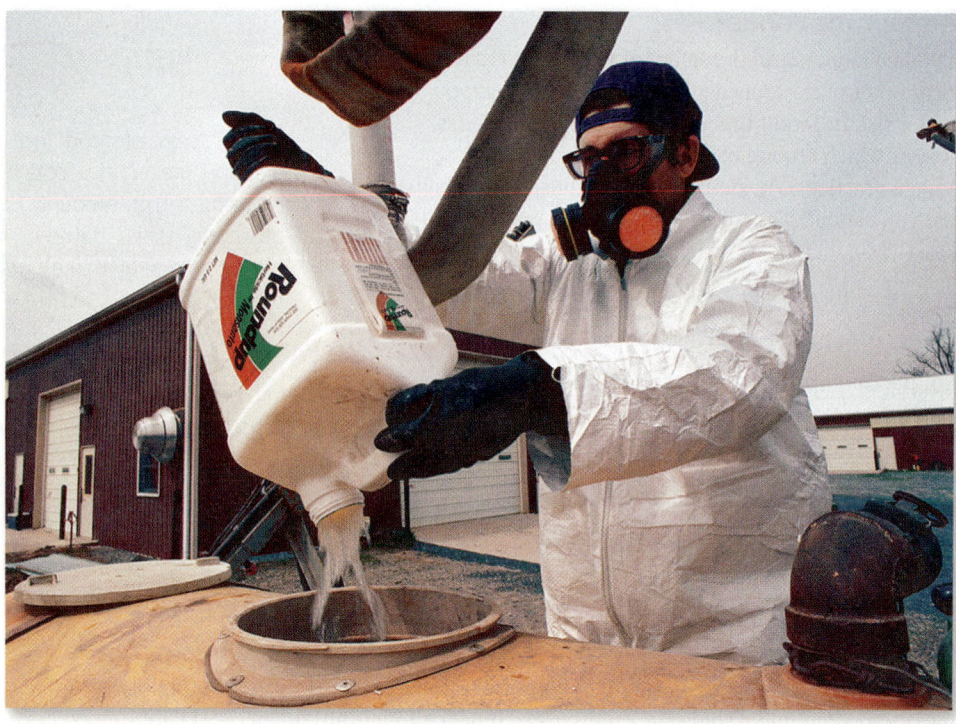

This farmworker is wearing protective gear as he handles a pesticide.

Source: Photo by Tim McCabe, USDA Natural Resources Conservation Service

TASTY Tidbits

The Environmental Working Group (EWG) is a nonprofit organization that includes scientists who use data from government sources to protect consumers. The EWG uses the results of government testing to make a list that ranks produce according to amounts of pesticide residues. In 2019, strawberries were at the top of the list because they had the highest pesticide residue levels. Avocados were among the produce that contained the lowest pesticide residues. To access the produce list, visit www.ewg.org/foodnews/dirty-dozen.php.

11.2g What About Pesticides in Food?

Pesticides can contaminate foods, especially produce. A **pesticide** is any substance that people use to control or kill unwanted insects, weeds, rodents, fungi, or other organisms. The use of pesticides in modern farming practices has helped increase crop yields, reduce food costs, and protect the quality of many agricultural products. However, many pesticides leave small amounts (pesticide residues) in or on treated crops, including fruits, vegetables, and grains, even when they're applied correctly. Concentrations of pesticide residues often decrease as food crops are washed, stored, processed, and prepared. Nevertheless, some of these substances may remain in fresh produce, such as apples or peaches, as well as in processed foods, such as canned applesauce or peaches.

AGE Fotostock/Pixtal

The Environmental Protection Agency (EPA) regulates the proper use of pesticides. The agency can limit the amount of a pesticide that's applied on crops, restrict the frequency or location of the pesticide's application, or require the substance be used only by specially trained, certified persons. The EPA also sets **pesticide tolerances,** maximum amounts of pesticide residues that can be in or on each treated food crop.

How Safe Are Pesticides?

The potential harmful effects of a pesticide in food depend on

- the particular chemical's toxicity,
- how much of it is eaten and how often, and
- a person's life stage and age. Pregnant women, children, those who are sick, and older adults may be more vulnerable to pesticides than others.[40]

Tolerable legal amounts of pesticide residues on or in foods are extremely small. However, it's possible that regular exposure to small amounts of these chemicals may enable the substances to accumulate in the body and produce toxicity or initiate cancer. Environmental health experts will continue to monitor the effects of pesticides on humans.

pesticide substance that people use to kill or control unwanted insects, weeds, or other organisms

pesticide tolerances maximum amounts of pesticide residues that can be in or on each treated food crop

Module 11.3

Dietary Adequacy: A Global Concern

11.3 - Learning Outcomes

After reading Module 11.3, you should be able to

1. Define all of the **key terms** in this module.
2. List factors that contribute to undernutrition in developing countries.
3. Describe how undernutrition during pregnancy and childhood can affect pregnant women and/or their children.
4. Describe efforts to increase the supply of nutritious food in countries where undernutrition is widespread.
5. Identify major federally subsidized food programs in the United States.
6. Discuss how biotechnology and sustainable agricultural methods can improve the environment.
7. Discuss proposed steps that consumers and farmers can take to help protect the environment.

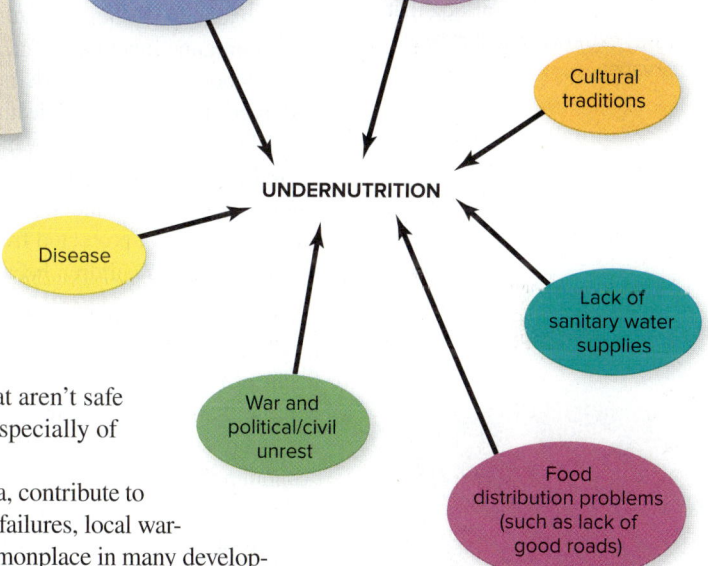

Stockbyte/Getty Images

11.3a Undernutrition

Undernutrition occurs when long-term energy and nutrient intakes are insufficient to meet an individual's needs. According to the World Health Organization, over 820 million people were chronically hungry in 2018.[41] A person who is chronically hungry doesn't consume enough food energy to be physically active. Throughout the world, 2 billion people consume diets that aren't safe and nutritionally adequate.[41] Chronic hunger and micronutrient deficiencies, especially of vitamin A, iron, and iodine, are often features of undernutrition.[42]

Regional food shortages, especially in developing countries of Asia and Africa, contribute to undernutrition. Such shortages can result from traditional dietary practices, crop failures, local warfare, and political instability and corruption. Poverty and undernutrition are commonplace in many developing countries. Impoverished people must also cope with infectious diseases, overcrowded and unsafe housing conditions, and polluted water supplies **(Fig. 11.11)**. The following section provides some general information about undernutrition; Unit 10 discussed overnutrition. Unit 7 includes information about protein malnutrition.

Undernutrition During Pregnancy

Undernutrition can be very harmful when it occurs during periods of rapid growth, such as pregnancy, infancy, and childhood. Women who are undernourished during pregnancy are more likely to die while giving birth than pregnant women who are adequately nourished. Furthermore, malnourished pregnant women have a high risk of giving birth to infants that are born prematurely. These babies often suffer from breathing problems and have low birth weights—conditions that increase their risk of dying during their first year of life.

Undernutrition During Infancy

As explained in Module 11.1, breast milk is the best food for young infants because it's sanitary, is nutritionally adequate, and provides babies with immunity to some infectious diseases. Throughout the world, only about 40% of babies consume only breast milk during their first 6 months of life.[43] Infant formulas are nutritious substitutes for breast milk, but they are generally more expensive. To extend infant formulas, poor parents in developing countries often add excessive amounts of water. This practice dilutes the nutritional value of the formula and

Figure 11.11 Factors that contribute to undernutrition. Many factors, including war, disease, and overpopulation, contribute to undernutrition.

undernutrition state of health that occurs when long-term energy and nutrient intakes are insufficient to meet an individual's needs

What IS That?

Although the kiwano (*Cucumis metuliferusis*) is native to southern Africa, this odd-looking cousin of the cucumber is grown in California. The green pulpy seeds can be scooped out of the rind and eaten as a snack or added to salads. Kiwano is a good source of plant protein (almost 4 g), iron (2.3 mg), and vitamin C (11 mg). The pulp, however, has a slimy texture and not much flavor. In Africa, kiwano is generally considered to be an edible weed that is not eaten unless other foods are unavailable.

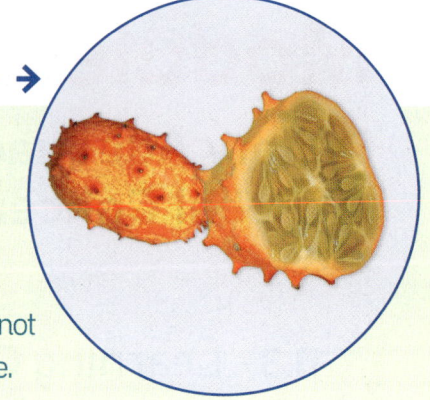

kwashiorkor form of protein-energy malnutrition that occurs when a child is abruptly weaned from breast milk and consumes inadequate amounts of high-quality protein

marasmic kwashiorkor form of protein-energy malnutrition that's characterized by edema and wasting

marasmus severe form of protein-energy malnutrition that causes extreme weight loss; starvation

increases the likelihood of contaminating it with disease-causing microbes. In infants, the diarrhea that results from drinking formula mixed with unsanitary water can rapidly cause loss of body water (dehydration) and death.

Dietitians and physicians recommend that infants be breastfed exclusively for the first 6 months of life. Ideally, babies should continue to receive breast milk in addition to solid foods well into their second year, especially in places where clean water is unavailable. Protein malnutrition typically occurs soon after impoverished children are weaned abruptly from breast milk and introduced to far-less-nourishing solid foods.

Undernutrition During the Preschool Years

In chronically undernourished children, nutrient deficiencies are responsible for delayed physical development, poor physical growth, impaired intellectual development, blindness, and premature death. The brain grows rapidly during the first 5 years of life. When undernutrition occurs during this period, the effects can be devastating to the child's brain and result in permanent learning disabilities. Additionally, chronically undernourished children tend to be shorter ("stunted")—if they survive to adulthood. Chronic undernutrition also depresses the body's immune functioning, increasing the risk of death from infectious diseases, such as measles, especially in childhood. Each year, undernutrition contributes to 45% of deaths of children throughout the world.[43] The vast majority of childhood deaths associated with undernutrition occurs among poor populations in developing countries, particularly in sub-Saharan Africa and parts of Asia.

In the United States and other developed countries, children are usually well nourished and vaccinated against common childhood diseases, including measles. In poorer nations, however, many children are malnourished and not protected from the virus that causes measles. Measles is a life-threatening illness for malnourished children because their immune systems don't function normally.

What's Protein-Energy Malnutrition? Protein-energy malnutrition (PEM) affects people whose diets lack adequate amounts of protein as well as energy. Kwashiorkor, marasmic kwashiorkor, and marasmus are forms of PEM. **Kwashiorkor** (*qwash'-ee-or'-kor*) primarily occurs in developing countries where mothers commonly breastfeed their infants until they give birth to another child. The older youngster, who's usually a toddler, is fairly healthy until abruptly weaned from its mother's milk to make way for the younger sibling. Although the toddler may obtain adequate energy by consuming a traditional diet of cereal grains, the diet lacks enough complete protein to meet the youngster's high needs. The signs and symptoms of kwashiorkor occur as a result of the child's poor diet.

Children with kwashiorkor have stunted growth; unnaturally blond, sparse, and brittle hair; and patches of skin that have lost their normal coloration. The children also have swollen cheeks, arms, legs, and bellies that make them look well fed, but their appearance is misleading. During starvation, levels of proteins in blood that maintain proper fluid balance decline, resulting in edema (see Unit 7). The edema makes the protein-deficient child look plump and overfed instead of thin and undernourished.

In many cases, the child suffering from kwashiorkor doesn't obtain enough energy and eventually develops **marasmic kwashiorkor**, a condition characterized by edema and *wasting* (**Fig. 11.12**). Wasting is the loss of organ and muscle proteins as the body tears down these tissues to obtain amino acids for energy.

Severe PEM causes extreme weight loss and a condition called **marasmus** (*mah-raz'-mus*), which is commonly referred to as starvation. Obvious signs of marasmus are weakness and wasting. People suffering from marasmus avoid physical activity to conserve energy, and they're often irritable. The following section describes efforts that can reduce the occurrence of PEM in the world.

11.3b World Food Crisis: Finding Solutions

Reducing protein-energy malnutrition through food aid programs is a major goal of the United Nations. The World Food Program and United Nations Children's Fund (UNICEF) are agencies within the United Nations that provide high-quality food for undernourished populations. UNICEF also supports the development and

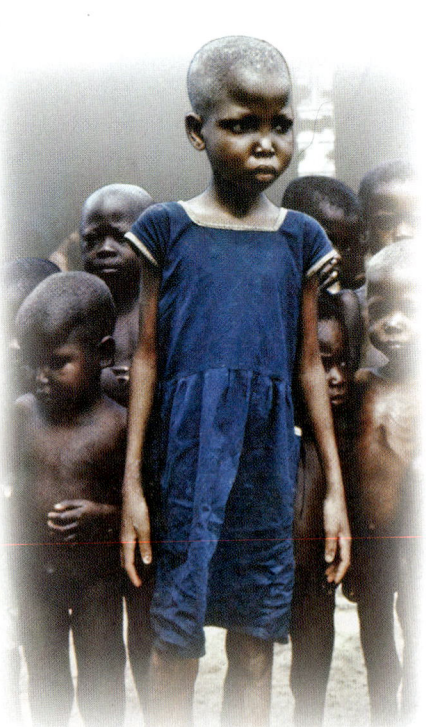

Figure 11.12 This photo of undernourished children was taken during a civil war in Nigeria (late 1960s).

Whole kiwano, Cut kiwano: Wendy Schiff; Kwashiorkor: Source: Centers for Disease Control and Prevention/Dr. Lyle Conrad

distribution of ready-to-use, therapeutic food (RUTF) to treat severe undernutrition among young children in developing countries. Plumpy'nut, for example, is an energy- and nutrient-dense paste made from a mixture of peanuts, powdered milk, oil, sugar, vitamins, and minerals. During processing, the paste is placed in foil packets to keep the food clean and make it easy to transport to remote places without refrigeration. In 2018, UNICEF's efforts helped save the lives of about 3 million starving children.[44]

11.3c Does Undernutrition Occur in the United States?

You may be surprised to learn that some people are undernourished in wealthy, developed nations such as the United States. Poverty is often responsible for undernutrition in any country. In 2017, 12.3% of the U.S. population was living at or below the U.S. Department of Health and Human Services poverty guideline.[45] In 2019, the poverty guideline was $25,750 for a family or household of 4 persons.[46]

Most American households are **food secure,** which means the people in those households have access to and can purchase sufficient food to lead healthy, active lives. In 2017, food insecurity was reported in about 12% of all households in the United States.[47] **Food insecurity** describes individuals or families who are concerned about running out of food or not having enough money to buy more food. People who are unemployed, work in low-paying jobs, or have excessive medical and housing expenses often experience food insecurity. Food insecurity may also affect older adults who live on fixed incomes, especially if they're forced to choose between purchasing nutritious food and buying life-extending medications.

Table 11.10 lists major federally supported food programs in the United States. Such programs provide food for people in need. However, not every eligible food-insecure person has access to or takes advantage

food secure describes households in which the residents have access to and can purchase sufficient food to lead healthy, active lives

food insecurity describes individuals or families who are concerned about running out of food or not having enough money to buy more food

TABLE 11.10 — MAJOR FEDERALLY SUBSIDIZED FOOD PROGRAMS IN THE UNITED STATES

Program	General Eligibility Requirements	Description
Supplemental Nutrition Assistance Program (formerly called the Food Stamp Program)	Low-income individuals and families who meet certain requirements and limitations	Participants use an Electronic Benefit Transfer (debit) card to purchase allowable food items.
Commodity Supplemental Food Program	Certain low-income groups, including pregnant women, young children, and older adults	In some states, state agencies distribute USDA surplus foods to eligible people.
Special Supplemental Nutrition Program for Women, Infants, and Children (WIC)	Low-income pregnant or breastfeeding women, infants, and children under 5 years of age who are at nutritional risk	Participants receive checks or vouchers to purchase milk, cheese, fruit juice, certain cereals, infant formula, and other specific food items at grocery stores. Nutrition education is also provided.
National School Lunch Program	Low-income children of school age	Certain schools receive subsidies from the government to provide free or reduced-price nutritionally balanced lunches.
School Breakfast Program	Low-income children of school age	Certain schools receive subsidies from the government to provide free or reduced-price nutritionally balanced breakfasts.
Child and Adult Care Food Program	Children enrolled in organized childcare programs and seniors in adult care programs	Sites receive reimbursement for nutritious meals supplied to participants.
The Nutrition Program Congregate Meals for the Elderly	Age 60 or older (no income guidelines)	Sites provide free, nutritious noon meals. Participants can contribute money for cost of the meal.
Home-Delivered Meals (Meals on Wheels)	Age 60 or older but unable to leave home	At least 5 days a week, volunteers deliver a noon meal to the participant's home. Meal is free, or participant can contribute money for the cost of the meal.
Food Distribution Program on Indian Reservations	Low-income American Indian or non-Indian households on reservations; members of federally recognized Native-American tribes	Distribution of monthly food packages. This program is an alternative to the Supplemental Nutrition Assistance Program and includes nutrition education component.

of the aid. For more information about the federal government's nutrition assistance programs, visit www.nutrition.gov/food-assistance-programs.

There are actions you can take to help relieve the problem of hunger in your community. You can stimulate student interest by researching the extent of food insecurity in the area and then writing an article about the situation for the campus newspaper. You can help food-insecure people directly by volunteering to prepare or serve food at a soup kitchen or homeless shelter in your community. You can also initiate and coordinate a canned food drive on your campus to benefit a local food pantry.

11.3d Feeding the World, Protecting Natural Resources

The world's population is estimated to be over 7 billion people. If the present rate of population growth doesn't slow, an estimated 9.7 billion people will be living on Earth in 2050.[48] By 2050, agricultural efforts will need to double their current level of production to meet the population's demand for more food.[49]

Our current system of food production relies primarily on conventional agricultural methods. In general, conventional farming requires considerable amounts of water and pesticides that can harm our environment. Irrigation systems often remove fresh water from rivers and other natural sources at a faster rate than it's restored. This activity reduces water flow to many communities. The water that runs off conventional farms can carry precious topsoil with it and pesticides that pollute waterways. Such farming methods also release greenhouse gases, especially carbon dioxide and methane, which contribute to global warming. Furthermore, the need for new farmland often requires cutting down trees so that forests can be converted to croplands. The loss of forests eliminates wild animal and plant habitats. About 40% of the Earth's land (excluding Greenland and Antarctica) is used for food production; very little suitable land remains to be farmed.[49] What can be done to feed the world's population without destroying the Earth's natural resources?

Cutting down forests and replacing them with new farmlands often harms the environment.

Barry Barker/McGraw-Hill Education

What's Sustainable Agriculture?

Sustainable agriculture involves farming methods that meet the demand for more food without depleting natural resources and harming the environment. The challenge is finding ways to have farmers and ranchers make the conversion from primarily conventional farming techniques to sustainable agriculture. Farming needs to be profitable for farmers and ranchers, so any switch from conventional to sustainable agricultural methods must not reduce their profit margins.

To solve many of the problems created by conventional agricultural methods, an international team[49] developed the following five points for establishing a universal policy that would help sustain agriculture:

- *Stop expanding agricultural activity, especially into tropical forests and grasslands.*
- *Find ways to improve crop yields on existing farms.*
  - Biotechnology in agriculture has led to the development of crops that supply higher yields, resist pests, or are tolerant of drought conditions. **Biotechnology** involves the use of living things—plants, animals, microbes to manufacture new products. *Genetically-modified organisms (GMOs)* are specific living things, such as pesticide-resistant corn and vitamin A–rich rice, that scientists have developed by changing the organisms' DNA. The USDA, however, does not recognize the term "genetically modified organism" for labeling purposes. (See the What IS That? feature in section 11.2b.)

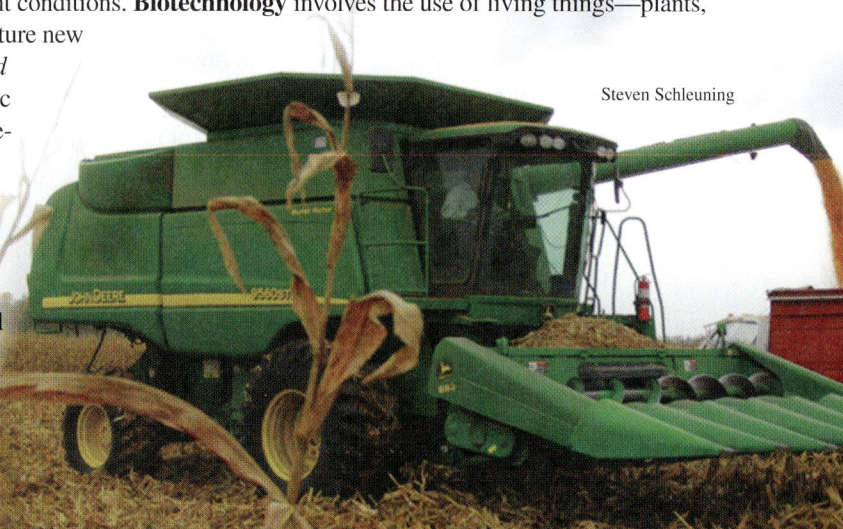

Steven Schleuning

sustainable agriculture farming methods that don't deplete natural resources while meeting the demand for food

biotechnology use of living things to manufacture new products

- By increasing food production or modifying the nutritional content of foods, biotechnology offers a way of reducing the world food crisis.

- ***Find ways to use natural resources and pesticides more efficiently.***
  - Use irrigation systems that apply water directly to a plant's base instead of spraying it into the air, where much of the water evaporates.
  - Rely more on nonchemical methods of pest management or **integrated pest management (IPM)**. IPM involves using a variety of methods for controlling pests while limiting damage to the environment. IPM methods include growing pest-resistant crops, using certain helpful insects to control crop-destroying bugs, and trapping adult insect pests before they can reproduce (**Fig. 11.13**).

- *Eat less meat.* Sixty percent of the world's crops (primarily grains) are grown for human consumption.[49] Most of the remaining crops are used to feed cattle and other farm animals. It takes about 30 pounds of grains to produce each pound of hamburger.[49] By eating less meat, especially beef, more grains could be produced to feed people. Grass-fed beef also spares grains for human consumption because grass isn't eaten by people.

- *Reduce food waste.* About 30% of food is wasted.[49] In many instances, the food spoils before you can eat it or it's thrown out as garbage. Reducing portion sizes and better menu planning can reduce the amount of food that you waste each day.

Taking Action

Poverty and hunger have always plagued humankind; the causes of poverty and hunger are complex and, therefore, are difficult to eliminate. Nevertheless, certain social, political, economic, and agricultural changes can reduce the number of people who are chronically hungry. In the short run, wealthy countries can provide food aid to keep impoverished people from starving to death. Families and small farmers in underdeveloped nations need to learn new and more efficient methods of growing, processing, preserving, and distributing nutritious regional food products. Additionally, governments can support programs that encourage breastfeeding and fortify locally grown or commonly consumed foods with vitamins and minerals that are often deficient in local diets.

In the long run, population control is critical for preserving the Earth's resources for future generations. Impoverished parents in poor countries often have many children because they expect only a few to survive and reach adulthood. When people are financially secure, adequately nourished, and well educated, they tend to have fewer, healthier children. Thus, long-term ways to slow population growth include providing well-paying jobs, improving public education, and increasing access to health care services.

U.S. Department of Agriculture (USDA)

Figure 11.13 **Helpful insect.** The spined soldier bug (left) makes a meal of a Mexican bean beetle larva. Bean beetle larvae are pests that can damage snap beans and soybeans.

integrated pest management (IPM) nonchemical methods of agricultural pest management

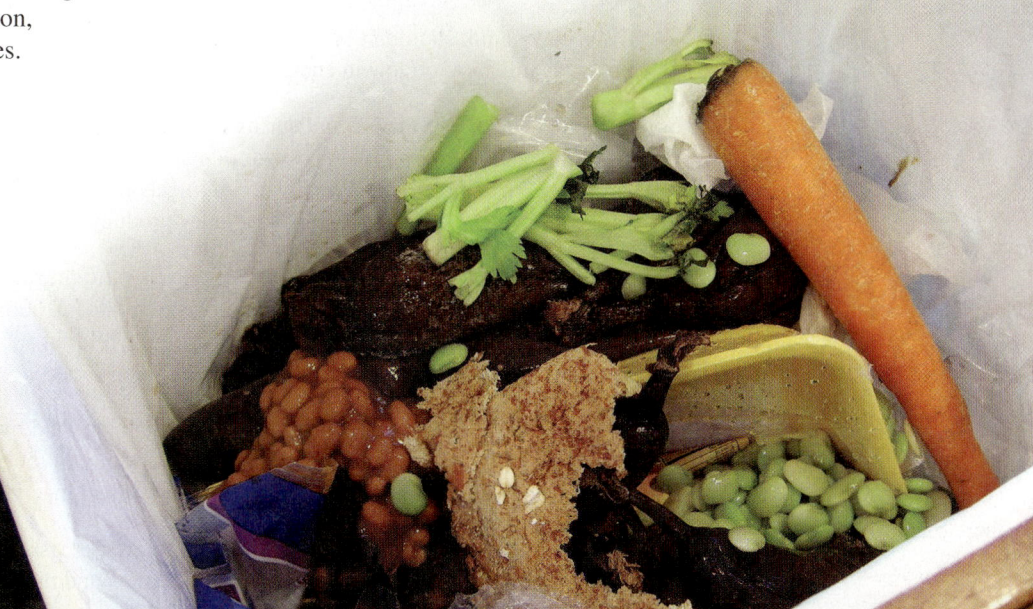

What steps can you take to reduce the amount of food that you waste?

Wendy Schiff

In a Nutshell

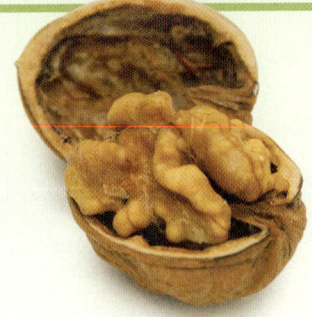

Module 11.1 Nutrition for a Lifetime

- The first trimester of pregnancy is a critical stage of prenatal development. The placenta transfers nutrients and oxygen from the mother's bloodstream to the embryo/fetus. The placenta also transfers wastes from the embryo/fetus to the mother's bloodstream, so her body can eliminate them.

- During pregnancy, a woman's body undergoes major physical changes that enable her body to nourish and maintain the developing embryo/fetus, as well as produce milk for her infant after its birth. Depending on the trimester, an expectant woman's requirements for energy, protein, and many other nutrients are greater than her needs prior to pregnancy.

- The amount of weight a woman should gain during pregnancy depends on her prepregnancy weight and the number of fetuses she's carrying. Women who gain excess weight during pregnancy are likely to retain the extra pounds after giving birth.

- Rapid weight gain, especially after the fifth month of pregnancy, could be a sign of gestational hypertension. If a woman with gestational hypertension develops convulsions, her condition is called eclampsia. In the United States, eclampsia is the second-leading cause of death among pregnant women.

- During the first 4 to 6 months of life, a healthy baby doubles its birth weight, and by 1 year of age, an infant's birth weight has tripled. Additionally, an infant's length increases by 50% during its first year of life. If an infant's diet lacks adequate energy and nutrients, the baby's growth may slow or even stop.

- Prolactin stimulates specialized cells in breasts to form milk. Oxytocin signals breast tissue to "let down" milk. The let-down reflex enables milk to travel in ducts to the nipple area.

- Breastfeeding offers several advantages for the infant and its mother. Colostrum contains antibodies, immune system cells, and a substance that encourages the growth of *Lactobacillus bifidus* in the infant's GI tract. Breastfed infants, especially those who are exclusively breastfed, have lower risks of allergies and gastrointestinal, respiratory, and ear infections than do formula-fed infants.

- Although iron-fortified infant formulas are nutritionally adequate and safe, their nutrient compositions aren't identical to human milk. Infant formulas don't supply immune system factors that are in breast milk. Human milk may contain inadequate amounts of vitamin D and the minerals iron and fluoride.

- Healthy babies are physically mature enough to consume solid baby foods by about 4 to 6 months of age. Breastfeeding can be combined with providing a variety of tolerated foods.

- Whole cow's milk shouldn't be fed to infants until they're 1 year of age. Fat-reduced cow's milk and fat-free cow's milk are too low in energy to be given to most children until they're 2 years of age.

- The rapid growth rate that occurs during a child's first 12 months of life tapers off quickly during the preschool years. When a child's growth rate slows, the youngster's appetite decreases because he or she doesn't need as much food. When planning meals for children, caregivers should emphasize nutrient-dense foods, such as lean meats, low-fat dairy products, whole-grain cereals, fruits, nuts, and vegetables.

- During adolescence, the child experiences puberty and the adolescent growth spurt. To provide the energy and nutrients needed to support such rapid growth rate, an adolescent's food intake increases accordingly. Nutrition-related problems that often affect young children and adolescents are iron deficiency, poor calcium intakes, and obesity.

- The aging process begins at conception and is characterized by numerous predictable physical changes, including the need for fewer calories later in life. Many of the undesirable physical changes associated with growing old are the result of a lifetime of physical inactivity.

- Compared to younger persons, older adults have greater risk of nutritional deficiencies. Diets of older adults often provide inadequate amounts of vitamins and minerals.

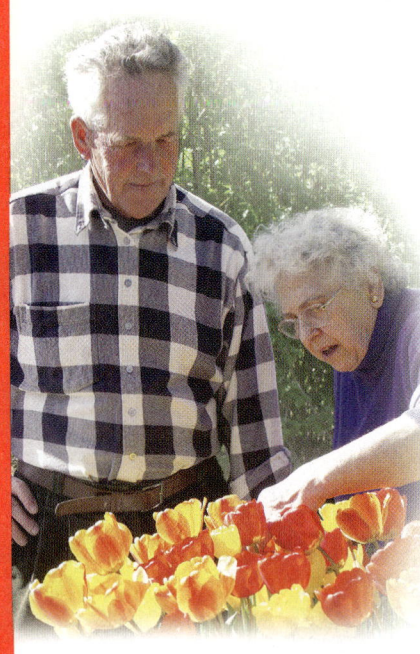

Pixtal/AGE Fotostock

- Factors that can influence an older person's nutritional status include medications, lack of social support, low income, lack of mobility, and tooth loss. People who have impaired cognitive and physical functioning may be unable to make decisions regarding planning nutritious meals, as well as to shop for and prepare food.

Module 11.2 How Safe Is My Food?

- Food-borne illness occurs when pathogens or their toxic by-products enter food and they're consumed. The United States has one of the safest food supplies in the world. The FDA and the USDA are the key federal agencies that protect consumers by regulating the country's food industry.

- Food-borne pathogens include bacteria, viruses, molds, protists, and parasitic worms. Food-borne pathogens may infect your digestive tract, inflaming the tissues. Some food-borne pathogens multiply in your intestinal tract, enter your bloodstream, and cause general illness when they invade other tissues. Other pathogens contaminate food and secrete poisons that irritate your intestinal tract and cause food intoxication. Protein-rich foods are more likely to support the growth of food-borne pathogens than other foods.

- Signs and symptoms of food-borne illness typically include vomiting, diarrhea, and intestinal cramps. Influenza is a respiratory tract infection, so it's inaccurate to call a bout of diarrhea and intestinal cramps the "stomach flu."

- Pathogens are found throughout your environment. Poor personal hygiene practices and improper food handling frequently result in food-borne illness. Failing to cook and store foods properly can also increase the likelihood of food-borne illness. According to the USDA, the "danger zone" for high-risk foods is between 40°F and 140°F. Cooking foods to the proper temperature destroys food-borne viruses and bacteria. Chilling food slows the growth of microbes.

- Pesticides can contaminate foods, especially produce. Concentrations of pesticide residues often decrease as food crops are washed, stored, processed, and prepared. The EPA regulates the proper use of pesticides and sets pesticide tolerances.

Module 11.3 Dietary Adequacy: A Global Concern

- Undernutrition occurs when long-term energy and nutrient intakes are insufficient to meet an individual's needs. Poverty and undernutrition are common in countries where people must cope with infectious diseases, overcrowded and unsafe housing conditions, and polluted water supplies.

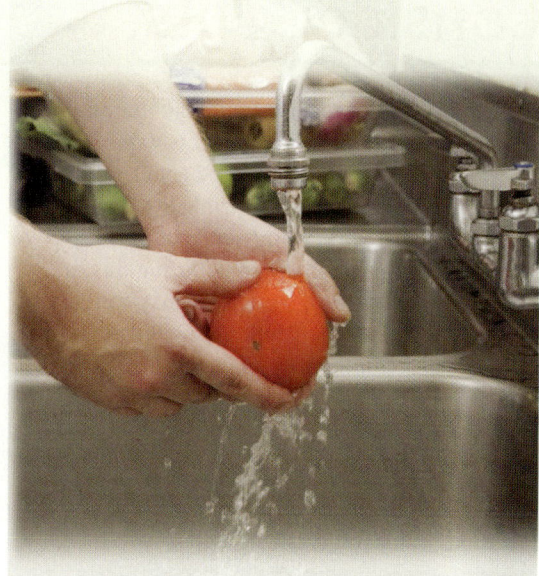
UpperCut Images/SuperStock

- In chronically undernourished children, nutrient deficiencies are responsible for stunted physical growth, delayed physical development, reduced immune system function, blindness, impaired intellectual development, and premature death. The vast majority of childhood deaths associated with undernutrition occur among poor populations in developing countries, particularly in parts of Africa and Asia.

- Undernourished pregnant women are more likely to die while giving birth than are adequately nourished pregnant women. Furthermore, malnourished pregnant women have a high risk of giving birth prematurely.

- In developing countries, poor parents often add excessive amounts of water to infant formula, which dilutes the nutritional value of the formula and increases the likelihood of contaminating it with disease-causing microbes. Babies should continue to receive breast milk in addition to solid foods well into their second year, especially in places where clean water is unavailable. Protein malnutrition typically occurs soon after impoverished children are weaned abruptly from breast milk and introduced to far-less-nourishing solid foods.

- In 2017, 12.3% of the U.S. population lived at or below the poverty guidelines. Food insecurity affected about 12% of all households in the United States in 2017. In the United States, several federally supported food programs provide food for people in need.

- An estimated 9.7 billion people will be living on Earth in 2050. Agricultural efforts will need to double their current level of production to meet the population's demand for more food. Our current system of food production relies primarily on conventional agricultural methods that use considerable amounts of water and pesticides and create greenhouse gases.

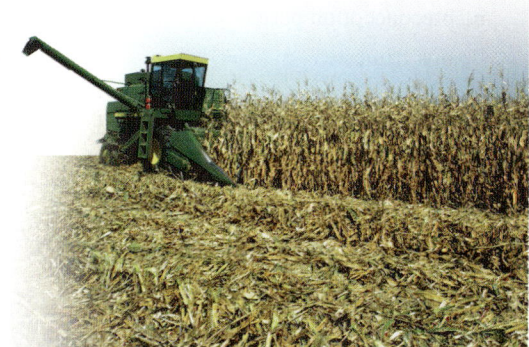
Glow Images

- Sustainable agriculture involves farming methods that meet the demand for more food without depleting natural resources and harming the environment. Steps that are recommended to solve the problems created by conventional agricultural methods include stopping the expansion of agricultural activity into tropical forests and grasslands; improving crop yields, for example by using biotechnology in agriculture; being more efficient with the use of natural resources and pesticides; eating less meat; and reducing food waste.

- Certain social, political, economic, and agricultural changes can reduce the number of people who are chronically hungry. Population control is critical for preserving the Earth's resources for future generations. Long-term ways to slow population growth include providing well-paying jobs, improving public education, and increasing access to health care services.

Consider This...

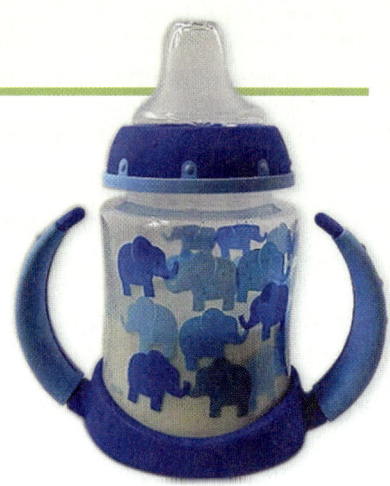

Wendy Schiff

1. One of your friends just found out that she is pregnant. Although her BMI is within the healthy range, she's concerned about gaining too much weight during pregnancy. What advice would you provide your friend concerning the need to gain some weight during this life stage? If your friend's prepregnancy weight was 125 pounds, how much weight would be appropriate for her to gain during pregnancy?

2. Your pregnant friend wants your advice concerning whether she should breastfeed or formula-feed her baby. After reading Unit 11, what information would you provide to help your friend decide to breastfeed?

3. Olivia is a healthy 2-month-old baby. Olivia's mother, Kara, wants to replace Olivia's iron-fortified infant formula with the same fresh fluid 2% milk that she drinks. What advice would you give to Kara concerning the appropriateness of making such a decision?

4. Are your parents, grandparents, and/or great-grandparents still alive? If any of your ancestors died before they were 60 years of age, can you identify their causes of death and factors that contributed to their deaths? What lifestyle changes can you make now that can help you achieve a longer, healthier lifetime?

5. Consider your usual food preparation and storage practices. From what you learned after reading Unit 11, list any practices you have that are unsafe.

6. What steps can you take to reduce the amount of food that you waste?

Test Yourself

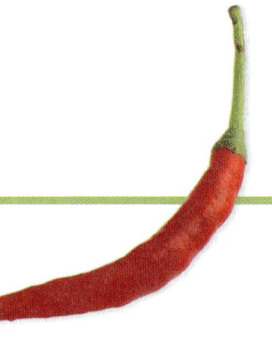

Select the best answer.

1. The embryo/fetus develops most of its organs during the
    a. preconception period.
    b. first trimester.
    c. second trimester.
    d. third trimester.

2. Preeclampsia is a form of _____ that can develop during pregnancy.
    a. hypertension
    b. diabetes
    c. hypertriglyceridemia
    d. anemia

3. A healthy infant who weighs 6.5 pounds at birth can be expected to weigh _____ pounds by her first birthday.
    a. 13.0   c. 19.5
    b. 16.5   d. 23.5

4. Breastfed infants are _____ than babies who are fed infant formula.
    a. more likely to have diarrhea
    b. less likely to have sickle cell disease
    c. more likely to have respiratory infections
    d. less likely to have ear infections

5. Which of the following factors can influence an older adult's nutritional status?
   a. Illnesses
   b. Medications
   c. Income level
   d. All of the above are correct.

6. Food-borne illnesses are usually characterized by
   a. flu-like signs and symptoms.
   b. coughing, sneezing, and respiratory inflammation.
   c. abdominal cramps, diarrhea, and vomiting.
   d. megaloblastic anemia and nervous system defects.

7. Which of the following practices doesn't help reduce the growth of food-borne pathogens?
   a. Washing hands before preparing food
   b. Keeping cold foods cold and hot foods hot
   c. Cooking foods to proper internal temperatures
   d. Storing cooked meat at room temperature

8. Which of the following temperatures is recommended for storing chilled foods in a refrigerator?
   a. 40°F
   b. 50°F
   c. 60°F
   d. 70°F

9. The _____ Program enables eligible low-income participants to use a special debit card to purchase food at authorized stores.
   a. Nutritious Food Purchase
   b. Supplemental Nutrition Assistance
   c. Healthy Diets for All
   d. Eat Better for Less

10. Which of the following actions is not a solution to the problems created by conventional agricultural methods?
    a. Cut down tropical forests to make way for more farmland.
    b. Improve crop yields through biotechnological advancements.
    c. Use integrated pest management methods.
    d. Eat less red meat.

11. Which of the following factors doesn't contribute to undernutrition?
    a. Long-term drought conditions that result in crop failures
    b. Civil unrest or wars that disrupt food production and supply routes
    c. Cultural practices that limit giving protein-rich foods to women and children
    d. Farming methods that rely on growing pest-resistant crops

12. Rachel's 85-year-old grandmother lives by herself in a major city. She has severe arthritis, which limits her ability to shop for groceries and prepare nutritious meals. Which of the following programs is sponsored by the U.S. government and would be helpful for Rachel's grandmother?
    a. WIC
    b. Meals on Wheels
    c. Healthy Diets for Needy Seniors
    d. UNICEF

Answers: 1. b 2. a 3. c 4. d 5. d 6. c 7. d 8. a 9. b 10. a 11. d 12. b

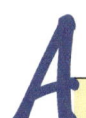

Answer This (Module 11.1d)

27 inches

References ➡ See Appendix D.

Design elements: Spiral notebook paper background, Stacked paper with clip background, Marginal note clip, and Culture & Cuisine globe icon: ©McGraw-Hill Education; In a Nutshell walnut: ©McGraw-Hill Education/Mark A. Dierker, photographer; Test Yourself red pepper: Iconotec/Glow Images

Appendixes

Appendix A	English-Metric Conversion and Metric-to-Household Units	A-2
Appendix B	Daily Values (DVs) Table	A-3
Appendix C	The Basics of Energy Metabolism	A-4
Appendix D	References	A-6
Appendix E	Dietary Reference Intake (DRI) Tables	A-21
Appendix F	Modifying Recipes for Healthy Living	A-27

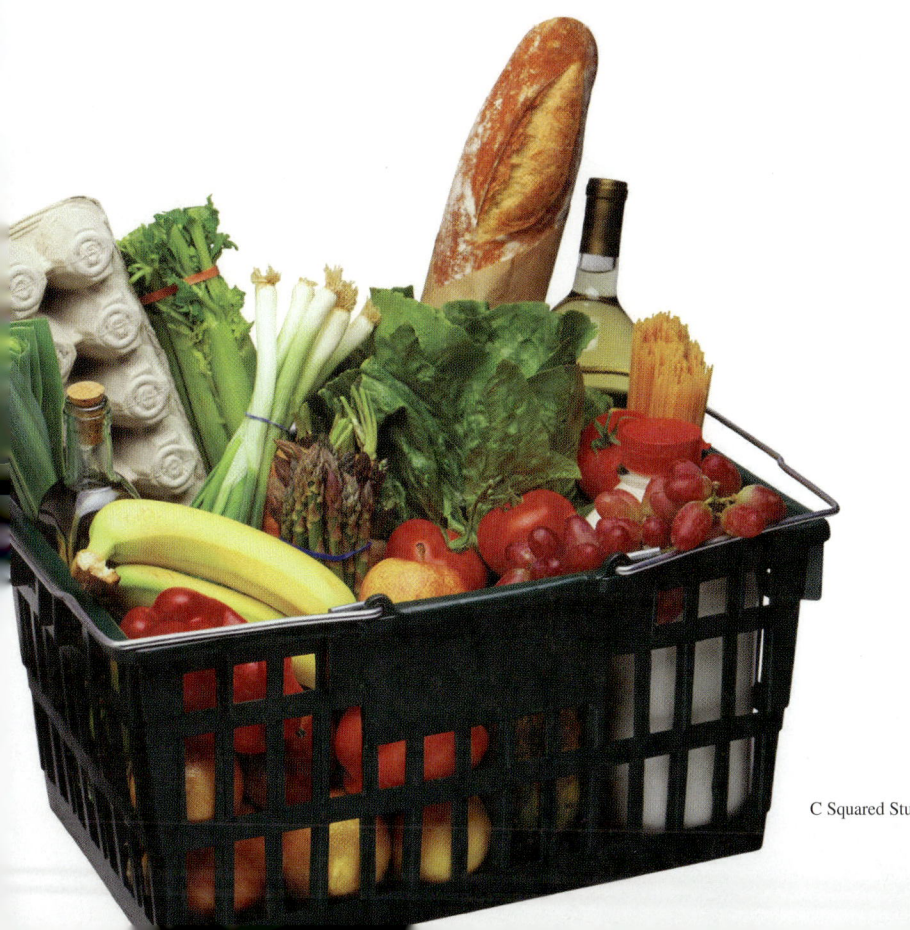

C Squared Studios/Getty Images

Appendix A

English-Metric Conversion and Metric-to-Household Units

Length			Weight		
English (USA)		Metric	English (USA)		Metric
inch	=	2.54 cm (centimeter)	ounce	=	28.35 g
foot	=	0.30 m (meter)	pound	=	0.45 kg
0.039 inch	=	millimeter (mm)	2.2 lb	=	kilogram
0.390 inch	=	centimeter (cm)			
39.4 inches	=	meter (m)			

Volume			Volume		
English (USA)		Metric	English (USA)		Metric
teaspoon	=	5 milliliters (ml)	1.06 quart	=	liter
tablespoon	=	15 ml			
fluid ounce	=	30 ml			
quart	=	0.95 liter (L)			
cup	=	237 ml			

Household Units			Household Units		
3 teaspoons (tsp)	=	1 tablespoon (Tbsp)	1 cup	=	8 fluid ounces
4 Tbsp	=	¼ cup	1 cup	=	½ pint
5 Tbsp + 1 tsp	=	⅓ cup	2 cup	=	1 pint
8 Tbsp	=	½ cup	4 cup	=	1 quart
16 Tbsp	=	1 cup	2 pints	=	1 quart
			4 quarts	=	1 gallon

Ingram Publishing/SuperStock

Appendix B

Daily Values (DVs) Table

Source: Modified from the FDA.

Dietary Component	Unit of Measure	Current Daily Values for People over 4 Years of Age
Total fat*	g	78
Saturated fatty acids*	"	20
Protein*	"	50
Cholesterol	mg	300
Total carbohydrate*	g	275
Fiber	"	28
Added sugars	"	50
Vitamin A	mcg (RAEs)	900
Vitamin D	mcg	20
Vitamin E	mg	15
Vitamin K	mcg	120
Vitamin C	mg	90
Folate	mcg	400
Thiamin	mg	1.2
Riboflavin	"	1.3
Niacin	"	16
Vitamin B-6	"	1.7
Vitamin B-12	mcg	2.4
Biotin	mcg	30
Pantothenic acid	mg	5
Calcium	"	1300
Phosphorus	"	1250
Iodine	mcg	150
Iron	mg	18
Magnesium	"	420
Copper	"	0.9
Zinc	"	11
Sodium	"	2300
Potassium	"	4700
Chloride	"	2300
Manganese	"	2.3
Selenium	mcg	55
Chromium	"	35
Molybdenum	"	45

*These Daily Values are based on a 2000-kcal diet.

Appendix C

The Basics of Energy Metabolism

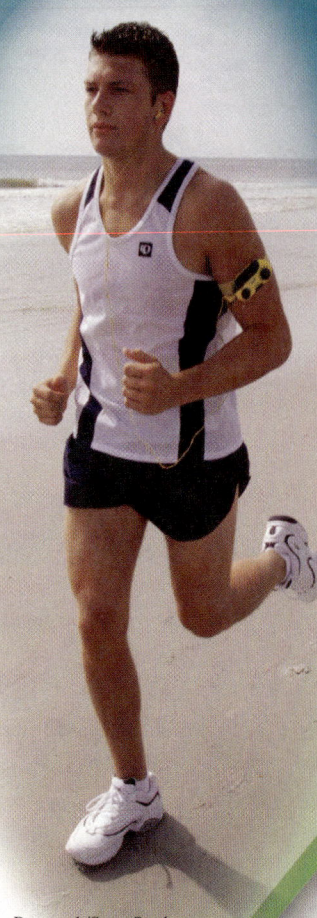

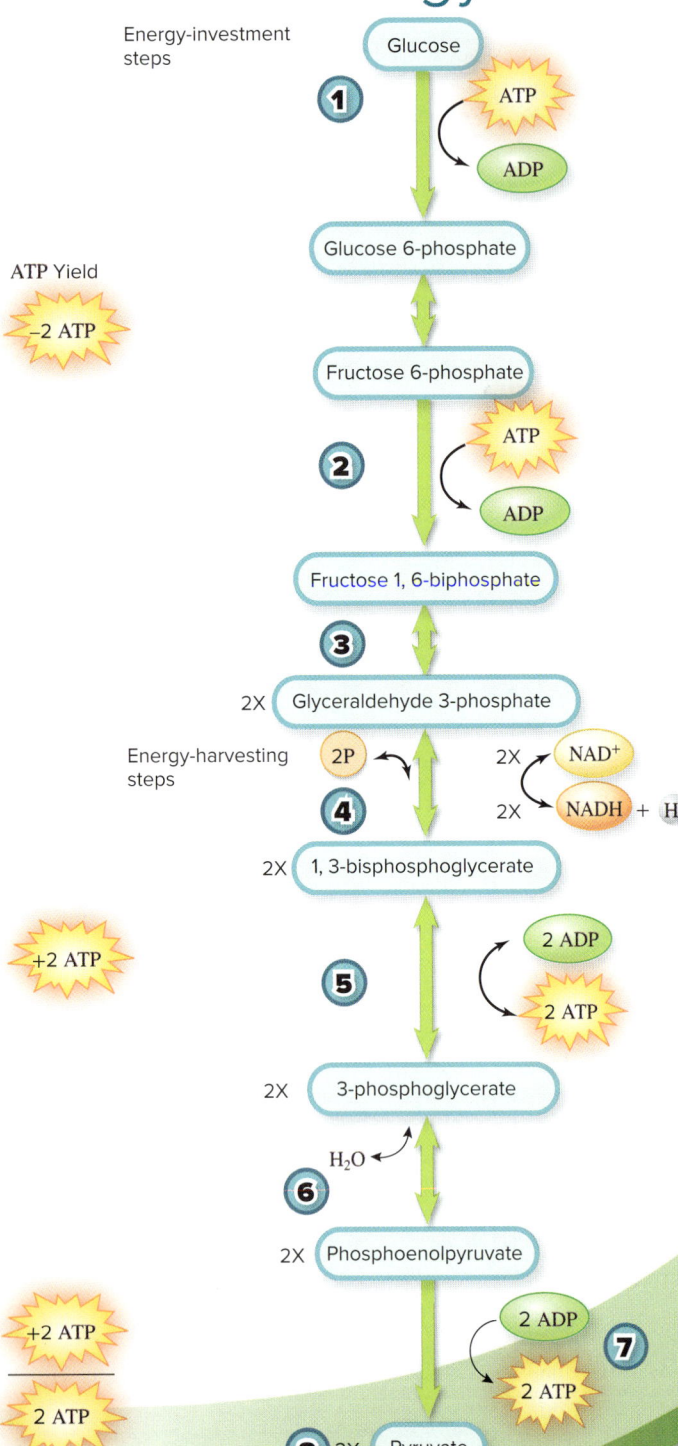

Energy-investment steps

ATP Yield

−2 ATP

Energy-harvesting steps

+2 ATP

+2 ATP
―――
2 ATP
(Net Gain ATP)

1. Adding phosphate to glucose using ATP produces an activated molecule.

2. Rearrangement, followed by a second addition of phosphate using ATP, produces fructose 1, 6-biphosphate.

3. The 6-carbon molecule is split into two 3-carbon-phosphate molecules.

4. Oxidation, followed by the addition of phosphate, produces 2 NADH + 2H$^+$ molecules and two 3-carbon-phosphate-phosphate molecules.

5. Removal of 2 phosphate groups by 2 ADP molecules produces 2 ATP molecules and two 3-carbon-phosphate molecules.

6. Removal of water produces two 3-carbon-phosphate molecules.

7. Removal of 2 phosphate groups by 2 ADP molecules produces 2 ATP molecules.

8. Pyruvate is the end product of this metabolic pathway.

Purestock/SuperStock

A-4

Appendix C The Basics of Energy Metabolism A-5

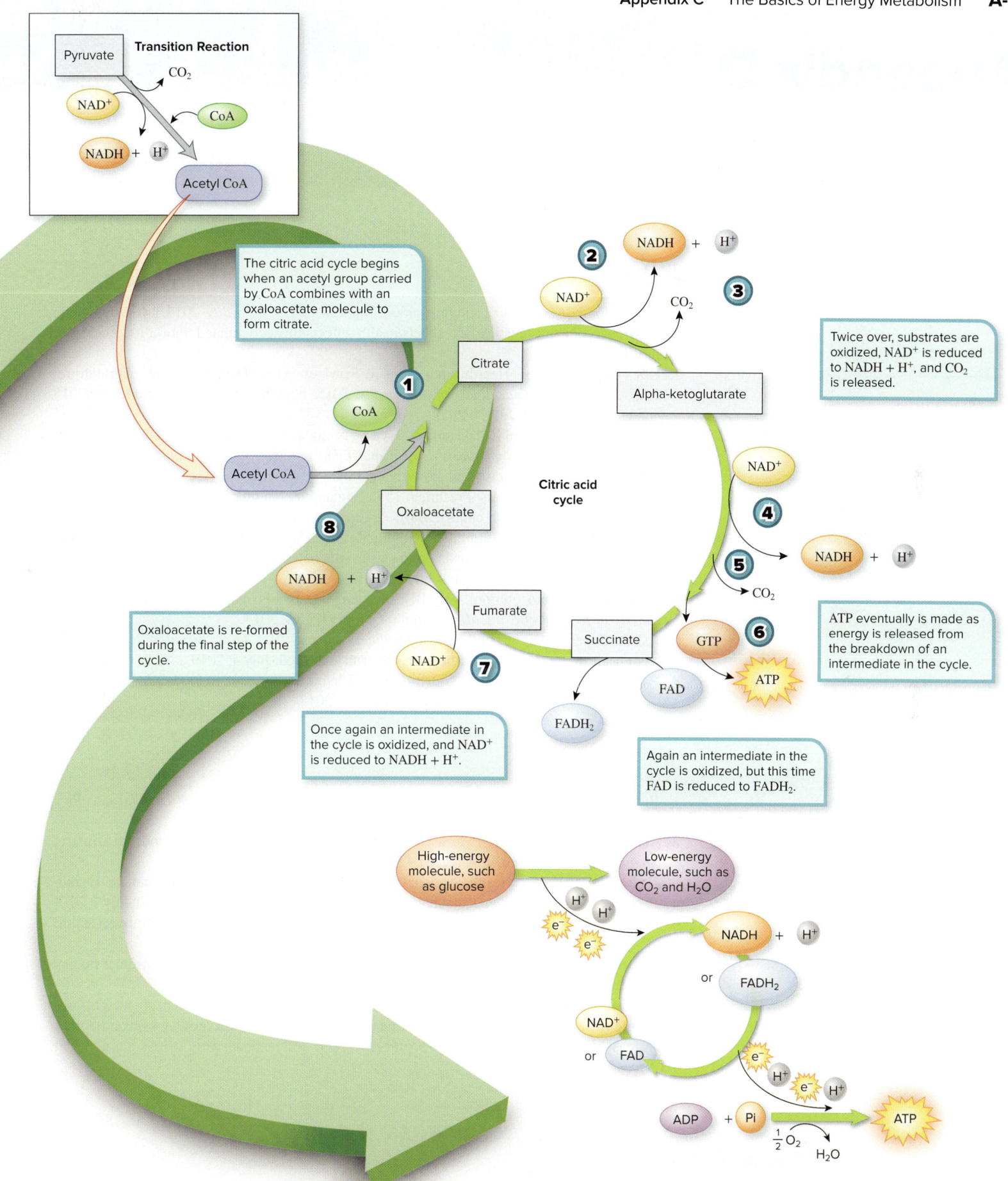

Appendix D

References

Unit 1

1. Centers for Disease Control and Prevention: *Tobacco-related mortality.* 2018. https://www.cdc.gov/tobacco/data_statistics/fact_sheets/health_effects/tobacco_related_mortality/ Accessed: July 4, 2019
2. U.S. Department of Health and Human Services, U.S. Department of Agriculture: *2015–2020 Dietary Guidelines for Americans.* 2015. http://health.gov/dietaryguidelines/2015/guidelines/ Accessed: July 4, 2019
3. U.S. Department of Health and Human Services, National Institutes of Health, Office of Dietary Supplements: *Dietary Supplement Health and Education Act of 1994. Public Law 103-417, 103rd Congress.* https://ods.od.nih.gov/About/DSHEA_Wording.aspx Accessed: July 4, 2019
4. Vadeboncoeur C and others: Freshman 15 in England: A longitudinal evaluation of first year university student's weight change. *BMC Obesity* 3:45, 2016.
5. U.S. Department of Agriculture, Agricultural Research Service: *Solid fats and added sugars in foods.* 2017. https://www.ars.usda.gov/news-events/news/research-news/2015/solid-fats-and-added-sugars-in-foods/ Accessed: July 4, 2019
6. Drewnowski A and Fulgoni VL (III): Nutrient density: Principles and evaluation tools. *American Journal of Clinical Nutrition* 99(suppl):1223S, 2014.
7. Ask the Experts: Dragon fruit. *Berkeley Wellness.* January 2011. https://www.berkeleywellness.com/healthy-eating/nutrition/article/dragon-fruit Accessed: July 4, 2019
8. Position of the Academy of Nutrition and Dietetics: Functional foods. *Journal of the Academy of Nutrition and Dietetics* 113(8):1096, 2013.

Unit 2

1. Benedetti F and others: How placebos change the patient's brain. *Neuropsychopharmacology* 36(1):339, 2011.
2. Marshall BJ and others: Pyloric *Campylobacter* infection and gastroduodenal disease. *Medical Journal of Australia* 142(8):439, 1985.
3. National Institutes of Health, National Center for Complementary and Integrative Health: *Pomegranate.* 2017. https://nccih.nih.gov/health/pomegranate/at-a-glance Accessed: July 4, 2019
4. National Institutes of Health, National Center for Complementary and Integrative Health: *Ginger.* 2016. https://nccih.nih.gov/health/ginger Accessed: July 4, 2019
5. Federal Trade Commission: *Miracle health claims.* 2011. https://www.consumer.ftc.gov/articles/0167-miracle-health-claims Accessed: July 4, 2019
6. Federal Trade Commission: Marketer who promoted a green coffee bean weight-loss supplement agrees to settle FTC charges. 2015. https://www.ftc.gov/news-events/press-releases/2015/01/marketer-who-promoted-green-coffee-bean-weight-loss-supplement Accessed: July 21, 2019

Unit 3

1. Institute of Medicine: *Dietary Reference Intakes for vitamin C, vitamin E, selenium, and carotenoids.* Washington, DC: National Academies Press, 2000.
2. Oregon State University, Linus Pauling Institute, Micronutrient Information Center: *Vitamin C.* 2018. https://lpi.oregonstate.edu/mic/vitamins/vitamin-C Accessed: July 4, 2019
3. National Academies of Sciences, Engineering, and Medicine: *Dietary Reference Intakes for Sodium and Potassium.* Washington, DC: The National Academies Press, 2019.
4. Barr SI and others: Interpreting and using the Dietary Reference Intakes in dietary assessment of individuals and groups. *Journal of the American Dietetic Association* 102(6):780, 2002.
5. U.S. Department of Agriculture: *ChooseMyPlate.gov.* https://www.choosemyplate.gov /Accessed: July 4, 2019
6. *Draft guidance for industry and FDA staff: Whole grain label statements.* 2006. https://www.fda.gov/food/guidanceregulation/guidancedocumentsregulatoryinformation/ucm059088.htm Accessed: July 4, 2019
7. U.S. Department of Agriculture, ChooseMyPlate.gov: *All about the fruit group.* 2018. https://www.choosemyplate.gov/fruit Accessed: July 4, 2019
8. U.S. Department of Agriculture, ChooseMyPlate.gov: *Tips: Focus on whole fruits.* https://www.choosemyplate.gov/fruits-tips Accessed: July 4, 2019
9. U.S. Department of Agriculture, ChooseMyPlate.gov: *All about oils: What are oils?* 2016. https://www.choosemyplate.gov/oils Accessed: July 4, 2019
10. U.S. Department of Agriculture: *Introduction to organic practices.* 2015. https://www.ams.usda.gov/publications/content/introduction-organic-practices Accessed: July 4, 2019
11. Johansson E and others: Contribution of organically grown crops to human health. *International Journal of Environmental Research and Public Health* 11:3870, 2014.
12. U.S. Department of Agriculture, Choosemyplate.gov: *Nutritional needs during pregnancy.* 2015. https://www.choosemyplate.gov/moms/pregnancy-nutritional-needs Accessed: July 4, 2019
13. National Institutes of Health, National Library of Medicine, MedlinePlus: Weight loss and alcohol. 2018. https://medlineplus.gov/ency/patientinstructions/000889.htm Accessed: July 4, 2019
14. U.S. Departments of Health and Human Services and Agriculture: *2015–2020 Dietary Guidelines for Americans.* 2015. https://health.gov/dietaryguidelines/2015/guidelines/ Accessed: July 17, 2018
15. U.S. Food and Drug Administration: *How to understand and use the Nutrition Facts label.* 2018. https://www.fda.gov/food/ingredientspackaginglabeling/labelingnutrition/ucm274593.htm. Accessed: July 4, 2019
16. U.S. Government Publishing Office, Electronic Code of Federal Regulation: *Title 21: Food and drugs, part 101–food labeling, subpart A—general provisions, §101.14 Health claims: General requirements.* https://www.ecfr.gov/cgi-bin/text-idx?SID=1aec8849e2bf8bd210e518715257e6ff&mc=true&node=se21.2.101_114&rgn=div8 Accessed: July 4, 2019
17. National Center for Complementary and Integrative Health: *Using dietary supplements wisely.* Updated January 2019. https://nccih.nih.gov/health/supplements/wiseuse.htm Accessed: July 4, 2019
18. National Center for Complementary and Integrative Health: *Vitamins and minerals.* 2018. https://nccih.nih.gov/health/vitamins Accessed: July 4, 2019
19. Clarke TC and others: Trends in the use of complementary health approaches among adults: United States, 2002–2012. *National health statistics reports; no 79.* Hyattsville, MD: National Center for Health Statistics. 2015.
20. National Center for Complementary and Integrative Health: *Use of complementary health approaches in the U.S., National Health Interview Survey, Why do people use certain complementary approaches?* 2012. https://nccih.nih.gov/research/statistics/NHIS/2012/wellness Accessed: July 4, 2019

21. National Center for Complementary and Integrative Health: *Herbs at a Glance: Echinacea.* 2016. https://nccih.nih.gov/health/echinacea/ataglance.htm Accessed: July 4, 2019
22. *Statista: Revenue of vitamins & nutritional supplements production in the United States from 2018 and 2019 (in billion U.S. dollars).* https://www.statista.com/statistics/235801/retail-sales-of-vitamins-and-nutritional-supplements-in-the-us/ Accessed: July 4, 2019
23. Huang H-Y and others: The efficacy and safety of multivitamin and multimineral supplement use to prevent cancer and chronic disease in adults: A systematic review for a National Institutes of Health State-of-the-Science Conference. *Annals of Internal Medicine* 145(5):372, 2006.

Unit 4

1. Besnard P: Taste of fat: A sixth taste modality? *Physiological Reviews* 96(1):151, 2016.
2. National Institutes of Health, U.S. National Library of Medicine, MedlinePlus: Choking—adult or child over 1 year. 2019. https://www.nlm.nih.gov/medlineplus/ency/article/000049.htm Accessed: July 4, 2019
3. Machado MV and Cortez-Pinto H: Diet, microbiota, obesity, and NAFLD: A dangerous quartet. *International Journal of Molecular Sciences* 1:17(4):pii: E481, 2016.
4. Hooman A and Hazen SL: Contribution of gut bacteria to lipid levels: Another metabolic role for microbes? *Circulation Research* 117:750, 2015.
5. Rao SSC and others: Brain fogginess, gas and bloating: A link between SIBO, probiotics and metabolic acidosis. *Clinical and Translational Gastroenterology* 9:162, 2018.
6. Bafeta A and others: Harms reporting in randomized controlled trials of interventions aimed at modifying microbiota: A systematic review. *Annals of Internal Medicine.* July 17, 2018.
7. National Institutes of Health, National Institute of Diabetes and Digestive and Kidney Diseases: *Constipation.* 2018. https://www.niddk.nih.gov/health-information/digestive-diseases/constipation Accessed: July 4, 2019
8. U.S. National Library of Medicine, MedlinePlus: *Diverticulosis.* 2017. https://medlineplus.gov/ency/article/007668.htm Accessed: July 4, 2019
9. National Institutes of Health, National Institute of Diabetes and Digestive and Kidney Diseases: *Diarrhea.* 2016. https://www.niddk.nih.gov/health-information/digestive-diseases/diarrhea Accessed: July 4, 2019
10. Mayo Clinic Staff: *Nausea and vomiting.* 2018. https://www.mayoclinic.org/symptoms/nausea/basics/definition/SYM-20050736?p=1 Accessed: July 4, 2019
11. National Institutes of Health, National Institute of Diabetes and Digestive and Kidney Diseases: *Acid reflux (GER & GERD) in adults.* 2014. https://www.niddk.nih.gov/health-information/digestive-diseases/acid-reflux-ger-gerd-adults Accessed: July 4, 2019
12. National Institutes of Health, National Institute of Diabetes and Digestive and Kidney Diseases: *Peptic ulcers (stomach ulcers).* 2014. https://www.niddk.nih.gov/health-information/digestive-diseases/peptic-ulcers-stomach-ulcers Accessed: July 4, 2019
13. National Institutes of Health, National Institute of Diabetes and Digestive and Kidney Diseases: *Gallstones.* 2017. https://www.niddk.nih.gov/health-information/digestive-diseases/gallstones/definition-facts Accessed: July 4, 2019
14. National Institutes of Health, National Institute of Diabetes and Digestive and Kidney Diseases: *Irritable bowel syndrome (IBS).* 2017. https://www.niddk.nih.gov/health-information/digestive-diseases/irritable-bowel-syndrome Accessed: July 4, 2019
15. U.S. National Library of Medicine, MedlinePlus: *Irritable bowel syndrome.* 2017. https://medlineplus.gov/ency/article/000246.htm Accessed: July 4, 2019
16. National Institutes of Health, National Institute of Diabetes and Digestive and Kidney Diseases: *Ulcerative colitis and colon cancer.* 2014. https://www.niddk.nih.gov/health-information/health-topics/digestive-diseases/ulcerative-colitis/Pages/facts.aspx#10 Accessed: July 4, 2019
17. American Cancer Society: *Colorectal cancer.* 2018. https://www.cancer.org/cancer/colon-rectal-cancer.html Accessed: July 4, 2019

Unit 5

1. U.S. Department of Agriculture, Economic Research Service: *Sugar and sweeteners yearbook tables, U.S. sugar supply and use.* Tables 51, 52, and 53. July 2019. https://www.ers.usda.gov/data-products/sugar-and-sweeteners-yearbook-tables.aspx Accessed: October 21, 2019
2. Centers for Disease Control and Prevention: *Attention deficit/hyperactivity disorder.* 2018. https://www.cdc.gov/ncbddd/adhd/index.html Accessed: July 4, 2019
3. Horton J: The truth about agave. 2014. *WebMD.* https://www.webmd.com/diet/features/the-truth-about-agave#1 Accessed: July 4, 2019
4. U.S. Food and Drug Administration: *High-intensity sweeteners.* 2014. https://www.fda.gov/Food/IngredientsPackagingLabeling/FoodAdditivesIngredients/ucm397716.htm Accessed: July 4, 2019
5. *Academy of Nutrition and Dietetics: Sugar substitutes: How much is too much?* 2018. https://www.eatright.org/food/nutrition/dietary-guidelines-and-myplate/sugar-substitutes-how-much-is-too-much Accessed: July 4, 2019
6. Crézé C and others: The impact of caloric and non-caloric sweeteners on food intake and brain responses to food: A randomized crossover controlled trial in healthy humans. *Nutrients* 10:615, 2018.
7. Centers for Disease Control and Prevention: *Botulism: Prevention.* 2018. https://www.cdc.gov/botulism/prevention.html Accessed: July 4, 2019
8. U.S. Food and Drug Administration: Code of Federal Regulations: *21 CFR 172.804 Title 21, volume 3* (April 1, 2018). https://www.accessdata.fda.gov/scripts/cdrh/cfdocs/cfcfr/CFRSearch.cfm?fr=172.804 Accessed: March 26, 2019
9. Otten JJ and others, eds: *Dietary Reference Intakes: The essential guide to nutrient requirements.* Washington, DC: National Academies Press, 2006.
10. U.S. Department of Agriculture, Agricultural Research Service: *What we eat in America, NHANES 2015–2016: Nutrient intakes from food and beverages: Mean amounts consumed by individuals: By gender and age.* 2018. https://www.ars.usda.gov/northeast-area/beltsville-md-bhnrc/beltsville-human-nutrition-research-center/food-surveys-research-group/docs/wweia-data-tables/ Accessed: July 4, 2019
11. Micha R and others: Association between dietary factors and mortality from heart disease, stroke, and type 2 diabetes in the United States. *Journal of the American Medical Association* 317(9):912, 2017.
12. U.S. Departments of Agriculture and Health and Human Services: 2015–2020 *Dietary Guidelines for Americans.* 2015. http://health.gov/dietaryguidelines/2015/guidelines/ Accessed: July 4, 2019
13. U.S. Department of Agriculture, Agricultural Research Service: *National nutrient database for standard reference legacy release.* 2018. https://ndb.nal.usda.gov/ndb/search/list?home=true Accessed: June 30, 2019
14. American Diabetes Association: *Diagnosing diabetes and learning about prediabetes.* 2014. http://www.diabetes.org/are-you-at-risk/prediabetes/?loc=atrisk-slabnav Accessed: June 30, 2019
15. Bailey RL and others: Sources of added sugars in young children, adolescents, and adults with low and high intakes of added sugars. *Nutrients* 10(1):102, 2018.
16. Bray GA and Popkin BM: Dietary sugar and body weight: Have we reached a crisis in the epidemic of obesity and diabetes? *Diabetes Care* 37:950, 2014.
17. Ludwig DS and others: Dietary carbohydrates: Role of quality and quantity in chronic disease. *The British Medical Journal* 361:k2340, 2018. June 13, 2018.
18. DiNicolantonio JJ and others: Added fructose as a principal driver of non-alcoholic fatty liver disease: A public health crisis. *Open Heart* 4:e000631, 2017.
19. National Institutes of Health, Institute of Diabetes and Digestive and Kidney Diseases: *Nonalcoholic fatty liver disease & NASH.* 2016. https://www.niddk.nih.gov/health-information/liver-disease/nafld-nash Accessed: July 4, 2019
20. Centers for Disease Control and Prevention, Diabetes: *Prevalence of both diagnosed and undiagnosed diabetes.* 2018. https://www.cdc.gov/diabetes/data/statistics-report/diagnosed-undiagnosed.html Accessed: July 4, 2019

21. Centers for Disease Control and Prevention, Diabetes Home: *Prediabetes: Your chance to prevent type 2 diabetes.* May 2019. https://www.cdc.gov/diabetes/basics/prediabetes.html Accessed: July 4, 2019
22. McCulloch DC: *Patient education:* Diabetes mellitus type 1: Overview (beyond the basics). *UpToDate.* Waltham, MA: UpToDate Inc. 2018. https://www.uptodate.com/contents/diabetes-mellitus-type-1-overview-beyond-the-basics?view=print Accessed: July 4, 2019
23. Centers for Disease Control and Prevention, Diabetes Home: *Who's at risk?* May 2019. https://www.cdc.gov/diabetes/basics/risk-factors.html Accessed: July 4, 2019
24. National Institute of Diabetes and Digestive and Kidney Diseases: *Pregnancy if you have diabetes.* 2017. https://www.niddk.nih.gov/health-information/diabetes/diabetes-pregnancy Accessed: July 4, 2019
25. National Institutes of Health, Institute of Diabetes and Digestive and Kidney Diseases: *The A1c test & diabetes.* 2018. https://www.niddk.nih.gov/health-information/diabetes/overview/tests-diagnosis/a1c-test Accessed: July 4, 2019
26. Forouhi NG and others: Dietary and nutritional approaches for prevention and management of type 2 diabetes. *The BMJ* 361:k2234, 2018.
27. Atkinson FS and others: International tables of glycemic index and glycemic load values: 2008. *Diabetes Care* 31(12):2281, 2008.
28. Venn BJ and Green TJ: Glycemic index and glycemic load: Measurement issues and their effect on diet-disease relationships. *European Journal of Clinical Nutrition* 61(Suppl 1): S122–S131, 2007.
29. Mayo Clinic Staff: *Hypoglycemia.* ND. https://www.mayoclinic.org/diseases-conditions/hypoglycemia/symptoms-causes/syc-20373685?p=1 Accessed: July 4, 2019
30. National Institutes of Health, Institute of Diabetes and Digestive and Kidney Diseases: *Lactose intolerance: Eating, diet, & nutrition for lactose intolerance.* 2018. https://www.niddk.nih.gov/health-information/digestive-diseases/lactose-intolerance/eating-diet-nutrition Accessed: July 4, 2019
31. Kim Y and Choi CH: Role of fructose malabsorption in patients with irritable bowel syndrome. *Journal of Neurogastroenterology and Motility* 24(2):161, 2018.
32. Colombel JF and others: Functional gastrointestinal symptoms in patients with inflammatory bowel disease: A clinical challenge. *Clinical Gastroenterology and Hepatology.* August 9, 2018. pii: S1542-3565(18)30810-3.
33. Position of the Academy of Nutrition and Dietetics: Health implications of dietary fiber. *Journal of the Academy of Nutrition and Dietetics* 115(11):1861, 2015.

Unit 6

1. U.S. Departments of Health and Human Services and Agriculture: *2015–2020 Dietary Guidelines for Americans.* 2015. http://health.gov/dietaryguidelines/2015/guidelines/ Accessed: July 5, 2019
2. U.S. Food and Drug Administration: *Final determination regarding partially hydrogenated oils (removing trans fat).* 2018. https://www.fda.gov/food/ingredientspackaginglabeling/foodadditivesingredients/ucm449162.htm Accessed: July 5, 2019
3. Federal Trade Commission: *FTC settlement prohibits marketers of children's vitamins from making deceptive health claims about brain and eye development.* 2010. https://www.ftc.gov/news-events/press-releases/2010/12/ftc-settlement-prohibits-marketers-childrens-vitamins-making Accessed: July 5, 2019
4. Zeisel, SH: Nutrition in pregnancy: The argument for including a source of choline. *International Journal of Women's Health* 5:193, 2013.
5. Murphy SL and others: Mortality in the United States, 2017. *NCHS Data Brief*, No. 328. Hyattsville, MD: National Center for Health Statistics. 2018.
6. American Heart Association: *Understanding blood pressure readings.* 2017. https://www.heart.org/en/health-topics/high-blood-pressure/understanding-blood-pressure-readings Accessed: July 5, 2019
7. Lubrano V and Balzan S: Consolidated and emerging inflammatory markers in coronary artery disease. *World Journal of Experimental Medicine* 5(1):21, 2015.

8. Centers for Disease Control and Prevention: *Heart disease risk factors.* 2015. https://www.cdc.gov/heartdisease/risk_factors.htm Accessed: July 5, 2019
9. Sachs FM and others: Dietary fats and cardiovascular disease: A presidential advisory from the American Heart Association. *Circulation* 136:e1–e23, 2017.
10. Micha R and others: Association between dietary factors and mortality from heart disease, stroke, and type 2 diabetes in the United States. *Journal of the American Medical Association* 317(9):912, 2017.
11. National Institutes of Health, National Center for Complementary and Integrative Health: *Herbs at a glance: Garlic.* 2016. https://nccih.nih.gov/health/garlic/ataglance.htm Accessed: July 5, 2019
12. März W and others: HDL cholesterol: Reappraisal of its clinical relevance. *Clinical Research in Cardiology* 106(9):663, 2017.
13. U.S. Department of Agriculture, Agricultural Research Service: *What we eat in America, NHANES 2015–2016.* 2018. https://www.ars.usda.gov/northeast-area/beltsville-md-bhnrc/beltsville-human-nutrition-research-center/food-surveys-research-group/docs/wweia-data-tables/ Accessed: July 5, 2019
14. U.S. Departments of Health and Human Services and Agriculture: Chapter 1, Key elements of healthy eating patterns: A closer look inside healthy eating patterns: Oils. *2015–2020 Dietary Guidelines for Americans.* 2015. https://health.gov/dietaryguidelines/2015/guidelines/chapter-1/a-closer-look-inside-healthy-eating-patterns/ Accessed: July 5, 2019
15. National Institutes of Health, National Center for Complementary and Integrative Health: *Omega-3 supplements: In depth.* 2018. https://nccih.nih.gov/health/omega3/introduction.htm Accessed: July 5, 2019
16. Zamora-Ros R and others: Moderate egg consumption and all-cause and specific-cause mortality in the Spanish European Prospective into Cancer and Nutrition (EPIC-Spain) study. *European Journal of Nutrition.* Published online June 15, 2018.
17. Soliman GA: Dietary cholesterol and the lack of evidence in cardiovascular disease. *Nutrients* 10(6):780, 2018.
18. Zhong VW and others: Associations of dietary cholesterol or egg consumption with incident cardiovascular disease and mortality. *Journal of the American Medical Association* 321(11):108, 2019.

Unit 7

1. U.S. Department of Agriculture, Agricultural Research Service: *What we eat in America, NHANES 2015–2016.* 2018. https://www.ars.usda.gov/northeast-area/beltsville-md-bhnrc/beltsville-human-nutrition-research-center/food-surveys-research-group/docs/wweia-data-tables/ Accessed: July 4, 2019
2. *U.S. Departments of Agriculture and Health and Human Services: 2015-2020 Dietary Guidelines for Americans.* 2015. Appendix E3-3.2. https://health.gov/dietaryguidelines/2015-scientific-report/15-appendix-E3/e3-2.asp Accessed: July 4, 2019
3. U.S. Departments of Agriculture and Health and Human Services: *2015–2020 Dietary Guidelines for Americans.* 2015. http://health.gov/dietaryguidelines/2015/guidelines/ Accessed: July 4, 2019
4. Oelke EA and others: *Quinoa. Alternative field crops manual.* University of Wisconsin-Extension, University of Minnesota: Center for Alternative Plant & Animal Productions, and the Minnesota Extension Service. (ND) https://www.hort.purdue.edu/newcrop/afcm/quinoa.html Accessed: July 4, 2019
5. Reinhart RJ: *Gallup.com: Snapshot: Few Americans vegetarian or vegan.* August 1, 2018. https://news.gallup.com/poll/238328/snapshot-few-americans-vegetarian-vegan.aspx Accessed: July 4, 2019
6. Appleby PN and Key TJ: The long-term health of vegetarians and vegans. *Proceedings of the Nutrition Society* 75(3):287, 2016.
7. Academy of Nutrition and Dietetics: Position of the Academy of Nutrition and Dietetics: Vegetarian diets. *Journal of the Academy of Nutrition and Dietetics* 116(12):1970, 2016.

8. Kocaoglu C and others: Cerebral atrophy in a vitamin B12-deficient infant of a vegetarian mother. *Journal of Health, Population and Nutrition* 32(2):367, 2014.
9. Cuenca-Sánchez M and others: Controversies surrounding high-protein diet intake: Satiating effect and kidney and bone health. *Advances in Nutrition* 6(3):260, 2015.
10. Zeratsky K: *Are high-protein diets safe for weight loss?* 2018. Mayo Clinic. https://www.mayoclinic.org/healthy-lifestyle/nutrition-and-healthy-eating/expert-answers/high-protein-diets/faq-20058207 Accessed: July 4, 2019
11. Position of the Academy of Nutrition and Dietetics, Dietitians of Canada, and the American College of Sports Medicine: Nutrition and athletic performance. *Journal of the Academy of Nutrition and Dietetics* 116(3):501, 2016.
12. Witard WC and others: Protein considerations for optimizing skeletal muscle mass in healthy young and older adults. *Nutrients* 8:181, 2016.
13. Naclerio F and Larumbe-Zabala E: Effects of whey protein along or as part of a multi-ingredient formulation on strength, fat-free mass, or lean body mass in resistance-trained individuals: A meta-analysis. *Sports Medicine* 46(1):125, 2016.
14. World Health Organization: *UNICEF/WHO/World Bank Group Joint Child Malnutrition Estimates: Key findings of the 2018 edition.* 2018. http://www.who.int/nutgrowthdb/2018-jme-brochure.pdf?ua=1 Accessed: July 4, 2019
15. Food and Agriculture Organization of the United Nations: *Edible insects: Future prospects for food and feed security.* 2013. http://www.fao.org/docrep/018/i3253e/i3253e.pdf Accessed: July 4, 2019
16. Anagnostou K and Orange JS: The value of food allergy prevention in clinical practice in pediatrics: Targeting early life. *Children (Basel)* 5(2):23, 2018.
17. National Institute of Allergy and Infectious Disease: *Food allergy.* 2018. https://www.niaid.nih.gov/diseases-conditions/food-allergy Accessed: July 4, 2019
18. Larson K and others: Introducing allergenic food into infants' diets: Systematic review. *MCN American Journal of Maternal and Child Nursing* 42(2):72, 2017.
19. Casella G and others: Non celiac gluten sensitivity and diagnostic challenges. *Gastroenterology and Hepatology from Bed to Bench* 11(3):197, 2018.
20. National Institutes of Health, National Institute of Diabetes and Digestive and Kidney Diseases: *Definition and facts for celiac disease.* 2016. https://www.niddk.nih.gov/health-information/digestive-diseases/celiac-disease/definition-facts Accessed: July 4, 2019

Unit 8

1. U.S. Department of Agriculture, Agricultural Research Service: *What we eat in America, NHANES 2015–2016.* 2018. https://www.ars.usda.gov/northeast-area/beltsville-md-bhnrc/beltsville-human-nutrition-research-center/food-surveys-research-group/docs/wweia-data-tables/ Accessed: July 4, 2019
2. World Health Organization: Micronutrient deficiencies: *Vitamin A deficiency.* (ND) http://www.who.int/nutrition/topics/vad/en/index.html Accessed: July 4, 2019
3. National Institutes of Health, Office of Dietary Supplements: *Vitamin A: Factsheet for professionals.* 2018. https://ods.od.nih.gov/factsheets/VitaminA-HealthProfessional/ Accessed: July 4, 2019
4. National Institutes of Health, Office of Dietary Supplements: *Vitamin D: Factsheet for professionals.* 2018. https://ods.od.nih.gov/factsheets/VitaminD-HealthProfessional/ Accessed: July 4, 2019
5. Wacker M and Holick MF: Sunlight and vitamin D: Global perspective for health. *Dermato-Endocrinology* 5(1):51, 2013.
6. National Institutes of Health, Office of Dietary Supplements: *Vitamin E.* 2018. https://ods.od.nih.gov/factsheets/VitaminE-HealthProfessional/ Accessed: July 4, 2019
7. National Institutes of Health, Office of Dietary Supplements: *Vitamin K.* 2018. https://ods.od.nih.gov/factsheets/VitaminK-HealthProfessional/ Accessed: July 4, 2019
8. National Institutes of Health, MedlinePlus: *Niacinamide.* 2018. https://medlineplus.gov/druginfo/natural/1534.html Accessed: July 4, 2019

9. National Institutes of Health, LiverTox, Clinical and research information on drug-induced liver injury: *Drug record: Niacin*. 2019. https://livertox.nih.gov/Niacin.htm#casereport Accessed: July 4, 2019
10. Ellsworth MA and others: Acute liver failure secondary to niacin toxicity. *Case Reports in Pediatrics* Article ID 692530, 3 pages, 2014.
11. National Institutes of Health, Office of Dietary Supplements: *Vitamin B6*. 2018. https://ods.od.nih.gov/factsheets/VitaminB6-HealthProfessional/ Accessed: July 4, 2019
12. Oregon State University, Linus Pauling Institute, Micronutrient Information Center: *Vitamin B12*. 2015. https://lpi.oregonstate.edu/mic/vitamins/vitamin-B12 Accessed: July 4, 2019
13. Dali-Youcef N. and Andrès R: An update on cobalamin deficiency in adults. *Quarterly Journal of Medicine* 102(1):17, 2009.
14. Centers for Disease Control and Prevention: *Data & statistics on spina bifida*. 2018. http://www.cdc.gov/ncbddd/spinabifida/data.html Accessed: September 25, 2018
15. National Institutes of Health, Office of Dietary Supplements: *Vitamin C*. 2018. https://ods.od.nih.gov/factsheets/VitaminC-HealthProfessional/ Accessed: July 4, 2019
16. Oregon State University, Linus Pauling Institute, Micronutrient Information Center: *Vitamin C*. 2018. https://lpi.oregonstate.edu/mic/vitamins/vitamin-C Accessed: July 4, 2019
17. National Institutes of Health, National Cancer Institute: *Cancer statistics*. 2018. https://www.cancer.gov/about-cancer/understanding/statistics Accessed: July 4, 2019
18. National Institutes of Health, National Cancer Institute: *Risk factors for cancer*. 2015. https://www.cancer.gov/about-cancer/causes-prevention/risk Accessed: July 4, 2019
19. Colditz GA and Sutcliffe S: The preventability of cancer. *JAMA Oncology*. Published online May 19, 2016.
20. National Institutes of Health, National Cancer Institute: *Cancer causes and prevention: Obesity*. 2015. https://www.cancer.gov/about-cancer/causes-prevention/risk/obesity Accessed: July 4, 2019
21. National Institutes of Health, National Cancer Institute: *Alcohol and cancer risk*. 2018. https://www.cancer.gov/about-cancer/causes-prevention/risk/alcohol/alcohol-fact-sheet Accessed: July 4, 2019
22. American Cancer Society, Summary of the ACS Guidelines on Nutrition and Physical Activity: *Common questions about diet and cancer*. 2016. https://www.cancer.org/healthy/eat-healthy-get-active/acs-guidelines-nutrition-physical-activity-cancer-prevention/common-questions.html Accessed: July 4, 2019
23. National Institutes of Health, National Cancer Institute: *Chemicals in meat cooked at high temperatures and cancer risk*. 2017. https://www.cancer.gov/about-cancer/causes-prevention/risk/diet/cooked-meats-fact-sheet Accessed: July 4, 2019

Unit 9

1. Oregon State University, Linus Pauling Institute, Micronutrient Information Center: *Fluoride*. 2015. https://lpi.oregonstate.edu/mic/minerals/fluoride Accessed: July 5, 2019
2. Arias CF and others: Bone remodeling: A tissue-level process emerging from cell-level molecular algorithms. *PLoSONE* 13(9):e0204171, 2018.
3. U.S. Department of Agriculture, Agricultural Research Service: *What we eat in America, NHANES 2015–2016*. 2018. https://www.ars.usda.gov/northeast-area/beltsville-md-bhnrc/beltsville-human-nutrition-research-center/food-surveys-research-group/docs/wweia-data-tables/ Accessed: July 5, 2019
4. Office of Dietary Supplements, National Institutes of Health: *Dietary supplement fact sheet: Calcium*. 2018. https://ods.od.nih.gov/factsheets/Calcium-HealthProfessional/ Accessed: July 5, 2019
5. National Osteoporosis Foundation: *What is osteoporosis and what causes it?* ND. https://www.nof.org/patients/what-is-osteoporosis/ Accessed: July 5, 2019
6. National Institutes of Health, Osteoporosis and Related Bone Diseases National Resource Center: *Osteoporosis: Peak bone mass in women*. 2018. https://www.bones.nih.gov/health-info/bone/osteoporosis/bone-mass Accessed: July 5, 2019

7. National Institutes of Health, National Institute of Arthritis and Musculoskeletal and Skin Diseases: *Osteoporosis overview*. 2018. https://www.bones.nih.gov/health-info/bone/osteoporosis/overview Accessed: July 5, 2019
8. Centers for Disease Control and Prevention, Community Water Fluoridation: *2014 national water fluoridation statistics*. 2016. https://www.cdc.gov/fluoridation/statistics/2014stats.htm Accessed: July 5, 2019
9. National Institutes of Health, Office of Dietary Supplements: *Potassium*. March 2019. https://ods.od.nih.gov/factsheets/Potassium-HealthProfessional/#change Accessed: July 5, 2019
10. Cleveland Clinic: *Salt substitutes*. ND. https://my.clevelandclinic.org/health/articles/17452-salt-substitutes Accessed: July 5, 2019
11. American Heart Association, News: *Cardiovascular diseases affect nearly half of American adults, statistics show*. January 31, 2019. https://www.heart.org/en/news/2019/01/31/cardiovascular-diseases-affect-nearly-half-of-american-adults-statistics-show Accessed: July 5, 2019
12. Centers for Disease Control and Prevention, High Blood Pressure: *Risk factors*. 2014. https://www.cdc.gov/bloodpressure/risk_factors.htm Accessed: February 12, 2019
13. U.S. Departments of Agriculture and Health and Human Services: *2015–2020 Dietary Guidelines for Americans*. 2015. https://health.gov/dietaryguidelines/2015/guidelines/ Accessed: July 5, 2019
14. American Heart Association: *How much sodium should I eat per day?* 2018. http://www.heart.org/en/healthy-living/healthy-eating/eat-smart/sodium/how-much-sodium-should-i-eat-per-day Accessed: July 5, 2019
15. American Heart Association: *Sodium*. 2018. https://www.heart.org/en/healthy-living/healthy-eating/eat-smart/sodium Accessed: July 5, 2019
16. National Institutes of Health, Office of Dietary Supplements: *Iron*. 2018. https://ods.od.nih.gov/factsheets/Iron-HealthProfessional/#h5 Accessed: July 5, 2019
17. Oregon State University, Linus Pauling Institute, Micronutrient Information Center: *Iron*. 2016. https://lpi.oregonstate.edu/mic/minerals/iron Accessed: July 6, 2019
18. National Institutes of Health, MedlinePlus: *Iron deficiency anemia*. 2018. https://medlineplus.gov/ency/article/000584.htm Accessed: July 6, 2019
19. American Red Cross: *Eligibility requirements: Requirements by donation type*. ND. https://www.redcrossblood.org/donate-blood/how-to-donate/eligibility-requirements.html Accessed: July 6, 2019
20. Office of Dietary Supplements, National Institutes of Health: *Magnesium*. 2018. https://ods.od.nih.gov/factsheets/Magnesium-HealthProfessional/ Accessed: July 6, 2019
21. Oregon State University, Linus Pauling Institute, Micronutrient Information Center: *Selenium*. 2015. https://lpi.oregonstate.edu/mic/minerals/selenium Accessed: July 6, 2019
22. Office of Dietary Supplements, National Institutes of Health: *Copper*. 2019. https://ods.od.nih.gov/factsheets/Copper-HealthProfessional/ Accessed: July 18, 2019
23. Oregon State University, Linus Pauling Institute, Micronutrient Information Center: *Iodine*. 2015. https://lpi.oregonstate.edu/mic/minerals/iodine Accessed: July 6, 2019
24. Mayo Clinic: *What's the difference between sea salt and table salt? Nutrition and healthy eating*. 2016. http://www.mayoclinic.org/healthy-lifestyle/nutrition-and-healthy-eating/expert-answers/sea-salt/faq-20058512 Accessed: July 6, 2019
25. National Institutes of Health, Office of Dietary Supplements: *Zinc*. March 2019. https://ods.od.nih.gov/factsheets/Zinc-HealthProfessional Accessed: July 6, 2019
26. Office of Dietary Supplements, National Institutes of Health: *Chromium*. 2018. https://ods.od.nih.gov/factsheets/Chromium-HealthProfessional/#h5 Accessed: July 6, 2019
27. McKinley M and others: *Anatomy & physiology: An integrative approach*. 3rd ed. Boston: McGraw-Hill Publishing Company, 2018.
28. Valtrin H: "Drink at least eight glasses of water a day." Really? Is there evidence for "8×8"? *American Journal of Physiological Regulation and Integrative Comparative Physiology* 283:R993, 2002.
29. Food and Nutrition Board, Institute of Medicine: *Dietary Reference Intakes for water, potassium, sodium, chloride, and sulfate*. Washington, DC: National Academies Press, 2004.
30. Shah MK and others: Hypernatremia in the geriatric population. *Clinical Interventions in Aging* 9:1987, 2014.

31. Killer SC and others: No evidence of dehydration with moderate daily coffee intake: A counterbalanced cross-over study in a free-living population. *PLoS ONE* 9(1):e84154, 2014.
32. Mayo Clinic Staff: *Hangovers*. 2017. https://www.mayoclinic.org/diseases-conditions/hangovers/symptoms-causes/syc-20373012 Accessed: July 6, 2019
33. Mayo Clinic: *Hyponatremia*. 2018. http://www.mayoclinic.org/diseases-conditions/hyponatremia/basics/symptoms/con-20031445 Accessed: July 6, 2019
34. Centers for Disease Control and Prevention: *Binge drinking*. 2018. https://www.cdc.gov/alcohol/fact-sheets/binge-drinking.htm Accessed: July 6, 2019
35. Centers for Disease Control and Prevention: *Fact sheets: Alcohol use and your health*. 2018. https://www.cdc.gov/alcohol/fact-sheets/alcohol-use.htm July 6, 2019
36. American Heart Association: *Alcohol and heart health*. 2014. https://www.heart.org/en/healthy-living/healthy-eating/eat-smart/nutrition-basics/alcohol-and-heart-health#.V0R7-fkrLIU Accessed: July 9, 2019

Unit 10

1. National Institutes of Health, National Heart, Lung, and Blood Institute: *Why is a healthy weight important?* ND. https://www.nhlbi.nih.gov/health/educational/lose_wt/index.htm Accessed: July 27, 2019
2. Fryar CD and others: Prevalence of overweight, obesity, and severe obesity among adults aged 20 and over: United States, 1960–1962 through 2015–2016. *National Center for Health Statistics, E-Stats*. September 2018. https://www.cdc.gov/nchs/data/hestat/obesity_adult_15_16/obesity_adult_15_16.pdf Accessed: July 27, 2019
3. Hales CM and others: Prevalence of obesity among adults and youth: United States, 2015–2016. *NCHS Data Brief*, No. 288, October 2017. https://www.cdc.gov/nchs/data/databriefs/db288.pdf Accessed: July 27, 2019
4. World Health Organization, Media Centre: *Obesity and overweight*. February 2018. http://www.who.int/en/news-room/fact-sheets/detail/obesity-and-overweight Accessed: July 27, 2019
5. Vegiopoulos A: Adipose tissue: Between the extremes. *The EMBO Journal* 36:1999, 2017.
6. Tandon P and others: Adipose morphology and metabolic disease. *Journal of Experimental Biology* 221:jeb164970, 2018.
7. Roubal PJ and others: A noninvasive mechanical treatment to reduce the visible appearance of cellulite. *Cutis* 98:393, 2016.
8. Centers for Disease Control and Prevention: *Adult obesity causes & consequences*. 2017. https://www.cdc.gov/obesity/adult/causes.html Accessed: July 27, 2019
9. Puhl RM and Heuer CA: Obesity stigma: Important considerations for public health. *American Journal of Public Health* 100(6):1019, 2010.
10. National Institutes of Health, National Heart, Lung, and Blood Institute: *Guidelines on overweight and obesity*: Electronic textbook. ND. https://www.nhlbi.nih.gov/health-pro/guidelines/current/obesity-guidelines/e_textbook/txgd/4142.htm Accessed: July 27, 2019
11. National Institutes of Health, National Heart, Lung, and Blood Institute: *Assessing your weight and health risk*. ND. http://www.nhlbi.nih.gov/health/educational/lose_wt/risk.htm Accessed: July 27, 2019
12. Lu HK and others: Hand-to-hand model for bioelectrical impedance analysis to estimate fat free mass in a healthy population. *Nutrients* 8(10) pii:E654, 2016.
13. Liu X and others: Prevalence and change of central obesity among US Asian adults: NHANES 2011–2014. *BMC Public Health* 17:678, 2017.
14. Kwon SC and others: Obesity and modifiable cardiovascular disease risk factors among Chinese Americans in New York City, 2009–2012. *Preventing Chronic Disease* 14, 160582, May 2017. https://www.cdc.gov/pcd/issues/2017/16_0582.htm Accessed: July 29, 2019
15. Garcia AL and others: Improved prediction of body fat by measuring skinfold thickness, circumferences, and bone breadths. *Obesity Research* 13:626, 2005.
16. Food and Nutrition Board, National Institute of Health: *Dietary Reference Intakes for energy, carbohydrate, fiber, fat, fatty acids, cholesterol, protein, and amino acids*. Washington, DC: National Academies Press, 2005.

17. Knudsen N and others: Small differences in thyroid function may be important for body mass index and the occurrence of obesity in the population. *Journal of Clinical Endocrinology & Metabolism* 90:4019, 2006.
18. Haugen HA and others: Variability of measured resting metabolic rate. *American Journal of Clinical Nutrition* 78:1141, 2005.
19. Hall KD and others: Energy balance and its components: Implications for body weight regulation. *American Journal of Clinical Nutrition* 95(4):989, 2012.
20. Berger S and Polotsky VY: Leptin and leptin resistance in the pathogenesis of obstructive sleep apnea: A possible link to oxidative stress and cardiovascular complications. *Oxidative Medicine and Cell Longevity* 2018:5137947. Published online February 20, 2018.
21. Herman P and others: Mechanisms underlying the portion-size effect. *Physiology & Behavior* 144:129, 2015.
22. Martin CB and others: Attempts to lose weight among adults in the United States, 2013–2016. *NCHS Data Brief,* No. 313, July 2018. https://www.cdc.gov/nchs/products/databriefs/db313.htm Accessed: July 27, 2019
23. National Institutes of Health, National Institute of Diabetes and Digestive and Kidney Diseases: *Choosing a safe and successful weight-loss program.* 2017. https://www.niddk.nih.gov/health-information/weight-management/choosing-a-safe-successful-weight-loss-program July 27, 2019
24. University of California–Los Angeles Health, RFO Weight Management Program: *Very low calorie diet (VLCD).* ND. https://www.uclahealth.org/clinicalnutrition/vlcd Accessed: July 27, 2019
25. American Council on Exercise: *Myths and misconceptions: Spot reduction and feeling the burn.* 2013. https://www.acefitness.org/education-and-resources/lifestyle/blog/3629/myths-and-misconceptions-spot-reduction-and-feeling-the-burn Accessed: July 27, 2019
26. Kraschnewski JL and others: Long-term weight loss maintenance in the United States. *International Journal of Obesity (London)* 34(11):1634, 2010.
27. National Weight Control Registry: *NWCR facts.* ND. http://www.nwcr.ws Accessed: July 27, 2019
28. Mayo Clinic, Weight loss: *Prescription weight loss drugs.* 2018. https://www.mayoclinic.org/healthy-lifestyle/weight-loss/in-depth/weight-loss-drugs/art-20044832?pg=2 Accessed: July 27, 2019
29. National Institutes of Health, National Institute of Diabetes and Digestive and Kidney Diseases, Weight-Control Information Network: *Bariatric surgery.* 2016. https://www.niddk.nih.gov/health-information/weight-management/bariatric-surgery Accessed: July 27, 2019
30. Lynn W and others: Laparoscopic Roux-en-Y gastric bypass is as safe as laparoscopic sleeve gastrectomy. Results of a comparative cohort study. *Annals of Medicine and Surgery (London)* 35:38, 2018.
31. Hota P and others: Laparoscopic adjustable gastric band erosion with intragastric band migration: A rare but serious complication. *Radiology Case Reports* 13(1):76, 2018.
32. Dyson P: Low carbohydrate diets and type 2 diabetes: What is the latest evidence? *Diabetes Therapy* 6:411, 2015.
33. Harvard T.H. Chan School of Public Health, The Nutrition Source: *Diet review: Intermittent fasting for weight loss.* ND. https://www.hsph.harvard.edu/nutritionsource/healthy-weight/diet-reviews/intermittent-fasting/ Accessed: July 27, 2019
34. Devalaraja S and others: Exotic fruits as therapeutic complements for diabetes, obesity and metabolic syndrome. *Food Research International* 44(7):1856, 2011.
35. Centers for Disease Control and Prevention, National Center for Health Statistics: *Prevalence of underweight among adults aged 20 and over: United States, 1960–1962 through 2015–2016.* 2017. https://www.cdc.gov/nchs/data/hestat/underweight_adult_15_16/underweight_adult_15_16.htm Accessed: July 27, 2019
36. American Psychiatric Association: *Diagnostic and statistical manual of mental disorders,* 5th ed. Arlington, VA: American Psychiatric Publishing, 2013.
37. National Eating Disorders Association: *What are eating disorders?* ND. https://www.nationaleatingdisorders.org/what-are-eating-disorders Accessed: February 17, 2019

38. National Institutes of Health, National Institute of Diabetes and Digestive and Kidney Diseases: *Binge eating disorder.* 2016. https://www.niddk.nih.gov/health-information/weight-management/binge-eating-disorder/definition-facts Accessed: July 27, 2019
39. O'Brien KM and others: Predictors and long-term health outcomes of eating disorders. *PLoS One* 12(7):e0181104, 2017.
40. National Institutes of Health, National Library of Medicine, MedlinePlus: *Bulimia.* March 2018. https://medlineplus.gov/ency/article/000341.htm Accessed: July 27, 2019
41. National Institutes of Health, National Library of Medicine, MedlinePlus: *Anorexia.* Updated March 2018. https://www.nlm.nih.gov/medlineplus/ency/article/000362.htm Accessed: July 27, 2019
42. Campbell K and Peebles R: Eating disorders in children and adolescents: State of the art review. *Pediatrics* 134(3):582, 2014.
43. American College of Obstetricians and Gynecologists, Committee Opinion No. 702: *Female athlete triad.* 2017. https://www.acog.org/Clinical-Guidance-and-Publications/Committee-Opinions/Committee-on-Adolescent-Health-Care/Female-Athlete-Triad Accessed: July 27, 2019
44. Office of Disease Prevention and Health Promotion, Health.gov: *Top 10 things to know about the second edition of the Physical Activity Guidelines for Americans.* Updated February 16, 2019. https://health.gov/paguidelines/second-edition/10things/ Accessed: February 16, 2019
45. National Heart Lung and Blood Institute: Physical activity and your heart: *Types of physical activity.* ND. https://www.nhlbi.nih.gov/health-topics/physical-activity-and-your-heart#Types Accessed: July 27, 2019
46. U.S. Department of Health and Human Services, 2018 Physical Activity Guidelines Advisory Committee: *Physical activity guidelines advisory committee scientific report.* 2018. https://health.gov/paguidelines/second-edition/report.aspx Accessed: July 28, 2019
47. National Heart Lung and Blood Institute: Physical activity and your heart: *Recommendations for physical activity.* ND. https://www.nhlbi.nih.gov/health-topics/physical-activity-and-your-heart#Types Accessed: July 27, 2019
48. Position of the Academy of Nutrition and Dietetics, Dietitians of Canada, and the American College of Sports Medicine: Nutrition and athletic performance. *Journal of the Academy of Nutrition and Dietetics* 116(3):501, 2016.
49. Economos CD and others: Nutritional practices of elite athletes: Practical recommendations. *Sports Medicine* 16:381, 1993.
50. National Collegiate Athletic Association: *Heat and hydration: How to maximize performance hydration.* ND. http://www.ncaa.org/sport-science-institute/heat-and-hydration Accessed: February 17, 2019
51. National Library of Medicine, MedlinePlus: *Heat emergencies.* 2017. https://medlineplus.gov/ency/article/000056.htm Accessed: July 27, 2019
52. Substance Abuse and Mental Health Services Administration: *The Dawn Report: 1 in 10 energy drink-related emergency department visits results in hospitalization.* March 13, 2014. http://www.samhsa.gov/data/sites/default/files/spot124-energy-drinks-2014.pdf Accessed: July 27, 2019

Unit 11

1. Otten JJ and others, eds, Institute of Medicine: *Dietary Reference Intakes: The essential guide to nutrient requirements.* Washington, DC: National Academies Press, 2006.
2. Martin JA and others: Births: Final data for 2017. *National Vital Statistics Reports* 67(8):1, 2018.
3. Centers for Disease Control and Prevention, Reproductive Health, Maternal and Infant Health: *Infant mortality.* March 2019. https://www.cdc.gov/reproductivehealth/MaternalInfantHealth/InfantMortality.htm Accessed: July 27, 2019
4. National Institutes of Health, National Heart, Lung, and Blood Institute: *Your guide to anemia.* 2011. http://www.nhlbi.nih.gov/files/docs/public/blood/anemia-yg.pdf Accessed: July 27, 2019

5. March of Dimes: *Weight gain during pregnancy*. January 2019. http://www.marchofdimes.org/pregnancy/weight-gain-during-pregnancy.aspx Accessed: July 27, 2019
6. Position of the Academy of Nutrition and Dietetics: Obesity, reproduction, and pregnancy outcomes. *Journal of the Academy of Nutrition and Dietetics* 116(4):667, 2016.
7. McGrath RT and others: Large-for-gestational-age neonates in type 1 diabetes and pregnancy: Contribution of factors beyond hyperglycemia. *Diabetes Care* 41(8):1821, 2018.
8. National Institutes of Health, National Heart, Lung, and Blood Institute, MedlinePlus: *Preeclampsia*. 2018. https://www.nlm.nih.gov/medlineplus/ency/article/000898.htm Accessed: July 27, 2019
9. World Health Organization: *Maternal mortality*. 2018. http://www.who.int/news-room/fact-sheets/detail/maternal-mortality Accessed: July 27, 2019
10. Lessen R and Kavanagh K: Position of the Academy of Nutrition and Dietetics: Promoting and supporting breastfeeding. *Journal of the Academy of Nutrition and Dietetics* 115(3):444, 2015.
11. American Academy of Pediatrics: Policy statement: Breastfeeding and the use of human milk. *Pediatrics* 129(3):e827, 2012.
12. Woldu MA and others: Consumption of unmodified cow's milk and the risk of iron deficiency anemia in infants and toddlers and its management. *International Journal of Pharmaceutical Sciences and Research* 5(1):51, 2013.
13. Centers for Disease Control and Prevention: *Breastfeeding report card: United States, 2018*. 2018. https://www.cdc.gov/breastfeeding/data/reportcard.htm Accessed: July 27, 2019
14. Ballard O and Morrow AL: Human milk composition: Nutrients and bioactive factors. *Pediatric Clinics of North America* 60(1):49, 2013.
15. U.S. Food and Drug Administration: *Once baby arrives from food safety for moms to be*. 2018. https://www.fda.gov/Food/ResourcesForYou/HealthEducators/ucm089629.htm Accessed: July 27, 2019
16. Fewtrell M and others: Complementary feeding: A position paper by the European Society for Paediatric Gastroenterology, Hepatology, and Nutrition (ESPGHAN) Committee on Nutrition. *Journal of Pediatric Gastroenterology and Nutrition* 64(1):119, 2017.
17. Fleischer DM and others: Adverse reactions to foods committee report: primary prevention of allergic disease through nutritional interventions: Guidelines for healthcare professionals. *Journal of Allergy and Clinical Immunology: In Practice* 1:29, 2013. https://www.aaaai.org/Aaaai/media/MediaLibrary/PDF%20Documents/Libraries/Preventing-Allergies-Healthcare-15.pdf Accessed: July 27, 2019
18. Centers for Disease Control and Prevention: *When, what, and how to introduce solid foods*. 2018. https://www.cdc.gov/nutrition/infantandtoddlernutrition/foods-and-drinks/when-to-introduce-solid-foods.html Accessed: July 27, 2019
19. American Academy of Allergy Asthma & Immunology: *Prevention of allergies and asthma in children*. ND. https://www.aaaai.org/conditions-and-treatments/library/allergy-library/prevention-of-allergies-and-asthma-in-children Accessed: July 27, 2019
20. Togias A and others: Addendum guidelines for the prevention of peanut allergy in the United States: Report of the National Institute of Allergy and Infectious Diseases–sponsored expert panel. *Allergy and Clinical Immunology* 139:29, 2017.
21. Perkin MR and others: Association of early introduction of solids with infant sleep: A secondary analysis of a randomized clinical trial. *JAMA Pediatrics* 172(8):e180739, 2018.
22. Macdonald LE and others: A systematic review and meta-analysis of the effects of pasteurization on milk vitamins, and evidence for raw milk consumption and other health-related outcomes. *Journal of Food Protection* 74(11):1814, 2011.
23. Wang D and others: Snacking patterns in children: A comparison between Australia, China, Mexico, and the US. *Nutrients* 10:198, 2018.
24. Centers for Disease Control and Prevention: *Childhood overweight and obesity*. 2018. https://www.cdc.gov/obesity/childhood/index.html Accessed: July 27, 2019
25. Centers for Disease Control and Prevention: *Childhood obesity causes & consequences*. 2016. https://www.cdc.gov/obesity/childhood/causes.html Accessed: July 27, 2019
26. Li A and others: A genetic link between prepregnancy body mass index, postpartum weight retention, and offspring weight in early childhood. *Obesity* 25(1):236, 2017.

27. Herrick KA and others: TV watching and computer use in U.S. youth aged 12–15, 2012. *NCHS Data Brief* No. 157, July 2014.
28. Centers for Disease Control and Prevention: *Tips for parents—ideas to help children maintain a healthy weight.* 2018. https://www.cdc.gov/healthyweight/children/index.html Accessed: July 27, 2019
29. U.S. Census Bureau: *Quick facts.* ND. https://www.census.gov/quickfacts/fact/table/US/PST045217#PST045217 Accessed: July 28, 2019
30. National Academies of Sciences, Engineering, and Medicine: *Meeting the dietary needs of older adults: Exploring the impact of the physical, social, and cultural environment: Workshop summary.* 2016. Washington, DC: National Academies Press.
31. Deierlein AL and others: Diet quality of urban older adults aged 60–99: The cardiovascular health of seniors and built environment study. *Journal of the Academy of Nutrition and Dietetics* 114(2):279, 2014.
32. Centers for Disease Control and Prevention, Healthy Living: *Be food safe: Protect yourself from food poisoning.* Updated April 2019. https://www.cdc.gov/Features/BeFoodSafe /Accessed: July 28, 2019
33. National Academy of Sciences, Board on Agriculture and Natural Resource, Report in Brief: *Genetically engineered crops: Experiences and prospects.* 2016. http://nas-sites.org /ge-crops/2016/05/16/report-in-brief/ Accessed: July 28, 2019
34. U.S. Department of Agriculture, Food Safety and Inspection Service: *"Danger Zone" (40 °F–140 °F).* 2017. https://www.fsis.usda.gov/wps/portal/fsis/topics/food-safety-education /get-answers/food-safety-fact-sheets/safe-food-handling/danger-zone-40-f-140-f/ct_index Accessed: July 28, 2019
35. U.S. Department of Agriculture, Food Safety and Inspection Service: *Freezing and food safety.* 2013. https://www.fsis.usda.gov/wps/portal/fsis/topics/food-safety-education/get-answers/food-safety-fact-sheets/safe-food-handling/freezing-and-food-safety/CT_Index Accessed: July 28, 2019
36. U.S. Department of Agriculture, Agricultural Research Service: *Best ways to clean kitchen sponges.* 2017. https://www.ars.usda.gov/news-events/news/research-news/2007/best-ways-to-clean-kitchen-sponges/ Accessed: July 29, 2019
37. Miranda RC and Schaffner DW. Longer contact times increase cross-contamination of *Enterobacter aerogenes* from surfaces to food. *Applied and Environmental Microbiology* 82(21):6490, 2016.
38. U.S. Department of Agriculture, Food Safety and Inspection Service: *Cooking safely in the microwave oven.* 2013. https://www.fsis.usda.gov/wps/portal/fsis/topics/food-safety-education/get-answers/food-safety-fact-sheets/appliances-and-thermometers/cooking-safely-in-the-microwave/cooking-safely-in-the-microwave-oven Accessed: July 28, 2019
39. U.S. Department of Agriculture, Food Safety and Inspection Service: *Basics for handling food safely.* 2015. https://www.fsis.usda.gov/wps/portal/fsis/topics/food-safety-education /get-answers/food-safety-fact-sheets/safe-food-handling/basics-for-handling-food-safely /ct_index Accessed: July 28, 2019
40. National Pesticide Information Center: *Pesticides—what's my risk?* 2012. http://npic.orst .edu/factsheets/WhatsMyRisk.html Accessed: July 28, 2019
41. World Health Organization: *World hunger is still not going down after three years and obesity is still growing — UN report.* July 15, 2019. https://www.who.int/news-room/detail/15-07-2019-world-hunger-is-still-not-going-down-after-three-years-and-obesity-is-still-growing-un-report Accessed: July 28, 2019
42. World Health Organization: *Malnutrition: Key facts.* 2018. https://www.who.int/news-room /fact-sheets/detail/malnutrition Accessed: July 28, 2019
43. World Health Organization: *Infant and young child feeding: Key facts.* 2018. http://www.who .int/en/news-room/fact-sheets/detail/infant-and-young-child-feeding Accessed: July 28, 2019
44. United Nations Children's Fund: *Supply annual report 2018.* June 2019. https://www.unicef .org/reports/annual-report-2018 Accessed: July 28, 2019
45. U.S. Census Bureau: *Income and poverty in the United States: 2017.* September 2018. https:// www.census.gov/library/publications/2018/demo/p60-263.html Accessed: July 27, 2019

46. U.S. Department of Health and Human Services, Poverty Guidelines: *HHS poverty guidelines for 2019*. 2019. https://aspe.hhs.gov/poverty-guidelines Accessed: July 28, 2019
47. Coleman-Jensen A and others: *Household food security in the United States in 2017*. Economic Research Report No. (ERR-256), September 2018. https://www.ers.usda.gov/publications/pub-details/?pubid=90022 Accessed: July 27, 2019
48. United Nations: *World population projected to reach 9.7 billion by 2050*. July 2015. http://www.un.org/en/development/desa/news/population/2015-report.html Accessed: July 28, 2019
49. Foley JA: Can we feed the world & sustain the planet? *Scientific American* 305(5):60, 2011.

Appendix E
Dietary Reference Intake (DRI) Tables

Dietary Reference Intakes (DRIs): Recommended Intakes for Individuals, Vitamins
Food and Nutrition Board, Institute of Medicine, National Academies

Life Stage Group	Vitamin A (µg/d)[a]	Vitamin C (mg/d)	Vitamin D (µg/d)[b,c]	Vitamin E (mg/d)[d]	Vitamin K (µg/d)	Thiamin (mg/d)	Riboflavin (mg/d)	Niacin (mg/d)[e]	Vitamin B-6 (mg/d)	Folate (µg/d)[f]	Vitamin B-12 (µg/d)	Pantothenic Acid (mg/d)	Biotin (µg/d)	Choline (mg/d)[g]
Infants														
0–6 mo	400*	40*	10	4*	2.0*	0.2*	0.3*	2*	0.1*	65*	0.4*	1.7*	5*	125*
7–12 mo	500*	50*	10	5*	2.5*	0.3*	0.4*	4*	0.3*	80*	0.5*	1.8*	6*	150*
Children														
1–3 y	300	15	15	6	30*	0.5	0.5	6	0.5	150	0.9	2*	8*	200*
4–8 y	400	25	15	7	55*	0.6	0.6	8	0.6	200	1.2	3*	12*	250*
Males														
9–13 y	600	45	15	11	60*	0.9	0.9	12	1.0	300	1.8	4*	20*	375*
14–18 y	900	75	15	15	75*	1.2	1.3	16	1.3	400	2.4	5*	25*	550*
19–30 y	900	90	15	15	120*	1.2	1.3	16	1.3	400	2.4	5*	30*	550*
31–50 y	900	90	15	15	120*	1.2	1.3	16	1.3	400	2.4	5*	30*	550*
51–70 y	900	90	15	15	120*	1.2	1.3	16	1.7	400	2.4[h]	5*	30*	550*
>70 y	900	90	20	15	120*	1.2	1.3	16	1.7	400	2.4[h]	5*	30*	550*
Females														
9–13 y	600	45	15	11	60*	0.9	0.9	12	1.0	300	1.8	4*	20*	375*
14–18 y	700	65	15	15	75*	1.0	1.0	14	1.2	400[i]	2.4	5*	25*	400*
19–30 y	700	75	15	15	90*	1.1	1.1	14	1.3	400[i]	2.4	5*	30*	425*
31–50 y	700	75	15	15	90*	1.1	1.1	14	1.3	400[i]	2.4	5*	30*	425*
51–70 y	700	75	15	15	90*	1.1	1.1	14	1.5	400	2.4[h]	5*	30*	425*
>70 y	700	75	20	15	90*	1.1	1.1	14	1.5	400	2.4[h]	5*	30*	425*
Pregnancy														
14–18 y	750	80	15	15	75*	1.4	1.4	18	1.9	600[j]	2.6	6*	30*	450*
19–30 y	770	85	15	15	90*	1.4	1.4	18	1.9	600[j]	2.6	6*	30*	450*
31–50 y	770	85	15	15	90*	1.4	1.4	18	1.9	600[j]	2.6	6*	30*	450*
Lactation														
14–18 y	1200	115	15	19	75*	1.4	1.6	17	2.0	500	2.8	7*	35*	550*
19–30 y	1300	120	15	19	90*	1.4	1.6	17	2.0	500	2.8	7*	35*	550*
31–50 y	1300	120	15	19	90*	1.4	1.6	17	2.0	500	2.8	7*	35*	550*

mg = milligram, µg = microgram

NOTE: This table taken from the DRI reports; see www.nap.edu) presents Recommended Dietary Allowances (RDAs) in **bold type** and Adequate Intakes (AIs) in ordinary type followed by an asterisk (*). RDAs and AIs may both be used as goals for individual intake. RDAs are set to meet the needs of almost all (97 to 98%) individuals in a group. For healthy breastfed infants, the AI is the mean intake. The AI for other life stage and gender groups is believed to cover needs of all individuals in the group, but lack of data or uncertainty in the data prevents being able to specify with confidence the percentage of individuals covered by this intake.

[a] As retinol activity equivalents (RAEs). 1 RAE = 1 µg retinol, 12 µg β-carotene, 24 µg α-carotene, or 24 µg β-cryptoxanthin. To calculate RAEs from REs of provitamin A carotenoids in foods, divide the REs by 2. For preformed vitamin A in foods or supplements and for provitamin A carotenoids in supplements, 1 RE = 1 RAE.

[b] cholecalciferol. 1 µg cholecalciferol = 40 IU vitamin D.

[c] In the absence of adequate exposure to sunlight.

[d] As α-tocopherol. α-Tocopherol includes RRR-α-tocopherol, the only form of α-tocopherol that occurs naturally in foods, and the 2R-stereoisomeric forms of α-tocopherol (RRR-, RSR-, RRS-, and RSS-α-tocopherol) that occur in fortified foods and supplements. It does not include the 2S-stereoisomeric forms of α-tocopherol (SRR-, SSR-, SRS-, and SSS-α-tocopherol), also found in fortified foods and supplements.

[e] As niacin equivalents (NE). 1 mg of niacin = 60 mg of tryptophan; 0–6 months = preformed niacin (not NE).

[f] As dietary folate equivalents (DFE). 1 DFE = 1 µg food folate = 0.6 µg of folic acid from fortified food or as a supplement consumed with food = 0.5 µg of a supplement taken on an empty stomach.

[g] Although AIs have been set for choline, there are few data to assess whether a dietary supply of choline is needed at all stages of the life cycle, and it may be that the choline requirement can be met by endogenous synthesis at some of these stages.

[h] Because 10 to 30% of older people may malabsorb food-bound B-12, it is advisable for those older than 50 years to meet their RDA mainly by consuming foods fortified with B-12 or a supplement containing B-12.

[i] In view of evidence linking folate intake with neural tube defects in the fetus, it is recommended that all women capable of becoming pregnant consume 400 µg from supplements or fortified foods in addition to intake of food folate from a varied diet.

[j] It is assumed that women will continue consuming 400 µg from supplements or fortified food until their pregnancy is confirmed and they enter prenatal care, which ordinarily occurs after the end of the periconceptional period—the critical time for formation of the neural tube.

Adapted from the *Dietary Reference Intakes* series, National Academies Press. Copyright 1997, 1998, 2000, 2001, 2011, by the National Academy of Sciences. The full reports are available from the National Academies Press at www.nap.edu.

Dietary Reference Intakes (DRIs): Recommended Intakes for Individuals, Elements
Food and Nutrition Board, Institute of Medicine, National Academies

Life Stage Group	Calcium (mg/d)	Chromium (µg/d)	Copper (µg/d)	Fluoride (mg/d)	Iodine (µg/d)	Iron (mg/d)	Magnesium (mg/d)	Manganese (mg/d)	Molybdenum (µg/d)	Phosphorus (mg/d)	Selenium (µg/d)	Zinc (mg/d)
Infants												
0–6 mo	200*	0.2*	200*	0.01*	110*	0.27*	30*	0.003*	2*	100*	15*	2*
7–12 mo	260*	5.5*	220*	0.5*	130*	11	75*	0.6*	3*	275*	20*	3
Children												
1–3 y	**700**	11*	**340**	0.7*	**90**	**7**	**80**	1.2*	**17**	**460**	**20**	**3**
4–8 y	**1000**	15*	**440**	1*	**90**	**10**	**130**	1.5*	**22**	**500**	**30**	**5**
Males												
9–13 y	**1300**	25*	**700**	2*	**120**	**8**	**240**	1.9*	**34**	**1250**	**40**	**8**
14–18 y	**1300**	35*	**890**	3*	**150**	**11**	**410**	2.2*	**43**	**1250**	**55**	**11**
19–30 y	**1000**	35*	**900**	4*	**150**	**8**	**400**	2.3*	**45**	**700**	**55**	**11**
31–50 y	**1000**	35*	**900**	4*	**150**	**8**	**420**	2.3*	**45**	**700**	**55**	**11**
51–70 y	**1000**	30*	**900**	4*	**150**	**8**	**420**	2.3*	**45**	**700**	**55**	**11**
>70 y	**1200**	30*	**900**	4*	**150**	**8**	**420**	2.3*	**45**	**700**	**55**	**11**
Females												
9–13 y	**1300**	21*	**700**	2*	**120**	**8**	**240**	1.6*	**34**	**1250**	**40**	**8**
14–18 y	**1300**	24*	**890**	3*	**150**	**15**	**360**	1.6*	**43**	**1250**	**55**	**9**
19–30 y	**1000**	25*	**900**	3*	**150**	**18**	**310**	1.8*	**45**	**700**	**55**	**8**
31–50 y	**1000**	25*	**900**	3*	**150**	**18**	**320**	1.8*	**45**	**700**	**55**	**8**
51–70 y	**1200**	20*	**900**	3*	**150**	**8**	**320**	1.8*	**45**	**700**	**55**	**8**
>70 y	**1200**	20*	**900**	3*	**150**	**8**	**320**	1.8*	**45**	**700**	**55**	**8**
Pregnancy												
14–18 y	**1300**	29*	**1000**	3*	**220**	**27**	**400**	2.0*	**50**	**1250**	**60**	**12**
19–30 y	**1000**	30*	**1000**	3*	**220**	**27**	**350**	2.0*	**50**	**700**	**60**	**11**
31–50 y	**1000**	30*	**1000**	3*	**220**	**27**	**360**	2.0*	**50**	**700**	**60**	**11**
Lactation												
14–18 y	**1300**	44*	**1300**	3*	**290**	**10**	**360**	2.6*	**50**	**1250**	**70**	**13**
19–30 y	**1000**	45*	**1300**	3*	**290**	**9**	**310**	2.6*	**50**	**700**	**70**	**12**
31–50 y	**1000**	45*	**1300**	3*	**290**	**9**	**320**	2.6*	**50**	**700**	**70**	**12**

NOTE: This table presents Recommended Dietary Allowances (RDAs) in **bold type** and Adequate Intakes (AIs) in ordinary type followed by an asterisk (*). RDAs and AIs may both be used as goals for individual intake. RDAs are set to meet the needs of almost all (97 to 98%) individuals in a group. For healthy breastfed infants, the AI is the mean intake. The AI for other life stage and gender groups is believed to cover needs of all individuals in the group, but lack of data or uncertainty in the data prevents being able to specify with confidence the percentage of individuals covered by this intake.

Sources: *Dietary Reference Intakes for Calcium, Phosphorus, Magnesium, Vitamin D, and Fluoride* (1997); *Dietary Reference Intakes for Thiamin, Riboflavin, Niacin, Vitamin B-6, Folate, Vitamin B-12, Pantothenic Acid, Biotin, and Choline* (1998); *Dietary Reference Intakes for Vitamin C, Vitamin E, Selenium, and Carotenoids* (2000); *Dietary Reference Intakes for Vitamin A, Vitamin K, Arsenic, Boron, Chromium, Copper, Iodine, Iron, Manganese, Molybdenum, Nickel, Silicon, Vanadium, and Zinc* (2001); and *Dietary Reference Intakes for Calcium and Vitamin D* (2011). These reports may be accessed via **www.nap.edu**.

Adapted from the *Dietary Reference Intake* series, National Academies Press. Copyright 1997, 1998, 2000, 2001, and 2011 by the National Academy of Sciences. The full reports are available from the National Academies Press at **www.nap.edu**.

Dietary Reference Intakes (DRIs): Recommended Intakes for Individuals, Macronutrients
Food and Nutrition Board, Institute of Medicine, National Academies

Life Stage Group	Carbohydrate (g/d)	Total Fiber (g/d)	Fat (g/d)	Linoleic Acid (g/d)	α-Linolenic Acid (g/d)	Protein[a] (g/d)
Infants						
0–6 mo	60*	ND	31*	4.4*	0.5*	9.1*
7–12 mo	95*	ND	30*	4.6*	0.5*	11.0
Children						
1–3 y	**130**	19*	ND[b]	7*	0.7*	13
4–8 y	**130**	25*	ND	10*	0.9*	19
Males						
9–13 y	**130**	31*	ND	12*	1.2*	34
14–18 y	**130**	38*	ND	16*	1.6*	52
19–30 y	**130**	38*	ND	17*	1.6*	56
31–50 y	**130**	38*	ND	17*	1.6*	56
51–70 y	**130**	30*	ND	14*	1.6*	56
>70 y	**130**	30*	ND	14*	1.6*	56
Females						
9–13 y	**130**	26*	ND	10*	1.0*	34
14–18 y	**130**	26*	ND	11*	1.1*	46
19–30 y	**130**	25*	ND	12*	1.1*	46
31–50 y	**130**	25*	ND	12*	1.1*	46
51–70 y	**130**	21*	ND	11*	1.1*	46
>70 y	**130**	21*	ND	11*	1.1*	46
Pregnancy						
14–18 y	**175**	28*	ND	13*	1.4*	71
19–30 y	**175**	28*	ND	13*	1.4*	71
31–50 y	**175**	28*	ND	13*	1.4*	71
Lactation						
14–18 y	**210**	29*	ND	13*	1.3*	71
19–30 y	**210**	29*	ND	13*	1.3*	71
31–50 y	**210**	29*	ND	13*	1.3*	71

NOTE: This table presents Recommended Dietary Allowances (RDAs) in **bold type** and Adequate Intakes (AIs) in ordinary type followed by an asterisk (*). RDAs and AIs may both be used as goals for individual intake. RDAs are set to meet the needs of almost all (97 to 98%) individuals in a group. For healthy breastfed infants, the AI is the mean intake. The AI for other life stage and gender groups is believed to cover needs of all individuals in the group, but lack of data or uncertainty in the data prevents being able to specify with confidence the percentage of individuals covered by this intake.

[a]Based on 0.8g protein/kg body weight for reference body weight.
[b]ND = not determinable at this time.

Sources: *Dietary Reference Intakes for Energy, Carbohydrate, Fiber, Fat, Fatty Acids, Cholesterol, Protein, and Amino Acids* (2002). National Academies Press. Copyright 1997, 1998, 2000, 2001, by the National Academy of Sciences. This report may be accessed via **www.nap.edu**.

Adapted from the *Dietary Reference Intake* series, National Academies Press. Copyright 1997, 1998, 2000, 2001, by the National Academy of Sciences. The full reports are available from the National Academies Press at **www.nap.edu.**

Dietary Reference Intakes (DRIs): Recommended Intakes for Individuals, Electrolytes and Water
Food and Nutrition Board, Health and Medicine Division, National Academies

Life Stage Group	Sodium (mg/d)	Sodium CDRR[a]	Potassium (mg/d)	Chloride (mg/d)	Water (l/d)
Infants					
0–6 mo	110*	ND[b]	400*	180*	0.7*
7–12 mo	370*	ND[b]	860*	570*	0.8*
Children					
1–3 y	800*	Reduce intakes if above 1,200 mg/day[c]	2000*	1500*	1.3*
4–8 y	1000*	Reduce intakes if above 1,500 mg/day[c]	2300*	1900*	1.7*
Males					
9–13 y	1200*	Reduce intakes if above 1,800 mg/day[c]	2500*	2300*	2.4*
14–18 y	1500*	Reduce intakes if above 2,300 mg/day[c]	3000*	2300*	3.3*
19–30 y	1500*	Reduce intakes if above 2,300 mg/day	3400*	2300*	3.7*
31–50 y	1500*	Reduce intakes if above 2,300 mg/day	3400*	2300*	3.7*
51–70 y	1500*	Reduce intakes if above 2,300 mg/day	3400*	2000*	3.7*
> 70 y	1500*	Reduce intakes if above 2,300 mg/day	3400*	1800*	3.7*
Females					
9–13 y	1200*	Reduce intakes if above 1,800 mg/day[c]	2300*	2300*	2.1*
14–18 y	1500*	Reduce intakes if above 2,300 mg/day[c]	2300*	2300*	2.3*
19–30 y	1500*	Reduce intakes if above 2,300 mg/day	2600*	2300*	2.7*
31–50 y	1500*	Reduce intakes if above 2,300 mg/day	2600*	2300*	2.7*
51–70 y	1500*	Reduce intakes if above 2,300 mg/day	2600*	2000*	2.7*
> 70 y	1500*	Reduce intakes if above 2,300 mg/day	2600*	1800*	2.7*
Pregnancy					
14–18 y	1500*	Reduce intakes if above 2,300 mg/day[c]	2600*	2300*	3.0*
19–30 y	1500*	Reduce intakes if above 2,300 mg/day	2900*	2300*	3.0*
31–50 y	1500*	Reduce intakes if above 2,300 mg/day	2900*	2300*	3.0*
Lactation					
14–18 y	1500*	Reduce intakes if above 2,300 mg/day[c]	2500*	2300*	3.8*
19–30 y	1500*	Reduce intakes if above 2,300 mg/day	2800*	2300*	3.8*
31–50 y	1500*	Reduce intakes if above 2,300 mg/day	2800*	2300*	3.8*

NOTE: The table is adapted from the *DRI reports*. See **www.nap.edu**. Adequate Intakes (AIs) are followed by an asterisk (*). These may be used as a goal for individual intake. For healthy breastfed infants, the AI is the average intake. The AI for other life stage and gender groups is believed to cover the needs of all individuals in the group, but lack of data prevent being able to specify with confidence the percentage of individuals covered by this intake; therefore, no Recommended Dietary Allowance (RDA) was set. [a]CDRR = Chronic Disease Risk Reduction Intakes; [b]Not determined owing to insufficient strength of evidence for causality and intake-response; [c]Extrapolated from the adult CDRR based on sedentary Estimated Energy Requirements.

Sources: National Academies of Sciences, Engineering, and Medicine. *Dietary Reference Intakes for Sodium and Potassium*. The National Academies Press, Washington, DC, 2019; and *Dietary Reference Intakes for Water, Potassium, Sodium, Chloride, and Sulfate* (2005). These reports may be accessed via **www.nap.edu**.

Acceptable Macronutrient Distribution Ranges

	Range (percent of energy)		
Macronutrient	Children, 1–3 y	Children, 4–18 y	Adults
Fat	30–40	25–35	20–35
omega-6 polyunsaturated fats (linoleic acid)	5–10	5–10	5–10
omega-3 polyunsaturated fats[a] (α-linolenic acid)	0.6–1.2	0.6–1.2	0.6–1.2
Carbohydrate	45–65	45–65	45–65
Protein	5–20	10–30	10–35

[a]Approximately 10% of the total can come from longer-chain n-3 fatty acids.

Source: *Dietary Reference Intakes for Energy, Carbohydrate, Fiber, Fat, Fatty Acids, Cholesterol, Protein, and Amino Acids* (2002). The report may be accessed via **www.nap.edu**.

Adapted from the *Dietary Reference Intakes series*, National Academies Press. Copyright 1997, 1998, 2000, 2001, 2011, by the National Academy of Sciences. The full reports are available from the National Academies Press at **www.nap.edu**.

Dietary Reference Intakes (DRIs): Tolerable Upper Intake Levels (UL[a]), Vitamins
Food and Nutrition Board, Institute of Medicine, National Academies

Life Stage Group	Vitamin A (µg/d)[b]	Vitamin C (mg/d)	Vitamin D (µg/d)	Vitamin E (mg/d)[c,d]	Vitamin K	Thiamin	Riboflavin	Niacin (mg/d)[d]	Vitamin B-6 (mg/d)	Folate (µg/d)[d]	Vitamin B-12	Pantothenic Acid	Biotin	Choline (g/d)	Carotenoids[e]
Infants															
0–6 mo	600	ND[f]	25	ND	ND	ND	ND	ND	ND	ND	ND	ND	ND	ND	ND
7–12 mo	600	ND	38	ND	ND	ND	ND	ND	ND	ND	ND	ND	ND	ND	ND
Children															
1–3 y	600	400	63	200	ND	ND	ND	10	30	300	ND	ND	ND	1.0	ND
4–8 y	900	650	75	300	ND	ND	ND	15	40	400	ND	ND	ND	1.0	ND
Males, Females															
9–13 y	1700	1200	100	600	ND	ND	ND	20	60	600	ND	ND	ND	2.0	ND
14–18 y	2800	1800	100	800	ND	ND	ND	30	80	800	ND	ND	ND	3.0	ND
19–70 y	3000	2000	100	1000	ND	ND	ND	35	100	1000	ND	ND	ND	3.5	ND
>70 y	3000	2000	100	1000	ND	ND	ND	35	100	1000	ND	ND	ND	3.5	ND
Pregnancy															
14–18 y	2800	1800	100	800	ND	ND	ND	30	80	800	ND	ND	ND	3.0	ND
19–50 y	3000	2000	100	1000	ND	ND	ND	35	100	1000	ND	ND	ND	3.5	ND
Lactation															
14–18 y	2800	1800	100	800	ND	ND	ND	30	80	800	ND	ND	ND	3.0	ND
19–50 y	3000	2000	100	1000	ND	ND	ND	35	100	1000	ND	ND	ND	3.5	ND

[a] UL = The maximum level of daily nutrient intake likely to pose no risk of adverse effects. Unless otherwise specified, the UL represents total intake from food, water, and supplements. Due to lack of suitable data, ULs could not be established for vitamin K, thiamin, riboflavin, vitamin B-12, pantothenic acid, biotin, or carotenoids. In the absence of ULs, extra caution may be warranted in consuming levels above recommended intakes.
[b] As preformed vitamin A only.
[c] As α-tocopherol; applies to any form of supplemental α-tocopherol.
[d] The ULs for vitamin E, niacin, and folate apply to synthetic forms obtained from supplements, fortified foods, or a combination of the two.
[e] Beta-carotene supplements are advised only to serve as a provitamin A source for individuals at risk of vitamin A deficiency.
[f] ND = Not determinable due to lack of data of adverse effects in this age group and concern with regard to lack of ability to handle excess amounts. Source of intake should be from food only to prevent high levels of intake.

Sources: Dietary Reference Intakes for Calcium and Vitamin D (2011); Dietary Reference Intakes for Calcium, Phosphorus, Magnesium, Vitamin D, and Fluoride (1997); Dietary Reference Intakes for Thiamin, Riboflavin, Niacin, Vitamin B-6, Folate, Vitamin B-12, Pantothenic Acid, Biotin, and Chlorine (1998); Dietary Reference Intakes for Vitamin C, Vitamin E, Selenium, and Carotenoids (2000); and Dietary Reference Intakes for Vitamin A, Vitamin K, Arsenic, Boron, Chromium, Copper, Iodine, Iron, Manganese, Molybdenum, Nickel, Silicon, Vanadium, and Zinc (2001). These reports may be accessed via www.nap.edu.

Adapted from the Dietary Reference Intakes series, National Academies Press. Copyright 1997, 1998, 2000, 2001, 2011, by the National Academy of Sciences. The full reports are available from the National Academies Press at www.nap.edu.

Dietary Reference Intakes (DRIs): Tolerable Upper Intake Levels (UL[a]), Elements and Electrolytes[b]
Food and Nutrition Board, Institute of Medicine, National Academies

Life Stage Group	Boron (mg/d)	Calcium (g/d)	Copper (μg/d)	Fluoride (mg/d)	Iodine (μg/d)	Iron (mg/d)	Magnesium (mg/d)[c]	Manganese (mg/d)	Molybdenum (μg/d)	Nickel (mg/d)	Phosphorus (g/d)	Selenium (μg/d)	Vanadium (mg/d)[d]	Zinc (mg/d)	Sodium	Potassium	Chloride (mg/d)
Infants																	
0–6 mo	ND[e]	1	ND	0.7	ND	40	ND	ND	ND	ND	ND	45	ND	4	ND	ND	ND
7–12 mo	ND	1.5	ND	0.9	ND	40	ND	ND	ND	ND	ND	60	ND	5	ND	ND	ND
Children																	
1–3 y	3	2.5	1000	1.3	200	40	65	2	300	0.2	3	90	ND	7	ND	ND	2300
4–8 y	6	2.5	3000	2.2	300	40	110	3	600	0.3	3	150	ND	12	ND	ND	2900
Males, Females																	
9–13 y	11	3	5000	10	600	40	350	6	1100	0.6	4	280	ND	23	ND	ND	3400
14–18 y	17	3	8000	10	900	45	350	9	1700	1.0	4	400	ND	34	ND	ND	3600
19–70 y	20	2.5[f]	10,000	10	1100	45	350	11	2000	1.0	4	400	1.8	40	ND	ND	3600
>70 y	20	2	10,000	10	1100	45	350	11	2000	1.0	3	400	1.8	40	ND	ND	3600
Pregnancy																	
14–18 y	17	3	8000	10	900	45	350	9	1700	1.0	3.5	400	ND	34	ND	ND	3600
19–50 y	20	2.5	10,000	10	1100	45	350	11	2000	1.0	3.5	400	ND	40	ND	ND	3600
Lactation																	
14–18 y	17	3	8000	10	900	45	350	9	1700	1.0	4	400	ND	34	ND	ND	3600
19–50 y	20	2.5	10,000	10	1100	45	350	11	2000	1.0	4	400	ND	40	ND	ND	3600

[a] UL = The maximum level of daily nutrient intake that is likely to pose no risk of adverse effects. Unless otherwise specified, the UL represents total intake from food, water, and supplements. Due to lack of suitable data, ULs could not be established for arsenic, chromium, and silicon. In the absence of ULs, extra caution may be warranted in consuming levels above recommended intakes.

[b] Although silicon has not been shown to cause adverse effects in humans, there is no justification for adding silicon to supplements.

[c] The ULs for magnesium represent intake from a pharmacological agent only and do not include intake from food and water.

[d] Although vanadium in food has not been shown to cause adverse effects in humans, there is no justification for adding vanadium to food, and vanadium supplements should be used with caution. The UL is based on adverse effects in laboratory animals and this data could be used to set a UL for adults but not children and adolescents.

[e] ND = Not determinable due to lack of data of adverse effects in this age group and concern with regard to lack of ability to handle excess amounts.

[f] Upper Limit declines to 2 after age 50.

Sources: National Academies of Sciences, Engineering, and Medicine. *Dietary Reference Intakes for Sodium and Potassium*. The National Academies Press, Washington, DC, 2019; *Dietary Reference Intakes for Calcium and Vitamin D* (2011); *Dietary Reference Intakes for Calcium, Phosphorus, Magnesium, Vitamin D, and Fluoride* (1997); *Dietary Reference Intakes for Thiamin, Riboflavin, Niacin, Vitamin B-6, Folate, Vitamin B-12, Pantothenic Acid, Biotin, and Choline* (1998); *Dietary Reference Intakes for Vitamin C, Vitamin E, Selenium, and Carotenoids* (2000); *Dietary Reference Intakes for Vitamin A, Vitamin K, Arsenic, Boron, Chromium, Copper, Iodine, Iron, Manganese, Molybdenum, Nickel, Silicon, Vanadium, and Zinc* (2001); *Dietary Reference Intakes for Water, Potassium, Sodium, Chloride, and Sulfate* (2004); and *Dietary Reference Intakes for Sodium and Potassium* (2019). These reports may be accessed via www.nap.edu.

Adapted from the *Dietary Reference Intakes* series, National Academies Press. Copyright 1997, 1998, 2000, 2001, 2011, by the National Academy of Sciences. The full reports are available from the National Academies Press at www.nap.edu.

Appendix F

Modifying Recipes for Healthy Living

By making minor changes to a recipe, you can improve the product's nutritional quality and make it healthier. Table F-1 provides suggestions for common ingredient substitutions and indicates how the changes improve the nutritional quality of the products. Modifying the type of milk in a waffle recipe, for example, can decrease the product's fat content. As you modify recipes, keep the following tips in mind.

- Don't change every ingredient. Make one or two minor changes each time you try the recipe. For example, if you're making a cake for the first time, don't eliminate all the sugar and fat. These are ingredients that add flavor, color, texture, and moisture to the cake. A cake with no sugar or fat would be dry and almost tasteless.
- Recipes can often be made healthier simply by making minor changes, such as replacing solid fat with canola oil, eliminating some or all of the salt, or reducing the amount of sugar by 25%. You probably will not notice a significant difference in taste or quality if you use ¾ cup of sugar instead of 1 cup or ½ teaspoon of salt instead of 1 teaspoon. Appendix A provides information about household measures, such as cups and teaspoons.

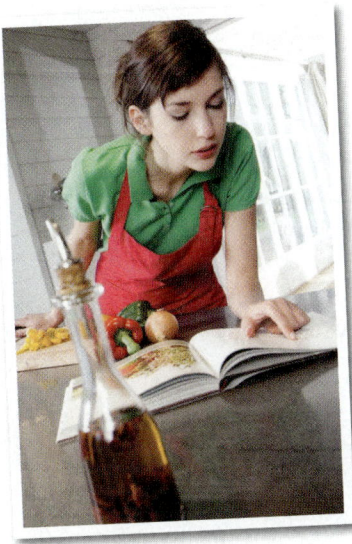

Onoky/Getty Images

Table F-1 Recipe Substitutions for Better Nutrition

Recipe Calls for	Modification or Substitution	Nutritional Effects of the Change
All-purpose (white) flour or bread flour	Use ½ whole-wheat flour and ½ all-purpose flour for each cup of all-purpose or bread flour.	Adds fiber
Butter or margarine (in baking)	Replace each quantity of butter or margarine with an equivalent amount of applesauce. Use ½ cup mashed cooked carrots, sweet potato, pumpkin, or squash for each 1 cup butter or margarine in baked goods.	Reduces calories and solid fat ("unhealthy fat"); adds some fiber and vitamins Reduces calories and solid fat; adds some fiber, vitamins, and phytochemicals
Cream	Use whole milk or half-and-half.	Reduces calories and solid fat
Cream cheese, regular	Use fat-free or reduced-fat ("Neufchatel") cream cheese.	Reduces calories and solid fat
Cheese, regular	Use low-fat or nonfat cheese. NOTE: Don't use nonfat cheese in cooked foods because it won't melt properly.	Reduces calories and solid fat
Enriched pasta or rice	Whole-grain pasta or brown rice. Mix ½ whole-grain pasta with ½ regular pasta.	Adds fiber
Eggs	Use 2 egg whites or ¼ cup egg substitute for each whole egg.	Reduces calories and solid fat
Evaporated milk	Use fat-free evaporated milk.	Reduces calories and solid fat
Condensed milk	Use fat-free evaporated milk. NOTE: Products won't be as sweet.	Reduces calories from solid fat and added sugar

A-27

Recipe Calls for	Modification or Substitution	Nutritional Effects of the Change
Fruit canned in heavy sugar syrup	Use fresh or frozen fruit. Use fruit canned in "own juice" or light syrup, or rinse sugar syrup from fruit before using.	Reduces calories and added sugar
Herbs with added salt (e.g., "garlic salt")	Use salt-free ground herbs and spices or fresh herbs and spices such as basil, cilantro, dill, oregano, or paprika.	Reduces sodium
Salt	Don't add to water before cooking vegetables or pasta. Don't add salt to foods before serving them.	Reduces sodium
Sour cream, regular	Use fat-free or low-fat sour cream. Use plain fat-free yogurt.	Reduces calories and solid fat
Sugar, white or brown	Reduce the amount of sugar by 25 to 50%. Use sugar-substitute that's appropriate for preparing baked products.	Reduces calories and sugar
Vegetable oil	Reduce amount by 25%. Use ¾ cup mashed cooked carrots, sweet potato, pumpkin, or squash for 1 cup oil in baked goods.	Reduces calories and adds "healthy" fat Reduces calories and fat and adds fiber, vitamins, and phytochemicals
Whole milk, 2% milk	Use fat-free or low-fat milk.	Reduces calories and solid fat

Glossary

A

absorption process by which substances are taken up from the digestive tract and enter the bloodstream or the lymph

absorptive cells digestive tract cells that absorb nutrients

Acceptable Macronutrient Distribution Ranges (AMDRs) macronutrient intake ranges that are nutritionally adequate and may reduce the risk of diet-related chronic diseases

accessory organs organs of the digestive system that assist digestive tract function

acid-base balance maintaining the proper hydrogen concentration of body fluids

added sugars sugars added to foods during processing or preparation

adenosine triphosphate (ATP) "energy currency" of cells

Adequate Intakes (AIs) dietary recommendations that assume a population's average daily nutrient intakes are adequate because no deficiency diseases are present

adipose cells fat cells; specialized cells that store fat

adolescent growth spurt period associated with puberty when a child's height and weight rapidly increase

aerobic conditions that include oxygen

aerobic exercise physical activities that involve sustained, rhythmic contractions of large muscle groups

aerobic metabolism metabolic pathways that require oxygen

alcohol (ethanol) a mind-altering depressant drug that's often classified as a food

alcohol abuser person who experiences problems at home, work, and school that are associated with his or her drinking habits

alcoholic person who is dependent on alcohol and experiences withdrawal signs and symptoms when he or she hasn't consumed the drug

alpha-linolenic acid an essential omega-3 fatty acid

alpha-tocopherol vitamin E

alternative sweeteners substances that are added to sweeten foods while providing few or no kilocalories

amino acids nitrogen-containing chemical units that comprise proteins

anabolic reactions chemical changes in cells that require energy to occur

anabolism metabolic processes that build larger substances from smaller ones

anaerobic conditions that lack oxygen

anaerobic metabolism metabolic pathway that functions without oxygen

anecdotes reports of personal experiences

angina chest pain that results from lack of oxygen to heart muscle tissue

anorexia nervosa (AN) severe psychological disturbance characterized by self-imposed starvation

antibodies proteins that help prevent and fight infection

antioxidant substance that protects cells and their components from being damaged or destroyed by harmful environmental and internal factors

appetite desire to eat appealing food

arachidonic acid (AA) omega-6 fatty acid derived from linoleic acid

ariboflavinosis riboflavin deficiency disease

arterial plaque lipid-filled patch that builds up within the wall of an artery, causing hardening of the artery

arteriosclerosis ("hardening of the arteries") condition that results from atherosclerosis

ascorbic acid vitamin C

atherosclerosis long-term disease process in which plaque builds up inside arterial walls

B

bacteria simple single-cell microorganisms

balance matching calorie intake with enough physical activity to maintain a healthy weight

bariatric medicine medical specialty that focuses on the treatment of obesity

basal metabolism the minimal number of calories the body uses for vital activities after fasting and resting for 12 hours

BE foods foods that contain detectable genetic material that's been modified by certain scientific methods

beriberi thiamin deficiency disease

beta-carotene carotenoid that the body can convert to vitamin A

bile substance needed for proper fat digestion

bile salts component of bile

bioavailability body's ability to absorb and use a nutrient

bioelectrical impedance technique of estimating body composition in which a device measures the conduction of a weak electrical current through the body

bioengineering scientific techniques that alter an organism's hereditary material

biotechnology use of living things to manufacture new products

blood alcohol concentration (BAC) estimated percentage of alcohol in blood

body mass index (BMI) numerical value that's used to relate body weight and risk of chronic health problems associated with excess body fat

bulimia nervosa (BN) eating disorder characterized by cyclic episodes of bingeing and calorie-restrictive dieting

C

caffeine naturally occurring stimulant drug

calcitonin hormone secreted by the thyroid gland when blood calcium levels are too high

cancer group of diseases characterized by abnormal cell behavior

carbohydrates class of nutrients that is a major source of energy for the body

carcinogen agent that causes cancer

cardiovascular disease (CVD) group of diseases that affect the heart and blood vessels

carotenodermia yellowish-orange dicoloration of the skin that results from excess beta-carotene in the body

carotenoids yellow, orange, and red pigments in fruits and vegetables

casein major protein in cow's milk

catabolic reactions chemical changes in cells that release energy

catabolism metabolic processes that break down larger substances into smaller ones

celiac disease chronic disease characterized by an autoimmune response in the small intestine to the protein gluten

cell smallest living functional unit in an organism

central-body obesity condition characterized by having a large amount of visceral fat and an "apple" shape

chemical digestion chemical breakdown of foods by substances secreted into the digestive tract

cholesterol sterol in animal foods that's made by your body

choline vitamin-like nutrient

chylomicron particle formed by small intestinal cells that transports lipids in the bloodstream

chyme mixture of gastric juice and partially digested food

cirrhosis hardening of tissues, such as the liver

coenzyme small molecule that interacts with an enzyme, enabling the enzyme to function

cofactor ion or small, non-protein molecule that helps an enzyme function

collagen fibrous protein that gives strength to connective tissue

colon major structure of the large intestine

colorectal cancer cancer that starts in either the colon or the rectum

colostrum initial form of breast milk that contains antibodies and immune system cells

complementary combinations mixing certain plant foods to provide all essential amino acids without adding animal protein

constipation bowel movements that occur less frequently than normal and/or are difficult to eliminate

control group group being studied that does not receive a treatment

cornea clear covering over the front of eyeball

cretinism condition that affects babies born to iodine-deficient women

cross-contamination unintentional transfer of pathogenic microbes from one food to another

D

Daily Values (DVs) set of nutrient intake standards developed for labeling purposes

deficiency disease state of health that occurs when a nutrient is missing from the diet

dehydration condition characterized by inadequate body water

diabetes mellitus (diabetes) group of serious chronic diseases characterized by abnormal glucose, fat, and protein metabolism

diastolic pressure pressure in an artery that occurs when the heart relaxes between contractions

diet usual pattern of food choices

dietary fiber (fiber) indigestible plant material; most types are polysaccharides

Dietary Reference Intakes (DRIs) various energy and nutrient intake standards for Americans

dietary supplement product that contains a vitamin, a mineral, an herb or other plant product, an amino acid, or a dietary substance that supplements the diet

digestion process by which large food components are mechanically and chemically broken down

digestive tract muscular tube that extends from the mouth to the anus

disaccharide simple sugar comprised of two monosaccharides

diuretic substance that increases urine production

diverticula small pouches that can form in the intestinal lining, especially the large intestine

DNA master molecule that has the instructions for making proteins

docosahexaenoic acid (DHA) omega-3 fatty acid derived from alpha-linolenic acid

double-blind study experimental design in which neither the participants nor the researchers are aware of each participant's group assignment

duodenum first segment of the small intestine

E

eating disorders psychological disturbances that lead to certain physiological changes and serious health complications

eclampsia condition that occurs when a woman with preeclampsia develops convulsions

edema accumulation of fluid in tissues

eicosapentaenoic acid (EPA) omega-3 fatty acid derived from alpha-linolenic acid

electrolytes minerals that have electrical charges when dissolved in water; ions

embryo human organism during the first 8 weeks after conception

empty calories calories from unhealthy fats, added sugars, and/or alcohol

emulsifier substance that helps fat-soluble and water-soluble compounds mix with each other

energy capacity to perform work

energy balance calorie intake equals calorie output

energy density energy value of a food in relation to the food's weight

energy intake calories from foods and beverages that contain macronutrients and alcohol

energy output calories cells use to carry out their activities

enrichment process of replacing some of the nutrients that were lost during a raw food's refinement

enzymes proteins that help chemical reactions occur

epiglottis flap of tissue that covers the entrance to the trachea (windpipe) to keep food from entering the lungs during swallowing

epithelial cells cells that form protective linings of the body

ergogenic aids foods, devices, dietary supplements, or drugs used to improve physical performance

esophagus tubular organ of the digestive tract that connects the back of the mouth with the stomach

essential amino acids amino acids the body cannot make or can't make enough to meet its needs

essential fatty acids lipids that must be supplied by the diet

essential nutrient nutrient that must be supplied by food

Estimated Average Requirement (EAR) amount of a nutrient that meets the needs of 50% of healthy people in a life stage/sex group

Estimated Energy Requirement (EER) average daily energy intake that meets the needs of a healthy person maintaining his or her weight

exercise physical activities that are usually planned and structured for a purpose

experiment a way of testing a scientific question

extracellular water fluid that surrounds cells or is in blood

extrusion reflex involuntary response in which a young infant thrusts its tongue forward when a solid or semisolid object is placed in its mouth

F

fad trendy practice that has widespread appeal for a period, then becomes no longer fashionable

fat-free mass lean tissues

fat-soluble vitamins vitamins A, D, E, and K

fatty acid chain of carbon atoms bonded to each other and to hydrogen atoms with an acid group on one end

Federal Trade Commission (FTC) federal agency that enforces consumer protection laws and investigates health claims

female athlete triad condition characterized by low energy intakes, abnormal menstrual cycles, and bone mineral irregularities

fetal alcohol spectrum disorder (FASD) condition characterized by abnormal physical and intellectual development that affects newborns of women who consumed alcohol during pregnancy

fetus human organism from 8 weeks after conception until birth

FODMAPs carbohydrates and sugar alcohols that the digestive tract doesn't digest and fully absorb

folic acid and **food folate** forms of folate

food insecurity describes individuals or families who are concerned about running out of food or not having enough money to buy more food

food intolerance negative physical reactions to eating a food that don't involve the immune system

food intoxication illness that results when poisons produced by certain microbes contaminate food and irritate the intestinal tract

food secure describes households in which the residents have access to and can purchase sufficient food to lead healthy, active lives

food-borne illness infection caused by microscopic disease-causing agents in food

fortification addition of any nutrient to food

free radicals chemically unstable factors that can damage or destroy cells

fructose monosaccharide in fruits, honey, and certain vegetables; "levulose" or "fruit sugar"

G

galactose monosaccharide that is a component of lactose

gastroesophageal reflux disease (GERD) chronic condition characterized by frequent heartburn

ghrelin protein that stimulates eating behavior

glucagon hormone that helps regulate blood glucose levels

glucose monosaccharide that is a primary fuel for muscles and other cells; "blood sugar"

gluten group of related proteins in wheat, barley, and rye

glycemic index (GI) measure of the body's blood glucose response after eating a food that supplies 50 g of digestible carbohydrates as compared to a standard amount of glucose or white bread

glycemic load (GL) value determined by multiplying the glycemic index of a carbohydrate-containing food by the amount of carbohydrate in a typical serving of the food

glycogen storage form of glucose in humans and other animals

goiter enlargement of thyroid gland

H

health claim statement that describes relationship between a food or food ingredient and reduced risk of a nutrition-related condition

heart attack loss of blood flow to a section of the heart muscle, causing the tissue to die

heartburn gnawing pain or burning sensation generally felt in the upper chest

heatstroke most dangerous form of heat-related illness

Heimlich maneuver life-saving technique for people who are choking

heme iron-containing portion of hemoglobin

heme iron form of iron that's well absorbed

hemoglobin iron-containing protein in red blood cells that transports oxygen to tissues

hemorrhoids clusters of small veins in the anal canal that can become inflamed and swollen

hepatitis inflammation of the liver

high-birth-weight (HBW) newborn generally weighing more than 8.8 pounds at birth

high-density lipoprotein (HDL) lipoprotein that transports cholesterol away from tissues and to the liver, where it can be eliminated

high-intensity ("artificial") sweeteners group of manufactured alternative sweeteners that are intensely sweet-tasting compared to sugar

high-quality protein protein that contains all essential amino acids in amounts that support the deposition of protein in tissues and the growth of a young person

homocysteine a toxic amino acid

hormones chemical messengers

hunger uncomfortable feeling that drives a person to consume food

hydration water status

hypertension abnormally high blood pressure levels that persist

hypoglycemia condition that occurs when the blood glucose level is abnormally low

I

ileum last segment of the small intestine

incubation period a length of time in which pathogens need to multiply in food or the digestive tract before they can cause illness

infant formula synthetic beverage that simulates human milk

insoluble fiber forms of dietary fiber that generally don't dissolve in water

insulin hormone that helps lower blood glucose levels

integrated pest management (IPM) nonchemical methods of agricultural pest management

intensity degree of effort used to perform a physical activity

intracellular water fluid that's inside cells

intrinsic factor (IF) substance produced in the stomach that helps vitamin B-12 absorption

iron deficiency anemia condition characterized by red blood cells that don't contain enough hemoglobin

irritable bowel syndrome (IBS) chronic condition characterized by frequent bouts of intestinal cramps with diarrhea or constipation

J

jejunum middle segment of the small intestine

K

ketone bodies chemicals that result from the incomplete breakdown of fat for energy

kilocalorie (kcal) or **Calorie** unit of measuring food energy

kwashiorkor form of protein-energy malnutrition that occurs when a child is abruptly weaned from breast milk and consumes inadequate amounts of high-quality protein

L

lactase enzyme that breaks down lactose into glucose and galactose

lactation milk production

lacteal lymphatic system vessel in a villus that absorbs most lipids

lactic acid compound formed from pyruvate during anaerobic metabolism

lactose disaccharide comprised of a glucose and a galactose molecule; "milk sugar"

lactose intolerance inability to digest lactose properly

lacto-ovovegetarian vegetarian who consumes milk products and eggs for animal protein

lactovegetarian vegetarian who consumes milk and milk products for animal protein

lecithin major phospholipid in food

legumes plants that produce pods with a single row of seeds

leptin hormone that reduces hunger and inhibits fat storage in the body

let-down reflex automatic physical response to a breastfeeding infant that enables milk to reach the nipple area

lifestyle way of living that includes diet, physical activity habits, use of tobacco and alcohol, and other typical patterns of behavior

linoleic acid an essential omega-6 fatty acid

lipases enzymes that break down lipids

lipids class of organic nutrients that generally don't dissolve in water (water insoluble)

lipoprotein structure that transports lipids through the bloodstream and lymph

low-birth-weight (LBW) infant generally weighing less than 5½ pounds at birth

low-density lipoprotein (LDL) lipoprotein that carries cholesterol to tissues

lower esophageal sphincter ring of muscle in the lower part of the esophagus; controls the opening between the esophagus and stomach

low-quality protein protein that lacks or has inadequate amounts of one or more of the essential amino acids

lymph fluid in the lymphatic system

M

macronutrients nutrients needed in gram amounts daily and that provide energy; carbohydrates, proteins, and fats

major minerals essential mineral elements required in amounts of 100 mg or more per day

malnutrition state of health that occurs when the body is improperly nourished

maltase enzyme that breaks down maltose into two glucose molecules

maltose disaccharide comprised of two glucose molecules; "malt sugar"

marasmic kwashiorkor form of protein-energy malnutrition that's characterized by edema and wasting

marasmus severe form of protein-energy malnutrition that causes extreme weight loss; starvation

mechanical digestion physical breakdown of foods

megadose generally defined as an amount of a vitamin or mineral that greatly exceeds the recommended amount

megaloblastic anemia condition characterized by fewer and abnormal red blood cells

metabolic rate body's rate of energy use a few hours after resting and eating

metabolism the sum of all chemical reactions occurring in living cells

micelle lipid-rich particle that is surrounded by bile salts; transports lipids to absorptive cells

micronutrients nutrients needed in microgram or milligram amounts (vitamins and minerals)

minerals elements in the Earth's rocks, soils, and natural water sources

moderation consuming foods in reasonable amounts

molds simple microbes that live on dead or decaying organic matter

monoglyceride single fatty acid attached to a glycerol backbone

monosaccharide simple sugar that is the basic molecule of carbohydrates

monounsaturated fatty acid fatty acid that has one double bond within the carbon chain

morning sickness nausea and vomiting associated with pregnancy

mucus slippery fluid that protects certain cells

myoglobin iron-containing protein in muscle cells that controls oxygen uptake from red blood cells

MyPlate USDA's dietary and menu planning guide

N

negative energy state calorie intake is less than calorie output

neural tube embryonic structure that eventually develops into the brain and spinal cord

non-alcoholic fatty liver disease (NAFLD) accumulation of fat in the liver that's not caused by alcohol consumption

nonessential amino acids group of amino acids that the body can make

nonexercise activity thermogenesis (NEAT) involuntary skeletal muscular activities such as fidgeting

nonheme iron form of iron in vegetables, grains, meats, and supplements

nutrient content claim statement that describes levels of nutrients in a packaged food

nutrient dense describes foods or beverages that contain more key beneficial nutrients in relation to total calories

nutrients life-sustaining chemicals in food that are necessary for proper body functioning

nutrition study of nutrients and how the body uses these substances

Nutrition Facts panel information on food packaging that indicates nutrition information per serving of the food

O

obesity condition characterized by an excessive and unhealthy amount of body fat

omega-3 fatty acid type of polyunsaturated fatty acid that has its first double bond at the number 3 carbon

omega-6 fatty acid type of polyunsaturated fatty acid that has its first double bond at the number 6 carbon

omnivore organism that can digest and absorb nutrients from plants, animals, fungi, and bacteria

organ collection of tissues that function in a related fashion

organ system group of organs that work together for a similar purpose

organic foods foods produced without the use of antibiotics, hormones, synthetic fertilizers and pesticides, genetic improvements, or ionizing radiation

organic nutrients nutrients that have carbon in their chemical structure

osteomalacia adult rickets; condition characterized by poorly mineralized (soft) bones

osteoporosis chronic disease characterized by bones with low mass and reduced structure

overweight having extra weight from bone, muscle, body fat, and/or body water

ovovegetarian vegetarian who eats eggs for animal protein

oxytocin hormone that causes the "let-down" response and the uterus to contract

P

pancreatic lipase digestive enzyme that removes two fatty acids from each triglyceride molecule

parathyroid hormone (PTH) hormone secreted by parathyroid glands when blood calcium levels are too low

partial hydrogenation food manufacturing process that adds hydrogen atoms to liquid vegetable oil, forming trans fats and saturated fats

pasteurization process that kills the pathogens in foods and beverages as well as many microbes responsible for spoilage

pathogens disease-causing microbes

peer review expert critical analysis of a research article before it's published

pellagra niacin deficiency disease

pepsin stomach enzyme that breaks down proteins into polypeptides

peptic ulcer a sore that occurs in the lining of the upper digestive tract

peptide bond chemical attraction that connects two amino acids together

peptides short chains of a few amino acids

peripheral vascular disease (PVD) atherosclerosis affecting a blood vessel that doesn't carry blood to the heart or brain

peristalsis type of muscular contraction of the digestive tract

pernicious anemia condition caused by the lack of intrinsic factor

pesticide substance that people use to kill or control unwanted insects, weeds, or other organisms

pesticide tolerances maximum amounts of pesticide residues that can be in or on each treated food crop

phospholipid type of lipid needed to make cell membranes and for proper functioning of nerve cells

physical activity movement resulting from contraction of skeletal muscles

physical fitness ability to perform moderate- to vigorous-intensity activities without becoming excessively fatigued

phytochemicals compounds made by plants that are not nutrients but may be healthful

pica craving nonfood items

placebo fake treatment, such as a sham pill, injection, or medical procedure

placebo effect positive response to a placebo

placenta organ of pregnancy that connects the uterus to the embryo/fetus via the umbilical cord

polypeptides chains of two or more amino acids

polysaccharides compounds comprised of several monosaccharides bonded together

polyunsaturated fatty acid fatty acid that has two or more double bonds within the carbon chain

positive energy state calorie intake is greater than calorie output

preeclampsia form of gestational hypertension

premature describes infant born before 37 weeks of pregnancy

prenatal period time between conception and birth; pregnancy

previtamin D inactive form of vitamin D

probiotics live and active cultures of beneficial microbes

prolactin hormone that stimulates milk production after delivery

proteins large, complex organic nutrients made up of amino acids

protists tiny, single-cell organisms that can have the characteristics of animals, plants, or fungi

provitamin A carotenoids that the body converts to vitamin A

puberty stage of life in which a person matures physically and is capable of reproduction

pyloric sphincter ring of muscle at the base of the stomach that controls the rate at which chyme leaves the stomach

pyruvate compound that results from anaerobic breakdown of glucose

Q

quackery practicing medicine without the proper training and licensing

R

Recommended Dietary Allowances (RDAs) daily nutrient recommendations that meet the needs of 97-98% of healthy people in a life stage/sex group

rectum lower section of the large intestine

requirement smallest amount of a nutrient that maintains a defined level of nutritional health

retinol (preformed vitamin A) form of vitamin A that's in animal sources of food

rickets vitamin D deficiency disorder in children

risk factor personal characteristic that increases a person's chances of developing a disease

S

saliva watery fluid secreted by the salivary glands that mixes with food in the mouth

salivary amylase enzyme secreted by the salivary glands that begins starch digestion in the mouth

satiety sense that enough food or beverages have been consumed to satisfy hunger

saturated fatty acid fatty acid that has only single bonds holding each carbon in the carbon chain together

scurvy vitamin C deficiency disease

semivegetarian or **flexitarian** person who eats eggs, fish, and dairy foods but generally avoids meat

set-point theory scientific notion that body fat content is genetically predetermined

skinfold thickness measurements technique of estimating body composition in which calipers are used to measure the width of skinfolds at multiple body sites

soluble fiber forms of dietary fiber that dissolve or swell in water

solvent substance in which other substances dissolve

spina bifida type of neural tube defect in which the spine doesn't form properly before birth and it fails to enclose the spinal cord

starch storage form of glucose in plants

stroke loss of blood flow to a region of the brain, causing the death of brain cells in that area

structure/function claim statement that describes the role a nutrient plays in maintaining a structure of the body or promoting a normal body function

subcutaneous fat layer of tissue that's under the skin and has more fat cells than other kinds of cells

sucrase enzyme that breaks down sucrose into a glucose and a fructose molecule

sucrose disaccharide comprised of a glucose and a fructose molecule; "table sugar"

sulfites group of sulfur-containing compounds in foods and often added to wines, potatoes, and shrimp as a preservative

sustainable agriculture farming methods that don't deplete natural resources while meeting the demand for food

systolic pressure maximum blood pressure within an artery that occurs when the heart contracts

T

teratogen agent that causes birth defects

testimonial personal endorsement of a product

thermic effect of food (TEF) energy used to digest foods and beverages as well as absorb and further process the macronutrients

thyroid hormone hormone that regulates the body's metabolic rate

tissues masses of cells that have similar characteristics and functions

Tolerable Upper Intake Level (Upper Level or UL) standard representing the highest average amount of a nutrient that's unlikely to be harmful when consumed daily

tolerance state that occurs when the liver adjusts to the usual amount of alcohol that's been consumed and metabolizes it more quickly

total body fat essential fat and storage fat tissue

total water intake refers to water obtained from metabolic and external sources

trace minerals essential mineral elements required in amounts that are less than 100 mg per day

trans fatty acids unsaturated fatty acids that have an unusual structure

treatment group group being studied that receives a treatment

triglyceride lipid that has three fatty acids attached to a three-carbon compound called glycerol; fats and oils

U

ulcerative colitis (UC) form of inflammatory bowel disease

undernutrition state of health that occurs when long-term energy and nutrient intakes are insufficient to meet an individual's needs

urea waste product of amino acid metabolism

U.S. Food and Drug Administration (FDA) federal agency that regulates claims on product labels

V

variety including many different nutrient-dense foods in your diet

vegans vegetarians who eat only plant foods

vegetarians people who eat plant-based diets

very-low-density lipoprotein (VLDL) lipoprotein that transports a high proportion of lipids in the bloodstream

villi (singular, **villus**) tiny, fingerlike projections of the small intestinal lining that participate in digesting and absorbing food

viruses microscopic agents that can cause infections

visceral fat adipose tissue that's under the abdominal muscles, which forms a protective apron over the stomach and intestines

vitamin organic micronutrient that can have a variety of functions in the body

vitamin precursors (provitamins, previtamins) substances in food or the body that cells can convert into active vitamins

W

water intoxication condition that occurs when too much water is consumed in a short time period or the kidneys have difficulty filtering water from blood

water-soluble vitamins thiamin, riboflavin, niacin, vitamin B-6, pantothenic acid, folate, biotin, vitamin B-12, and vitamin C

weaning gradual process of shifting from breastfeeding or bottle-feeding to drinking from a cup and eating solid foods

whole grains the entire, ground, cracked, or flaked seeds of cereal grains, such as wheat, buckwheat, oats, corn, rice, wild rice, rye, and barley

Index

A

AAP (American Academy of Pediatrics), 330
Abdominal fat, 280
Abdominal thrusts, 79, 79f
Absorption
    calcium, 235, 236
    defined, 75
    digestive system functions, 86f
    in large intestine, 84
    lipids, 83, 83f
    minerals and, 233
    proteins, 164, 165f, 166
    in small intestine, 81, 81f
    vitamin B-12, 213, 214f, 215
    of vitamins, 190
    of water-soluble nutrients, 82f
Absorptive cells, 81, 81f, 83f, 113f, 139f, 140, 140f, 165
Academy of Nutrition and Dietetics, 35, 37
Açai, 300
Acceptable Daily Intakes (ADIs), for high-intensity sweeteners, 109, 109t
Acceptable Macronutrient Distribution Ranges (AMDRs), 44, 149
    for carbohydrates, 44t
    for fats, 44t
    for proteins, 44t, 168, 174
Accessory organs, 76, 76f, 84
Acesulfame-K, 108t
Acetylcholine, 136
Acid-base balance, 162–163
Acidophilus, 64t
Acid reflux, 89–90, 94f
Activities of daily living, 305f
Added sugars, 105, 107t, 112, 117
Adenosine triphosphate (ATP), 96, 97, 306
Adequate Intakes (AIs), 44f
    defined, 44
    for fiber, 123
    for water, 260
ADHD (attention-deficit/hyperactivity disorder), 105
Adipose cells, 116, 141, 141f, 279–280, 279f
Adipose tissue. See Body fat
Adjustable gastric banding, 297–298, 298f
Administration for Community Living, 337
Adolescence, 334
Adolescent growth spurt, 334
Adrenaline, 121
Advertising
    food, 24, 32
    weight-loss, 300
Aerobic conditions, 306
Aerobic exercise, 305, 305f
Aerobic metabolism, 96

Aflatoxin, 222t
Agave nectar, 106, 118
Age
    See also Older adults
    metabolic rate and, 286–287
Age-Related Eye Disease Study (AREDS), 197
Age-related macular degeneration (AMD), 197, 197f
Aging process, 336, 337t
Agricultural Marketing Service, 339
Agriculture
    conventional, 351
    sustainable, 351–352
AI. See Adequate Intakes (AIs)
Air, swallowing, 123
Alanine, 163t
Albumin, 162
Alcohol, 263–269, 266t
    atherosclerosis and, 147
    binge drinking, 263
    blood alcohol concentration, 264–266, 264t, 265f
    body's processing of, 264
    calories in, 9
    as carcinogen, 222, 222t
    classification of drinkers, 263, 264t
    defined, 263
    as diuretic, 261, 268
    empty calories in, 53
    energy drinks and, 312
    fat production and, 141
    health and, 267, 268f
    health benefits of, 268, 269
    health problems related to, 268, 269, 269f
    help for abuse/dependence, 269
    nervous system effects of, 264t
    nutritional status and, 268
    poisoning, 266
    standard drink of, 263
    tolerance, 266
    triglycerides and, 146
    use disorders, 266
    zinc absorption and, 254
Alcohol abuser, 266
Alcoholics, 254, 266, 268
Alcoholics Anonymous, 269
Aflatoxin, 222t
Allergen labeling, 177f
Allergies, food, 176–177, 331, 332
Alli, 297
Allicin, 148
Almonds, 14, 170
Alpha-carotene, 11t

I-1

Alpha cells, 114
Alpha-linolenic acid, 10t, 131
Alpha-tocopherol, 201
    See also Vitamin E
Alternative sweeteners, 108–109, 108t
Aluminum, antacids and, 90
Alzheimer's disease, 192, 202
AMD (age-related macular degeneration), 197, 197f
AMDRs. *See* Acceptable Macronutrient Distribution Ranges (AMDRs)
American Academy of Pediatrics (AAP), 330
American Cancer Society, 35
American Diabetes Association, 118
American diet, 29, 55
American Heart Association, 243
American Red Cross, 247
Amino acids
    absorption and transport of, 165f, 166
    branched chain, 313t
    classification of, 163
    components of, 163, 163f
    converted into glucose, 116
    defined, 163
    essential, 10t, 163, 163t, 170
    excess, 167–168, 167f
    limiting, 170
    metabolism of, 211
    nonessential, 163, 163t
    peptide bonds between, 164, 164f
    supplements, 174
    using to build proteins, 166
Ammonia, 167f, 174
Amylase, salivary, 113
Anabolic reactions, 286
Anabolism, 96
Anaerobic conditions, 306
Anaerobic metabolism, 96
Anaphylactic shock, 176
Anecdotes, 24, 30, 34
Anemia
    iron deficiency, 246–247
    megaloblastic, 211, 215
    pernicious, 215
    sickle cell, 246f
    types of, 246
Angina, 144
Anisakis, 341t
Anorexia nervosa (AN), 302–303
Antacids, 90
Anthocyanins, 11t
Antibiotic-resistant bacteria, 51
Antibiotics, 88, 204
Antibodies, 162, 163
Antioxidants, 10, 192, 192f, 201f, 218
Anus, 76f
Appetite, 291
"Apple" body shape, 281
Arachidonic acid (AA), 133, 327
AREDS (Age-Related Eye Disease Study), 197
Arginine, 163t
Ariboflavinosis, 206, 207
Arsenic, 222t, 231, 231t
Arterial plaque, 143, 143f, 144

Arteries
    carotid, 144f
    hardening of, 144
Arteriosclerosis, 144
Arthritis, 250f
Artificial sweeteners, 108–109
Ascorbic acid, 218
    See also Vitamin C
Asian-Americans, 283
Asian Diet Pyramid, 55, 56f
Asian diets, 41, 283
Asparagine, 163t
Aspartame, 108t, 109
Aspartic acid, 163t
Atherosclerosis
    assessing risk for, 148–149
    defined, 142
    lipoproteins and, 144, 145f, 146
    process of, 142f–143f, 144
    reducing risk for, 147–148
    risk factors for, 146–147
Athletes
    dietary advice for, 307–311, 308t
    ergogenic aids for, 311–312, 313t
    female athlete triad, 303
    protein needs of, 174
    water needs of, 260
Atkins diet, 175
ATP (adenosine triphosphate), 96, 97, 306
Attention deficit/hyperactivity disorder (ADHD), 105
Autoimmune disease
    celiac disease, 71, 178
    defined, 178
    pernicious anemia, 215
    type 1 diabetes, 118
Avidin, 217f
Avocados, 50

B

Baby food, homemade, 332
BAC. *See* Blood alcohol concentration (BAC)
Bacteria, 339, 340t–341t
    diarrhea and, 88
    intestinal, 85
    probiotics, 17, 60, 85, 88, 93
"Bad foods," 13
Baking soda, 313t
Balance, in healthy diets, 15
Bariatric medicine, 297–298, 297f
Basal metabolism, 286
Beans, 168
Beef fat, 131, 132f
Bee pollen, 311
Beer belly, 280
Beets, 261f
BE food, 339
Belviq, 297
Benzene, 222t
Beriberi, 206, 207
Beta-alanine, 313t
Beta-carotene, 11t, 64t, 192, 194, 195, 196, 197
Beta cells, 114
Beta-hydroxy-beta-methylbutyrate (HMB), 313t

Bile, 84, 123, 190
Bile salts, 138, 139f, 141, 141f
Binge drinking, 263, 264t, 266
Binge-eating disorder, 302
Bioavailability, 233
Bioelectrical impedance, 284
Bioengineering, 339
Biological factors, influencing weight gain, 291
Biological therapy, 94
Biotechnology, 351–352
Biotin, 10t, 189t, 216, 217t
    deficiency, 217t
    food sources of, 206f, 217t
    functions of, 191f, 217t
    RDA for, 217t
    toxicity, 217t
    as water-soluble vitamin, 205
Birth weight, 323
Bisphenol A (BPA), 262, 262f
Bitter, 77
Bitter orange, 299t
Bleach, for sanitizing surfaces, 344
Blindness
    age-related macular degeneration and, 197
    night, 196
    preventing, 196
    vitamin A deficiency and, 196
Blogs, 35
Blood alcohol concentration (BAC), 264–266, 264t, 265f
Blood cells, 72f
    See also Red blood cells
Blood clots/clotting, 143f, 144, 203f
Blood donation, 247
Blood glucose
    diabetes and, 118, 119
    fasting levels of, 118
    glycemic index and, 120–121
    maintaining normal levels of, 114, 114f–115f
    monitoring levels of, 119
Blood pressure, 162
    See also Hypertension
    classification of, 242t
    diastolic, 242
    high, 144, 242–243
    systolic, 242
    tips for taking, 242f
Blood sugar. *See* Glucose
Blood thinners, 202
Blue agave, 106
BMI. *See* Body mass index (BMI)
Body
    energy sources for, 9f
    fluid compartments, 258, 258f
    organization of your, 72, 73f
    organ systems of, 74, 74t
    as remarkable machine, 95–97
Body composition
    adipose tissue and, 279–280
    metabolic rate and, 286
    sex differences in, 6f
Body fat
    See also Obesity; Overweight
    body composition, 6f
    body mass index and, 282–283
    cellulite, 281
    distribution, 280f, 281–282, 281f
    excess, 146, 281–282
    gaining. *See* Weight gain
    health problems related to, 281–282
    healthy amount of, 285
    kilocalories represented by, 289f, 290
    measuring, 284
    reducing. *See* Weight loss
    sex differences in, 280f, 281f
    subcutaneous fat, 280, 280f
    total body fat, 279
    visceral fat, 280, 280f, 282
    waist circumference measurement, 282
    weight classification by percentage of, 285t
Body image, 301
Body mass index (BMI)
    calculation of, 282
    categories, 283, 283t
    defined, 282
    limitations of, 283
Body weight. *See* Weight
"Boil order," 262
Bok choy, 236, 237
Bone health
    fluoride and, 240
    magnesium and, 248
    minerals for, 232f
    osteoporosis and, 203, 238–239
    vitamin D and, 198
    vitamin K and, 203
    vitamins for, 191f
Bone remodeling, 234
Bone tissue, 238f
Boron, 230f, 231t
Bottled water, 262
BPA (bisphenol A), 262, 262f
Bran, wheat, 15, 110
Branched chain amino acids, 313t
Brazil nuts, 250f
Breast cancer, 222
Breastfeeding
    benefits of, 327, 329–330, 349
    diet for, 329
    lactation, 327–329, 328f
    quitting too soon, 330
    vegan diet and, 173
    weaning from, 332
Breast milk, 327, 329–330
Broccoli, 236
Brown adipose cells, 279
Brown rice, 123
Brown sugar, 105t
Buffer, 163
Bulimia nervosa (BN), 302
Bulk food stores, 179
Butter, 147, 151
Butter fat, 131
Butylated hydroxyanisole (BHA), 134
Butylated hydroxytoluene (BHT), 134

B vitamins, 10t
  See also Vitamin B-1 (thiamin); Vitamin B-12 (cobalamin); Vitamin B-2 (riboflavin); Vitamin B-3 (niacin); Vitamin B-6 (pyridoxine); Pantothenic acid; Folate; Biotin
  deficiencies, 206–207
  food sources of, 206f
  requirement for, 42

C

Cadmium, 231
Caffeine, 10
  content of selected beverages, 314t
  defined, 312
  as diuretic, 261
  food sources of, 11t
  health effects of, 11t, 313t
  side effects, 313t
  toxicity, 312
Calcitonin, 234
Calcium, 10t, 53, 231t, 234–239
  absorption of, 235, 236
  constipation and, 90
  in dairy foods, 47
  deficiency, 234, 239t, 335
  food sources of, 230f, 234–237, 236f, 236t, 239t
  functions of, 232, 232f, 239t
  kidney stones and, 62
  megadoses of, 62
  MyPlate food sources of, 237f
  osteomalacia and, 200
  osteoporosis and, 201, 238–239
  RDA for, 239t
  regulating blood level of, 234, 235f
  storage of, 42
  supplements, 239
  toxicity, 239t
Calcium ascorbate, 218
Calcium carbonate, 239
Calcium citrate, 239
Calcium phosphate, 199
Calcium pyruvate, 313t
Calories
  calculating, 9
  defined, 8
  empty, 13, 14, 51, 101
  excess intake of, 117
  intake of, 286, 287
  output of, 286
  reducing intake of, 294
Campylobacter jejuni, 340t
Cancer
  carcinogens, 221, 222t
  colorectal, 93–94, 122
  defined, 221
  diet and, 222–223, 222t
  metastasized, 221
  obesity and, 222–223
  progression, 222f–223f
  risk factors for, 221–222
  risk reduction, 223
  vitamins and, 221–223
Canned fish, 235

Canned foods, 262
Canned fruit, 112
Capsaicin, 11t
Carbohydrate-restricted diets, 298
Carbohydrates, 6, 9, 100–127
  AMDR for, 44t
  athletes and, 309–310
  complex, 110
  defined, 102
  digestion of, 113–116, 113f
  for exercise recovery, 310
  fiber, 110–111
  foods rich in, 309t
  functions, 7t
  health and, 117–123
  intake of, 309–310
  intolerance, 122
  loading, 309
  obesity and, 117
  as primary fuel, 307
  RDA for, 116
  recommended intake of, 112
  simple, 103–105
  tooth decay and, 122
Carcinogens, 221, 222t
Cardiovascular disease (CVD), 134, 142–153
  angina, 144
  arteriosclerosis, 144
  atherosclerosis, 142, 142f–143f, 144, 146–149
  calcium and, 239
  deaths from, 143
  heart attack, 144
  hypertension, 144
  obesity and, 283
  reducing risk for, 147–148
  risk factors for, 146–147
  stroke, 144
  treatment options, 153
Cardiovascular system, 74t
Caro, Isabelle, 302f
Carotenodermia, 196
Carotenoids, 194, 196
Carotid arteries, 144f
Casein, 331
Catabolic reactions, 286
Catabolism, 96
Cattle, 352
Cause and effect, 29
Celiac disease, 71, 178
Cell(s), 72, 73f
  absorptive, 13f, 81, 81f, 83f, 139f, 140, 140f, 165
  adipose, 141, 279–280, 279f
  alpha, 114
  beta, 114
  defined, 8
  energy use by, 95–97, 102, 116
  epithelial, 194, 196
  fat, 116, 141, 141f
  functions, 8f
  malignant, 93, 221, 221f
  membrane, 258
  muscle, 72f, 73f

Index   I-5

Cell(s) (*continued*)
    proteins and, 162
    red blood, 116, 166, 211, 212f, 232f, 246, 246f
    types of, 72f
Cellulite, 281
Cellulose, 110
Centers for Disease Control and Prevention (CDC), 347
Centi-, 9t
Central-body obesity, 281, 282, 283
Central nervous system, 97
Cereals, 123
Charcoal-grilled meats, 223
Chemical digestion, 75
Chemical messengers, 51
Chemotherapy, 94
Child and Adult Care Food Program, 351t
Childhood nutrition, 334–336
Children
    adolescent growth spurt, 334
    with anemia, 247
    fostering positive eating behaviors in, 335
    nutrition-related concerns in, 335–336
    obesity in, 336
    physical activity for, 336
    protein and energy needs of, 173
    puberty, 334
    stunting in, 175, 350
    undernutrition in, 350
    vegetarian/vegan, 173
Chinese-Americans, 283
Chinese cabbage, 236, 237
Chinese children, 334
Chitosan, 299t
Chloride, 10t, 231t, 256t
    as electrolyte, 232
    functions of, 232f
Chlorophyll, 248
Choking, first aid for, 79, 79f
Cholesterol, 130, 134
    See also Lipoproteins
    absorption and transport of, 140, 145f
    bile and, 123
    carbon atoms in, 134f
    cardiovascular disease and, 122, 144
    classification of blood levels, 148t
    content in foods, 135t
    defined, 134
    fiber and, 111, 124
    functions of, 134–135
    gallstones and, 91
    intake recommendations, 149–150
    oxidized LDLs, 146, 146f
Choline, 10t, 136, 189t, 216, 217t
    deficiency, 217t
    food sources of, 206f, 217t
    functions of, 191f, 217t
    RDA for, 217t
    toxicity, 217t
Chondroitin, 60, 64t
Chromium, 10t, 231t, 299t, 313t
    deficiency, 255t, 256
    food sources of, 230f, 254, 255t

    functions of, 254, 255t
    RDA for, 255t
    toxicity, 255t, 256
Chronic diseases, 29, 336
    defined, 4
    risk factors for, 4–5
    vitamin E supplements and, 202
Chutney, 56
Chylomicrons, 83, 83f, 140, 140f, 144
Chyme, 80, 84
Cigarette smokers, 44, 220
Circulatory system, effects of aging on, 337t
Cirrhosis, 118, 268, 269f
Clostridium botulinum, 109, 340t
Clostridium perfringens, 340t
Clots/clotting, 143f, 144, 203f
Cobalt, 231
Coconut oil, 134, 151
Cod liver oil, 64t, 187, 193f, 198
Coenzyme Q_{10}, 64t, 313t
Coenzymes, 205, 205f, 206, 211, 232
Cofactors, 232
Coffee, 261, 265
Cognitive behavioral therapy, 303
Colds, 218
Cold storage time limits, 346t
Collagen, 162, 218
Collard greens, 236
Colon, 84
Colon cancer, 93
Colon cleansing, 92
Colonics, 92
Colorectal cancer, 93–94, 93f
    fiber and, 122
    risk factors for, 94
    signs and symptoms of, 93–94
    treatment options, 94
Colostrum, 327
Commodity Supplemental Food Program, 351t
Complementary combinations, 171, 171f
Complete proteins, 170
Complex carbohydrates, 110
Cones, 196f
Congeners, 261
Conjugated linoleic acid, 299t
Constipation, 87, 90, 94f
Consumer protection laws, 32, 35
Contrave, 297
Control group, 26, 27
Conventional farming, 351
Conventional wisdom, 24
Cooking. *See* Food preparation
Coomes, Olivia, 161, 174
Copper, 10t, 231t
    deficiency, 251, 251t
    food sources of, 230f, 251, 251t
    functions of, 232f, 251, 251t
    RDA for, 251t
    toxicity, 251t
Corn, 110, 191
Cornea, 196
Corn oil, 132f

Cow's milk, 331
Cravings, 325
C-reactive protein, 147
Creatine, 313t
Cretinism, 253
Croker, Amanda, 58, 187
Cross-contamination, 342
Cruciferous vegetables, 195
Cryptosporidium, 341t
Culture, food choices and, 15, 29, 56, 85, 110, 151, 176, 191, 233, 283, 334
Cured meats, 346t
Curry, 56
Cutting boards, food safety and, 342, 344
Cyclamates, 109
Cysteine, 163t
Cystic fibrosis, 190, 204

D

Daily Values (DVs), 58–59, 61, A-3
Dairy, 47, 235
    calcium in, 45, 47, 235, 236f, 237f
    Dietary Guidelines for, 52t
    "full-fat," 148
    minerals in, 230f
    MyPlate guidelines, 55f
    one-ounce equivalents, 47f
    potassium in, 241f
    vitamins in, 193f, 206f
"Danger zone," 342
DASH diet, 243
Death
    from cardiovascular disease, 143
    leading causes of, 5f
    from pellagra, 207
Deci-, 9t
Deficiencies
    biotin, 217t
    calcium, 234, 239t, 335
    choline, 217t
    copper, 251, 251t
    fluoride, 239t
    folate, 211, 215–216, 216t
    iodine, 253, 255t
    iron, 246–247, 249t, 335
    magnesium, 248, 249t
    niacin, 206, 207, 209t
    pantothenic acid, 217t
    potassium, 240, 243t
    protein, 175
    selenium, 250, 251t
    sodium, 243t
    thiamin, 206, 207, 209t
    vitamin, 187, 188, 195–196, 200–202, 206–207
    vitamin A, 195–196, 197t
    vitamin B-6, 211t
    vitamin B-12, 211, 215–216, 216t
    vitamin C, 220, 220t
    vitamin D, 187, 200–201, 201t
    vitamin E, 202, 203t
    vitamin K, 204, 204t
    zinc, 254, 254t
Deficiency disease, 10
Dehydration, 88, 261, 311
Dementia, 207
Dental fluorosis, 240, 240f
Dermatitis, 207
Developing countries, 349
DHA (docosahexaenoic acid), 131, 133, 150, 327
Diabetes mellitus
    classification of, 119t
    defined, 118
    monitoring, 119
    during pregnancy, 119
    prevention of, 120–121
    as risk factor for CVD, 146
    type 1, 118
    type 2, 118, 119
Diarrhea, 88, 94f, 207
Diastolic pressure, 242
Dietary adequacy, 253, 349–353
Dietary fiber, 53, 110–111, 111t
Dietary Guidelines for Americans, 52–54, 52t
    2015–2020 version, 52–54
    applying, 54t
    on cholesterol, 150
    on essential fatty acids, 150
    on iron, 247
    key recommendations, 53
    on potassium, 240
    on protein, 168
    on saturated fats, 149–150
    on sodium, 243
    on trans fats, 134
    very-low-fat, 298
Dietary guides, 55
    See also MyPlate
Dietary Reference Intakes (DRIs), 43f
    See also Recommended Dietary Allowances (RDAs)
    Acceptable Macronutrient Distribution Ranges (AMDRs), 44, 149
    Adequate Intakes (AIs), 44
    carbohydrates, 112
    defined, 42–43
    Estimated Average Requirement (EAR), 43
    Estimated Energy Requirement (EER), 43
    Recommended Dietary Allowances (RDAs), 43–44
    tables, A-21–A-26
    Tolerable Upper Intake Level (UL), 44
Dietary Supplement Health and Education Act (DSHEA), 60
Dietary supplements. *See* Supplements
Dietetics, 37
Diet(s)
    Asian, 41
    cancer and, 222–223, 222t
    DASH, 243
    defined, 4
    diet-related carcinogens, 222t
    fad, 298–299
    features of healthy, 15
    gluten-free, 178t
    high-protein, 174, 175
    low-carbohydrate, 298
    meal planning, 45–56
    paleo, 175
    plant-based, 233
    requirements and recommendations for, 42–44
    very-low-calorie, 294

Diet(s) (continued)
  very-low-fat, 298
  Western, 29
Digestion
  of carbohydrates, 113–116, 113f
  chemical, 75
  defined, 75
  of lipids, 138–141, 138f–139f
  mechanical, 75
  overview of, 75
  of proteins, 164–168, 164f–165f, 166f
  of vitamins, 190
Digestive enzymes, 138
Digestive system, 74t, 75–86
  digestive tract, 76–85, 76f
  effects of aging on, 337t
  summary of, 86f
Digestive system disorders
  acid reflux, 89–90
  bile, 91
  colorectal cancer, 93–94
  common sites of, 94f
  constipation, 87
  diarrhea, 88
  gallstones, 91, 91f
  gastroesophageal reflux disease (GERD), 89–90, 94f
  hemorrhoids, 87, 87f
  irritable bowel syndrome, 92
  peptic ulcers, 90
  ulcerative colitis, 92–93
  vomiting, 88
Digestive tract, 76–85, 76f
  accessory organs of, 76, 76f, 84
  defined, 75
  esophagus, 78, 78f
  fiber and, 122
  large intestine, 84–85, 85f
  major organs of, 76, 76f
  mouth, 77
  small intestine, 81, 81f
  stomach, 80, 80f
Dipeptides, 164
Disaccharides, 104
Disclaimers, 35
Disease
  autoimmune, 178
  chronic, 4–5, 29, 336
  deficiency, 10
  food-borne, 13, 85
  genetic susceptibility to, 29
  vitamin-deficiency, 188
Disordered eating, 301
Diuretics, 261, 268
Diverticula, 87, 87f, 94f
DNA, 166, 211, 339
Docosahexaenoic acid (DHA), 131, 133, 150, 327
Double-blind study, 26
Dragon fruit, 17
DRIs. See Dietary Reference Intakes (DRIs)
Drunk driving, 263
Dry eye, 196
Duodenum, 81, 81f
DVs (Daily Values), 58–59, 61, A-3

E

EAR (Estimated Average Requirement), 43, 43f
Eating disorders
  anorexia nervosa, 302–303
  binge-eating disorder, 302
  bulimia nervosa, 302
  causes of, 301
  defined, 301
  female athlete triad, 303
  risk factors for, 301
  treatment for, 303
Echinacea, 62, 64t
Eclampsia, 326, 327
E. coli bacteria, 88, 340t
Edamame, 137f
Edema, 162, 162f, 163
EER (Estimated Energy Requirement), 43, 287
Eggs, 137, 143, 153, 217f, 343, 346t
Egg substitutes, 153
Eicosapentaenoic acid (EPA), 131, 133
Electrolytes, 232, 259, 260, 310
Electrons, 192
Embryo, 322
Emergency food supply, 347, 347t
Emotional stress, 147
Empty calories, 13, 14, 51, 101
Emulsifier, 137
Endocrine system, 74t
  effects of aging on, 337t
Endosperm, 15
Enemas, 92
Energy
  defined, 95
  Estimated Energy Requirement (EER), 43
  from fat or carbohydrates, 307, 307f
  food, 8
  glucose for, 116
  metabolic energy needs, 286–287
  metabolism, 95–97, 97f
  needs of athletes, 307, 308t
  negative energy state, 290, 290f, 291
  for physical activity, 287–288
  positive energy state, 290, 290f
  protein-energy malnutrition (PEM), 350
  sources, 9f
Energy balance, 289–291, 289f, 290f
Energy bars, 310
Energy density, 14, 14f
Energy drinks, 261, 312
Energy intake, 286
Energy metabolism, 95–97, 97f, A-4
Energy output (energy expenditure), 286, 287, 294
Energy sources, 9f
English-Metric conversion, A-2
Enrichment, 46
Environmental factors, influencing weight gain, 291–292
Environmental Protection Agency (EPA), 150, 262, 348
Environmental Working Group (EWG), 348
Enzymes, 162
  coenzymes, 211, 232
  defined, 77
EPA (Environmental Protection Agency), 150, 262, 348

Epiglottis, 78, 78f
Epinephrine, 121
Epithelial cells, 194, 196
Epoxy resins, 262, 262f
Ergogenic aids, 311–312, 313t
Erthritol, 108
Esophagus, 76, 76f, 78, 78f, 86f
Essential amino acids, 163, 163t, 170
Essential fat, 279
Essential fatty acids, 131, 133, 133f, 150
Essential nutrients, 10, 10t
Estimated Average Requirement (EAR), 43, 43f
Estimated Energy Requirement (EER), 43, 287
Estrogen, 222, 238, 303
Ethanol, 263
    See also Alcohol
Evening primrose oil, 64t
Exercise
    See also Physical activity
    aerobic, 305, 305f
    carbohydrates for recovery after, 310
    defined, 304
    fueling, 306–307
    health benefits of, 304
    to prevent osteoporosis, 239
    resistance, 174, 305
    for weight loss, 294, 295
Experiments, 24
Extracellular water, 258
Extrusion reflex, 332

F

Fad, defined, 298
Fad diets, 298–299
Family history, 5
Farmers' markets, 179
FAS (fetal alcohol syndrome), 269
FASD (fetal alcohol spectrum disorder), 269, 269f
Fast-food industry, 134, 179
Fast foods, 180
Fasting, 299
Fat (adipose) cells, 116, 141, 141f, 279–280, 279f
Fat, body. See Body fat
Fat-free mass, 279
Fat-free milk, 47, 151
Fats, 6, 9, 10t, 128–159
    See also Lipids
    absorption and transport of, 140
    AMDR for, 44t
    diets high in, 48
    digestion of, 138–141, 138f–139f
    excess, 141
    functions, 7t
    intake recommendations, 149–150
    liquid, 131
    as primary fuel, 307
    solid, 51, 53, 131, 147, 152
    trans, 53, 133–134, 133f, 149
    types of, 148
Fat-soluble nutrients, 83f
Fat-soluble vitamins, 189, 189t, 193–204, 193f

Fatty acids, 130, 130f
    effects on LDLs and HDLs, 149f
    essential, 131, 133, 133f, 150
    in fats and oils, 132t
    monounsaturated, 149f
    omega-3, 131, 150, 150t, 173
    omega-6, 131, 150
    polyunsaturated, 149f
    saturated, 53, 131, 132t, 148, 149f
    sources of reliable, 149f
    unsaturated, 131, 132t
"Fatty liver," 267
FDA. See Food and Drug Administration (FDA)
Feces, 84–85
Federally subsidized food programs, 351t
Federal nutrition assistance programs, 350–351, 351t
Federal Trade Commission (FTC), 32, 35, 134
Female athlete triad, 303
Fermentation, 85
Fetal alcohol spectrum disorder (FASD), 269, 269f
Fetal alcohol syndrome (FAS), 269
Fetus, 322
Fiber, 102, 110–111, 110f
    colorectal cancer and, 122
    content of common foods, 111t
    digestive tract and, 122
    health and, 122–123
    heart health and, 122–123
    increasing intake of, 123
    insoluble, 111, 111t
    soluble, 111, 111t
    weight control and, 123
Fibrin, 162
First Amendment freedoms, 31
Fish, 50, 235, 346t
Fish oil supplements, 60, 64t, 150
Flatulence, 85, 123
Flaxseed, 64t
Flaxseed oil, 64t
Flexibility exercise, 305f
Flexitarians, 172
Flu, 340
Fluid balance, 162, 259, 259f
Fluid compartments, 258, 258f
Fluids, replenishing, 310–311
Fluoride, 231t, 239–240
    deficiency, 239t
    food sources of, 239t
    functions of, 232f, 239t
    RDA for, 239t
    toxicity, 239t
Fluorosis, 240, 240f
FODMAPs, 122
Folate (including folic acid), 10t, 189t, 211, 211–216
    deficiency, 211, 215–216, 216t
    food sources of, 206f, 212, 213t, 216t
    function of, 191f
    functions of, 211, 212f, 216t
    during pregnancy, 324t
    RDA for, 216t
    toxicity, 216t
    as water-soluble vitamin, 205

Food advertising, 291–292
Food allergies, 176–177, 331, 332
Food and Drug Administration (FDA)
    artificial sweeteners and, 109
    bottled water and, 262, 332
    BPA regulation and, 262
    disclaimers and, 35
    food-borne illness and, 347
    food labels and, 57, 58, 59
    food safety and, 338
    nutrition information and, 31, 37
    partially hydrogenated oils and, 133
    stevia and, 106
    supplements and, 60, 61–62
    trans fat labeling and, 134
    weight-loss medications and, 297
Food-borne illnesses, 13, 85
    common sources of, 340t–341t
    defined, 338
    prevention of, 342–346
    from restaurants, 347
    signs and symptoms of, 340, 340t–341t
Food choices, factors affecting, 4f
Food costs, 179–180
Food cravings, 325
Food energy, 8
    See also Energy
Food folate, 211
    See also Folate
Food groups
    combination foods, classification of, 51
    dairy foods, 47
    fruits, 49
    grains, 45–46
    introduction to, 45–51
    MyPlate, 55
    proteins, 48
    vegetables, 50
Food guides, 16
Food insecurity, 351
Food intolerances, 177
Food intoxication, 339
Food irradiation, 347
Food labels
    allergen information on, 177f
    claims on, 59
    Daily Values (DVs), 58–59
    food allergies and, 177
    ingredient list, 106
    Nutrition Facts panel, 57–58, 57f
Food poisoning, 339
Food preparation
    cleanliness and, 344
    dangerous practices, 342f
    heart healthy tips, 150–153
    preventing food-borne illnesses and, 342–344
    weight loss and, 295
Food processing
    mineral content and, 233
    salt added during, 241
Food production, 351–352
Food Pyramids, 55, 56f

Food(s)
    See also specific foods
    advertising, 291–292
    bacteria in, 339, 340t–341t
    as best source of nutrients and phytochemicals, 15
    bioengineered, 339
    carbohydrate-rich, 309t
    cholesterol content of, 135t
    emergency supply of, 347, 347t
    energy dense, 14
    functional, 17, 17f
    glycemic index of, 120–121, 121f
    "good" and "bad," 13–14
    irradiation of, 347
    junk, 13, 117
    nutrient-dense, 13–14, 14f
    organic, 51
    pesticides in, 348
    processed, 15, 117
    proteins in, 169–171, 169t
    solid, 332–333
    staple, 110
Food safety, 338–348
    contaminated surfaces and, 345
    cutting boards and, 342, 344
    pesticides, 348
    potential dangers, 338–339
    restaurant foods and, 347
    role of government agencies in, 338
    rules, 346
    temperature guide for, 342f
    USDA recommended safe minimum internal temperatures, 342–343, 343t
Food secure, 351
Food Stamp Program, 351t
Food storage, 345, 346t
Food waste, 352
Formula feeding, 330–331, 349–350
Fortification, 46
Fractures, 238
Framingham Heart Study, 27
Free radicals, 10, 146, 146f, 192f, 201, 201f, 218
Freezing food, 343, 345
Freshman fifteen, 12
Frey, McKenzie, 277
Fructose, 103, 106
    See also High-fructose corn syrup
Fruit juices, 49, 112, 310, 333
Fruits, 180
    calcium in, 237f
    canned, 112
    examples, 49
    minerals in, 230f
    MyPlate guidelines, 55f
    nutritional content of, 49
    one-ounce equivalents, 49f
    potassium in, 241f
    as snacks, 53
    storing, 53
    vitamins in, 193f, 206f
FTC. *See* Federal Trade Commission (FTC)
Functional foods, 17, 17f
Fungi, 339

G

Galactose, 103
Gallbladder, 76, 76f, 81, 84f
Gallstones, 91, 91f, 94f
Garcinia cambogia, 299t
Garlic, 62, 64t
Gastric bypass surgery, 297–298, 297f
Gastritis, 26
Gastroesophageal reflux (GER), 89
Gastroesophageal reflux disease (GERD), 89–90, 94f
Gastrointestinal (GI) tract, 75
Genetically modified organisms (GMOs), 339, 351
Genetic factors, influencing weight gain, 291
Genetic mutations, 166
Genetic susceptibility, 29
Gestational diabetes, 119
Gestational hypertension, 326
Ghee, 151
Ghrelin, 291
GI (glycemic index), 120–121, 120f, 121f
Giardia, 341t
Gimmicks, 298
Ginger, 29, 64t
Ginkgo biloba, 62, 65t
Ginseng, 65t, 311, 312, 313t
Globesity, 279
Glucagon, 114, 114f–115f, 162
Glucomannan, 299t
Glucosamine, 60, 65t
Glucose, 97, 104
    See also Blood glucose
    defined, 103
    for energy, 116, 116f
    as essential nutrient, 10t
    food sources of, 103
    recycling, 306f
Glutamic acid, 163t
Glutamine, 163t
Gluten, 71, 178
Gluten-free diet, 178t
Glycemic index (GI), 120–121, 120f, 121f
Glycemic load, 120f, 121
Glycine, 163t
Glycogen, 110, 110f, 116
Glycogen loading, 309
Goat's milk, 333
Goiter, 252, 252f
"Good foods," 13
Government agencies, food safety and, 338
Grains, 45–46, 171
    calcium in, 237f
    Dietary Guidelines on, 53
    enriched, 46
    examples of, 46
    fortified, 46
    minerals in, 230f
    MyPlate guidelines, 55f
    one-ounce equivalents, 46f
    potassium in, 241f
    refined, 15, 15f, 45
    vitamins in, 193f, 206f
    whole, 45, 123

Grams, 9
Grapefruit juice, 337f
Green superfood supplements, 23
Green tea, 65t, 299t
Grocery shopping tips, 180, 295
Ground meat, 344, 345
Growth spurt, 334
Guarana, 312
Guar gum, 299t
Guava, 219
Gums, 110
Gut microbiome, 85

H

Hair, effects of aging on, 337t
Hand washing, 343
Hangovers, 261
"Hardening of the arteries," 144
HDLs (high-density lipoproteins), 144, 144f, 145, 145f, 148t
Health
    alcohol and, 267, 268f
    carbohydrates and, 117–123
    proteins and, 174–178
Health claims
    on food labels, 59
    unproven, 32, 33, 34, 35
Health on the Net, 35
Healthy diets, 15
Heart attack, 144
Heartburn, 89, 90
Heart disease, 5, 129, 134, 143
    See also Cardiovascular disease (CVD)
Heart health
    alcohol and, 269
    fiber and, 122–123
    fish oil supplements and, 150
    food selection and preparation tips for, 150–153
    Mediterranean Diet and, 148
Heat cramps, 311t
Heat exhaustion, 311t
Heat-related illness, 311, 311t
Heatstroke, 311, 311t
Heavy drinkers, 264t
Heimlich maneuver, 79, 79f
Helicobacter pylori (*H. pylori*), 26
Heme, 210
Heme iron, 244
Hemicellulose, 110
Hemoglobin, 119, 210, 244
Hemorrhoids, 87, 87f, 94f
Hepatitis, 118, 268, 269f
Hepatitis A (HAV), 341t
Herbal supplements, 12, 60, 337
    safety of, 62
Heterocyclic amines, 223
High-birth-weight, 325
High-density lipoproteins (HDLs), 144, 144f, 145, 145f, 148t
High-fructose corn syrup, 101, 105, 105t, 106, 112
High-intensity sweeteners, 108–109
High-protein diet, 174, 175
High-quality protein, 170
Hinduism, 56

Histidine, 10t, 163t
Hoodia, 299t
Homocysteine, 210, 211
Honey, 105t, 109, 118, 333
Hormones, 51, 96, 162
Human intervention studies, 26
Human milk, 330–331, 331t, 349
    See also Breastfeeding
Hunger, 291
Hydration, 258, 259
Hydrochloric acid (HCl), 80, 216
Hydrogen ions, 163
Hydroxycitric acid (HCA), 299t
Hyperactivity, 105
Hypertension, 144
    causes of, 243
    classification of, 242t
    defined, 242
    gestational, 326
    sodium intake and, 243
    treatment for, 243
Hypoglycemia, 121–122

I

IBS (irritable bowel syndrome), 92, 94f
Ileum, 81, 81f
Immune system, 74t
    effects of aging on, 337t
Incomplete proteins, 170
Incubation period, 340
Indian cuisine, 56
Indian reservations, food distribution program on, 351t
Infant formulas, 322, 330–331, 331t, 349–350
Infant nutrition, 327–333
    formula feeding, 330–331, 349–350
    lactation, 327–330
    solid foods, 332–333
    undernutrition, 349–350
Infants
    foods and beverages to avoid feeding, 333
    high-birth-weight, 325
    low-birth-weight, 323
    premature, 323, 323f
    weaning, 332
Inflammatory bowel disease (IBD), 92
Influenza, 340
Ingredient list, 106
Insects, 176
Insoluble fiber, 111, 111t
Insulin, 114, 114f–115f, 118, 162
Insulin resistance, 118, 119, 146
Integrated pest management (IPM), 352
Integumentary system, 74t
Intensity, 304–305
Intermittent fasting, 299
Internet, nutrition information on, 34–35
Intestinal bacteria, 85
Intestinal gas, 85, 123
Intracellular water, 258
Intrinsic factor (IF), 214, 214f
Iodide, 252

Iodine, 10t, 231t
    deficiency, 253, 255t
    excess, 253
    food sources of, 230f, 252, 252t, 255t
    functions of, 232f, 252, 255t
    RDA for, 255t
    toxicity, 255t
Iodized salt, 253
Ions, 259f
IPM (integrated pest management), 352
Iron, 10t, 53, 231t
    deficiency, 246–247, 249t, 335
    food sources of, 230f, 244, 245f, 245t, 247, 249t
    functions of, 232f, 244, 249t
    heme iron, 244
    increasing intake of, 247
    megadoses of, 62
    nonheme iron, 244
    during pregnancy, 324t
    RDA for, 249t
    in spinach, 244
    storage of, 42
    supplements, 246
    toxicity, 249t
Iron cookware, 247
Iron deficiency anemia, 246–247
Irradiation, 347
Irritable bowel syndrome (IBS), 92, 94f
Isoflavonoids, 11t
Isoleucine, 10t, 163t

J

Jejunum, 81, 81f
Juices, 49, 112, 333
Junk food, 13, 117

K

Kale, 195, 236
Kava, 62, 65t
Kefir, 88
Keratin, 162
Ketoacidosis, 116
Keto diet, 175
Ketone bodies, 116, 299
Kidneys, 260, 261
Kidney stones, 62, 174, 201, 220, 261
Kilo-, 9t
Kilocalories (kcal), 8, 9
Kimchi, 85
Kiwano, 350
Kwashiorkor, 350

L

Labels. *See* Food labels
Lactase, 113, 122
Lactation, 322
    See also Breastfeeding
    process, 328–329, 328f
Lacteal, 81, 140
Lactic acid, 306f
Lactobacillus, 64t
Lactobacillus bifidus, 327
Lacto-ovovegetarians, 172

Lactose, 104, 105
Lactose intolerance, 122, 238
Lactovegetarians, 172
La Leche League, 330
Large intestine, 76, 76f, 84–85, 85f, 86f
Larynx, 78f
Lavender, 65t
LDLs (low-density lipoproteins), 144, 144f, 145, 145f, 146, 146f
Lead, 231
Lecithin, 136, 137f
Leftovers, 345, 346t
Legumes, 169, 171, 233
Leptin, 291
Let-down reflex, 328–329
Leucine, 10t, 163t
Lifestyle, 5, 16, 153
Lignin, 110
Limiting amino acids, 170
Linoleic acids, 10t, 131, 131f, 327
Lipases, 138
Lipids, 6, 128–159
   See also Cholesterol; Fats; Fatty acids; Oils
   absorption and transport of, 83, 140
   cholesterol, 134–135, 134f
   classification of blood levels, 148t
   defined, 130
   digestion of, 138–141, 138f–139f
   functions, 7t
   phospholipids, 135–137, 136f
   role of, 130
   triglycerides, 130
Lipoproteins, 140
   See also High-density lipoproteins (HDLs); Low-density lipoproteins (LDLs)
   atherosclerosis and, 144, 145f, 146
   composition and size of, 144f
Listeria monocytogenes, 340t
Liters, 9
Lithium, 231t
Liver, 76, 76f, 84f, 86f, 116
   cirrhosis, 118, 268, 269f
   "fatty liver," 267
   hepatitis, 118, 268, 269f
   non-alcoholic fatty liver disease (NAFLD), 118
Livestock, 352
Local farmers, 179
Locusts, 176
Loperamide, 88
Low-birth-weight (LBW), 323
Low-carbohydrate diets, 298
Low-density lipoproteins (LDLs), 144, 144f, 145, 145f, 146, 146f, 148t
Lower esophageal sphincter, 80, 80f
Low-fat milk, 47
Low-quality protein, 170
Lubricants, 162
Lutein, 11t, 194
Lycopene, 11t, 194
Lymph, 81, 140
Lymphatic system, 74t, 83f, 140
   effects of aging on, 337t
Lysine, 10t, 163t

M

Macronutrients, 9
   See also Carbohydrates; Fats; Protein(s)
   intakes, 112f
Macular degeneration, 197
Maculas, 197
Magnesium, 10t, 231t, 232
   deficiency, 248, 249t
   food sources of, 230f, 248, 248t, 249f, 249t
   functions of, 232f, 248, 249t
   RDA for, 249t
   side effects, 90
   toxicity, 248, 249t
Major minerals, 231
Malignant cells, 93, 221, 221f
Malnutrition, 12, 350
Maltase, 113
Maltose, 104
Manganese, 10t, 231t, 232f, 256t
Mannitol, 108
Maple syrup, 105t
Marasmic kwashiorkor, 350
Marasmus, 350
Margarine, 151
Marshall, Barry, 26
Meal planning, 45–56, 179
   food groups, 45–51
Meals on Wheels, 351t
Meats
   cold storage time limits for, 346t
   cooking at high temperature, 223
   eating less, 352
   high-fat, 48
   lean, 150
   processed, 41, 222t
   red, 170
   tips for purchasing, 180
Meat substitutes, 170
Meat thermometer, 343f
Mechanical digestion, 75
Medical history, 4–5
Medical professionals
   mistrust of, 30–31
   nutrition information from, 36–37
Medications
   prescription, 337
   weight-loss, 297
Mediterranean Diet, 148, 150
Mediterranean Diet Pyramid, 55, 56f
MedWatch program, 63
Megadose, 62
Megaloblastic anemia, 211, 215
Melatonin, 60, 65t
Menopause, 238
Menu planning, 295
Mercury, 231
Metabolic energy needs, 286–287
   calculating, 287
Metabolic rate
   basal, 286
   defined, 286
   influences on, 286–287

Metabolic water, 259
Metabolism
   aerobic, 96
   amino acid, 211
   anaerobic, 96
   basal, 286
   basics, 95–97, 97f
   catabolism, 96
   defined, 8
   energy, 95–97, 97f, A-4
   thrifty, 291
Methionine, 10t, 163t, 211
Metric conversions, A-2
Metric prefixes, 9t
Metric-to-household units, A-2
Mexican cuisine, 15
Micelle, 139, 139f
Micro-, 9t
Microgram, 9
Micronutrients, 9, 16
   See also Minerals; Vitamins
Microwave cooking, 345
Middle-age spread, 280
Mild cognitive impairment, 202
Milk, 14f, 47, 122, 151
Milk of magnesia, 248
Milli-, 9t
Milligram, 9
Minerals, 6, 10t, 229–256
   See also specific types
   absorption of, 233
   defined, 229
   food sources of, 230, 230f
   functions of, 7t, 229, 231–232, 231t, 232f
   major, 231
   supplements, 12, 60, 62, 233
   trace, 231
Misinformation. *See* Nutrition information and misinformation
Moderate drinkers, 264t
Moderate-intensity activity, 305f
Moderation, 15
Molasses, 105t
Molds, 339
Molecules, 75
Molybdenum, 10t, 231t
"Money back" guarantees, 34
Monk fruit extracts, 108t
Monoglyceride, 139
Monosaccharides, 103
Monounsaturated fatty acids, 131, 131f, 132f, 149f
Moreno, Marisa, 3
Morning sickness, 324–325
Motor vehicle accidents, 268
Mouth, 76, 76f, 77, 86f
Mucilage, 110
Mucin, 162
Mucus, 80
Multivitamin/multimineral (MV/M) supplements, 60, 63, 173, 233
Muscle cells, 72f, 73f
Muscle-strengthening exercises, 174
Muscular system, 74t
   effects of aging on, 337t

Mutations, 166
Myoglobin, 244
MyPlate, 55, 55f, 55t, 112, 168
   calcium and, 237f
   children's section of, 335
   fat-soluble vitamins and, 193f
   iron and, 245f
   magnesium and, 249f
   minerals and, 230f
   older adults and, 337
   potassium and, 241f
   water-soluble vitamins and, 206f
   zinc and, 254f
MyPyramid Plan, 55

N

NAFLD (non-alcoholic fatty liver disease), 118
Nails, effects of aging on, 337t
Nasal cavity, 78f
National Academy of Sciences, 339
National Bioengineered Food Disclosure Law, 339
National Heart, Lung, and Blood Institute, 278
National Institute on Aging, 337
National Osteoporosis Foundation, 35
National School Lunch Program, 351t
National Weight Control Registry, 296
Natural disasters, 347
Natural resources, 351–352
NatureSmart LLC, 134
NBTY, Inc., 134
Negative energy state, 290, 290f, 291
Negative thought patterns, 296
Neotame, 108t
Nerve cells, 72f
Nervous system, 74t
   effects of aging on, 337t
   major organs, 74t
   primary functions of, 74t
Neural tube, 215
Neural tube defects, 215, 215f
Nguyen, Damian, 229
Niacin. *See* Vitamin B-3 (niacin)
Niacinamide, 206
Nickel, 231, 231t
Night blindness, 196
Nitrate, 313t
Nitrogen, 168
Non-alcoholic fatty liver disease (NAFLD), 118
Non-celiac gluten sensitivity, 178
Nonessential amino acids, 163, 163t
Nonexercise activity thermogenesis (NEAT), 288
Nonheme iron, 244
Nonnutrients, 10
Norovirus, 341t
Nursing bottle syndrome, 122
Nut butters, 153
Nutrient content claims, 59
Nutrient-dense food, 13–14, 14f
Nutrients
   added to foods, 46
   classes of, 6
   defined, 3

Nutrients (*continued*)
   essential, 10
   fat-soluble, 83f
   food as best source of, 15
   functions, 6, 7t, 8
   macronutrients, 9
   micronutrients, 9
   organic, 6
   safe intake of, 16, 16f
   water-soluble, 82f
Nutrient supplements. *See* Supplements
Nutrition
   basics, 6–12
   childhood, 334–336
   defined, 3
   global issues in, 349–353
   infant, 327–333
   key concepts, 13–17, 13t
   for older adults, 336–337
   in pregnancy, 323–325, 324t
   in prenatal period, 322–323
   reasons to learn about, 4–5
Nutrition experts, 33, 36–37
Nutrition Facts panel, 57–58, 57f
Nutrition information and misinformation
   anecdotes, 24, 30, 34
   on Internet, 34–35
   mistrust of medical professionals and, 30–31
   from nutrition experts, 36–37
   popular sources of, 33
   reasons for misinformation, 31–32
   "red flags" of misinformation, 33–34, 34f
   requirements and recommendations, 42–44
   skeptical consumerism and, 32–33
   sources of reliable, 36–37
   testimonials, 24, 34
Nutrition Program Congregate Meals for the Elderly, 351t
Nutrition research
   cause and effect in, 29
   conflicting findings from, 28
   experiments, 24
   Framingham Heart Study, 27
   human intervention studies, 26
   population studies, 27, 29
   research bias and, 28
   science-based evidence, 24–27
Nutritive sweeteners, 106
Nuts, 14, 50, 123, 170, 233

O

Obesity, 12
   cancer and, 222–223
   carbohydrates and, 117
   central-body, 281, 282, 283
   childhood, 336
   defined, 278
   epidemic of, 278–279
   health problems related to, 278, 281–282
   map of, in U.S., 279f
   medical treatments for, 297–298
   prevalence of, 278t
Office of Dietary Supplements, 63

Oils, 53, 55
   See also Lipids
   food group, 50
   partially hydrogenated, 133–134
   vegetable, 50, 53
Older adults
   body fat in, 285
   dehydration in, 261
   magnesium deficiency in, 248
   metabolic rate in, 286–287
   nutrition-related concerns, 337
   nutrition for, 336–337
   nutrition resources for, 337
   osteoporosis in, 238
   physical inactivity and, 337
   vitamin B-12 deficiency in, 216
   weight loss in, 337
Oleic acid, 131f
Olive oil, 132f, 151
Olives, 50
Omega-3 fatty acids, 131, 150, 150t, 173
Omega-3 supplements, 60
Omega-6 fatty acids, 131, 150
Omega end, 130
Omnivore, 75, 75f
Organic foods, 51
Organic nutrients, 6
Organism, 73
Organs, 73
Organ systems
   of body, 74, 74t
   defined, 73
Orlistat, 297
Osteomalacia, 200
Osteoporosis, 203, 238–239
Overfat, 278
   See also Obesity; Overweight
Overnutrition, 12
Overweight
   See also Obesity
   defined, 278
   epidemic of, 278–279
   health problems related to, 278, 281–282
   prevalence of, 278t
Ovovegetarians, 172
Oxalate, 220
Oxalic acid, 233, 236
Oxidized LDLs cholesterol, 146, 146f
Oxytocin, 328, 329

P

Paleo diet, 175
Palm oil, 134, 151
Pancreas, 76, 76f, 81, 84f, 86f, 114
Pancreatic lipase, 138, 139f
Pantothenic acid (vitamin B-5), 10t, 189t, 216, 217t
   deficiency, 217t
   food sources of, 206f, 217t
   functions of, 191f, 217t
   RDA for, 217t
   toxicity, 217t
   as water-soluble vitamin, 205

V

Valerian, 62, 65t
Valine, 10t, 163t
Vanadium, 231t
Variety, 15
Vegans, 172, 173, 216
Vegetable oils, 50, 53
Vegetables, 50, 180
    calcium in, 237f
    cruciferous, 195
    minerals in, 230f
    MyPlate guidelines, 55f
    one-ounce equivalents, 50
    potassium in, 241f
    vitamins in, 193, 206f
Vegetarianism, 172–173, 173t
Vermin, 342
Very-low-calorie diets, 294
Very-low-density lipoproteins (VLDLs), 140, 144f, 145f, 146
Very-low-fat diets, 298
Villi/villus, 81, 81f, 82f
Viruses, 339, 341t
Visceral fat, 280, 280f, 282
Vitamin A, 10t, 162, 189t, 194–197
    deficiency, 195–196, 197t
    food sources of, 194–195, 195t, 197t
    functions of, 191f, 192, 194, 197t
    megadoses of, 62
    preformed, 194
    provitamin A, 194
    RDA for, 197t
    sources of, 193f
    summary of, 197t
    toxicity, 196, 197t
    vision and, 196, 196f
Vitamin B-1 (thiamin), 10t, 189t
    deficiency, 206, 207, 209t
    food sources of, 206f, 207, 207t, 209t
    functions of, 191f, 209t
    RDA for, 209t
    toxicity, 209t
    as water-soluble vitamin, 205
Vitamin B-2 (riboflavin), 10t, 189t
    deficiency, 206, 207, 209t
    food sources of, 206f, 207, 208t, 209t
    functions of, 191f, 209t
    RDA for, 209t
    toxicity, 209t
    as water-soluble vitamin, 205
Vitamin B-3 (niacin), 10t, 189t, 191
    deficiency, 206, 207, 209t
    food sources of, 206f, 207, 208t, 209t
    functions of, 191f, 209t
    megadoses of, 62, 206, 209
    RDA for, 209t
    toxicity, 209, 209t
    as water-soluble vitamin, 205
Vitamin B-5. *See* Pantothenic acid (vitamin B-5)
Vitamin B-6 (pyridoxine), 10t, 189t
    deficiency, 211t
    food sources of, 206f, 210, 210t, 211t
    functions of, 191f, 210, 211t
    megadoses of, 62
    RDA for, 211t
    toxicity, 210, 211t
    as water-soluble vitamin, 205
Vitamin B-12 (cobalamin), 10t, 173, 189t, 211–216
    absorption of, 213, 214f, 215
    deficiency, 211, 215–216, 216t
    food sources of, 206f, 212, 213t, 216t
    functions of, 191f, 211, 212f, 216t
    RDA for, 216t
    toxicity, 216t
    as water-soluble vitamin, 205
Vitamin C, 10t, 189t, 218–220
    cold viruses amd, 218
    deficiency, 220, 220t
    food sources of, 206f, 219, 219t, 220t
    functions of, 191f, 192, 218, 220t
    iron absorption and, 244
    megadoses of, 62
    RDA for, 44, 220t
    requirement for, 42
    toxicity, 220, 220t
    as water-soluble vitamin, 205
Vitamin D, 10t, 53, 189t, 198–201, 201
    deficiency, 187, 200–201, 201t
    as fat-soluble vitamin, 198
    food sources of, 199, 199t, 201t
    functions of, 191f, 199, 199f
    geography and, 200f
    megadoses of, 62
    previtamin D, 198, 198f
    production of, by body, 198f
    RDA for, 201t
    sources of, 193f
    storage of, 42
    summary of, 201t
    sunlight and, 200
    supplements, 239
    toxicity, 201t
Vitamin E, 10t, 189t, 201–203
    antioxidant activity of, 201, 201f
    deficiency, 202, 203t
    food sources of, 202, 202t, 203t
    functions of, 191f, 192
    RDA for, 203t
    sources of, 193f
    summary of, 203t
    supplements, 62, 202
    toxicity, 202, 203t
Vitamin K, 10t, 189t, 203–204
    AI for, 204t
    blood clotting and, 203f
    deficiency, 204, 204t
    food sources of, 204, 204t
    functions of, 191f, 203, 203f
    sources of, 193f
    summary of, 204t
    toxicity, 204t
Vitamin precursors, 188

Vitamins, 6, 186–227
    See also specific vitamins
    absorption of, 190
    cancer and, 221–223
    classification of, 189, 189t
    conserving in your food, 190
    deficiencies, 187, 188, 195–196, 200–201, 202, 206–207
    defined, 188
    digestion of, 190
    as essential nutrients, 10, 10t
    fat-soluble, 189, 189t, 193–204, 193f
    functions, 7t, 191–192, 191f
    power player, 206–207
    supplements, 12, 60, 62, 173, 202, 221, 233, 239
    toxicities, 189
    water-soluble, 189, 189t, 205–220
Vomiting, 88, 94f

W

Waist circumference, 282
Warfarin, 203
Warren, Rubin, 26
Warrington, Neill, 101, 118
Washington, Theresa, 321
Wasting, 350
Water, 6, 257–262
    bottled, 262
    in conventional agriculture, 351
    daily water balance, 259, 260f
    dehydration, 261
    as essential nutrient, 10, 257
    excess, 261
    fluid balance, 259, 259f
    fluid compartments and, 258, 258f
    in food and beverages, 257, 257t
    functions of, 7t, 258
    hydration, 258, 259
    losses, 260–261
    metabolic, 259
    requirements for, 260, 261
    Safe Drinking Water Act, 262
    tap, 262
    total water intake, 259, 260f
Water intoxication, 261, 311
Water-soluble nutrients, 82f
Water-soluble vitamins, 189, 189t, 205–220
Weaning, 332
Websites, nutrition information on, 34–35
Weight, 53
    See also Obesity; Overweight; Weight gain; Weight loss
    body mass index, 282–283, 283t
    classification by percentage of body fat, 285t
    factors influencing, 286–292
    underweight, 175, 300
Weight control, fiber and, 123
Weight gain, 277
    carbohydrates and, 117
    in college, 12
    excess fat and, 141
    factors influencing, 291–292
    kilocalories and, 290–291
    during pregnancy, 325–327, 325t, 326f
    for underweight people, 300
    water, 260
Weight loss, 277
    advertising hype and, 300
    from dehydration, 261
    goal setting for, 294
    high-protein diet and, 175
    key factors for success, 294–296
    kilocalories and, 290–291
    lifestyle changes for, 294
    medically sound, 293
    medications for, 297
    in older adults, 337
    reasonable rate of, 294
    successful, 296
    supplements, 299, 299t
    surgeries, 297–298, 297f
    unreliable methods of, 298–300
West, Karlin, 71
Wester, Mary, 23
Western diet, 29, 55, 172
Wheat bran, 15, 110
Wheat germ, 137f
Whey, 175
White adipose cells, 279, 279f, 280
White flour, 15f
White granulated sugar, 105t
Whole grains, 15, 45, 123
Whole milk, 47
Withdrawal, alcohol, 266
World food crisis, 350–351
World Food Program, 350
World Health Organization (WHO), 175, 279, 349
World population, 351
Worms, parasitic, 339, 341t

X

Xylitol, 108

Y

Yogurt, 85
Yohimbe, 299t

Z

Zeaxanthin, 194
Zetia, 153
Zinc, 10t, 231t, 232
    deficiency, 254, 255t
    excess, 254
    food sources of, 230f, 253, 253t, 254f, 255t
    functions of, 232f, 253, 255t
    RDA for, 255t
    toxicity, 255t
    Upper Level for, 254